Kidney and Urinary Tract Diseases in the Newborn

Aftab S. Chishti • Shumyle Alam
Stefan G. Kiessling
Editors

Kidney and Urinary Tract Diseases in the Newborn

Springer

Editors
Aftab S. Chishti
Division of Pediatric Nephrology
Hypertension and Renal Transplantation
Kentucky Children's Hospital
University of Kentucky
Lexington, KY
USA

Stefan G. Kiessling
Division of Pediatric Nephrology
Hypertension and Renal Transplantation
Kentucky Children's Hospital
University of Kentucky
Lexington, KY
USA

Shumyle Alam
Urogenital Center
Division of Pediatric Urology
Cincinnati Children's Medical Center
Cincinnati, OH
USA

ISBN 978-3-662-52077-2 ISBN 978-3-642-39988-6 (eBook)
DOI 10.1007/978-3-642-39988-6
Springer Heidelberg New York Dordrecht London

Printed on acid-free paper

Springer is part of Springer Science+Business Media (www.springer.com)

Preface

Physicians have always been fascinated by the complexity and intricacy of fetal organogenesis including the development of the genitourinary tract. The individual developmental stages, though complicated and still incompletely understood, usually occur without interruptions. On the other hand, newborns can face a wide variety of anomalies of the urinary tract including structural and mechanistic, spanning from acute and reversible to chronic and progressive pathology.

Advances in our understanding of pathophysiologic concepts of disease and the use of new diagnostic modalities have led to increased and early detection of a variety of conditions. In addition, increased experience and new therapeutic interventions are commonly associated with improved outcome in this particularly vulnerable patient population. This has caused a shift in certain areas to now increased interest in neonatal conditions and their possible impact on adult disease.

Care of newborns and infants with congenital kidney and urinary tract disease is complex and requires the expertise of multiple specialists, including nephrologists, urologists, neonatologists as well as other pediatric specialists depending on the condition.

This inaugural edition of "Kidney and Urinary Tract Diseases in Neonates and Infants", a first of its kind as it solely focuses on neonates and infants, attempts to provide a comprehensive overview of common medical and surgical entities that are seen in newborns and tries to be a "hands-on" resource for clinicians working with this particular patient population.

Though a first edition can never be perfect, we think to have included a variety of chapters covering the vast majority of clinical entities providers will encounter in their clinical work.

All chapters are written by experts in the field and the editors are extremely grateful for the time and effort that each contributor has provided to make this endeavor possible and, hopefully, successful.

Any task as complex as the completion of a book publication requires sets of helpful hands in the background. The editors therefore especially appreciate the constant support and guidance of Ms. Joni Fraser as without her help the publication would not have been possible.

Lexington, KY, USA — Aftab S. Chishti
Cincinnati, OH, USA — Shumyle Alam
Lexington, KY, USA — Stefan G. Kiessling

Contents

Development of the Kidney and Lower Urinary Tract

1

Joana Rosa Pereira dos Santos and Tino D. Piscione

1.1 Introduction

Congenital abnormalities of the kidney and urinary tract (CAKUT) are the cause of 30–50 % of end-stage renal disease in young children [307]. CAKUT are represented by a heterogeneous group of renal, ureter, and bladder malformations across a wide range of clinical severity (Table 1.1). The incidence of renal and urinary tract anomalies in humans is 0.3–1.6 per 1,000 live born and stillborn infants [359]. Renal malformations account for 20–30 % of all solid-organ birth defects detected by antenatal sonography during pregnancy [273]. Thirty percent of cases occur in association with extrarenal malformations [359] and may be found as part of over 100 congenital syndromes (Table 1.2) [173].

This chapter approaches CAKUT from an embryological perspective with emphasis on morphologic, cellular, and molecular events in normal urinary tract development. The science of human embryology relates to form and process of tissue development and integrates molecular, cellular, and structural factors within a dynamic spatiotemporal framework. A clear understanding of human embryology provides a foundation for understanding structure-function relationships within a given tissue or organ. It also renders insight into the pathological basis of congenital malformation resulting from perturbations in normal organ development and leads to the recognition of associated malformations within the same organ system (e.g., genitourinary system) when developmental mechanisms are shared between tissues (e.g., kidney and ureter). Consequently, the principles of urinary tract embryology described in this chapter are fundamental to the diagnosis and clinical management of CAKUT in fetuses and newborns and crucial to understanding the long-term impact of CAKUT on overall health.

Developmental events in kidney, ureter, and bladder morphogenesis are highly conserved across vertebrate species [75]. The use of model organisms such as mice, zebrafish, and frogs has been invaluable for defining gene expression patterns in the embryonic urinary tract system and for providing a spatiotemporal framework upon which to study gene function. Understanding relationships between gene expression and function has been greatly facilitated by the creation of a molecular atlas of gene expression for the developing urinary tract, which can be accessed online through the GenitoUrinary Development Molecular Anatomy Project (GUDMAP; http://www.gudmap.org/index.html) [117]. Gene function has been largely elucidated through the anal-

J.R.P. dos Santos, MD (✉)
T.D. Piscione, MD, PhD, FRCP©
Division of Nephrology,
Department of Pediatrics,
The Hospital for Sick Children,
555 University Ave, Toronto, ON,
Canada M5G 1X8
e-mail: joana.dossantos@sickkids.ca

A.S. Chishti et al. (eds.), *Kidney and Urinary Tract Diseases in the Newborn*,
DOI 10.1007/978-3-642-39988-6_1, © Springer-Verlag Berlin Heidelberg 2014

Table 1.1 Examples of renal, ureter, and bladder malformations

Renal malformations
Renal agenesis
Renal hypoplasia
Renal dysplasia
Renal duplication
Horseshoe kidney
Renal ectopia (e.g., pelvic kidney)
Cross-fused ectopia
Cystic kidney diseases
Polycystic kidney disease (autosomal dominant, autosomal recessive)
Multicystic dysplastic kidney
Medullary cystic kidney
Nephronophthisis
Ureteral malformations
Ureteral agenesis
Ureteral duplication
Ureteropelvic junction obstruction
Ureteral stricture (distal to the ureteropelvic junction)
Hydroureter (nonobstructive)
Ectopic ureter
Ureterocele
Bladder malformations
Bladder exstrophy
Bladder diverticulum
Vesicoureteral reflux

Table 1.2 Human congenital malformation syndromes associated with CAKUT

Syndromes with cystic dysplasia	
Apert	Meckel-Gruber
Bardet-Biedl	Meckel syndrome, type 7
Branchio-oto-renal	Melnick-Needles
Campomelic dysplasia	Pallister-Hall
Cornelia de Lange	Patau (trisomy 13)
Down (trisomy 21)	Senior-Loken
Edwards (trisomy 18)	Tuberous sclerosis
Jeune asphyxiating thoracic dystrophy	von Hippel-Lindau
	Zellweger
Syndromes with polycystic kidneys	
Congenital rubella	Peutz-Jeghers
Ehlers-Danlos	Pyloric stenosis
Kaufman-McKusick	Roberts
Noonan	Short rib-polydactyly, types II, III, and IV
	Zellweger
Syndromes with horseshoe kidney	
Abruzzo-Erickson	Pallister-Hall
Bowen-Conradi	Pyloric Stenosis
Cerebro-oculo-facio-skeletal (Pena-Shokeir)	Roberts
Facio-cardio-renal (Eastman-Bixler)	Trisomy 18 (Edwards)
Focal Dermal Hypoplasia (Goltz-Gorlin)	Trisomy 21 (Down)
Oral-cranial-digital (Juberg-Hayward)	Turner
Syndromes with unilateral renal agenesis	
Acro-renal-mandibular	Ivemark
Adrenogenital (21-OH-ase deficiency)	Klippel-Feil
Alagille	Lacrimo-auriculo-dento-digital
Cardiofacial	Larsen
Cat-Eye	Lenz microphthalmia
Cerebro-oculo-facio-skeletal (Pena-Shokeir)	Mayer-Rokitansky
Chondroectodermal dysplasia (Ellis-van Creveld)	Miller-Dieker, lissencephaly
Coffin-Siris	Oculo-auriculo-vertebral dysplasia (Goldenhar)
Congenital rubella	Olfactogenital dysplasia (Russell-Silver)
Fetal alcohol	Spondylocostal dysostosis

ysis of embryonic mouse mutant phenotypes generated either by targeted mutagenesis, which disrupts gene function universally, or by conditional mutagenesis, which renders in loss of gene function in a cell-specific or time-dependent manner [159]. This chapter will make reference to genetic studies in mice to gain insight into morphogenetic, molecular, and cellular mechanisms which underlie normal development of the human kidney, ureter, and bladder. By convention, text references to human genes will be noted in capitalized italics whereas mouse genes are in sentence case italics [262].

This chapter is subdivided into broad categories representing stereotypic processes in urinary tract formation. These include descriptions of the

Table 1.2 (continued)

Syndromes with renal and/or ureteral duplications	
Achondrogenesis	Congenital Rubella
Acrocephalosyndactyly (Saethre-Chotzen)	Denys-Drash
Acro-renal (Dieker-Opitz)	Fetal Alcohol
Adrenogenital (21-OH-ase deficiency)	Klippel-Feil
Bowen-Conradi	Noonan
Branchio-oto-renal	Oculo-auriculo-vertebral dysplasia (Goldenhar)
Braun-Bayer	Rubinstein-Taybi
Cerebro-oculo-facio-skeletal (Pena-Shokeir)	Trisomy 21
	Turner
Syndromes with hydroureter or hydronephrosis	
Apert	Johanson-Blizzard
Campomelic Dysplasia	Kaufman-McKusick
Chondroectodermal dysplasia (Ellis-van Creveld)	Larsen
Coffin-Siris	Menkes
Cornelia de Lange	Noonan
DiGeorge	Pyloric stenosis
Fetal Alcohol	Spondylocostal dysostosis
	Wolfram
Syndromes with renal ectopia	
Cardiofacial	Marfan
Cerebro-cost-mandibular	Mayer-Rokitansky
Craniosynostosis-radial aplasia (Baller-Gerold)	Oculo-auriculo-vertebral dysplasia (Goldenhar)
Denys-Drash	Pallister-Hall
Klippel-Feil	Seckel
	Spondylocostal dysostosis
Syndromes with renal hypoplasia	
Branchio-oto-renal	Ivemark
Campomelic Dysplasia	Poland
Cornelia de Lange	Pyloric Stenosis
Fetal Alcohol	Seckel
	Townes-Brock
Syndromes with bladder exstrophy	
Syndactyly, type IV (Haas)	

Reproduced with modifications from Clarren [63], with permission

early embryonic origins of the kidneys, ureters, and bladder, as well as descriptions of later events involved in renal collecting duct and nephron morphogenesis, ureter formation, and bladder development. Within each subdivision, attention is given to genetic or molecular control mechanisms essential for executing key developmental programs. Specific references to urinary tract morphogenesis in embryonic mice are made when orthologous events in humans have not been fully characterized. Consequently, the information in this chapter serves as a framework for understanding the breadth and complexity of anatomical and functional defects of the urinary system that present clinically in the fetus and newborn infant.

1.2 Embryonic Origins of the Urinary System

1.2.1 Overview of the Early Urinary Tract Embryology

The mammalian urinary system has embryologic cellular origins in the mesodermal and endodermal germ layers of the post-gastrulation embryo [76]. Mesodermal derivatives comprise all epithelial cell types of the mature nephron, renal pelvis, and ureter, as well as non-epithelial cell types including glomerular endothelial and mesangial cells, renal parenchymal interstitial cells (also known as stromal cells), ureteral and bladder smooth muscle cells, and adipocytes and connective tissue-producing fibrocytes of the renal capsule and ureter and bladder adventitia. Endodermal tissue, on the other hand, gives rise to the luminal epithelial cells of the bladder and urethra. Kidney and ureter development requires the initial formation of a mesoderm-derived embryonic structure known as the nephric duct (also known as the Wolffian duct or mesonephric duct). Conversely, bladder development is preceded by formation of the urogenital sinus. The following sections (Sects. 1.2.2 and 1.2.3) describe formation of the nephric duct and urogenital sinus, respectively. Table 1.3 compares the chronology of human and mouse urinary tract development.

Table 1.3 Embryonic time table for nephrogenesis: human versus mouse

	Human	Mouse
Pronephros		
First appearance	22 days	9 days
Regresses by	25 days	10 days
Mesonephros		
First appearance	24 days	10 days
Regresses by	16 weeks	14 days
Metanephros appears	28–32 days	11 days
Collecting tubules and nephrons	44 days	13 days
Glomeruli	8–9 weeks	14 days
Nephrogenesis ceases	34–36 weeks	4–7 days after birth
Length of gestation	40 weeks	19 days

Reproduced with modifications from Woolf et al. [364], with permission from Elsevier

1.2.2 Nephric Duct Morphogenesis

Mesoderm-derived ancestors of the kidneys and ureters originate from within a narrow strip of tissue termed intermediate mesoderm (IM) which is located bilaterally on each side of the embryonic midline. IM is evident in human fetuses by week 4 of gestation based on the appearance of the nephric duct [139]. In mice, IM is detected by embryonic day 8.5 (E8.5) based on tissue-specific patterns of gene expression [76, 336]. IM extends bilaterally in an anteroposterior, or rostral-caudal, direction from the level of the twelfth somite at the embryonic midsection to the cloaca, which is a midline embryonic structure located in the embryonic hind region [139]. During week 4 of human fetal gestation (E9.0 in mice), IM is induced along its anteroposterior axis to form a paired set of single-cell-layered epithelial tubes which are the nephric ducts. Fully formed nephric ducts extend the full length of IM and deviate at its posterior end towards the midline to insert into the cloaca (see Sect. 1.2.3).

While the nephric duct is formed, surrounding intermediate mesoderm (referred to as mesenchyme) is induced to undergo epithelial transformation. This inductive process results in the sequential generation of three morphologically unique nephrogenic primordia – the pronephros, mesonephros, and metanephros – which connect to the anterior, mid-, and posterior sections of the nephric duct, respectively (Fig. 1.1) [75]. The pronephros is a primitive paired organ characterized by a single glomerular and tubular filtrative unit (Fig. 1.1a). In lower-order animals such as amphibians and fish, the pronephros functions as a transient embryonic excretory organ. Conversely, in higher-order mammals including humans, pronephric structures are transiently represented by nonfunctioning rudimentary tubules which degenerate by apoptosis [86, 286]. The mesonephros is a more sophisticated filtrative system characterized by several well-developed glomerular- and tubular-like structures that connect directly to the nephric duct at its midsection (Fig. 1.1b). In adult fish and amphibians, the mesonephros replaces the pronephros as the definitive filtrative organ [75]. In humans, mesonephric development begins late in the fourth week of gestation and results in the transient production of fetal urine [118, 242]. By week 5, most mesonephric tissue undergoes degeneration while the remaining tissues in males contribute to the formation of the reproductive system, including the efferent ductules of the testis, vas deferens, epididymis, and seminal vesicle. In female fetuses, the mesonephros regresses although vestigial structures may persist and are represented clinically as Gartner's duct cysts, epoophoron, and paroophoron [226]. As mesonephric degeneration takes place, IM surrounding the posterior nephric duct (termed metanephric mesenchyme) is induced to form the metanephros, which represents the nascent mammalian kidney (Fig. 1.1c). Induction of metanephric mesenchyme (MM) is dependent on outgrowth of an epithelial diverticulum from the nephric duct termed the ureteric bud (UB) which occurs at approximately week 5 of human fetal gestation (E10.5 in mice). Invasion of MM by the UB initiates a series of reciprocal inductive interactions that triggers formation of the adult mammalian kidney and ureters. Detailed descriptions of kidney and ureter morphogenesis are provided in Sects. 1.3 and 1.4.

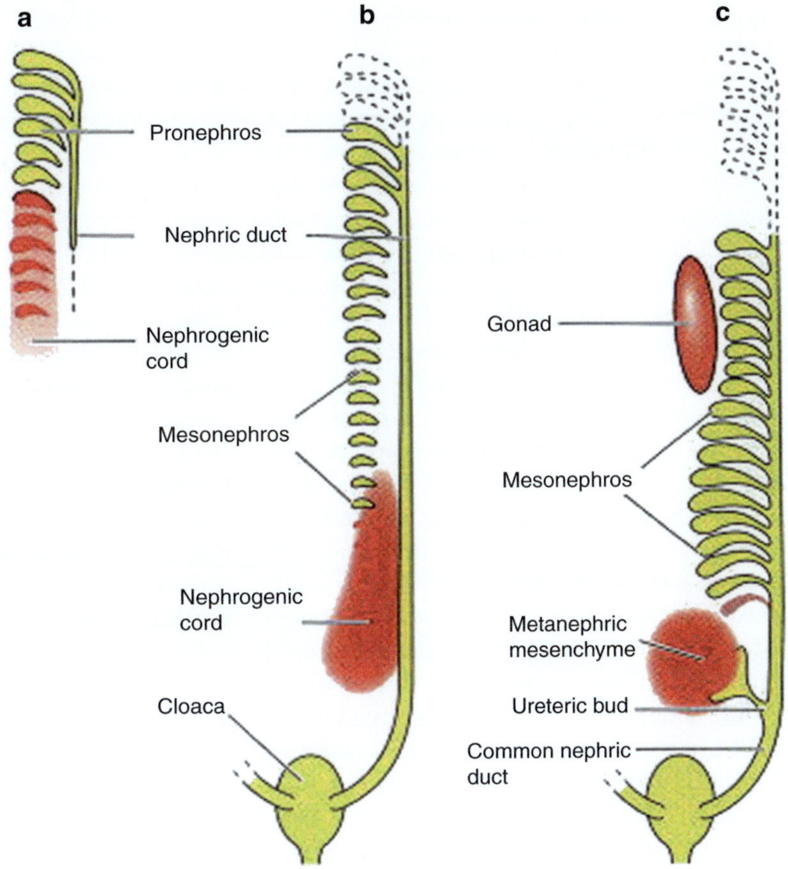

Fig. 1.1 Formation of nephrogenic primordia. (**a**) The nephrogenic cord and pronephros. (**b**) The mesonephros. (**c**) The metanephros

1.2.2.1 Molecular Pathways Involved in Nephric Duct Morphogenesis

Genetic studies in mice point to critical roles played by four transcription factor genes – *Lhx1*, *Pax2*, *Pax8*, and *Osr1* – in specifying IM for kidney and ureter development. *Lhx1* (Lim homeobox protein 1) encodes a member of the Lim family of homeodomain proteins which are essential to forming anterior embryonic structures [311]. *Pax2* and *Pax8* are paired box domain DNA-binding proteins which function as master regulators of tissue development in several organ systems, including kidney [26]. *Lhx1*, *Pax2*, and *Pax8* mRNAs are among the earliest gene transcripts detected in IM [26]. All three genes ultimately show mRNA expression in nephric duct cells, and their functions are essential to normal nephric duct formation. Mice lacking *Lhx1* function fail to form nephric ducts [336], whereas mice homozygous for a null *Pax2* mutation form posteriorly truncated nephric ducts [34, 335]. Combined inactivation of *Pax2* and *Pax8* results in complete absence of the nephric duct [26], suggesting that Pax family members have overlapping functions in anterior regions of IM. Combined *Pax2/8* function may be important for demarcating IM from lateral plate and paraxial mesoderm since *Pax2* mRNA are exclusively detected at the boundaries of these mesodermal compartments at stages prior to nephric duct formation [336]. Expression of *Pax2* and *Pax8* in this region appears to be under the positive control of bone morphogenetic protein 4 (BMP4; encoded by the *Bmp4* gene) which is secreted by cells in adjacent lateral plate mesoderm and in overlying ectoderm [142, 143, 236]. Negative control over these inductive interactions appears to be provided by other as-yet undefined factors secreted by nearby somites [190].

Osr1 encodes an odd-skipped related zinc-finger DNA-binding protein and is required to specify IM for kidney development [141]. *Osr1* is expressed in IM surrounding the nephric duct along its entire length and is excluded from nephric duct cells. Mice lacking *Osr1* function form nephric ducts but lack kidneys, which suggest that *Osr1* plays an important role in specifying posterior IM for kidney development.

Hox genes encode a large family of homeodomain proteins and are organized into related gene subgroups or clusters sharing functions that coordinate regional expression of other genes involved in axial patterning of a wide range of embryonic tissues [71]. Two mouse hox gene clusters – *Hox4* and *Hox11* – have been implicated in establishment of anterior and posterior IM cell identity, respectively, along the early embryonic AP axis. A role for *Hox4* genes in promoting anterior IM cell fate is suggested by the mRNA expression pattern for *Hoxb4* which is detected in early mesoderm at the anterior boundary of prospective IM [9]. The notion that *Hox4* genes establish an anterior code for IM is supported by studies in cultured chick embryos which revealed an anterior shift in expression of IM-specific markers *Lhx1* and *Pax2* within chick mesoderm when the anterior limits of *Hoxb4* expression were experimentally manipulated [263]. Conversely, evidence in mice suggests that *Hox11* cluster genes (*Hoxa11*, *Hoxc11*, and *Hoxd11*) control posterior IM cell fate and promote differentiation of cells within this region along a metanephric cell lineage. In a study which involved the use of tissue-specific promoter sequences in transgenic mice to expand mesodermal expression of *Hoxd11* anteriorly into a region of IM normally fated for mesonephros development, ectopically activating *Hoxd11* in this region resulted in transformation of mesonephric tubules into a more metanephric phenotype [212]. This observation suggested that *Hox11* cluster genes are necessary for instructing IM cells to differentiate along a metanephric cell fate instead of a mesonephric cell fate. Hox11 genes also appear to be required for enabling posterior IM cells to respond appropriately to inductive cues which initiate kidney and ureter development. This is revealed in compound mutant mice when either combinations of two or all three paralogous *Hox11* genes are mutated, which results in severe kidney hypoplasia or complete agenesis of kidneys and ureters, respectively [356]. In vitro, proteins encoded by *Hox11* genes form a DNA-binding complex with proteins encoded by *Pax2* and the Eyes absent 1 (*Eya1*) proteins and directly activate the expression of key metanephric regulators, glial-derived neurotrophic factor (*Gdnf*) and sine oculis homeobox 2 (*Six2*) (see Sect. 1.3.3.1) [105]. Consequently, the complete absence of kidneys and ureters in *Hox11* triple mutant mice is likely due to a failure of *Hox11* genes to appropriately activate the expression of other genes critical for initiating urinary tract development.

1.2.3 Urogenital Sinus Morphogenesis

The urogenital sinus is an embryonic structure which originates as a sub-compartment of the cloaca. The cloaca is an endoderm-derived transient hollow structure located midline in the embryonic hind region. It connects bilaterally with the posterior ends of the paired nephric ducts (Fig. 1.2). In humans, the cloaca is formed by the third week of fetal gestation from confluence of the allantois and hindgut [267]. The allantois precedes the umbilicus as the conduit for embryonic gas and solute exchange with the placenta, while the hindgut ultimately forms distal colonic structures including the rectum and the upper part of the anal canal. Between weeks 6 and 7, the cloaca is subdivided into dorsal and ventral chambers by a fold of mesodermal tissue which projects into the cloacal cavity and creates a transverse ridge known as the cloacal septum (also known as the urorectal septum; Fig. 1.2a). The dorsal chamber generates the anorectal canal which communicates with the hindgut and ultimately develops into the rectum and anus. The ventral chamber forms the urogenital sinus which is connected at its anterior end to the allantois via

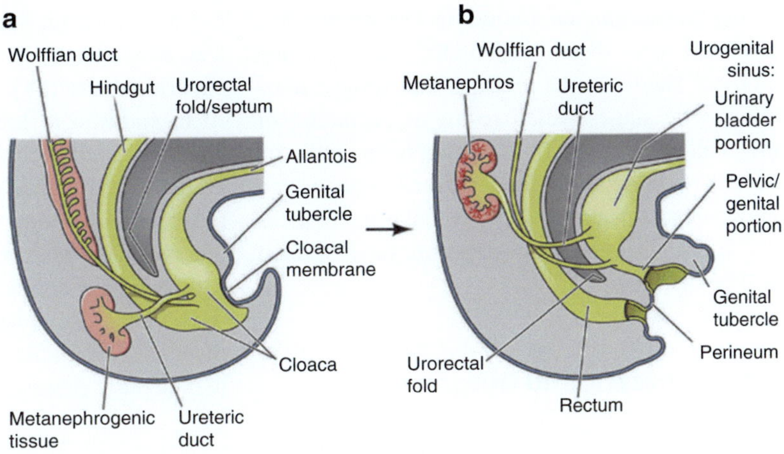

Fig. 1.2 Development of the urogenital sinus. (**a**) The cloaca and its anatomical location relative to other early embryonic urogenital tissues. (**b**) The primitive bladder forms from the anterior portion of the urogenital sinus. The posterior portion contributes to the formation of the urethra and external genital organs (Reproduced from Tasian et al. [331], Copyright 2010, with permission from Elsevier)

the vesico-allantoic canal or urachus (Fig. 1.2b). By week 12, the vesico-allantoic canal closes completely and remains as the median umbilical ligament in the fully developed fetus. Failure of this obliteration may result in urachal remnants which may present in the newborn infant as a vesico-umbilical fistula, vesico-urachal diverticulum, urachal sinus, and urachal cyst [317]. Once cloacal septation is completed by week 7, the urogenital sinus is further subdivided into upper and lower zones of endodermal cell differentiation [171]. Endodermal cells lining the upper zone of the urogenital sinus differentiate into bladder epithelium, while lower-zone urogenital sinus cells give rise to urethral epithelial cells. Morphogenetic and molecular processes involved in bladder development will be discussed in Sect. 1.5.

Failure to initiate or complete cloacal septation during fetal development has severe clinical consequences and is thought to underlie the pathogenesis of a wide range of urogenital and anorectal human malformations [170, 249]. Morphogenetic and molecular mechanisms underlying cloacal septation are poorly understood. Several processes have been implicated, including regional changes in mesenchymal cell proliferation along the cloacal periphery [306] which may be responsible for generating the tissue folds associated with septation [135, 229, 341]. Genetic studies in mice with gene disruptions affecting Sonic Hedgehog signaling have shown that this pathway is essential to the process of partitioning the cloaca into urogenital and anorectal sub-compartments [56, 116, 252]. Activating Sonic Hedgehog signaling seems to be necessary for stimulating cloacal mesenchyme cell proliferation as removing *Shh* function prior to cloacal septation associated with reduced levels of mesenchymal cell proliferation along the anterior and lateral cloacal margins, which resulted in anorectal and genitourinary defects [267, 306].

1.3 Embryology of the Kidney

1.3.1 Overview of Kidney Morphogenesis

The mammalian kidney develops as a result of reciprocal inductive interactions between the ureteric bud, which is an epithelial outgrowth of the caudal nephric duct, and the metanephric mesenchyme, which is represented by a region of undifferentiated mesodermal cells surrounding the caudal nephric duct. Cellular descendants of the ureteric bud contribute to formation of the renal collecting system, which includes both cortical and medullary collecting ducts, the epithelial lining of the renal calyces and pelvis, and also the urothelial lining of the ureter. Conversely, metanephric mesenchymal cells engage in a complex morphogenetic program which involves mesenchymal-to-epithelial transformation and cellular differentiation and results in formation of all nephron segments, including the glomerulus, proximal and distal convoluted tubules, and loops of Henle. In the sections that follow, morphogenetic stages which result in formation of the collecting system and nephron will be described. In addition, the functions of genes and molecules known to control normal renal branching morphogenesis and nephron development will be discussed.

1.3.2 Ureteric Bud Outgrowth

Outgrowth of the ureteric bud (UB) from the nephric duct heralds the onset of kidney development. The UB forms in response to inductive signals provided by metanephric mesenchyme (MM). These signals induce the UB to elongate and extend towards MM. In humans, UB outgrowth occurs during week 5 of fetal gestation and in mice, at embryonic day 10.5 (E10.5) [261, 298]. Defects in ureteric bud induction are likely to underlie CAKUT phenotypes such as unilateral or bilateral renal aplasia which result from complete failure of UB outgrowth or in duplex kidney which occurs as a result of supernumerary UB formation [256].

The cellular basis of UB outgrowth was recently investigated in murine kidney organ culture using time-lapse imaging to follow the fate of nephric duct cells labeled with a fluorescent marker [60]. The first sign of UB formation is the appearance of an epithelial swelling on the dorsal surface of the posterior nephric duct. This morphologic event is associated with local increases in nephric duct epithelial cell proliferation and restructuring of the nephric duct luminal surface from a simple, single-layered epithelium to a pseudostratified epithelium. The significance of epithelial pseudostratification in this region prior to UB outgrowth is unknown. Similar restructuring of epithelial cell domains has been shown to occur in other developing organ systems where epithelial budding takes place, including liver, thyroid, and mammary gland [24, 93]. It is thought that converting the future budding site from a simple to pseudostratified epithelium might render a higher density of cells for rapid expansion within this region in order to form the UB, although this notion has not been confirmed experimentally [68].

In addition to local changes in cell number, changes in epithelial cell shape and movement are noted to precede regional swelling in the posterior nephric duct. Evidence in mice suggests that cellular rearrangements are essential for enriching the epithelial domain where budding will take place with cells that are capable of responding to inductive signals from surrounding metanephric mesenchyme [60].

1.3.3 Molecular Control of Ureteric Bud Outgrowth

Induction of UB outgrowth depends on molecular interactions between secreted peptides produced by MM cells with receptors on the surface of UB cells. These inductive interactions are under the control of transcriptional networks acting within MM or UB cells to coordinate gene expression and regulate the capacity of UB cells to respond to inductive cues within a precise spatiotemporal framework. This section summarizes the roles played by selected genes and molecular pathways in UB outgrowth as revealed through mutational analyses in mice and, where applicable, in humans.

1.3.3.1 Positive Control of UB Outgrowth

Glial-derived neurotrophic factor (GDNF) and two members of the fibroblast growth factor (FGF) family of signaling peptides, FGF7 and FGF10, are secreted growth factors which play important roles in UB outgrowth. In mouse kidney organ culture, recombinant GDNF, FGF7, and FGF10 proteins are each shown to be potent in vitro inducers of ureteric bud outgrowth [197, 268, 288]. At stages which precede UB outgrowth, endogenous GDNF and FGF10 are secreted by MM cells which surround the posterior nephric duct [197, 288]. These peptides exert their actions by binding and activating cell surface receptor tyrosine kinases (RTKs) expressed on the surface of posterior nephric duct and nascent UB cells. GDNF binds an RTK encoded by the Ret proto-oncogene (*Ret*) in complex with the GDNF family receptor alpha 1 (*Gfrα1*) co-receptor [38, 82]. Fibroblast growth factor receptor 2 (*Fgfr2*) is the candidate RTK receptor for FGF10 given its expression within the nephric duct and UB [343, 379].

RTK activation initiates downstream signaling through a number of pathways including Ras-ERK/MAPK, phospholipase C gamma (PLCγ)/Ca++, and phosphoinositidyl-3-kinase (PI3K) [179]. Ret and Fgfr2 receptor activation results in the expression of *Etv4* and *Etv5* (Fig. 1.3), which are genes that encode two members of the E-26 (ETS) family of transcription factors. ETS proteins are involved in a wide variety of functions including the regulation of cellular differentiation, cell cycle control, cell migration, cell proliferation, apoptosis, and angiogenesis [237]. During kidney development, *Etv4* and *Etv5* function as genetically downstream of *Gdnf* and *Ret*. Their activities are necessary for regulating expression of other genes essential to UB outgrowth [179].

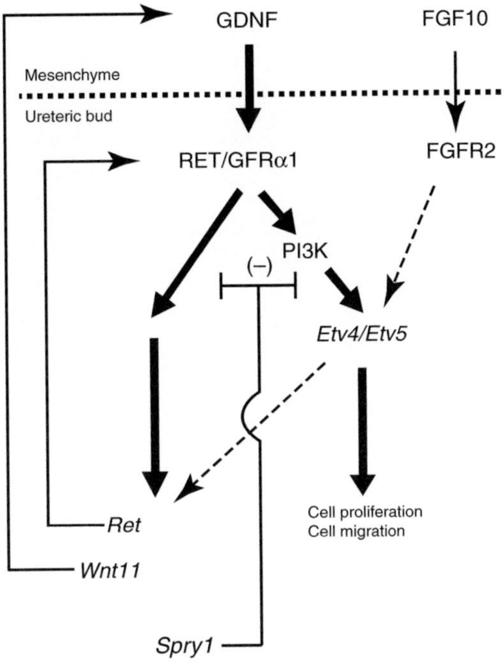

Fig. 1.3 Model of the role for *Etv4* and *Etv5* in a gene network controlling ureteric bud branching morphogenesis. GDNF secreted by metanephric mesenchyme signals to the ureteric bud through a RET/GFRα1 receptor complex to activate the expression of a number of genes, including *Etv4* and *Etv5*, which promote ureteric bud growth and branching. Positive effects on branching may be mediated through cell proliferation and cell migration. Expression of *Etv4* and Etv5 requires PI3K activity. A weaker contribution to the regulation of *Etv4/5* expression may be provided by FGF10, acting via FGFR2. Positive regulation of this network is provided by *Wnt11*, which lies downstream of GDNF-RET signaling. Negative regulation is provided by *Spry1* which antagonizes RET signaling post-ligand activation. *Bold arrows* depict strong effects. *Dashed arrows* denote weak or possible effects (Reproduced from Costantini [68], with permission)

Complete loss of *Gdnf* or *Ret* function in vivo in mice leads to UB outgrowth failure and results in renal and ureter agenesis in 70–80 % of affected littermates [38, 253, 293, 303, 304]. Renal agenesis phenotypes were also generated in mice with homozygous null mutations in genes that encode transcription factors *Sall1*, *Eya1*, *Pax2*, and *Hox11* homeodomain proteins which are required for normal *Gdnf* expression [33, 34, 356, 366, 367] (Fig. 1.4, left panel). Table 1.4 provides a list of gene mutations which cause renal agenesis in mice. Conversely, mutations in genes that normally limit the domain of GDNF expression, such as *Slit2*, *Robo2*, and *Foxc2*, result in the formation of multiple UBs, leading to duplex ureters and kidneys [107, 166] (Fig. 1.4, right panel).

Additional control over UB outgrowth is provided by mechanisms which regulate *Ret* expression in nephric duct cell and nascent UB cells. During normal kidney development, *Ret* expression in the embryonic mouse nephric duct is positively regulated by *Pax2* and *Pax8*. In vitro, Pax2 and Pax8 proteins activate *Ret* transcription by binding directly to the *Ret* gene promoter [65]. The UB fails to form in mice with homozygous null *Pax2* mutations and in mice with compound homozygous null mutations in *Pax2* and *Pax8* due to severe defects in nephric duct formation [26]. However, genetic studies in heterozygous *Pax* mutants suggest that *Ret* expression in the nephric duct is highly sensitive to the level of *Pax2* gene activity. This was revealed in mice heterozygous for a null *Pax2* mutation, which demonstrate renal hypoplasia and lower levels of *Ret* expression compared with mice heterozygous for a null *Ret* mutation, which have normal

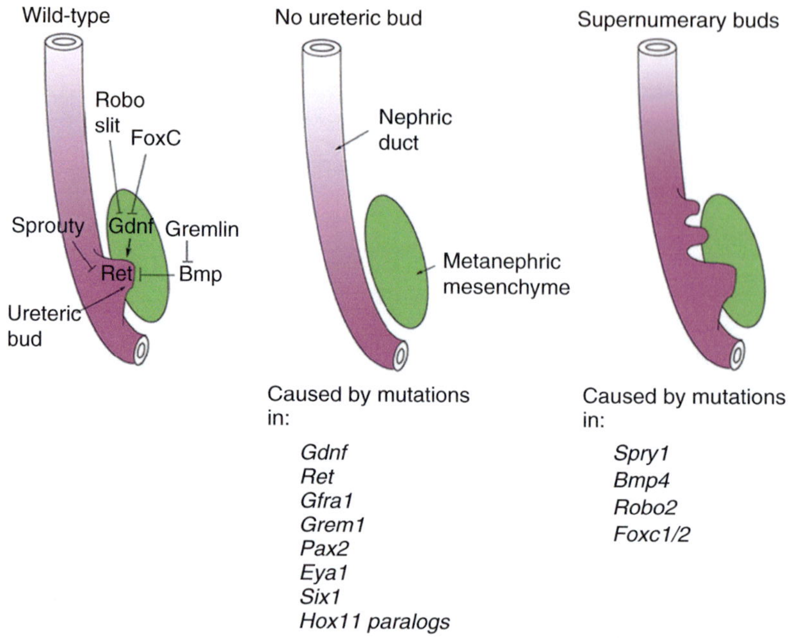

Fig. 1.4 Signals that promote or suppress ureteric bud outgrowth. *Left panel* highlights a subset of molecular interactions that control normal ureteric bud outgrowth by negatively regulating the stimulatory actions of Gdnf and Ret. *Pink area* represents the nephric duct. Green area denotes metanephric mesenchyme. *Middle* and *right panels* illustrate the effect on ureteric bud outgrowth in mice following genetic disruption. Below the images in the *middle* and *right panels* are listed a subset of gene mutations which result in failure to induce a ureteric bud (*middle panel*) or supernumerary budding (*right panel*). See Sect. 1.3.3.1–2 for details (Reproduced with modifications from Dressler [76], with permission)

kidneys [65]. A more severe phenotype was generated in compound mutant mice heterozygous for null mutations in both *Pax2* and *Ret*, which displayed a high frequency of unilateral or bilateral renal agenesis [65]. Collectively, these data suggest that one important function of *Pax2* in nephric duct morphogenesis is to establish the expression domain of *Ret*.

Gata-binding protein 3 (*Gata3*) encodes a zinc finger transcription factor with a role in maintaining *Ret* expression during nephric duct morphogenesis and UB outgrowth. Genetic studies in mice suggest that *Gata3* functions within a regulatory pathway that lies downstream of beta-catenin (encoded by *Ctnnb1*), a cytoplasmic protein with DNA-binding properties which functions as a transcription factor in the presence of Wnt-mediated signals [108]. At stages that precede UB outgrowth, *Gata3* is necessary to maintain *Ret* expression in the caudal nephric duct, which is essential for nephric duct extension towards the cloaca. Nephric ducts of mice lacking *Gata3* function are deficient for *Ret* and show severe nephric duct cell proliferation and differentiation defects [108, 109]. Some nephric duct cells located rostral to the presumptive budding zone maintain *Ret* expression, which leads to ectopic UB formation. This observation suggests that one role for *Gata3* may be to coordinate the recruitment of cells with high levels of Ret to the presumptive budding zone.

The mechanism by which GDNF-Ret signaling causes UB outgrowth is not entirely known. The effects of Ret receptor activation on bud formation may be in response to chemotactic effects of GDNF on nascent UB cells. This is revealed in two reports showing chemoattractant properties for GDNF in vitro on cultured kidney cells [328, 329]. Another study involving chimeric mice made up of a mosaic of cells with varying levels of *Ret* activity suggested that *Ret* is necessary to recruit highly sensitized nephric duct cells to the

Table 1.4 Mouse models of renal agenesis

Gene	Type of protein	Defects in humans	References
Involved in nephric duct formation			
Pax2 and Pax8	Transcription factor	Renal coloboma syndrome	[26, 295, 335]
Gata3	Transcription factor	HDR syndrome	[109, 342]
Lhx1	Transcription factor	–	[157, 247, 336]
Involved in ureter budding			
GDNF-Ret/GFRα1 pathway components			
Gdnf	Secreted molecule, neurotrophin family	Hirschsprung disease	[8, 210, 253, 293]
Ret	Receptor tyrosine kinase	Hirschsprung disease	[83, 303]
GFRα1	GPI-linked neurotrophin receptor	Hirschsprung disease	[38, 88]
Required for GDNF expression			
Eya1	Transcription factor	Branchio-oto-renal	[1, 366]
Hox11 paralogs	Transcription factor	–	[356]
Sall1	Transcription factor	Townes-Brocks syndrome	[160, 232]
Six2	Transcription factor	–	[367]
Pax2	Transcription factor	Renal coloboma syndrome	[34]
Osr1	Transcription factor	–	[141]
Required for Ret expression			
Gata3	Transcription factor	HDR syndrome	[108, 109, 342]
Ctnnb1 (β-catenin)	Transcriptional co-activator, Wnt pathway	–	[188]
Emx2	Transcription factor	–	[204]
Involved in metanephric mesenchyme induction			
WT1	Transcription factor	Denys-Drash	[165]

Reproduced with modifications from Uetani and Bouchard [340], with permission
HDR hypoparathyroidism-deafness-renal anomalies syndrome

site of ureteric budding so that they can readily respond to GDNF [60] (Fig. 1.5).

The role of FGF proteins on UB induction is less clear. In vitro, recombinant FGF7 and FGF10 proteins were capable of inducing UB outgrowth in isolated nephric duct organ cultures [185]. The stimulatory effects of FGF proteins on UB outgrowth were augmented by co-incubating cultures with an inhibitor of TGF-β signaling, suggesting that the nephric duct is normally desensitized to FGFs by local inhibitory feedback. Since *Fgf7* mRNA are not expressed in MM at stages preceding UB outgrowth, *Fgf10* is the more likely candidate for activating FGFR-mediated inductive responses in vivo. Targeted deletion of *Fgf10* results, however, in mice which form UBs but display later defects in UB branching [60]. A similar phenotype was generated in mice with inactivating mutations in *Fgfr2* conditionally limited to the UB cell lineage, which are able to form a UB but show defects in UB branching that lead to renal hypoplasia [316, 379], suggesting that other mechanisms (viz., GDNF-RET signaling) are able to compensate for loss of FGF signaling in these mutants. A recent study showed that complete penetrance of UB agenesis was generated in *Fgf10*$^{-/-}$ mutants by introducing a single null allele for GDNF [60]. Taken together, these studies strongly suggest that GDNF is the dominant inducer of UB outgrowth whereas FGF10 has a weaker role, possibly due to local variances in gene expression or inhibitory feedback on RTK signaling [60].

1.3.3.2 Negative Control of UB Outgrowth

Experimentally, the nephric duct is competent to respond to ectopic GDNF via RET and initiate ureteric bud formation and branching at multiple

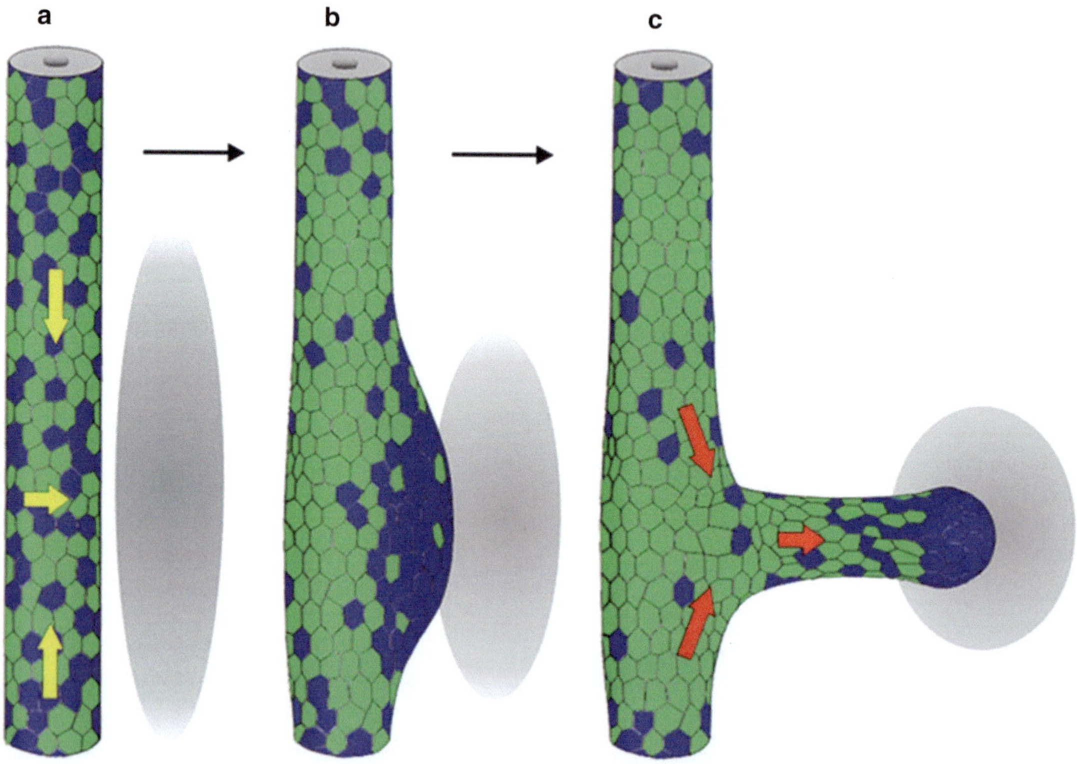

Fig. 1.5 Model for the rearrangement of nephric duct cells at different stages of ureteric bud formation. (**a**) Pre-ureteric bud induction. (**b**) Onset of ureteric bud induction. (**c**) Ureteric bud outgrowth and early elongation. *Blue* and *green areas* represent nephric duct cells with high and low relative levels of RET activity, respectively. *Shaded regions* denote nephrogenic mesenchyme. *Yellow arrows* in (**a**) illustrate the convergence of cells with high levels of RET activity along the long axis of the posterior nephric duct. *Red arrows* in (**c**) demonstrate the recruitment of cells with high levels of Ret signaling to the ureteric bud tip (Reproduced from Chi et al. [60], Copyright 2009, with permission from Elsevier)

sites along its anteroposterior axis [250, 288]. This propensity for random budding may underlie the cause of renal malformations that result when either more than one UB is formed (e.g., duplex kidney) or when induction occurs in the wrong position along the nephric duct's anteroposterior axis (e.g., VU reflux). Consequently, a number of inhibitory mechanisms are used to control the stimulatory response of nephric duct cells to inductive signaling and ensure that UB outgrowth is limited to a single site.

Sprouty proteins provide inhibitory control over signaling pathways activated by GDNF and FGF. Sprouty proteins are intracellular peptides which are known to antagonize RTK signaling downstream of ligand-receptor interactions [84]. In the developing kidney, Sprouty1 (*Spry1*) expression is induced downstream of GDNF-RET signaling in nephric duct and nascent UB cells. Sprouty2 (*Spry2*) and Sprouty4 (*Spry4*) are additional family members expressed in UB cells following outgrowth [377], which suggests that Sprouty proteins also exert negative feedback inhibition at later stages of UB morphogenesis.

At the UB outgrowth stage, *Spry1* plays a role in repressing the nephric duct's response to GDNF and FGF10 and controlling their stimulatory effects on the nephric duct [68]. This inhibitory role was revealed genetically in a series of two reports involving complex analyses of mouse mutants with single or combined loss-of-function mutations in *Spry1*, *Gdnf*, and *Fgf10*. Loss of *Spry1* function in mice resulted in renal malformations including multiple ureters, multiplex

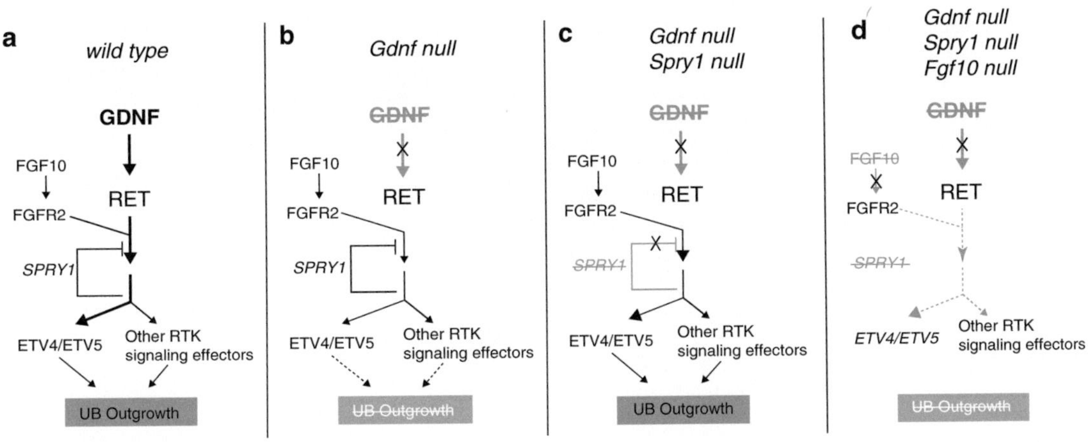

Fig. 1.6 Summary of results from genetic studies in mice supporting a model for *Gdnf* and *Fgf10* cooperating in the induction of ureteric bud outgrowth under the inhibitory control of *Spry1*. (**a**) Wild-type scenario. GDNF acts as the principal inducer (depicted by *bold arrows*) by activating RET, resulting in the upregulation of genes which stimulate ureteric bud outgrowth. FGF10 provides a substantially weaker effect via FGFR2. *Spry1* exerts inhibitory control by antagonizing RTK signaling. (**b**) When *Gdnf* is genetically inactivated, FGF10 is incapable of overcoming the inhibitory effects of *Spry1* on FGFR2 signaling, resulting in failed ureteric bud outgrowth. (**c**) The stimulatory effects of FGF10 on ureteric bud outgrowth are unmasked in mice lacking *Gdnf* by additionally removing *Spry1*, thereby rescuing ureteric bud outgrowth failure in *Gdnf* null mice. (**d**) Confirmation that FGF10 is providing the inductive cue in *Gdnf*/*Spry1* double null mice is provided by additionally removing Fgf10 function, which prevents formation of a ureteric bud (Reproduced with modifications from Michos et al. [197])

kidneys, and hydroureter [14, 15]. These features were associated with ectopic ureteric bud induction, increased expression of *Gdnf* in the metanephric mesenchyme, and expanded expression of GDNF-RET target genes (viz., *Wnt11*). The presence of multiple ureters and the occurrence of renal and ureteral duplications in *Spry1* $^{-/-}$ mice represented a loss of negative control over the stimulatory actions of GDNF. Reducing the *Gdnf* gene dosage in *Spry1* $^{-/-}$ mutant mice by 50 % was sufficient to restore control over UB outgrowth and eliminate the formation of supernumerary buds [14], indicating that inhibitory molecular mechanisms which control GDNF-RET signaling activity are critical to the formation of a normal, single ureteric bud. In another study, the effect of inactivating *Spry1* in mice with complete loss of *Gdnf* function (*Gdnf* $^{-/-}$ mice) was examined (Fig. 1.6). Removing *Spry1* function in mice lacking *Gdnf* was sufficient to rescue renal agenesis and result in generation of a single ureteric bud (Fig. 1.6), likely because the nephric duct now became sensitized to the inductive effects of *Fgf10* [197]. Additionally removing *Fgf10* in *Spry1* $^{-/-}$, *Gdnf* $^{-/-}$ compound mutant mice resulted in renal agenesis [197], which served as evidence that *Fgf10* was capable of fulfilling the role of inducer in the absence of Gdnf only when *Spry1*-mediated inhibition was lifted. A number of studies suggest that angiotensin II signaling may be involved in regulating the levels of *Spry1* mRNA expression in the developing UB, although the local response to angiotensin II in UB cells appears to be dependent on which angiotensin receptor, AT1R or AT2R, is activated [372, 373]. These data support the existence of negative feedback mechanism involving *Spry1* and activation of angiotensin signaling which controls UB outgrowth by regulating which nephric duct cells will respond to GDNF- and FGF10-mediated signals.

Bone morphogenetic protein-4 (*Bmp4*) also negatively regulates UB outgrowth and is locally suppressed by Gremlin 1 (*Grem1*), allowing budding to occur in the correct position. *Bmp4* belongs to a family of genes that encode signaling peptides secreted by MM and UB cells in the embryonic mouse kidney and shown to regulate various stages of kidney development [39]. Kidney organ culture studies have revealed inhibitory roles for BMP4 and other BMP family members including BMP2 and BMP7 in ureteric bud branching morphogenesis [42, 255, 259, 274]. At stages prior to UB induction, *Bmp4* mRNA are expressed broadly in mesenchymal cells surrounding the nephric duct [29, 80, 199]. The expression domain for *Bmp4* partially overlaps with the expression of *Grem1*, which encodes an extracellular antagonist that sequesters secreted BMPs and reduces local BMP signaling activity [199]. The role of *Bmp4* as a negative regulator of UB outgrowth is suggested by the appearance of ureteral duplication and severe hydronephrosis in mutant mice heterozygous for a null *Bmp4* allele [206]. In contrast, *Grem1-deficient* mouse embryos display renal agenesis, presumably due to unopposed inhibitory actions of BMP4 on the nephric duct [199]. At the molecular level, *Grem1* is necessary to maintain and propagate the expression of *Wnt11* in the UB tips, which promotes *Gdnf* expression in MM via a positive feedback mechanism. This infers that BMP4 functions within an inhibitory feedback mechanism that suppresses UB induction by antagonizing the local effect of GDNF-RET signaling on the nephric duct [206].

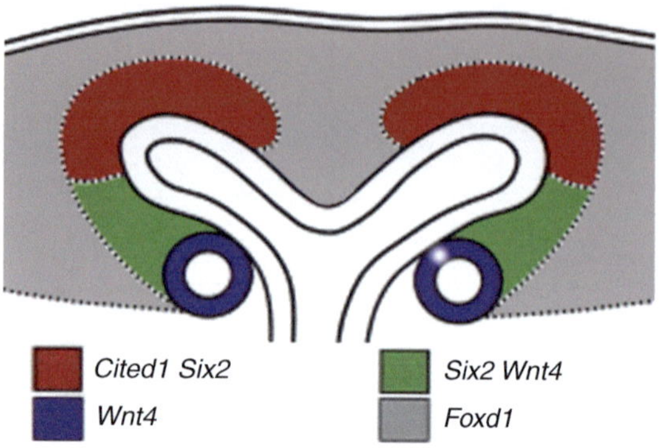

Fig. 1.7 *Six2*, *Cited1*, *Wnt4*, and *Foxd1* gene expression domains in condensed mesenchyme. Depicted is a graphic representation of condensed mesenchyme at the tips of two ureteric bud branches, signifying that metanephric mesenchyme induction has occurred. Cells with high levels of *Six2* and *Cited1* expression (*red area*) represent a subpopulation of condensed mesenchyme cells that are self-renewing and undifferentiated. These cells give rise to a second cell subpopulation within condensed mesenchyme (*green area*) which feature upregulation of *Wnt4* and downregulation of *Cited1*. These cells represent progenitor cells that are fated to undergo cell differentiation and generate all specialized epithelial cells of the mature nephron. Downregulation of *Six2* in cells which express *Wnt4* (*blue area*) signifies the transition from a mesenchymal to an epithelial cell phenotype. Surrounding mesenchymal condensates and epithelial progenitors are stromal cells which require *Foxd1* expression and are necessary for normal nephron development (Reproduced with modifications from Mugford et al. [214], Copyright 2009, with permission from Elsevier)

1.3.4 Induction of Metanephric Mesenchyme

Prior to UB induction (E9.5 in mice), MM is characterized by a population of undifferentiated, non-polarized cells which are dispersed loosely along the ventral caudal nephric duct and marked by the expression of *Osr1* [76]. At this stage of development, *Osr1*-positive (*Osr1* $^{+}$) cells in mice represent a multipotent cell population which are the precursors for epithelial, stromal, and vascular tissue elements in the mature kidney [27]. With advancing gestational age, *Osr1* $^{+}$ cells become progressively restricted in their fate as progenitors of nephron epithelial cells [213] and are transformed into a tightly associated, polarized cell population that forms primitive tubules. Further differentiation of epithelial cell types within these primitive tubules occurs in a spatially organized proximal-distal pattern, resulting in formation of the glomerular and tubular segments of the mature nephron.

Invasion of MM by the UB marks a critical stage in the divergence of mesenchymal cell fate. Upon contact with the UB, the MM condenses to form a discrete zone 4–5 cells thick around the ampulla of the advancing UB [12, 155]. The appearance of condensed mesenchyme (CM) around the tip of the UB signifies that MM induction has occurred. Based on patterns of gene expression, CM is subdivided into two cell populations. One population is comprised of undifferentiated rapidly proliferating cells which are marked by upregulated expression of transcriptional regulators *Six2* and Cbp/p300-interacting transactivator 1 (*Cited1*) (Fig. 1.7) and are thought to represent a pool of self-renewing multipotent epithelial progenitors [28, 158]. The second group is a subpopulation of the first and represents cells which have embarked on the pathway towards epithelial differentiation along an epithelial lineage and are marked by the upregulated expression of the secreted peptide wingless-type MMTV integration site family, member 4 (*Wnt4*) and downregulated expression of *Cited1* [214] (Fig. 1.7). A third population of MM cells is marked by the expression of the forkhead box D1 transcription factor *Foxd1* (Fig. 1.7), which surrounds cap condensates and is thought to give rise to interstitial or stromal cells [122, 214, 308]. Stromal cells secrete extracellular matrix and growth factors and are thought to provide a supportive framework around the developing nephrons and collecting system. Genetic fate mapping studies in mice suggest a common origin for nephron epithelial and stromal lineages which diverges just before UB induction [28, 158, 213]. However, conflicting reports on stromal lineage have shown that some stromal cells originate in paraxial mesoderm [110] or migrate into the developing kidney as neural crest precursors once UB has invaded MM [287, 297].

1.3.5 Control Mechanisms Involved in Mesenchymal Induction

Metanephric mesenchyme condensation occurs in response to a Wnt signal, likely Wnt9b, secreted by the UB. The kidneys of mouse embryos lacking *Wnt9b* are rudimentary and devoid of nephrons [48]. The renal defect is characterized by developmental arrest at the stage where the UB invades metanephric mesenchyme and branches to form a T-shaped structure. Consequently, loss of *Wnt9b* prevents mesenchymal condensation from occurring and blocks initiation of tubulogenesis.

Wnt9b induces the expression of *Wnt4* in cap mesenchyme, which initiates the program that converts mesenchyme to epithelial cells [48]. This interaction appears to be mediated by canonical signaling pathways involving beta-catenin. In one study, the inductive functions of *Wnt9b* were prevented by removing beta-catenin in condensed mesenchyme cells of embryonic mice by conditional mutagenesis [244]. In the same study, activating beta-catenin through overexpression of a constitutively active, stabilized form in MM functionally rescued the inductive defects in *Wnt9b* and *Wnt4* mutants and was capable of initiating the tubulogenic program for epithelial cell differentiation. These data strongly implicate canonical signaling pathways in carrying out the initial functions of *Wnt9b* protein during MM induction and nephron epithelial cell differentiation. However, there appears to be a need to attenuate canonical Wnt signaling once induction has taken place since normal epithelial tubules do not form in embryonic mouse kidneys when activated beta-catenin continues to be overproduced in MM [244]. Consequently, the tubulogenic response to Wnt signaling following MM induction is likely to involve noncanonical signaling mechanisms.

Six2, *Sall1*, and *Wt1* are three transcription factor-encoding genes which are implicated in maintaining a sufficient number of self-renewing nephron progenitor cells to generate all the nephrons that ultimately comprise the mature kidney. *Six2* is a homeodomain transcriptional regulator [158, 308], *Sall1* encodes for a mammalian spalt-like homeotic gene [160, 232], and *Wt1* encodes a zinc finger transcription factor with both a DNA- and RNA-binding properties [348]. Dominant mutations in *SALL1* are the cause of Townes-Brock syndrome (OMIM: 107480), which features renal hypoplasia, dysplasia, or vesicoureteral reflux in addition to anal and limb anomalies [160, 292]. Denys-Drash syndrome (OMIM: 194080) is an autosomal dominant disorder caused by inactivating mutations for *WT1* and characterized by gonadal dysgenesis, diffuse mesangial sclerosis, and increased risk of Wilms tumor [67, 177].

During embryonic mouse kidney development, *Six2*, *Sall1*, and *Wt1* are expressed at low levels in uninduced mesenchyme and upregulated in condensed mesenchyme [158, 160, 232, 308, 370]. *Six2* plays a major role in maintaining the multipotency of nephron progenitors, while *Sall1* and *Wt1* appear to have a more important role in progenitor cell survival. The kidneys of mice homozygous for *Six2* loss-of-function mutations are small and malformed and exhibit ectopic nephron formation along the tips and stalks of ureteric bud branches [308]. The nephrogenic defect in *Six2* mutant mice is attributed to premature epithelial cell differentiation, presumably in response to uncontrolled *Wnt9b* activity, which exhausts the progenitor pool and results in fewer nephrons. In contrast, in the absence of *Sall1* and *Wt1*, MM undergoes apoptosis resulting in unilateral or bilateral renal agenesis in two-thirds of *Sall1* knockout mice [232] and bilateral renal agenesis in 100 % of mice homozygous for inactivating *Wt1* mutations [165].

The functional properties of *Sall1* in kidney development were assessed in an in vitro colony-forming assay. When cultured in the presence of an inducing signal (viz., Wnt4), isolated MM from wild-type mice formed colonies which were reconstituted in organ culture into kidney-like tissues with glomerular and tubular components [239]. Molecular studies on these cultured rudiments revealed expression of epithelial cell markers for glomeruli, proximal and distal tubules, and loops of Henle. In contrast, although MM cells from *Sall1*-deficient mice were able to form colonies and induce the expression of tubulogenic genes, colony size was significantly smaller, suggesting that the dominant role of *Sall1* is to promote progenitor cell survival. Additional support for a survival role was provided by the analysis of MM induction in organ culture, which showed that isolated mesenchyme from *Sall1* mutant mice retained their competence to respond to an inducer but resulted in the formation of smaller tubules [232]. Other genes involved in promoting mesenchymal survival include bone morphogenetic protein 7 (*Bmp7*) [79, 104], *Pax2* [333], and *Fgfr2* [260].

Wt1 is required for MM survival and appears to be necessary for induced mesenchyme to condense around the UB following induction. Evidence in favor of these roles is suggested by the analysis of MM induction when *Wt1* function is removed either by genetic deletion in vivo [165] or by morpholino knockdown in embryonic kidney organ culture [120]. When cultured ex vivo, isolated mesenchyme from *Wt1*-deficient mice failed to aggregate in response to inducing signals from wild-type UB and subsequently underwent apoptosis [73]. A similar result was achieved by co-culturing wild-type kidney explants in the presence of WT1 morpholinos, which modify gene function by preventing translation. Instead of forming a tightly packed cap around the UB, MM was loosely arranged around UB tips in morpholino-treated explants. It was suggested that this finding may be due to defects in cytoskeletal rearrangements or in the formation of focal adhesion complexes on the basis of transcriptional profiling of *Wt1* targets in normal embryonic mouse kidney tissue [120]. Additional targets of *Wt1* which were revealed by this analysis included several MM survival genes with promoters that bind WT1 protein, including *Pax2*, *Sall1*, *Bmp7*, and *Fgfr2* [120]. Thus, one function of *Wt1* may be to regulate cellular events such as cell survival and cell-cell adhesion in a concerted manner which promotes nephron cell fate.

1.3.6 Development of the Collecting System

1.3.6.1 Overview of Collecting Duct Morphogenesis

The collecting duct system refers to the cortical and medullary collecting ducts, the renal calyces, and the renal pelvis of the mature kidney [261, 298]. Development of the collecting duct system involves an embryonic process termed renal branching morphogenesis, which refers to growth and branching of the UB [130]. This process is dependent on reciprocal inductive interactions between MM and UB cells within the embryonic kidney. As a developmental process, branching morphogenesis is essential to the formation of several tissues including kidney, lung, mammary tissue, exocrine pancreas, and salivary glands (reviewed in Hu and Rosenblum [130]). In kidney development, renal branching morphogenesis may be considered as a sequence of related events, which include (1) outgrowth of the ureteric bud, (2) iterative branching of the ureteric bud and derivation of its daughter collecting ducts, (3) patterning of the cortical and medullary collecting duct system, and (4) formation of the pelvicalyceal system.

In human kidney development, renal branching morphogenesis commences between the fifth and sixth week of fetal gestation [261]. In mice, this process is initiated at E11.5 when the ureteric bud invades the metanephric mesenchyme and forms a T-shaped, branched structure [298]. This T-shaped structure subsequently undergoes further iterative branching to generate approximately 8 branch generations in the embryonic mouse kidney [51, 298] and 15 generations of branching in the human fetal kidney [261]. In humans, the first 9 generations of ureteric bud branching are completed by approximately the 15th week of fetal gestation [261]. Throughout this time, new nephrons are induced at the newly formed tips of ureteric bud branches through reciprocal inductive interactions with surrounding metanephric mesenchyme. By the 20th–22nd week, ureteric bud branching is completed, and the remainder of collecting duct development occurs by extension of peripheral (or cortical) segments and remodeling of central (or medullary) segments [261]. During these final stages of UB morphogenesis, new nephrons continue to form predominantly through the induction of approximately four to seven nephrons around the tips of terminal collecting duct branches which have completed their branching program while retaining the capacity to induce formation of multiple new nephrons [261, 298].

1.3.6.2 Cellular Events Involved in UB Branching Morphogenesis

Throughout normal kidney development, the branching UB recapitulates a sequence of morphogenetic events. This sequence is characterized by (1) expansion of the advancing ureteric bud branch at its leading tip (called the ampulla); (2) remodeling of the ampulla, leading to the formation of new UB branches; and (3) growth and elongation of the newly formed branch segment (referred to as the branch "stalk" or "trunk").

Insight into cellular events that take place in UB morphogenesis has been provided by studies of embryonic mouse kidney development in organ culture using time-lapse imaging to follow the fate of UB cells labeled with a visible marker (e.g., enhanced green fluorescent protein; EGFP) in the developing UB as it grows and branches [174, 310, 351]. From these studies, it is evident that cells at the UB tips undergo a burst of cell proliferation which causes regional expansion two to three times the diameter of the parental trunk, leading to ampulla formation [310, 351] (Fig. 1.8a–c). Once the ampulla forms, there is significant cell movement within the ampulla resulting in asymmetric redistribution of highly proliferating cells to the very tips of the UB branch and cells with lower rates of proliferation closer to the branch trunk [310]. Simultaneously, branch formation occurs by an as-yet uncharacterized morphogenetic process of remodeling which causes the ampulla to bifurcate (Fig. 1.8d–f). Studies show that rapidly dividing cells remain at the leading edge of the newly formed branch as they advance forward, whereas cells with lower rates of proliferation remain behind and are incorporated into the trunk [310] (Fig. 1.8g). Based on gene expression patterns, tip cells are viewed as progenitor cells for the formation of new branches throughout kidney development since these cells tend to express genes associated with growth and cell proliferation [49, 179, 300]. For the most part, trunk cells are represented by gene expression patterns associated with the acquisition of specialized functions such as acid-base homeostasis and water balance [22]. Some trunk cells, however, retain the potential to generate new branches, as suggested by patterns of lateral branching (described below).

The majority of UB bifurcations are symmetrical wherein the ampulla flattens and extends in two opposite directions. Asymmetrical patterns of branching have been demonstrated in embryonic mouse kidney organ culture (e.g., trifid branching, which occurs when three daughter branches arising from one ampulla, and lateral branching, which results from de novo branch formation arising from a UB truncal segment) [351]. Morphometric analyses of individual branch growth parameters have revealed a conserved hierarchical pattern of diminishing final length for successive UB branch generations such that sixth-generation branches are shorter

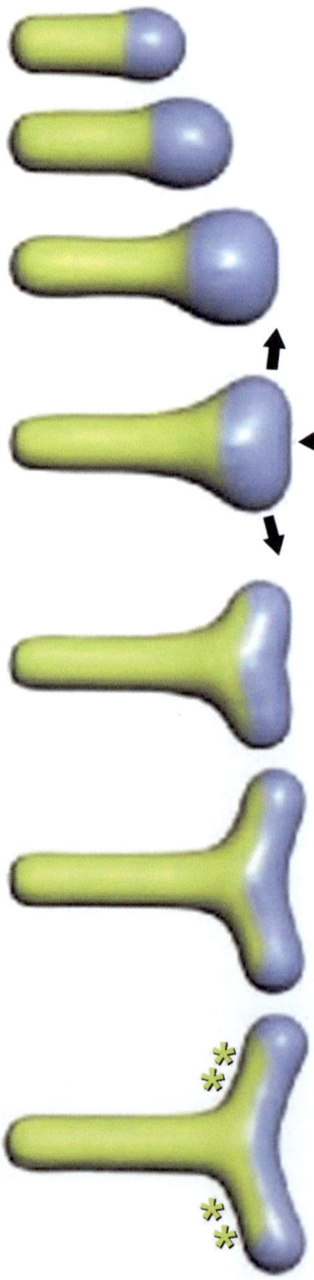

Fig. 1.8 A model for the fate of tip and trunk cells during ureteric bud elongation and branching. (**a**) Shown is a ureteric bud branch segment. The *yellow area* denotes cells residing within the branch trunk. The *blue area* represents cells within the ureteric bud branch tip. At subsequent stages of growth and branching (**b**)–(**g**), *yellow* and *blue regions* denote cells which are derived from the original primary branch trunk and tip segments. (**b**) and (**c**) The trunk elongates through an internal mechanism. Tip cells (*blue*) proliferate under the influence of GDNF/Ret signaling to form the enlarged ampulla. (**d**) The ampulla and the adjacent trunk epithelium are remodeled by an as-yet uncharacterized mechanism which leads to branch bifurcation (**e**). (**f**) and (**g**) Elongation of the newly formed branch generates a new, secondary branch segment with its own trunk and tip zones. Cells which originated as primary branch trunk cells (*yellow*) occupy the proximal sides (adjacent to the *asterisks*) of the two new secondary branch trunks. Cells from the primary branch ampulla (*blue*) form the two new tips and the distal epithelium of the secondary branch trunks (Reproduced from Shakya et al. [310], Copyright 205, with permission from Elsevier)

than fifth-generation branches, etc. [351]. However, in kidney organ culture, asymmetric branching has been described such that branches forming in the posterior region of kidney explants elongate at a slower growth rate compared with branches formed in anterior regions [42]. Presumably, mechanisms that promote asymmetrical branch growth may be important to achieving the final nonspherical shape of the fully formed, mature kidney [51, 351].

1.3.6.3 Molecular Mechanisms that Stimulatory Renal Branching Morphogenesis

GDNF-RET signaling is shown in vivo and in vitro to be a major stimulus for subsequent ureteric bud branching [250, 309]. The ability of *Gdnf* to stimulate UB branching in vivo is revealed by the demonstration of multiple branched ureteric buds in transgenic mice which express *Gdnf* ectopically along the full length of the nephric duct [309]. In response to RET receptor activation, UB tip cells secrete Wnt11 (Fig. 1.9), which acts on MM cells to maintain *Gdnf* expression and thereby promote branching through positive feedback [186]. Signaling responses to GDNF are negatively regulated by Sprouty genes as demonstrated in organ culture experiments with embryonic kidney explants from *Spry1* mutant mice, which show increased sensitivity to GNDF [14]. In addition, loss of *Spry1* function was also associated with increased MM expression of *Wnt11* and *Gdnf* which resulted in an increased number and diameter of UB branches [60, 152, 250], illustrating that negative feedback mechanisms are an important determinant of normal UB branch patterning.

The functional role of GDNF-RET signaling in branching morphogenesis is not well understood. Recombinant GDNF has been shown to be a potent stimulant of UB cell proliferation in organ culture studies [250], leading to the assumption that *Gdnf* stimulates UB branching by promoting UB cell proliferation within the ampulla. It is unlikely, however, that stimulating cell proliferation alone is sufficient to induce

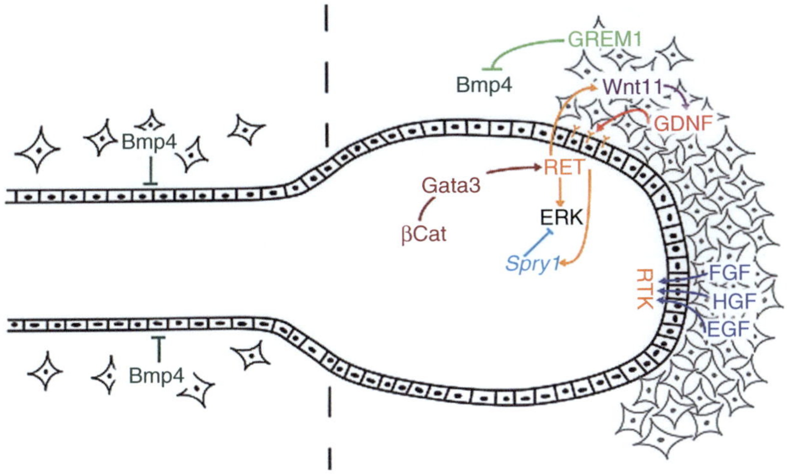

Fig. 1.9 Molecular interactions between stimulatory and inhibitory signals in control of ureteric bud branching morphogenesis. Shown is a sketch of a ureteric bud branch tip surrounded by loose mesenchyme around its truncal segment (*left*) and condensed mesenchyme at the leading edge of the ampulla (*right*). GDNF-RET signaling activity is localized to the branch tip. Wnt11, a molecular target of GDNF-RET, is secreted by branch tip cells and acts on surrounding metanephric mesenchyme to maintain *Gdnf* expression. RET activation in tip cells also upregulates expression of *Spry1*, which feeds back negatively on RET to modulate GDNF-RET signaling activity within the ampulla. Other RTK signaling pathways such as FGF, EGF, and HGF provide additional stimulatory control over branching. BMP4, expressed in mesenchymal cells surrounding the branch trunk exert an inhibitory effect on branching. Gremlin, expressed in mesenchyme around the branch tip, antagonizes BMP4 and facilitates ureteric bud branching by negating local inhibitory effects of BMP4 (Reproduced from Michos [196], Copyright 2009, with permission from Elsevier)

branching since mitotic cells are found in all regions of the ampulla [195]. It is possible that activating RET is necessary to induce cell movements in the ampulla that promote branching [310], much in the way that RET is essential for cellular rearrangements that drive UB outgrowth [60]. The availability of high-resolution imaging systems combined with transgenic technologies that enable tracking the future destination of UB cells will likely provide the means to better understand the mechanistic basis of GDNF-RET signaling on branching.

In vitro studies show that recombinant GDNF alone is not sufficient to induce robust branching in isolated ureteric bud culture [269, 288], suggesting that parallel signaling mechanisms are also involved in controlling ureteric bud branching. Several in vivo and in vitro reports suggest that FGF signaling has direct effects on the UB branching. Following UB outgrowth, several FGFs and their RTK receptor counterparts are expressed in the developing mouse kidney, including ligand-encoding genes *Fgf2*, *Fgf7*, *Fgf8*, and *Fgf10*, as well as receptor genes *Fgfr1* and *Fgfr2*, isoform IIIb (*Fgfr2IIIb*) [43, 268, 270]. All members of the FGF family of ligands are capable of exerting effects on UB growth and cell proliferation as demonstrated in organ culture experiments when isolated UB are exposed to recombinant FGF proteins [268]. These in vitro observations are consistent with in vivo reports describing decreased ureteric bud branching, decreased cell proliferation, and increased ureteric bud apoptosis in Fgf7 and Fgf10 knockout mice and in mouse mutants following conditional deletion of the *Fgfr2* in the ureteric bud lineage [260].

Different FGF family members exert unique spatial effects on ureteric bud cell proliferation in vitro. For example, FGF10 preferentially stimulates cell proliferation at the ureteric bud tips, whereas FGF7 induces cell proliferation in a nonselective manner throughout the developing collecting duct system [268]. These data suggest that multiple FGF family members may function in complex morphogenetic programs that control three-dimensional growth of the developing collecting duct system. FGF7 is also shown to induce the expression of the Sprouty gene, *Spry2*, in developing collecting ducts in vitro [59]. Consequently, FGF7 may participate in a negative feedback loop that controls UB branching by regulating *Gdnf* and *Wnt11* expression.

Two additional RTK ligands hepatocyte growth factor (HGF) and epidermal growth factor (EGF) represent two additional RTK ligands which are expressed in the developing kidney and have been shown to act synergistically in promoting UB branching during mouse kidney development [138, 290, 363]. HGF and EGF proteins bind their respective RTK, MET and EGFR, and activate downstream signaling through PI3K, ERK, and a number of other RTK-mediated pathways [149]. HGF has been shown to promote UB branching in kidney organ culture [45, 209], yet inactivating *Met* function exclusively in the UB lineage using a conditional knockout approach resulted in only a modest decrease in UBB and a 30 % reduction in nephron number [138]. Since *Egfr* is upregulated in Met-deficient UB cells and recombinant EGF can partially rescue UB branching in these Met mutant kidneys, it has been suggested that HGF/MET and EGF/EGFR signaling play complementary roles in UB morphogenesis [138]. Complementary functions for *Met* and *Egfr* were revealed in vivo by combining UB-specific deletion of *Met* with a hypomorphic *Egfr* mutation, which resulted in embryos with small kidneys and severely reduced UB branching [138]. The interaction between HGF/MET and EGF/EGFR serves as an example for molecular cross talk between other RTK signaling mechanisms, including pathways activated by FGF-FGFR interactions, that may act cooperatively with GDNF/RET to control UB branching morphogenesis (Fig. 1.9).

1.3.6.4 Inhibitory Pathways Involved in Control of Renal Branching Morphogenesis

Negative regulators of UB branching include activin A and TGFβ1 [37, 64, 259, 279, 291], semaphorins 3a and 4D (Sema3a and Sema4D) [163, 338], and several BMP family members (reviewed in Cain et al. [39]) based on evidence of their abilities to inhibit branch formation in

UB organ or cell culture models or in mouse genetic mutants which cause downstream signaling to be blocked or attenuated in UB cells.

Bone morphogenetic proteins represent a large group of signaling peptides which share a conserved signaling mechanism. BMP signaling involves ligand binding to receptor complexes that include serine threonine kinase receptors called activin-like kinases (ALKs) and downstream signaling through receptor-activated SMAD proteins, which become phosphorylated upon ligand-receptor binding and translocate to the nucleus to control transcription of several target genes involved in cell adhesion and differentiation [39]. Modulation of this pathway may be provided by interactions between BMP-ALK receptor complexes with extracellular molecules which may either augment signaling (e.g., glypican-3 heparan sulfate proteoglycans; *Gpc3*) [44, 121, 140] or attenuate signaling (e.g., gremlin; *Grem1*) [199] depending on context.

BMP ligands *Bmp-2*, *-4*, *-5*, *-6*, and *-7* and Alk receptors Alk-3 and -6 are expressed in the developing kidney in distinct but partially overlapping domains [72, 80, 103, 345]. Genetic studies suggest that *Alk3* is the dominant signaling receptor in the UB since inactivating *Alk3* specifically in the UB cell lineage by conditional mutagenesis results in medullary hypoplasia and cortical cysts [119] while the embryonic kidneys of *Alk6-deficient* mice are normal [371]. Kidney organ culture studies have revealed inhibitory roles for BMP-2, -4, and -7 in ureteric bud branching morphogenesis ex vivo [42, 255, 259, 274]. The kidneys of *Bmp7*-deficient mouse embryos are small which is associated with decreased UB branching and nephron formation [79, 104]. The renal phenotype in this mutant is attributed, however, to a cell survival defect within the mesenchymal compartment causing the loss of mesenchyme-derived factors that promote UB branching rather than a direct effect on UB cells.

Embryonic mice that carry germline null mutations in *Bmp2* or *Bmp4* die before kidney development begins, thus precluding an analysis of their individual roles in nephrogenesis [81, 360, 376]. The presence of one *Bmp2* null allele does not seem to affect UB branching since the kidneys of $Bmp2^{+/-}$ heterozygotes appear normal [121]. However, an inhibitory function for *Bmp2* was revealed by additionally removing the enhancing function of glypican-3 (*Gpc3*) in *Bmp2* heterozygous mutant mice, which resulted in an abnormal increase in UB branching and cell proliferation [121].

Understanding the role of *Bmp4* in UB branching through in vivo analysis of *Bmp4* heterozygotes is made complex because *Bmp4* heterozygous null mice display a broad spectrum of kidney and ureter malformations [206]. An inhibitory function for *Bmp4* in regulating UB branching is suggested by studies in kidney explants from wild-type mice, in which recombinant BMP4 protein suppressed kidney growth, UB branching, and nephron formation in a dose-dependent manner [37, 42, 274]. Modulating the level of BMP4 activity in vivo is shown to alter the three-dimensional architecture of UB branching as revealed when antagonists of BMP signaling (viz., *Cer1* (cerberus homolog 1) and *Grem1*) are dysregulated in embryonic mice [58, 228]. BMP antagonism appears to function by coordinating the inhibitory activities of BMP4 (and possibly BMP2) with the stimulatory effects of GDNF and WNT11, thus providing a mechanism for spatial patterning of UB branching [58, 199].

Recent studies have shown that Sonic Hedgehog signaling is required to pattern UB branching during kidney development. In the embryonic kidney, *Shh* is initially expressed exclusively in the UB and later is restricted in its expression to the ureter epithelial and medullary collecting ducts [374]. An early requirement for *Shh* in UB induction was revealed by the analysis of mice with germline null *Shh* mutation [374]. These mice exhibited severe developmental abnormalities which included bilateral renal aplasia or the presence of a single dysplastic kidney. Dysplastic kidneys from these mutants showed decreased levels of *Pax2* and *Sall1*, implying that Sonic Hedgehog signaling is necessary to regulate genes that promote UB induction. In addition, removing *Shh* activity resulted in downregulation of the levels of Gli proteins which normally activate transcription (i.e., Gli activator) in the face of Gli3 proteins which normally repress transcription (i.e., Gli3 repressor). Eliminating *Gli3* function in *Shh* mutant mice rescued kidney development and restored *Pax2* and *Sall1* levels. This analysis suggests that one early role of *Shh* in kidney development is to counterbalance the inhibitory influence of Gli3 repressor activity at the time of UB induction. This notion of balancing Gli activator and repressor functions is later important in establishing cortical and medullary domains within the collecting duct system as shown in mice when Sonic Hedgehog signaling is inappropriately activated in the developing renal cortex. Ectopic HH signaling was induced in the renal cortex of mice with targeted inactivation of *Ptc1* in the UB cell lineage, which resulted in decreased UB branching and caused renal hypoplasia [41]. The branching defect in *Ptc1* conditional mutants was associated with decreased levels of *Gdnf, Ret*, and *Wnt11* expressions, which were restored in *Ptc1* mutant mice by additionally overexpressing a constitutively active form of Gli3 repressor protein in these mutants [41]. These data suggest that a gradient of HH signaling activity exists within the developing kidney which is characterized by low levels of Gli activator function and high levels of Gli3 repressor in the cortex. This pattern of Hedgehog activity appears to be necessary for setting up gene expression patterns in the renal cortex which promote UB branching and repress branching in the medulla.

1.3.6.5 Development of the Renal Medulla and Pelvicalyceal System

Between weeks 22 and 34 of human fetal gestation [261], or at E15.5 in embryonic mice [298], the renal cortex and medulla of the developing kidney become morphologically distinct. The cortex contains all glomerular, proximal, and distal tubular tissue elements as well as adjoining segments of the descending and ascending loops of Henle and cortical collecting ducts. It is organized as a relatively compact, outer rim of tissue and represents about 70 % of total kidney volume at birth [51]. The renal medulla lies deep to the cortex. It is comprised of longitudinal arrays of collecting ducts and loops of Henle which are interspersed with peritubular capillaries that surround both tubular tissues.

During embryonic kidney development, distinct morphologic differences emerge between collecting ducts located in the medulla compared to those located in the renal cortex during this stage of kidney development. Medullary collecting ducts are organized into elongated, relatively unbranched linear arrays which converge centrally to form the papilla. In contrast, collecting ducts located in the renal cortex actively induce metanephric mesenchyme until nephrogenesis is complete. The most central segments of the collecting duct system that are formed from the first five generations of ureteric bud branching undergo remodeling by increased ductile growth and dilatation to form the pelvis and calyces (reviewed in Al-Awqati and Goldberg [4]). The renal pelvis is lined by UB-derived epithelium and is surrounded by smooth muscle at its confluence with the proximal ureter. The calyces, in turn, represent extensions of the renal pelvis which surround the papilla.

The developing renal cortex and medulla exhibit distinct axes of growth. The renal cortex grows along a circumferential axis, resulting in a tenfold increase in volume while preserving compact organization of cortical tissue around the developing kidney [51]. In this manner, developing glomeruli and tubules maintain their relative position in the renal cortex with respect to the external surface of the kidney or renal capsule. Preserving this spatial relationship between developing nephrons and the renal capsule appears to be crucial as revealed by defective nephron development in mice that fail to form a renal capsule [169].

In contrast to the circumferential pattern of growth exhibited by the developing renal cortex, the developing renal medulla expands 4.5-fold in thickness along a longitudinal axis perpendicular to the axis of cortical growth [51]. This pattern of growth is attributed to elongation of outer medullary collecting ducts [51]. Elongation of medullary collecting ducts is governed by oriented cell division (OCD), a process which involves aligning cell mitotic spindles with the long axis of a structure [98]. OCD leads to duct elongation without a change in lumen diameter. Conversely, cystic dilatation of ducts occurs when OCD is disrupted [98, 284].

Signaling mechanisms implicated in control of OCD include planar cell polarity and Wnt signaling. Fat4 is a single-pass transmembrane protein and component of the planar cell polarity signaling pathway which is required for OCD as demonstrated in *Fat4*-deficient mice. Targeted disruption of *Fat4* in embryonic mice caused randomization of OCD in developing collecting ducts, which resulted in the formation of dilated collecting ducts and cystic kidneys [284]. The Wnt7 signaling molecule, encoded by *Wnt7b*, is expressed in UB trunk cells and is necessary for CD elongation which takes place during formation of the medulla and papilla [375]. When *Wnt7b* function is lost in UB-derived cells by conditional inactivation, CDs that form the medulla and papilla become grossly dilated [375]. *Wnt9b*, which is expressed in UB tip cells and which plays an important role in MM induction, is later expressed in medullary CD cells where it acts to control OCD through an autocrine signaling mechanism [150]. The role of *Wnt9b* in this process is reflected by the occurrence of cysts and disruption of OCD in collecting ducts of mice when *Wnt9b* is deleted from UB-derived cells [150].

Development of the medulla coincides with the appearance of stromal cells between the 7th and 8th generations of ureteric bud branches [51]. It is suggested that stromal cells provide stimulatory cues which promote growth of medullary collecting ducts [51]. Additional support for this hypothesis is provided by analyses of mutant mice lacking stromal transcription factors Pod1 (also known as TCF21) [69, 272] or Foxd1 [11, 69, 122, 272], which demonstrate defects in medullary collecting duct patterning.

Mutations in a number of genes that encode molecular components of the renin-angiotensin system, which is best known for its role in controlling renal hemodynamics, cause abnormalities in the development of the renal calyces and pelvis. Mice homozygous for a null mutation in the angiotensinogen gene (*Agt*) demonstrate progressive widening of the calyx and atrophy of the papillae and underlying medulla [230]. Identical defects occur in homozygous mutants for the angiotensin receptor-1 (*Agtr1*) gene [208]. The underlying defect in these mutants appears to be decreased cell proliferation of the smooth muscle cell layer lining the renal pelvis, resulting in decreased thickness of this layer in the renal pelvis and proximal ureter. Mutational inactivation of *Agtr2* (encoding angiotensin receptor-2) results in a range of anomalies including vesicoureteral reflux, duplex kidney, renal ectopia, ureteropelvic or ureterovesical junction stenoses, renal dysplasia or hypoplasia, multicystic dysplastic kidney, or renal agenesis [231]. *Agtr2* null mice demonstrate a decreased rate of apoptosis of the cells around the ureter, suggesting that *Agtr2* also plays a role in morphogenetic remodeling of the ureter.

1.3.6.6 Terminal Differentiation of Collecting Ducts

Ureteric bud epithelial cell differentiation results in the formation of two functionally distinct mature cell types – principal cells and intercalated cells. Principal cells (PC) are characterized by the expression of aquaporin-2 water channels (encoded *Aqp2*) and are necessary for water homeostasis [22]. Intercalated cells (IC) are required for acid-base balance and excrete either hydrogen ions (alpha-intercalated cells) or bicarbonate (beta-intercalated cells) [347]. In the mature kidney, PCs and ICs are relatively distributed throughout the entire collecting duct system in a manner such that the ratio of PC to IC increases towards the papilla [22]. In the developing kidney, immature PCs and ICs initially express functional markers for both mature cell types [22]. Terminal differentiation results in PCs and ICs acquiring gene expression patterns that reflect their cell type-specific functions.

A number of signaling mechanisms that have been implicated in controlling the relative ratio of PCs to ICs during collecting duct development include the forkhead transcription factor gene, *Foxi1*, Notch signaling, and Wnt signaling. *Foxi1* is required for IC cells to form as *Foxi1* null mice displayed embryonic kidneys with collecting ducts lacking in IC cells without abnormal formation of PC cells [22]. A mechanism involving activation of Notch receptor signaling appears to favor the formation of PCs over ICs as the ratio of PC/IC is reduced in mice when Notch signaling is perturbed [147, 193]. Wnt signals play a role in patterning cell types within the collecting duct system by maintaining UB cells in an immature state. This was shown in mice by deleting beta-catenin (*Ctnnb1*) in the UB lineage, which resulted in premature cell differentiation as revealed by the ectopic expression of mature CD cell markers (e.g., ZO1 and aquaporin-2; *Aqp2*) in UB tip cells [32, 137, 188]. In addition, *Wnt7b*, which is expressed in branch trunks, appears to promote the formation of PC cells by regulating collecting duct elongation and OCD [375].

1.3.7 Nephron Development

1.3.7.1 Overview of Nephron Development

In humans, the first functioning nephrons are formed by week 9 and excrete urine by week 12. By 34–36 weeks gestation, fetal nephrogenesis is completed, following which no new nephrons are formed [126, 261]. Total nephron number varies tenfold in humans with normal kidney function and is reported to range from 200,000 to 2,000,000 [129, 131]. Environmental and genetic factors can impact on total nephron number [127, 211], and low nephron number at birth is associated with the development of hypertension and renal disease in adulthood [30, 31, 183]. Infants with low birth weight as a result of intrauterine growth retardation and premature birth are particularly susceptible to adult renal disease since low birth weight correlates strongly with reduced nephron endowment (Table 1.5) [74, 131, 278].

Table 1.5 Susceptibility factors for hypertension and renal disease in humans associated with low nephron number [181]

Susceptibility factor	References
Low birth weight	[125, 187, 278]
Preterm birth	[125, 278]
Short stature	[129, 238, 315]
Reduced kidney mass or volume	[234, 301, 321, 378]
Maternal gestational diabetes	[7, 225]

Nephron formation is initiated when a subpopulation of condensed mesenchyme cells is induced to enter a program of epithelial cell differentiation. This process of differentiation is termed mesenchymal-epithelial transformation (MET) and ultimately generates all epithelial cell types comprising the mature nephron, including the visceral and parietal epithelium of the glomerulus, the proximal convoluted tubule, the ascending and descending limbs of the loops of Henle, and the distal convoluted tubule [261, 298]. MET results in the conversion of loosely associated, non-polarized mesenchymal cells into tightly associated, polarized epithelial cells, which form primitive tubules. Tubule formation, or tubulogenesis, is characterized by the appearance of morphologically distinct epithelial structures (viz., pre-tubular aggregates, renal vesicles, comma-shaped bodies, and S-shaped bodies) which are generated throughout kidney development according to stereotypic sequence (Fig. 1.10). Pre-tubular aggregates are solid cell clusters which represent the progenitor cell subpopulation of condensed mesenchyme that is induced to differentiate along a nephron-specific epithelial cell lineage. Renal vesicles are hollow structures deriving from pre-tubular aggregates which are comprised of immature epithelial cells that begin to show patterns of nephron segment-specific gene expression. Comma-shaped bodies are transitional structures which convert renal vesicles into S-shaped bodies. S-shaped bodies are tubular structures which may be considered as primitive nephrons based on segment-specific differences in cellular morphology and gene expression. The following sections describe morphogenetic events which occur at each step of nephron development based on observations in human fetuses and mouse embryos [261, 298].

1.3.7.2 Early Stages of Nephron Development

Pre-tubular aggregates form as a localized oval-shaped cluster of cells separated from condensed mesenchyme situated near the base of the UB ampulla. Appearance of the pre-tubular

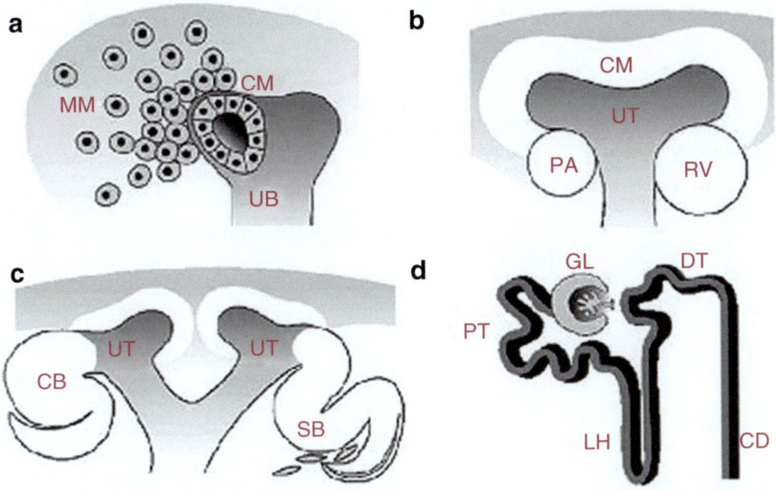

Fig. 1.10 Overview of nephron morphogenesis. (**a**) Metanephric mesenchyme (MM) responds to signals from the ureteric bud (UB) branch tip by condensing around its leading edge. Condensed mesenchyme (CM) contains self-renewing nephron progenitor cells which contribute to the generation of all glomerular and tubular epithelial cells of the mature nephron. (**b**) A subpopulation of CM proximal to ureteric bud branch form a pretubular aggregate (PTA). PTA cells subsequently undergo epithelial transformation and form a hollow structure, the renal vesicle (RV), which connects with its adjacent ureteric bud branch tip (UT). (**c**) Transitional structures are generated by the formation of a distal and proximal cleft within the RV, resulting in formation of a comma-shaped body (CB) and S-shaped body (SB). The distal cleft is invaded by endothelial cell precursors which form the glomerular capillary network. (**d**) The mature nephron is characterized by morphologically and functionally distinct epithelial segments: the glomerulus (GL), proximal convoluted tubule (PT), loop of Henle (LH), and distal convoluted tubule (DT). The nephron is connected at its distal end to the ureteric bud-derived collecting duct (CD) (Reproduced with modifications from Little et al. [176], Copyright 2010, with permission from Elsevier)

aggregate coincides with MET as mesenchymal cells within this cluster acquire a polarized, epithelial cell phenotype, including the formation of adherens junctions and a partial basement membrane [12, 101]. Simultaneous with epithelialization, an internal cavity forms within the pre-tubular aggregate, at which point the structure is called a renal vesicle. The initial renal vesicle is a spherical hollow ball which elongates and widens at the end which is distal to the UB ampulla. The renal vesicle subsequently abuts against the ampulla and forms a connection between these two structures, permitting the UB lumen to communicate with the internal cavity of the renal vesicle [12]. Fusion with the ampulla is a relatively late event in renal vesicle morphogenesis and requires restructuring of the UB cell basement membrane [101]. A completely patent lumen linking the primordial nephron to the UB is evident by the late comma-/early S-shaped body stage [101].

The establishment of glomerular and tubular domains (referred to as nephron segmentation) is initiated by the sequential formation of two clefts in the renal vesicle [261]. Creation of a lower cleft that termed the vascular cleft heralds formation of the comma-shaped body. The comma-shaped body is a transient structure that rapidly undergoes morphogenetic conversion into an S-shaped body following the appearance of an upper cleft. Segmentation is clearly distinguished in S-shaped bodies by the organization of cells into three distinct sub-compartments or limbs. The middle and upper limbs give rise to the proximal and distal tubular segments of the mature nephron, respectively, while visceral and parietal epithelia of the mature glomerulus derive from the lower limb [261, 298]. Prospective cells of the loop of Henle are thought to be first positioned at the junctional region of the middle and upper limbs of the S-shaped body [223].

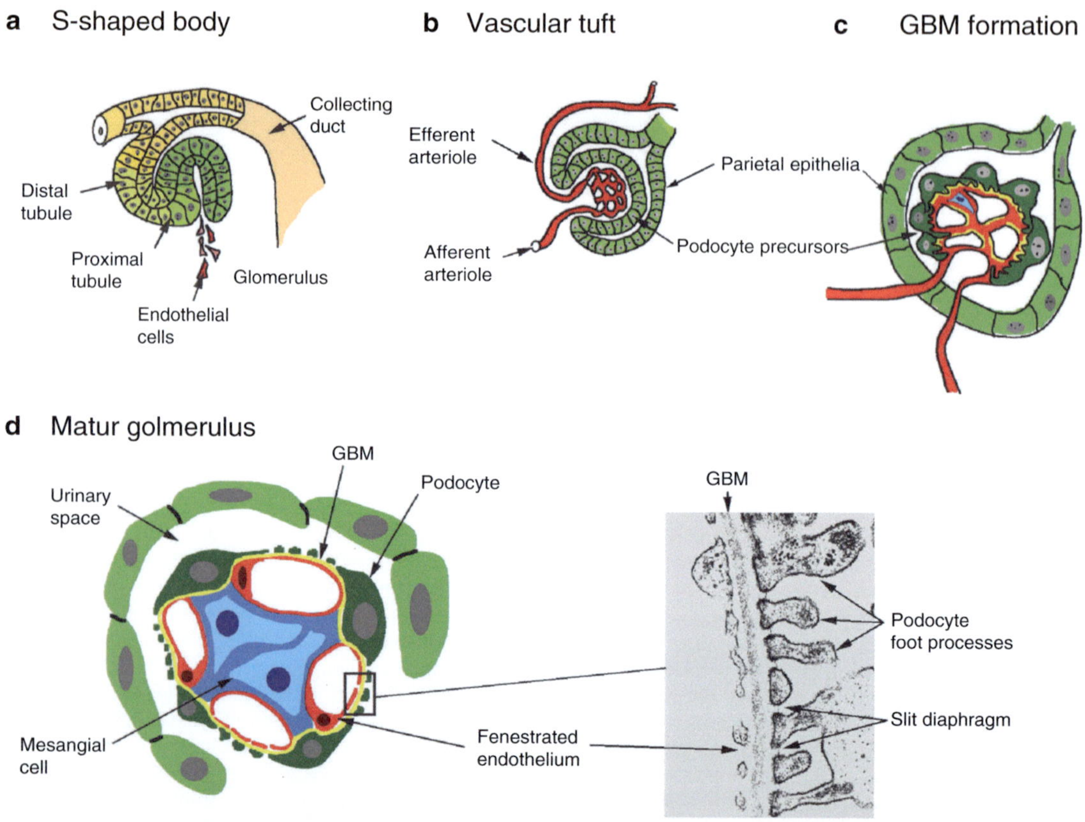

Fig. 1.11 Glomerular development. (**a**) Endothelial cells are recruited into the cup-shaped glomerular precursor region of the S-shaped body forming a primitive vascular tuft. (**b**) Podocyte precursors contact invading endothelial cells and begin to differentiate. In turn, endothelial cells form a primitive capillary plexus (capillary loop stage). (**c**) An interposed glomerular basement membrane forms between podocytes and endothelial cells. Parietal epithelial cells encapsulate the developing glomerulus. (**d**, *left panel*) Elaboration of podocyte primary and secondary cellular processes accompanies podocyte differentiation and formation of the glomerular filtration barrier. (**d**, *right panel*) A high-magnification electron micrograph showing the fenestrated endothelium, podocyte foot processes and slit diaphragms located between the interdigitating foot processes (Reproduced from Piscione and Waters [257], with permission)

As the vascular cleft broadens and deepens, the lower limb of the S-shaped body forms a cup-shaped unit (Fig. 1.11a). Epithelial cells lining the inner wall of this cup will ultimately generate visceral glomerular epithelial cells, or podocytes [164, 261]. Cells lining the outer wall of the cup form parietal glomerular epithelium, or Bowman's capsule. The vascular cleft also serves as an entry portal for the migration of endothelial and mesangial progenitor cells which subsequently differentiate and organize into the glomerular vascular tuft [89, 277]. Recruitment of endothelial and mesangial precursors into the vascular cleft coincides with the formation of a primitive vascular plexus and the deformation of the S-shaped body lower limb into a cup-like structure [261] (Fig. 1.11b). This denotes the capillary loop stage of glomerulogenesis.

The fetal origin of endothelial and mesangial cells is unknown. Endothelial and mesangial cells have been thought to share a similar origin based on experimental evidence involving autologous transplantation of embryonic kidney rudiments into adult renal cortex. These studies suggest that glomerular endothelial and mesangial precursors originate from a unique subpopulation of induced metanephric mesenchyme that does not differentiate along epithelial or stromal lineages [134, 275, 277]. This theory is supported by another study showing a conserved mechanism for both endothelial and mesangial precursor cell recruitment into the developing glomerulus [89]. However, conflicting evidence comes from experiments involving rodent fetal kidneys engrafted onto avian chorioallantoic membrane which support the potential role of angiogenesis in glomerular capillary tuft [296].

Cells residing along the inner surface of the lower S-shaped body limb represent nascent podocytes (Fig. 1.11a). At this stage, immature podocytes are proliferative and exhibit a columnar shape, apical cell attachments, and a single-layer basement membrane [164]. At the capillary loop stage, podocytes lose their mitotic capability [219] and begin to demonstrate a complex cellular architecture (Fig. 1.11d, left panel), including the formation of actin-based cytoplasmic extensions, or foot processes, and the formation of specialized intercellular junctions, termed slit diaphragms [100, 246] (Fig. 1.11d, right panel).

1.3.7.3 Nephron Maturation

Maturation of glomerular and tubular segments of the developing nephron is characterized by morphological changes reflecting growth. The most striking changes occur in the proximal convoluted tubule and loop of Henle, which show increased tortuosity with maturation and elongation, respectively [261]. At a cellular level, proximal tubular epithelial cells transition from a columnar to a cuboidal cell phenotype and develop microvilli on their apical surfaces [92]. Proximal tubule growth is reflected by a gradual increase in tubular diameter and length and is dependent on oriented cell division [324]. At birth, the human kidney exhibits variation in proximal tubule length from the outer to inner cortex, which becomes uniform by approximately 1 month of postnatal life [97]. From a functional perspective, proximal tubule length correlates strongly with sodium reabsorption such that immature proximal tubules have a limited capacity to reabsorb filtered sodium [322].

The descending and ascending limbs of the primitive loop of Henle are first recognizable as a U-shaped structure in the periphery of the developing renal cortex [221, 223]. Maturation of the primitive loop involves elongation of both ascending and descending limbs through the corticomedullary boundary. Longitudinal growth of the medulla contributes to lengthening of the loops of Henle such that all but a small percentage of the loops of Henle extend below the corticomedullary junction in full-term newborn infants [261]. As the kidney increases in size postnatally, the loops of Henle further elongate and reach the inner two-thirds of the renal medulla in the mature kidney.

Continued maturation of the loop of Henle is accompanied by specialization of descending and ascending limb epithelial cells as they acquire unique transport functions [224]. Regional specification of cell function is essential to the kidney's urine-concentrating mechanism as differential transport of urine water and solutes along its descending and ascending limbs, respectively, contributes to generation of an interstitial medullary tonicity gradient. Maintenance of this interstitial tonicity gradient is functionally coupled to urine concentration by rendering a favorable gradient within the medulla for water reabsorption from collecting ducts. Consequently, longer loops are more capable of generating steeper medullary tonicity gradients, hence favoring an increased urine-concentrating capacity. The clinical significance of this relationship is best illustrated in extremely premature newborn infants who have small kidneys that feature short loops of Henle owing to the reduced distance between the renal capsule and the renal papilla. Consequently, the urine-concentrating capacity of the premature kidney is limited by generation of a shallow medullary tonicity gradient.

Glomerulogenesis is completed in human fetuses by 36 weeks gestation in accordance with cessation of nephrogenesis. At birth, superficial glomeruli are chronologically the last to be formed and are significantly smaller than juxtamedullary glomeruli, which are the earliest formed glomeruli [97]. Subsequent growth and maturation involves hypertrophy, with glomeruli reaching adult size by 3 ½ years of age [97]. Glomerular hypertrophy likely plays an important role in glomerular filtration rate (GFR) maturation in term infants who have completed kidney development and enter postnatal life with their full complement of glomeruli [282]. Other factors affecting glomerular function in the newborn term and preterm infant are renal blood flow, which increases at birth [156, 344], and glomerular filtration barrier surface area, which expands progressively from birth to adulthood [97].

The glomerular filtration barrier is a physiologic module comprised of glomerular capillary endothelial cell fenestrations, slit diaphragms which are modified cell-cell junctions between adjacent podocyte foot processes, and the glomerular basement membrane which lies interposed between podocytes and glomerular capillary endothelium (reviewed in Kreidberg [164]; Pavenstadt et al. [246]). The capillary loop stage of glomerulogenesis marks a critical time point in glomerular maturation since it is at this stage that endothelial fenestrations form and podocytes transition from an immature to mature cellular phenotype [89, 164].

1.3.7.4 Genes Implicated in Mesenchymal-to-Epithelial Transformation and Nephron Development

Throughout embryonic kidney development, undifferentiated nephron epithelial progenitor cells are marked by high levels of expression for *Cited1* and *Six2* in condensed mesenchyme surrounding the UB tips. Mesenchymal-to-epithelial transformation (MET) coincides with an initial decrease in the expression of *Cited1* and a subsequent progressive decline in *Six2* expression within a subpopulation of cells which will eventually form pre-tubular aggregates. It is not known what regulates these changes in *Cited1* and *Six2* expression, although a decline in *Cited1* expression within condensed mesenchyme cells seems to be necessary for epithelial transformation to occur [214].

In response to Wnt9b, cells with declining *Six2* activity show upregulated expression of a number of genes necessary for the formation of epithelial tubes, including *Fgf8*, *Wnt4*, and *Lhx1* [244] (Fig. 1.12). *Fgf8* and *Wnt4* are essential for initiating the epithelial cell differentiation as demonstrated by the epithelialization defects in embryonic kidneys of *Fgf8* and *Wnt4* mutants, which show kidney development arrest at the PTA stage [106, 251, 323]. *Lhx1* is not essential for the initial stages of epithelialization since PTA is evident in kidneys of *Lhx1* embryonic mutant mice before kidney development is halted at the RV stage [157]. Molecular studies have revealed that *Fgf8* is expressed earlier than *Wnt4* and is required for the expression of *Wnt4* and *Lhx1* in induced MM [106, 251]. Once MET is initiated, Wnt4 maintains its own expression and likely functions in a cell-autonomous fashion [151]. The initial functions of Wnt proteins during MET are thought to be dependent on canonical signaling mechanisms involving beta-catenin. Activation of this pathway is likely transient since sustained beta-catenin activity within *Cited1*-negative, *Six2*-positive, *Wnt4*-positive cells is shown to prevent epithelial tubule formation in

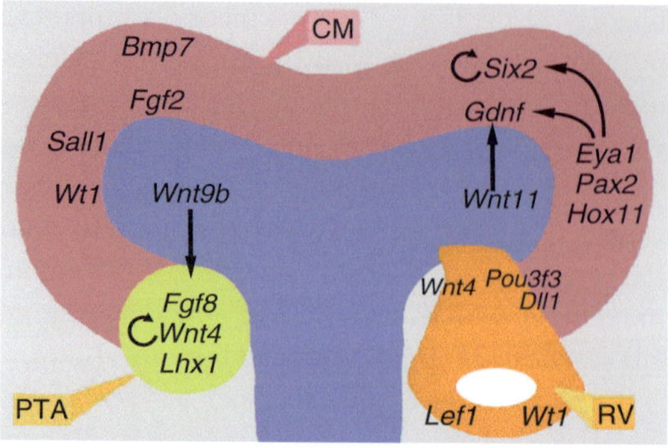

Fig. 1.12 Genes involved in regulating mesenchymal-to-epithelial transformation and establishment of proximal and distal nephron cell fates during early nephron development. Shown is a schematic representation of a branched ureteric bud (*blue area*) with condensed mesenchyme (CM; *pink area*) surrounding the *branch tips*. A pre-tubular aggregate (PTA; *yellow area*) and renal vesicle (RV; *orange area*) are also represented. The diagram illustrates expression domains of genes involved in several stages of early nephron morphogenesis: mesenchyme induction (*Gdnf*, *Eya1*, *Pax2*, *Hox11* paralogs, *Wnt9b*), nephron progenitor cell self-renewal and/or survival (*Six2*, *Sall1*, *Bmp7*, *Wt1*, and *Fgf2*), epithelial transformation (*Fgf8*, *Wnt4*, *Lhx1*), and early nephron segmentation (*Wnt4*, *Lef1*) and the formation of proximal and distal nephron segments (*Wt1*, *Dll1*, *Pou3f3*) (Reproduced with modifications from Little et al. [176], Copyright 2010, with permission from Elsevier)

transgenic mice [244]. Several reports suggest that epithelial cell differentiation and tubulogenesis depend on noncanonical Wnt/planar cell polarity (PCP) signaling pathways [36, 330]. This transition in Wnt signaling may involve *Dkk1*, an inhibitor of canonical Wnt signaling, which is upregulated in Wnt4-expressing cells as they transition from pre-tubular aggregates to renal vesicles [101].

Nephron segmentation refers to the process which establishes gene expression domains that promote the formation of glomerular and tubular epithelial cells along the proximal-distal axis of the developing nephron. As early as the renal vesicle stage, proximal-distal expression domains are established as illustrated by the complementary gene expression of patterns of *Wnt4* and *Lef1* (encoding lymphoid enhancer-binding protein 1) (Fig. 1.12), which is a downstream target of Wnt signals [214]. Expression studies show that *Wnt4* is localized to distal RV cells which are closest to the UB, while proximal RV cells which are furthest from the UB express *Lef1*. Other genes which define the "distal domain" include the POU domain homeobox gene *Pou3f3* (aka *Brn1*), which is required for the formation of loops of Henle [221], and Delta-like 1 (*Dll1*) and Jagged1 (*Jag1*), which are membrane-associated proteins that activate Notch receptor signaling and are implicated in setting up the proximal-distal axis during early nephron development [55]. Conversely, proximal domain markers include *Wt1*, which is necessary for normal podocyte development [112], and *Tmem100*, which encodes a transmembrane protein whose function in kidney development is unknown [101].

Establishing and/or maintaining segment-specific patterns of epithelial cell differentiation during early nephron development is dependent on the functions of *Lhx1* and genes encoding members of the Notch signaling pathway. *Lhx1* appears to control the decision between adopting a glomerular and a tubular epithelial cell fate. This role was revealed in a chimeric study involving the analysis of embryos comprised of a mosaic of wild-type cells and cells deficient in *Lhx1* activity [157]. This study showed that *Lhx1* function was dispensable for the formation of glomerular epithelial cells as only wild-type cells (i.e., cells with full *Lhx1* activity) were detected within proximal and distal tubular segments of the mature nephron, whereas glomerular epithelial cells (i.e., podocytes and cells of Bowman's capsule) were comprised of a mosaic of wild-type cells and Lhx1-deficient cells [157]. Analyses of temporal patterns of gene expression within the developing kidney reveal that the onset of *Lhx1* expression in cells of pre-tubular aggregates follows the induction of *Fgf8* and *Wnt4* and is subsequently expressed in all cells of renal vesicles as these structures progress along their morphogenetic sequence [157]. *Lhx1* promotes the expression of *Pou3f3* and *Dll1*, which have explicit roles in segment-specific epithelial cell differentiation. *Pou3f3* is essential for formation of loops of Henle as well as terminal differentiation of distal tubule epithelial cells [221]. In contrast, *Dll1* is implicated in the formation of proximal tubules as embryonic mice with a hypomorphic mutation for *Dll1* showed a reduction in proximal tubules [55].

Proteins encoded by *Dll1* (Delta-like 1) and *Jag1* (Jagged1) belong to a family of membrane-bound ligands which bind and activate transmembrane Notch receptors on the surface of neighboring cells [312, 313]. Notch receptor activation regulates progenitor cell proliferation and differentiation in many organ systems (reviewed in Chiba [62]). The defect in proximal tubule formation exhibited by *Dll1* hypomorphic mutants is consistent with several reports showing that Notch signaling is essential for the formation of glomerular and proximal tubule segments of the nephron [55, 191]. Among genes which encode Notch signaling pathway molecules in mammals, *Notch1* and *Notch2* receptor genes and ligands *Jag1* and *Dll1* are expressed in RVs and S-shaped bodies in non-overlapping expression domains [54, 258]. Genetic studies show that *Notch2* is the dominant receptor since conditional deletion of *Notch2* in MM results in the formation of rudimentary nephrons comprised of cells expressing distal tubule markers and lacking podocytes and proximal tubule cells [55]. In contrast, a requirement for *Notch1* in proximal nephron formation was only revealed in *Notch1* conditional mutants when the gene dosage of *Notch2* is halved [324]. At later stages of tubular development, *Notch1* and *Notch2* cooperatively regulate OCD in developing proximal tubules, which is necessary to prevent cystic dilatation and malignant transformation to renal cell carcinoma-like tumors [324]. A role for Notch signaling in glomerular development was suggested by the analysis of a mouse model for Alagille syndrome caused by a hypomorphic mutation in *Notch2* [191, 192]. In humans, Alagille syndrome is characterized by a multisystem disorder featuring heart, eye, liver, skeletal, and renal defects with variable penetrance [5, 87]. The kidneys of mice with two hypomorphic *Notch2* alleles or one hypomorphic *Notch2* allele combined with one *Jag1* loss-of-function allele were hypoplastic and featured glomeruli arrested in their development at the capillary loop stage [191, 192]. The primary glomerulogenesis defect in these mice was attributed to failure to form the vascular tuft, although it was not clear from the analysis whether this resulted from a defect in the initial formation or differentiation of podocytes or, alternatively, abnormal migration of endothelial and mesangial cells into the vascular cleft. Thus, while Notch signaling appears to be critical for the formation of glomeruli and proximal tubules, additional studies are still required to determine what role, if any, Notch signaling plays in governing cell fate decisions which affect podocyte cell differentiation.

Mechanisms that control the differentiation of nephron epithelial cell progenitors into podocytes are poorly understood although evidence in nonmammalian urogenital systems, such as zebrafish and Xenopus, have implicated two transcription factor genes, *Foxc2* and *Wt1*, in this process [235, 358]. In the developing mouse kidney, *Foxc2* expression is first detected along the inner surface of the vascular cleft in comma-shaped bodies, which is the position occupied by podocyte progenitors during the morphological transition from comma-shaped body to S-shaped body [326]. Subsequently, *Wt1* expression is upregulated in the same cells at the S-shaped body stage [248]. The role of *Wt1* in podocyte differentiation is not evident through the analysis of *Wt1* knockout mice since development is arrested at MM induction [165]. However, a role for *WT1* in podocyte differentiation is suggested by the occurrence of diffuse mesangial sclerosis in humans with dominant mutations in *WT1* [67, 144, 177, 245]. Diffuse mesangial sclerosis is a congenital form of proteinuric glomerulopathy which is characterized by defects in podocyte differentiation [369] and is featured along with gonadal defects in humans with Denys-Drash (OMIM: 194080) and Frasier syndromes (OMIM: 136080), which are caused by dominant WT1 mutations [10, 67, 154]. The identical glomerular phenotype in mice is demonstrated in mice with targeted *Wt1* mutations genetically similar to the *WT1* mutation in humans with Denys-Drash syndrome [99, 112, 114, 245], which serves as additional evidence that *Wt1* has an important role in podocyte differentiation. Several studies have shown that *Wt1* acts as a transcriptional activator by binding to the promoters of a number of genes expressed in developing and mature podocytes including *Vegf*, *Nphs1* (encoding nephrin), and *Podxl* (podocalyxin) [111, 115, 243, 349]. Recent studies in zebrafish and Xenopus have suggested that functions of *Wt1*, *Foxc2*, and Notch signaling converge to regulate the expression of podocyte-specific genes [235, 358]. Further identification of genes whose promoters bind WT1 will be essential to our understanding of WT1 function in glomerular development [120].

Podocyte terminal differentiation relies on the function of a number of transcription factors, including those encoded by transcription factor 21 (*Tcf21*; also known as *Pod1*), LIM homeobox transcription factor 1 beta (*Lmx1b*), and the Kreisler leucine zipper homolog *Mafb*. In mice with loss-of-function mutations in *Tcf21*, *Lmx1b*, and *Mafb*, glomerulogenesis is disrupted, and podocytes show altered expression of structural genes (e.g., nephrin, collagen type IV) which become evident at the capillary loop stage (in the case of *Tcf21* mutant mice) or later (in the case of *Lmx1b* and *Mafb* mutants) [201, 272, 285]. In humans, *LMX1b* mutations are identified in patients with Nail-Patella syndrome, which is associated with focal segmental glomerulosclerosis [78].

Recruitment of endothelial and mesangial precursors and subsequent formation and assembly of the glomerular capillary tuft require vascular endothelial growth factor (VEGF) and platelet-derived growth factor-B (*Pdgfb*). VEGF is secreted by podocyte precursors of early S-shaped bodies and continues to be secreted by mature podocytes in postnatal life [153]. During early glomerulogenesis, VEGF promotes recruitment of angioblasts into the vascular cleft [337]. This process is tightly regulated as severe glomerular defects result in mice when the gene dosage of *Vegf* is genetically manipulated [89, 90].

Pdgfb is expressed by endothelial cells and binds to its receptor, PDGF receptor-beta (*Pdgfrb*) [175], on the surface of mesangial cell precursors to promote inward migration into the vascular cleft of S-shaped bodies. The function of this axis is required for proliferation and assembly of glomerular capillaries and mesangium as revealed by the absence of glomerular capillary tufts in mice deficient of either *Pdgfb* or *Pdgfrb* [168, 320].

During the S-shaped stage, podocyte progenitors express a primitive glomerular basement membrane which is composed predominantly of laminin-1 and α-1 and α-2 subchains of type IV collagen [202]. During glomerular development, composition of the glomerular basement membrane undergoes transition as laminin-1 is replaced by laminin-11, and α-1 and α-2 type IV collagen chains are replaced by α-3, α-4, and α-5 subchains [202]. As demonstrated in several mouse models, failure of these changes result in severe structural and functional defects [200, 203, 233].

1.3.7.5 Cessation of Nephrogenesis

At the morphologic level, the final stages of nephrogenesis are marked by a progressive absence of ureteric bud ampullae and a decline in the density of *Six2*-positive, *Cited1*-positive nephron epithelial progenitor cells within cap condensates [158]. The mechanism that triggers this change in progenitor cell self-renewal and differentiation is unknown. A recent report described three-dimensional modeling of the nephrogenic zone in postnatal mice and revealed that a rapid wave of mesenchymal cell differentiation occurs during the final stages of nephrogenesis with the induction of multiple nephrons around a single UB tip [283]. Thus, it is possible that mass induction exhausts the self-renewing progenitor cell pool, perhaps because the signal for self-renewal is no longer present in sufficient quantity [123]. In line with this view, nephrogenesis might be prolonged if progenitor cell self-renewal and/or survival was restored by providing the necessary signal or stimulus [123]. A study involving uninephrectomized fetal sheep showed that removing one kidney in utero accelerated the rate nephron induction in the remaining kidney [74], indicating that the developing kidney in some species may compensate for loss of nephron mass in utero. It is tempting to speculate, then, that nephrogenesis could be "rescued" in utero in humans by intervening prior to 34-week gestation in human fetuses with renal hypoplasia or in fetuses exposed to maternal factors (e.g., maternal malnutrition) that affect final nephron endowment [167, 187, 362, 380]. The evolution of functional genomics and high-throughput gene expression technologies has rapidly advanced our understanding of genes and pathways involved in starting and stopping nephrogenesis [35, 52, 305] in humans [124, 264]. Validating these studies through functional analyses should provide a clearer understanding of the mechanisms involved in establishing final nephron number.

1.4 Ureter Development

The mature ureter is a muscle-walled tube which acts as a conduit for urine flow from the kidney to the bladder. Its luminal surface is covered by a water-impermeable, stratified epithelium which is termed urothelium. Smooth muscle cells encompass the mature ureter along its proximal-distal length (Fig. 1.13) and propagate urine flow by peristalsis. In humans, ureteral malformations are represented by a heterogeneous group of anatomical defects, including ureteral agenesis, duplication, ectopia, and strictures, as well as ureteral dilatation (or hydroureter) which may be

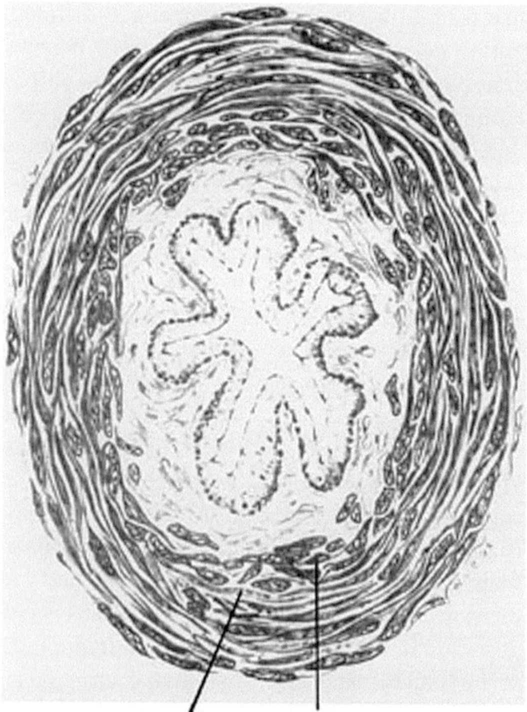

Fig. 1.13 Photomicrograph of a mature, human ureter in cross section at the mid-length. Longitudinal and spiral or circular smooth muscle layers are denoted (Reproduced from Woodburne [361], with permission)

associated either with urinary tract obstruction above or below the bladder or secondary to an intrinsic defect in smooth muscle peristalsis [205]. Traditional views on normal ureter development have stemmed largely from pathological descriptions of human fetal ureter defects from autopsy specimens [184]. Conventional concepts on ureter development have been challenged by the results of recent studies which have rendered new insights on normal and abnormal ureter morphogenesis [17, 61, 339]. Likewise, phenotypic analyses in mouse genetic mutants with ureteral malformations have been highly informative in clarifying developmental disruptions which underlie these anomalies. The following section reviews current concepts of ureter development in humans and draws inferences from studies in mice. This information serves as a foundation for understanding the pathophysiological basis of human congenital urinary tract obstruction syndromes.

1.4.1 Normal Ureter Morphogenesis

Normal ureter development follows a complex sequence of events initiated by UB outgrowth and elongation and succeeded by a process of maturation which involves smooth muscle and urothelial cell differentiation, distal ureter remodeling, and formation of a connection with the developing bladder (Fig. 1.14). Following UB outgrowth, the truncal segment of UB elongates and initiates a series of reciprocal interactions with surrounding mesenchyme that induces periureteral mesenchyme to differentiate into ureteral smooth muscle and UB cells to transform into urothelium. Initially, the ureter is separated from the primitive bladder (represented at this stage by the upper urogenital sinus) by the common nephric duct, which intervenes between the ureteric bud and the urogenital sinus. The common nephric duct subsequently degenerates, and the ureter separates from the nephric duct to form a connection to the bladder. A more detailed description of this process is provided in Sect. 1.5.2.

The initial stages of ureter development are common to both sexes. In humans, this occurs at approximately weeks 11–12 of gestation [189, 325] and E15.5 in mice [16]. Once the common nephric duct degenerates and the ureter separates to connect with the bladder, the disconnected nephric duct migrates posteriorly and unites with tissues derived from the lower urogenital sinus, which adopt different fates in males and females. In males, the paired nephric ducts enter the presumptive prostatic urethra and contribute to the bilateral formation of seminal vesicles and ejaculatory ducts. In females, the anterior nephric duct degenerates in response to a lack of androgen production. Posterior segments become incorporated into the Mullerian duct-derived lower third of the vagina and may persist in mature females as vestigial structures [23, 77, 276].

The newly formed ureter is represented by a single-cell-lined epithelial tube surrounded by a loose network of undifferentiated mesenchymal cells. Studies on first-trimester fetal autopsy specimens have revealed that the immature ureter is patent between gestation weeks 5 and 7 and then is periodically obstructed by epithelial cells

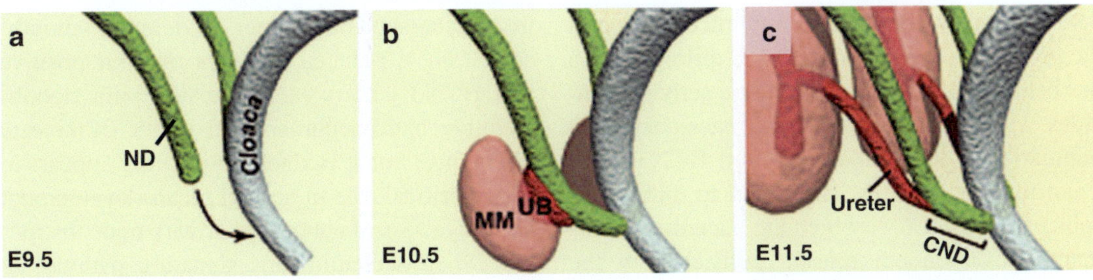

Fig. 1.14 Early stages of distal ureter morphogenesis. (**a**) Ureter formation requires that the nephric duct (ND) extend posteriorly to reach and fuse with the cloaca/urogenital sinus. (**b**) The ureteric bud (UB) develops as an outgrowth of the posterior nephric duct in response to signals emanating from the metanephric mesenchyme (MM). (**c**) The UB invades the MM and branches to form the collecting duct system. The section of ureteric bud located between the MM and ND differentiates into the ureter. The nephric duct segment located between the ureter and cloaca/urogenital sinus represents the common nephric duct. This segment is eliminated by apoptosis during distal ureter maturation (Reproduced with modifications from Uetani and Bouchard [340], with permission)

and proceeds through repetitive cycles of recanalization during the elongation phase of development [6, 281]. By gestation week 12, this process of recanalization is complete, and the normal ureter remains as a hollow tube for the rest of its development. The purpose of this cycle of obstruction and recanalization in human fetal ureter development is not known; however, these processes appear to be unique to ureter morphogenesis since they are not documented in other ureteric bud-derived structures, such as renal collecting ducts and the pelvicalyceal system [240, 241]. One suggestion is that this process may be required to transform the luminal of the nascent ureter from a single layer of cells into a stratified urothelium [182]. Between weeks 12 and 15, the immature ureter epithelium transforms from a monolayer to a pseudostratified epithelium which is characterized by the expression of apical proteins called uroplakins (in mice, encoded by *UpkII* or *UpkIIIa*) [162]. Uroplakins confer water impermeability to the urothelial surface. In humans, mutations in *UPKIIIA* have been associated with ureteral malformations including vesicoureteral reflux and multicystic dysplastic kidney (OMIM: 611559), the latter which is associated with a ureter that lacks a patent lumen [146, 302].

Between 5 and 8 weeks gestation, the fetal kidney ascends to its stereotypic position from the sacral region to the upper lumbar segments. Ureteral smooth muscle formation is evident by approximately week 12 of gestation in the human fetus [189, 325] (E15.5 in mice) [50, 374]. Initial events involve the aggregation and proliferation of periureteral mesenchymal cells which form condensations around the nascent ureters [374]. Condensates are subsequently induced to undergo smooth muscle cell differentiation and are characterized by an increase in smooth muscle actin, smooth muscle myosin heavy chain, and SM22, which is an early marker of smooth muscle cell differentiation [50, 374]. Smooth muscle cell differentiation is initiated in the region surrounding the proximal ureter and renal pelvis and continues in a proximal to distal manner until the entire ureter is covered by smooth muscle by week 22 [189, 325]. Differentiated smooth muscle cells are assembled into fibers which are arranged in spiral bundles around the developing ureter. By week 17, a second inner layer of smooth muscle is generated and assembled into longitudinal bundles. Longitudinal smooth muscle fibers are restricted to the region surrounding the distal two-thirds of the ureter and extend into the tunnel formed by the ureter as it passes through the dorsal bladder wall [218, 346].

Urine flow from the kidney to the bladder is an active process and is mediated by the peristaltic activity of ureter smooth muscle. Peristaltic activity is initiated within the region of the ureteropelvic junction (UPJ) and propagates distally along the length of the ureter in a coordinated fashion [66, 368]. During development, ureter peristalsis is evident by E15.5 in mice as soon as the process of smooth muscle cell differentiation has begun [70]. Onset of peristaltic activity coincides with the presence of two pacemaker cell populations – Cajal-like cells and HCN3 cells. Cajal-like cells show similarity to interstitial cells of Cajal (ICCs), which are pacemaker cells that control smooth muscle peristalsis in the intestinal tract [294]. ICCs and Cajal-like cells are marked by the cell surface expression of the receptor tyrosine kinase, c-kit [70, 334]. Cajal-like cells are found within the lamina propria and between smooth muscle fibers of the embryonic mouse renal pelvis and proximal ureter regions [40, 70, 133]. HCN3 cells are characterized by the activity of hyperpolarization-activated cation channels. These cells play a pivotal role in regulating cell excitability in cardiac and enteric nervous tissues [96, 365]. HCN3 cells are specifically localized to the UPJ, and their function in this region is thought to initiate unidirectional propagation of smooth muscle peristalsis from proximal to distal [133]. Based on immunohistochemistry, abnormal patterns of pacemaker cell distribution or number have been described in resected ureteral tissues from children with congenital UPJ obstruction, suggesting that the cause of this disorder may involve intrinsic defects in pacemaker cell differentiation, survival, or migration [161, 319]. A recent report described the occurrence of severe nonobstructive hydronephrosis and hydroureter accompanied by complete absence of c-kit-positive cells in the renal pelvis and proximal ureter in a mouse model of Pallister-Hall syndrome (OMIM: 146510) [40]. Pallister-Hall syndrome is a multisystem congenital disorder in humans with urinary tract malformations in approximately 60 % of cases [113, 136]. PHS has been mapped to the GLI3 locus [148], which encodes a transcription factor in the Sonic Hedgehog signaling pathway that has activator or repressor functions depending on it cleavage state [132]. In PHS, nonsense and frameshift mutations result in constitutive GLI3 repressor activity, which abrogates Sonic Hedgehog signaling [148]. When Sonic Hedgehog signaling was genetically inactivated in a tissue-specific manner by deleting smoothened (*Smo*), reduced numbers of c-kit positive and HCN3 cells were associated with nonobstructive hydronephrosis and ureter dyskinesia [40]. Thus, Sonic Hedgehog signaling appears to play a critical role in normal ureter development and may cause of congenital urinary tract obstruction when activating this signaling pathway is disrupted.

1.4.2 Molecular Control of Ureter Development

Ureter smooth muscle formation and urothelial cell maturation is coordinated by reciprocal inductive interactions between mesenchymal and epithelial compartments of the developing ureter. Early in ureter development, immature urothelial cells derived from the UB stalk secrete Sonic Hedgehog, which acts on peri-ureteral condensed mesenchyme through its cell surface receptor Patched1 to stimulate cell proliferation and induce expression of *Bmp4* [374]. Inactivating *Shh* in the mouse urinary tract delays ureteral smooth muscle cell differentiation [374]. Proximal ureter segments of *Shh* null mice show reduced amounts of smooth muscle whereas distal segments lack smooth muscle completely. *Bmp4* expression is completely lost in *Shh* mutant ureters, suggesting that one role of *Shh* is to maintain *Bmp4* expression in the ureteral mesenchyme [3].

Bmp4 is uniformly expressed in ureter mesenchyme at early developmental stages and becomes localized to areas of active smooth muscle cell differentiation [374]. In vitro, BMP4 protein promotes the differentiation of peri-ureteral mesenchyme into smooth muscle [29, 207, 274, 350]. In vivo, decreased BMP4 signaling either by gene deletion in peri-ureteral mesenchyme cells or by direct antagonism in organ culture with proteins that sequester BMP4 protein (e.g., noggin, gremlin) resulted in a gradual reduction of ureter smooth muscle [350]. These data serve as strong evidence that *Bmp4* plays a regulatory role in the formation of ureteral smooth muscle.

The ability of ureter mesenchyme to condense and respond to epithelial-derived cues during mouse ureter development depends on the gene function of *Tbx18*. *Tbx18* encodes a transcription factor belonging to a family which share a highly conserved DNA-binding region known as the T-box and act as activators or repressors depending on molecular context [220]. *Tbx18* is exclusively activated in distal ureter mesenchyme prior to condensation and before *Bmp4* expression is induced in this compartment [2]. When *Tbx18* function is lost due to gene disruption in mice, ureteral mesenchyme fails to condense, and mesenchymal *Ptc1* expression is significantly downregulated, rendering mutant mesenchyme unresponsive to *Shh* signals [2]. Moreover, urothelial cell expression of *Shh* is present but detected at lower than normal levels in *Shh* mutants, suggesting that the response of peri-ureteral mesenchymal cells to secreted *Shh* is dose dependent. Consequently, *Bmp4* activation is blocked in mutant mesenchyme, and *Tbx18*$^{-/-}$ mutant mice display severely dilated and truncated ureters that lack smooth muscle. *Tbx18* may also control local molecular cross talk between mesenchymal and epithelial cell populations that supports urothelial cell differentiation. This is revealed in *Tbx18*$^{-/-}$ mutants by showing that ureter epithelial cells fail to proliferate and differentiate into a functional urothelium, leading to the generation of a flat, single-layered urothelium devoid of uroplakin [2]. These data support the concept that growth and differentiation programs of ureter smooth muscle and urothelium are tightly coupled during ureter development [3].

Smooth muscle formation proceeds in a stereotypic manner from proximal to distal during normal ureter development. Sonic Hedgehog signaling is believed to promote this myogenic sequence by controlling mesenchymal cell proliferation along the proximal-distal axis of the developing ureter. The proliferative functions of *Shh* on peri-ureteral mesenchyme are first observed at the proximal end of the ureter, which initiates the myogenic program in that region before more distal regions. In the absence of *Shh*, smooth muscle formation is significantly delayed, such that the fewer mesenchymal cells form condensations and transform into smooth muscle at the proximal end of the ureter and smooth muscle formation is absent at the distal end of the ureter [374]. The effects of *Shh* on smooth muscle development may be dependent on *Bmp4* since *Bmp4* mRNA expression is lost in *Shh* mutants. Evidence from mouse embryonic organ culture studies suggests that *Bmp4* is sufficient to promote mesenchymal cell differentiation into a ureter-specific smooth muscle phenotype. This was demonstrated in experiments using agarose beads soaked in recombinant BMP4 which were placed ectopically near UB-derived renal collecting ducts. These studies showed that BMP4 was sufficient to induce ureter smooth muscle differentiation around collecting ducts, which secondarily caused renal collecting duct cells to express urothelial cell markers [29, 198].

Other genes implicated in proximal-distal ureter smooth muscle patterning include teashirt zinc finger homeobox 3 (*Tshz3*), which belongs to a family of transcription factors with roles in anterior-posterior patterning of embryonic tissues [91, 94]. *Tshz3* function is dispensable in early ureter myogenesis for mesenchymal condensation and proliferation events but is required later in proximal smooth muscle differentiation programs [50]. During normal development, *Tshz3* is expressed in the mesenchyme along the entire length of the ureter and is shown to be upregulated by recombinant BMP4 in organ culture ex vivo [50]. Mice homozygous for a null *Tshz3* mutation exhibit nonobstructive hydroureter and akinetic ureters which lack evidence of smooth muscle cell differentiation within the proximal regions of the ureter yet display normal ureter smooth muscle cell differentiation distally. The defect in *Tshz3* null mice is thought to lie downstream of *Shh* and *Bmp4* since *Ptc1* and *Bmp4* expressions are unaffected in condensed proximal mesenchyme and exogenous BMP4 is incapable of rescuing proximal ureter smooth muscle differentiation in *Tshz3* mutant ureter organ culture.

1.5 Development of the Bladder

1.5.1 Normal Bladder Morphogenesis

The mature urinary bladder is comprised of an inner epithelial cell layer (i.e., bladder urothelium) and an outer smooth muscle layer (anatomically referred to as detrusor muscle). Bladder urothelial cells are endoderm-derived and originate from the luminal epithelial cells from the upper zone of the definitive urogenital sinus. In contrast, bladder smooth muscle cells are mesodermal derivatives arising from surrounding splanchnic mesenchyme.

Mesenchyme encompassing the primordial bladder is spatially organized into three morphologically distinct cell layers: (1) an outer adventitial layer, (2) an inner subepithelial layer (which lies next to the basal surface of immature urothelium), and (3) an interposing subadventitial layer [46]. Cells within all three layers have been shown experimentally to be capable of differentiating into smooth muscle cells [13]. However, only mesenchymal cells within the adventitial and sub-adventitial layers undergo smooth muscle cell differentiation during normal bladder development. In contrast, cells residing within the subepithelial layer remain undifferentiated throughout development.

In the human fetus, bladder smooth muscle cell differentiation is variably reported to occur between 7- and 12-week gestation (E13.5 in mice) [102, 227, 314]. At 10 weeks, the primitive bladder has a distinct outer muscle layer consisting of a continuous sheet of closely packed cells [102]. By 11 weeks, muscle fibers of the bladder wall form a meshwork of interlacing smooth muscle bundles. With the exception of the bladder neck, bladder musculature in the human fetus consists of large smooth muscle bundles arranged as an intermingling network in the absence of distinct layers by week 12 of gestation [102]. In the bladder neck, smooth muscle is replaced by a layer of undifferentiated mesenchyme which is in continuity with similar cells surrounding the urethral wall. Between 12 and 14 weeks, a collar of circularly oriented smooth muscle forms around the bladder neck. At 18 weeks, a relatively thin layer of smooth muscle is distinguished in the region of the trigone and extends into the bladder neck to merge with urethral smooth muscle.

1.5.2 Molecular Mechanisms Involved in Bladder Development

Bladder smooth muscle cell differentiation occurs in response to inductive signals emanating from urothelial cells [13]. Expression studies implicate Sonic Hedgehog as a strong candidate for this role since *Shh* is expressed in developing bladder urothelium, and genes which are activated by Sonic Hedgehog signaling (e.g., *Ptc1*, *Gli1*, *Bmp4*) are expressed in adjacent mesenchyme [314]. In organ culture experiments, exogenous Sonic Hedgehog was shown to be sufficient to induce mesenchyme cell proliferation and smooth muscle cell differentiation in bladder mesenchymal explants which had been separated from urothelium [47]. These data are consistent with genetic studies in mice which showed dysregulated mesenchymal cell proliferation and decreased bladder smooth muscle cell differentiation in mice by eliminating the function of *Gli1* and *Gli2*, which are downstream effectors of activated Sonic Hedgehog signaling [56]. The proliferative effects of *Shh* are dose dependent as increasing concentrations of exogenous Sonic Hedgehog increased bladder size and mesenchymal cell number ex vivo [47]. These data are consistent with a model in which mesenchymal cells closest to bladder urothelium are induced to proliferate in response to high concentrations of Shh and thus maintain a pool of undifferentiated smooth muscle cell progenitors. However, the effect of *Shh* on smooth muscle cell differentiation may be a secondary phenomenon since blocking Sonic Hedgehog signaling in bladder explants had no effect on the expression of smooth muscle cell terminal differentiation markers once smooth muscle formation had already been initiated [314]. These data suggest that while *Shh* may be involved in initiating smooth muscle cell differentiation, other pathways are likely involved in maturation of bladder smooth muscle.

Based on expression studies, molecular cross talk between Sonic Hedgehog and BMP4 signaling may be important for radial patterning of smooth muscle during bladder development. Expression analyses in developing mouse bladder are consistent with Bmp4 being a target of Sonic Hedgehog signaling as high levels of *Bmp4* mRNA are detected in subepithelial mesenchyme of embryonic mouse bladder and follow the onset of *Gli1* and *Gli2* expression in this compartment by one day [178]. Conversely, lower levels of *Bmp4* mRNA coincide with reduced *Gli1* and *Gli2* mRNA levels in peripheral mesenchyme. It has been suggested that *Bmp4* opposes the mitogenic effects of Sonic Hedgehog signaling based on an analysis of embryonic bladders from *Gli2* knockout mice. Tissue analysis of these mutants showed ectopic smooth muscle formation in regions of the subepithelial mesenchyme layer in which *Bmp4* mRNA expression was lost [56]. Other factors, including TGF-beta and serum response factor (SRF), may be involved in regulating smooth muscle cell differentiation as their expressions coincide with upregulation of several smooth muscle cell differentiation markers, such as *SMAA*, *SMMHC*, smooth muscle protein 22-α (*SM22α*), and *calponin* [172].

1.5.3 Formation of the Ureterovesical Junction

The route taken by the ureter through the smooth muscle layer of the bladder trigone is critical to forming a competent anti-reflux mechanism (Fig. 1.15). It is designed in such a way that retrograde flow of urine to the ureters and kidney is prevented by effectively compressing the intramural ureter against the smooth muscle wall during bladder contractions. A non-refluxing ureterovesical junction (UVJ) necessitates the normal formation of a tunnel through which the ureter passes through the bladder wall, an appropriate angle of entry of the ureter into the bladder, a well-formed trigone, and a correctly positioned ureteral orifice within the trigone. The clinical condition in humans resulting from an incompetent anti-reflux mechanism is vesicoureteral reflux (VUR), which is one of the most common urinary tract disorders in young children with a reported incidence as high as 1 % of live births (reviewed in Murawski et al. [217]).

The traditional view of UVJ morphogenesis was largely based on pathological studies of autopsy specimens from fetuses with lower urinary tract anomalies [327, 355, 357]. The model arising from these studies described UVJ formation as resulting from fusion of the two common nephric ducts with the posterior wall of the developing bladder, thus creating the transmural tunnel

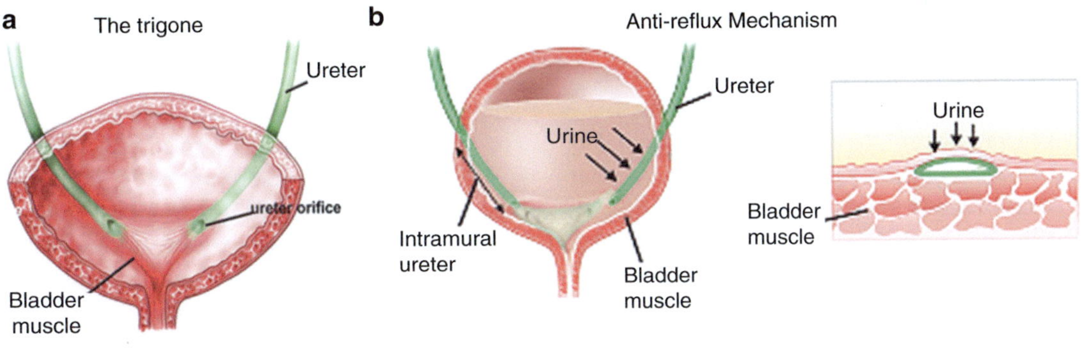

Fig. 1.15 Diagrammatic representation of the trigone and bladder anti-reflux mechanism. (**a**) The trigone is a triangular-shaped region located at the bladder base. It is bordered anterolaterally by bilateral ureteral orifices and posteriorly by the urethral orifice. (**b**) Schematic of the trigone and its connections with the ureters showing the intramural ureter segment that is normally compressed to prevent back-flow of urine to the ureters and kidneys. (**b**, *inset*) Schematic showing compression of the intramural ureter (Reproduced with modifications from Viana et al. [346], with permission)

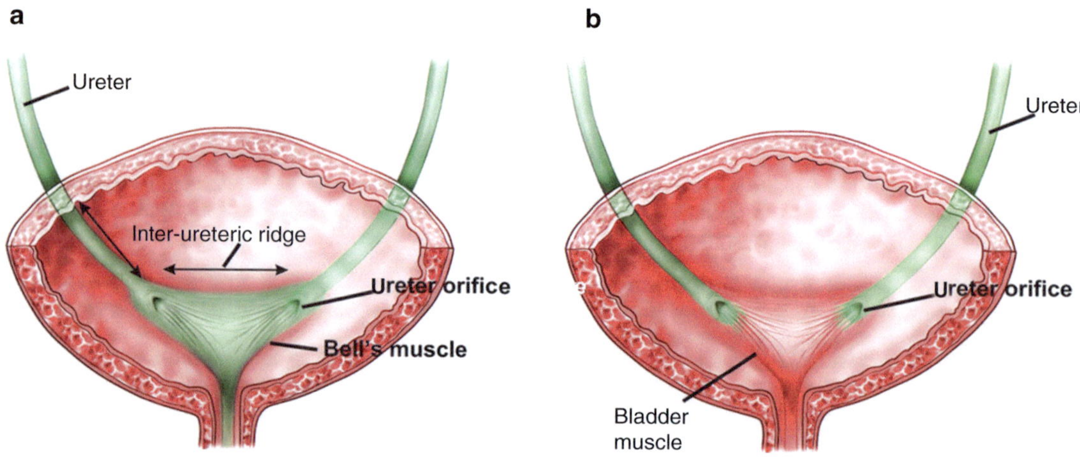

Fig. 1.16 Traditional and revised models of ureterovesical junction (UVJ) formation. Shown are schematic representations of the bladder, ureter, and trigone. Embryonic origins are illustrated by *green* (mesoderm-derived) and *red* (endoderm-derived) areas. (**a**) Traditional model of UVJ formation. The trigone forms in large part from ureteral fibers that fan out across the basal surface of the bladder generating the interureteric ridge and Bell's muscle. In this instance, the trigone is considered to form independently of the bladder. (**b**) Revised model of UVJ formation. The trigone and smooth muscle surrounding the intramural ureter are derived from bladder muscle. Ureteral fibers which extend into the bladder wall contribute a small amount to the intramural ureter tunnel (Reproduced with modifications from Viana et al. [346], with permission)

and the trigone [184, 357]. Based on this view, the outer muscle and inner epithelial layers of the bladder trigone were thought to share a similar mesodermal origin with the muscle and epithelial layers of the ureter (Fig. 1.16a). The traditional model of UVJ formation has been recently challenged by recent studies on distal ureter maturation in wild-type mice at multiple stages of embryonic development [16, 17, 339, 346]. Accordingly, a revised model of UVJ formation has emerged in which the trigone shares an endodermal origin with smooth muscle and epithelial layers of the developing bladder (Fig. 1.16b).

The first critical event in UVJ formation is degeneration of the common nephric duct. Elimination of the common nephric duct occurs as a result of cell apoptosis which occurs progressively once ureteric bud outgrowth takes place [17, 339] (Fig. 1.17a). As a consequence of common nephric duct degeneration, the nascent ureter approximates with the dorsal surface of the urogenital sinus (i.e., the primitive bladder) as ureter extends posteriorly towards the bladder and as the bladder grows and expands anteriorly towards the ureter [339]. At this stage, the distal end of the nascent ureter is observed to rotate 180° at the point where it connects to the nephric duct (Fig. 1.17b), which causes the distal ureter to make contact tangentially with the dorsal surface of the primitive bladder wall (Fig. 1.17c). The mechanism of ureter rotation around the nephric duct at this stage is unknown, although the rotation process appears to be facilitated by expansive growth of the primitive bladder [17]. The section of distal ureter which lies in contact with the bladder subsequently undergoes a second round of apoptosis. With that distal segment eliminated, the ureter becomes detached from the nephric duct, thus generating an open-ended tube which is connected to a single kidney proximally. The distal end of the newly formed ureter proper is subsequently observed to migrate towards the base of the bladder where it is properly oriented to penetrate the muscular exterior surface of the future trigone (Fig. 1.17d). Concomitantly, the nephric duct, which becomes detached from the newly formed ureter, remains in the region to connect with the urethra.

It is widely held that the location of ureteric budding along the long axis of the nephric duct determines the final position at which the ureter enters the bladder and results in vesicoureteral

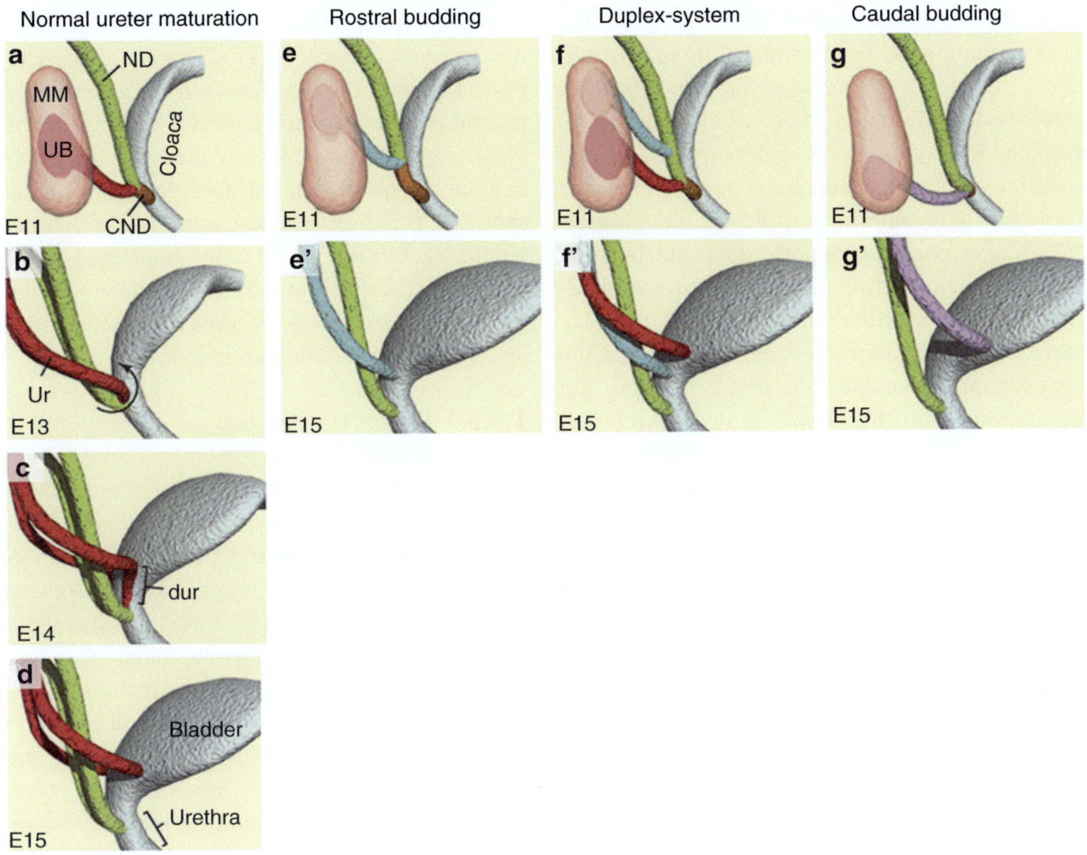

Fig. 1.17 Morphological events in distal ureter maturation and associated lower urinary tract malformations. (**a**)–(**d**) Normal distal ureter maturation and UVJ formation. (**a**) Following invasion of the metanephric mesenchyme (MM) by the newly formed ureteric bud (UB), the common nephric duct (CND; *brown*) is eliminated by apoptosis. (**b**) CND elimination brings the ureter in direct contact with the cloaca, or primordial bladder. Concomitantly, the ureter rotates around the long axis of the nephric duct (ND). (**c**) Ureter rotation orients the distal segment of the ureter towards the developing bladder. The distal-most segment of the ureter (dUr) lies against the exterior bladder surface and is also eliminated by apoptosis. (**d**) A new connection point between the ureter and the bladder is generated. (**e**) A rostral ectopic ureter (*blue*) forms in the absence of primary ureter. In this scenario, the CND is longer than usual. This results in a shorter segment of distal ureter meeting the bladder once ureter rotation takes place, and results (**e'**) in formation of an ectopic ureter that connects in the bladder neck, urethra, or remains attached to nephric duct. (**f**) In duplex systems, a second ureter (*blue*) is induced along the nephric duct, typically at a rostral position in reference to the primary ureter (*red*). (**f'**) Following distal ureter maturation, the rostral ectopic ureter connects below the primary ureter, either in the bladder neck, urethra or remains attached to nephric duct. (**g**) When caudal ureter budding occurs, the connection point between the ureter and nephric duct is very close to the cloaca. In this instance, the length of the CND is very short. (**g'**) The near absence of CND accelerates elimination of the distal ureter and positions the VUJ in an ectopic lateral position (Reproduced with modifications from Uetani and Bouchard [340]. With permission)

reflux when budding occurs ectopically [184]. This principle was put forward by Mackie and Stevens and is based on their pathological studies of urinary tract specimens from fetuses with congenital hydronephrosis. Based on their observations, they proposed that ureters entering the bladder ectopically in the region of the bladder neck would arise as the result of UB formation at a position which is anterior to the usual site of budding. Conversely, they postulated that UB formation at a posterior position would lead to ectopic ureters entering the bladder abnormally and closer to its apex. This model of abnormal UVJ formation has been validated by in vivo evidence from several mouse models of VUR (reviewed in Murawski et al. [217]) and may be explained by defects in ureter separation and rotation as described above. For example, UB formation at an anterior ectopic site would result in a longer common nephric duct and hence a greater distance between the site of ureteric budding and the primitive bladder (Fig. 1.17e). By increasing the distance between the UB and the growing primitive bladder, ureter rotation and separation from the nephric duct might be delayed and result in a low-lying insertion site [339] (Fig. 1.17e'). This is best exemplified in humans and mice with duplicated ureters which feature an anterior renal moiety connecting with a ureter that inserts ectopically into the bladder neck and which may be associated with hydroureter and hydronephrosis [184] (Fig. 1.17f and f'). Conversely, a posteriorly positioned UB site causes the ureter to reach the primitive bladder prematurely owing to a shorter common nephric duct and thus positions the ureter to inappropriately enter the bladder at a more lateral angle than normal [340] (Fig. 1.17g and g').

The mechanism by which the ureter passes through the trigone is poorly understood. Traditional beliefs on bladder embryology suggested that the intramural passage was generated from ureteral smooth muscle fibers extending into the bladder and stretching across the base of the bladder during trigone formation [327, 357]. This theory has been refuted by a recent study involving smooth muscle cell lineage analysis in transgenic mice, which strongly suggests that ureter-derived tissue plays a minor role in forming the intramural passage [346]. Using two transgenic mouse lines that selectively labeled derivatives of either ureteral mesenchyme or bladder mesenchyme, it was shown that the ureter contributed only a thin sheath of longitudinal smooth muscle fibers to the intramural passage through the trigone. The same report provided evidence that the process involved in forming the intramural tunnel is intrinsic to the bladder and is not dependent on the presence of a ureter. This was revealed in *Pax2* mutant mice, which lack ureters due to agenesis of the posterior nephric duct. In the absence of ureters, *Pax2* mutant mice displayed normal bladder development and showed normal patterns of smooth muscle organization in the trigone. Moreover, the trigone of *Pax2* mutants exhibited gaps in smooth muscle which corresponded to regions where the intramural tunnels would be formed. These gaps contained blood vessels that would normally follow the intramural ureter yet were devoid of ureter epithelium and ureter-derived smooth muscle [346].

1.5.3.1 Genes Implicated in UVJ Formation

Due to the variable penetrance of a number of gene mutations which disrupt early stages of urinary tract development (e.g., nephric duct morphogenesis, ureteric bud outgrowth), there exists the opportunity to define functions for these genes at later stages of development, including UVJ formation [217]. These genes include *Foxc1*, *Foxc2*, *Robo2*, *Bmp4*, and *Spry1*. As described in Sect. 1.3.3.1, *Foxc1*, *Foxc2*, and *Robo2* are involved in repressing mesenchymal *Gdnf* expression and thereby limiting the sites where RET is activated in the nephric duct [107, 166]. *Bmp4* and *Spry1* exert their inhibitory roles on GDNF-RET signaling activity by altering the sensitivity of nephric duct/UB cells to GDNF [14, 197, 206]. Mice with loss-of-function mutations in any one of these five genes exhibit inappropriate activation of GDNF-RET signaling in nephric duct cells which leads to the formation of supernumerary UBs or anterior displacement of the site of UB outgrowth [14, 107, 166, 206]. Ureters arising from anterior ectopic UBs in these mutants are severely dilated and insert below the bladder neck, as predicted by Mackie and Stevens [184]. Although VUR has only been associated with *ROBO2* mutations in humans (OMIM: 602431) [180], evidence from genetic studies in mice strongly support the possibility that other genes involved in regulating GDNF-RET signaling activity may be mutated in humans with VUR [217].

Defective regulation of *Ret* expression in the nephric duct has been shown to associate with VUJ malformation in mice. In the absence of *Ret* function, mouse kidney and ureter development is arrested and 80 % of mutants display renal and ureter agenesis [303, 304]. The remaining 20 % exhibited severe hydroureter and refluxing ureters that inserted abnormally below the bladder [61]. The defect in these *Ret* mutants is attributed to a failure to connect the nephric duct with the urogenital sinus until after the UB is formed. Morphologic analysis of nephric duct extension in *Ret* mutants revealed a defect in formation of cytoplasmic extensions which are thought to guide cells at the tip of the caudal nephric towards the urogenital sinus. *Ret* expression depends on retinoic acid signaling as revealed in *Aldh2* null mice, which display decreased Ret expression in the nephric duct and show a similar phenotype in nephric duct guidance [61]. In addition, *Ret* expression also depends on the function of *Gata3*. When *Gata3* function is removed in nephric duct cells by conditional deletion, embryos exhibit the same delay in uniting the nephric duct with urogenital sinus [61, 109]. *Gata3* expression is maintained in mice with mutations in genes involved in retinoic acid synthesis (e.g., *Aldh2* mutants), and *Aldh2* expression is unaffected in mutants [61]. Consequently, it is not known how Gata3 and retinoic acid signaling interact to control *Ret* expression.

Thirty percent of mice that carry the *Pax2^{1Neu}* mutation develop VUR which is associated with renal hypoplasia [25]. The *Pax2^{1Neu}* mutation in mice is a nonsense mutation and is orthologous to the *PAX2* mutation in humans with renal coloboma syndrome (OMIM: 120330), which is characterized by optic colobomas and a range of renal anomalies including VUR [295, 299]. Mice heterozygous for the *Pax2^{1Neu}* mutation demonstrate posteriorly placed UBs and ureters which penetrate the bladder aberrantly, resulting in a shortened intramural ureter [95]. The developmental defect in *Pax2^{1Neu}* heterozygous mutant mice is attributed to delayed separation of the ureter from the nephric duct which occurs independent of a defect in nephric duct elongation or *Ret* expression [25]. Moreover, ectopic positioning of the UB occurs without changes in *Gdnf* expression or dysregulated expression of genes which control the *Gdnf* expression domain, such as *Robo2*. Anterior budding is believed to be the primary cause of vesicoureteral reflux (VUR) in humans and mice [215]. However, at least two mouse models of VUR (i.e., *Pax2$^{1Neu/+}$* mice and the C3H/HeJ mouse strain [216]) have been linked causally to posterior UB positioning resulting in delayed UVJ formation. These studies suggest that strict adherence to the spatiotemporal relationships between ureteric budding and distal ureter morphogenesis may not be universally applied to the pathogenesis of VUR in all instances.

Elimination of the common nephric duct by apoptosis is viewed as a key step in coordinating subsequent remodeling events during distal ureter morphogenesis. Studies in mice show that when common nephric duct degeneration is either delayed or blocked completely, the developing ureter does not establish proper spatial relationships with the primitive bladder and defects in ureter separation and bladder insertion occur [17]. Vitamin A or retinoic acid signaling appears to be necessary to regulate apoptosis and trigger common nephric duct degeneration. Removing retinoic acid signaling genetically results in urinary tract obstruction and dilated ureters which insert ectopically below the bladder. This phenotype is demonstrated in mice with homozygous null mutations in *Aldh2* [17] as well as in compound mutant mice doubly homozygous for null mutations in *Rarα* and *Rarβ* [16], which encode retinoic acid receptors. *Aldh2* mutants showed a marked reduction in common nephric duct apoptosis [17], suggesting that retinoic acid signaling is necessary for elimination of the common nephric duct by regulating apoptosis in this region. As in all retinoic acid pathway mutants, the common nephric duct persists and ureter separation is delayed, leading to the conclusion that the regulatory function of retinoic acid-dependent signals on common nephric duct apoptosis is critical for proper ureter remodeling.

A recent study implicated genes encoding members of the leukocyte antigen-related (LAR) family of phosphatases as strong candidates to activate common nephric duct cell apoptosis. LAR phosphatases function by dephosphorylating activated tyrosine kinase receptors [265], including activated RET [271]. Protein tyrosine phosphatase, receptor type, F (*Ptprf*) and protein tyrosine phosphatase, receptor type, D (*Ptprd*) encode two LAR family members which are expressed in common nephric duct cells and are shown in vitro and in vivo to induce apoptosis by opposing RET activation [339]. In vivo analyses show that 52 % of mice with compound homozygous inactivating mutations in both *Ptprf* and *Ptprd* exhibited unilateral or bilateral urinary tract obstruction in addition to severe craniofacial abnormalities. Loss of LAR phosphatase function in these mutants suppressed apoptosis of common nephric duct cells and was associated with higher levels of phosphorylated RET as detected with specific antibodies. Detailed analyses of distal ureter morphogenesis in these mutants revealed significant remodeling defects that were associated with abnormal positioning of the UVJ below the bladder. In vitro studies in HEK cells further confirmed the functional relationships between LAR phosphatase activity and RET phosphorylation in the regulation of apoptosis. Since the UVJ phenotype in *Ptprf/Ptprd* double mutants is not fully penetrant, the mechanism for regulating apoptosis during ureter maturation must involve other genes which remain to be defined.

1.6 Human Urinary Tract Malformations and Genetic Associations

A number of urinary tract malformation syndromes display familial patterns of inheritance. For example, heterogeneous renal malformations are reported in 9 % of first-degree relatives of newborns with bilateral renal agenesis or bilateral renal dysgenesis [280]. Siblings of patients with VUR are reported to have a higher incidence of reflux than the normal population [57]. Hence, the occurrence of urinary tract malformations with familial patterns of inheritance in humans favors a genetic etiology. However, the majority of cases with isolated defects occur in patients without a familial pattern [280].

Candidate approaches have been used to screen patients or stillborn fetuses with isolated UT malformations for mutations in genes associated with syndromic malformations. In one study, a large European cohort of children with chronic kidney disease and severe renal hypoplasia and/or dysplasia was screened for mutations in *HNF1β*, *PAX2*, *SALL1*, *EYA1*, and *SIX1* [354]. These genes were selected on the basis of their associations with congenital syndromes that feature renal hypoplasia/dysplasia prominently. For instance, *HNF1β* mutations are known to cause renal cysts and diabetes syndrome (also known as MODY5; OMIM: 137920) [20, 21]. Human *PAX2* mutations are associated with renal coloboma syndrome, an autosomal dominant condition characterized in humans by optic nerve colobomas, hearing defects, and a spectrum of renal malformations including hypoplasia, renal agenesis, dysplasia, and VUR [295, 299]. *SALL1* mutations are found in patients with Townes-Brock syndrome (OMIM: 107480), which features anal, limb, and ear anomalies as well as renal hypoplasia, dysplasia, and VUR [160, 292]. *EYA1* and *SIX1* mutations have been identified in patients with branchio-oto-renal (OMIM: 113650), which presents with branchial arch, otic, and renal anomalies including unilateral or bilateral renal agenesis, hypoplasia, dysplasia as well as ureteral defects such as duplication or absence of ureter and megaureter [1]. In the European cohort study, *HNF1β* and *PAX2* mutations were detected in 15 % of all CKD subjects whereas *SALL1*, *EYA1*, and *SIX1* mutations were rarely detected in patients who did not have syndromic features [354]. Results from this study showed that mutations in *HNF1β* accounted for 25 % of mutations in patients with renal dysplasia or hypoplasia who manifest cysts, leading the authors to conclude that patients with cystic renal dysplasia should be screened for *HNF1β* mutations. Another study involving a multiethnic North American pediatric cohort reported an association for *HNF1β* mutations in 10 % of children with chronic kidney disease associated with unilateral renal agenesis or renal hypodysplasia [332]. The presence of *HNF1β* mutations has also been shown to exacerbate the phenotype of individuals with autosomal dominant polycystic kidney disease who carry mutations in PKD1 (polycystin-1) [19]. From a clinical perspective, it is possible that the presence of an *HNF1β* mutation may impart a higher risk of disease progression in patients with other types of urinary tract malformations.

Attention has been given to looking for mutations in genes encoding components of the GDNF-RET signaling cascade considering the strength of evidence for this pathway in normal urinary tract development in rodents [68]. In humans, heterozygous *RET* mutations cause Hirschsprung's disease (intestinal aganglionosis; OMIM# 142623) [83] and are reported rarely in patients with Hirschsprung's disease who also have renal hypoplasia and/or severe hydronephrosis [254]. A number of studies have reported low detection frequencies of *GDNF*, *RET*, and *GFRα1* mutations in cases of isolated UT malformation. In one study, *RET* mutations were reported in 8 of 29 stillborn fetuses (27.5 %) with unilateral or bilateral renal agenesis whereas no disease-causing mutations in *GDNF* or *GFRα1* were found in these cases [318]. Another study involving 105 fetuses with bilateral renal agenesis or hypodysplasia identified *RET* mutations in less than 7 % of cases and detected no *GDNF* mutations [145]. Similarly, a low detection rate for *GDNF* and *RET* mutations (<5 %) has been reported in a study involving 122 patients with UT malformations other than renal agenesis [53]. The explanation for detecting mutations in GDNF-RET pathway genes with such low frequency is not clear, although it is possible that there may be critical as-yet undefined differences between humans and mice regarding molecular control of UB outgrowth and branching events.

The pace of gene discovery in humans with isolated urinary tract malformations has been accelerated by the development of array-based analyses, whole exome sequencing, and genome-wide association studies (GWAS) [352, 353]. Despite technological advances in bioinformatics and high-throughput sequencing, it is estimated that a monogenic cause is identified in less than 20 % of patients with at least one recognizable urinary tract defect [128, 222, 289, 354]. Oligenic inheritance or gene modifier effects are likely to account for the remaining 80+% cases of children with isolated urinary tract malformations [354]. Table 1.6 lists a number of websites which are searchable databases for information on genetic associations with human disease.

Estimating the true prevalence of gene mutations in humans with severe urinary tract malformations

Table 1.6 Web resources for genetic associations with human disease

OMIM (Online Mendelian Inheritance in Man)	
Web address	http://www.ncbi.nlm.nih.gov/omim
Summary	Curated database cataloguing known gene-disease associations and providing clinical and molecular information on Mendelian disorders
HuGE Navigator (Human Genome Epidemiology Navigator)	
Web address	http://hugenavigator.net/HuGENavigator/home.do
Summary	Updated database in human genome epidemiology including population prevalence for genetic variants and disease-gene associations, gene-gene and gene-environment interactions, and interpretation of gene testing
DECIPHER (Database of Chromosomal Imbalances and Phenotype in Humans using Ensembl Resources)	
Web address	http://decipher.sanger.ac.uk/
Summary	Curated database cataloguing known gene-disease associations and providing clinical and molecular information on Mendelian disorders
GeneTests	
Web address	http://www.ncbi.nlm.nih.gov/sites/GeneTests/?db=GeneTests
Summary	Information center for clinical genetic testing including clinical and research lab directory
CTD (Comparative Toxicogenomics Database)	
Web address	http://ctdbase.org/
Summary	Searchable database providing information on known and predicted gene-disease and chemical-disease associations

is complicated by interactions between genetic, environmental, and nutritional factors. Environmental, drug, or toxin exposure, and maternal nutrition have all been associated with the occurrence of urinary tract malformation in humans and rodents [18, 85, 167, 266]. The strength of genotype-phenotype correlation may be further weakened by incomplete penetrance or variable expressivity, as reported for non-syndromic forms of CAKUT with autosomal dominant inheritance patterns [194, 352]. These factors must be taken into consideration when weighing the benefits of offering genetic testing to patients or relatives.

References

1. Abdelhak S, Kalatzis V, Heilig R, Compain S, Samson DCV, Weil D, Cruaud C, Sahly I, Leibovici M, Bitner-Glindizicz M, Francis M, Lacombe D, Vigneron J, Charachon R, Boven K, Bedbeder P, Van Regemorter N, Weissenbach J, Petit C (1997) A human homologue of the *Drosophila eyes absent* gene underlies Branchio-Oto-Renal (BOR) syndrome and identifies a novel gene family. Nat Genet 15:157–164
2. Airik R, Bussen M, Singh MK, Petry M, Kispert A (2006) Tbx18 regulates the development of the ureteral mesenchyme. J Clin Invest 116(3):663–674
3. Airik R, Kispert A (2007) Down the tube of obstructive nephropathies: the importance of tissue interactions during ureter development. Kidney Int 72(12): 1459–1467
4. Al-Awqati Q, Goldberg MR (1998) Architectural patterns in branching morphogenesis in the kidney. Kidney Int 54:1832–1842
5. Alagille D, Estrada A, Hadchouel M, Gautier M, Odievre M, Dommergues JP (1987) Syndromic paucity of interlobular bile ducts (Alagille syndrome or arteriohepatic dysplasia): review of 80 cases. J Pediatr 110(2):195–200
6. Alcaraz A, Vinaixa F, Tejedo-Mateu A, Fores MM, Gotzens V, Mestres CA, Oliveira J, Carretero P (1991) Obstruction and recanalization of the ureter during embryonic development. J Urol 145(2): 410–416
7. Amri K, Freund N, Vilar J, Merlet-Benichou C, Lelievre-Pegorier M (1999) Adverse effects of hyperglycemia on kidney development in rats: in vivo and in vitro studies. Diabetes 48(11): 2240–2245
8. Angrist M, Bolk S, Halushka M, Lapchak PA, Chakravarti A (1996) Germline mutations in glial cell line-derived neurotrophic factor (GDNF) and RET in a Hirschsprung disease patient. Nat Genet 14(3):341–344
9. Barak H, Rosenfelder L, Schultheiss TM, Reshef R (2005) Cell fate specification along the anterior-posterior axis of the intermediate mesoderm. Dev Dyn 232(4):901–914
10. Barbaux S, Niaudet P, Gubler M-C, Grünfeld J-P, Jaubert F, Kuttenn F, Fékété CN, Souleyreau-Therville N, Thibaud E, Fellous M, McElreavey K (1997) Donor splice-site mutations in WT1 are responsible for Frasier syndrome. Nat Genet 17: 467–470
11. Bard J (1996) A new role for the stromal cells in kidney development. Bioessays 18(9):705–707
12. Bard JB (2002) Growth and death in the developing mammalian kidney: signals, receptors and conversations. Bioessays 24(1):72–82
13. Baskin LS, Hayward SW, Young P, Cunha GR (1996) Role of mesenchymal-epithelial interactions in normal bladder development. J Urol 156(5):1820–1827
14. Basson MA, Akbulut S, Watson-Johnson J, Simon R, Carroll TJ, Shakya R, Gross I, Martin GR, Lufkin T, McMahon AP, Wilson PD, Costantini FD, Mason IJ, Licht JD (2005) Sprouty1 is a critical regulator of GDNF/RET-mediated kidney induction. Dev Cell 8(2):229–239
15. Basson MA, Watson-Johnson J, Shakya R, Akbulut S, Hyink D, Costantini FD, Wilson PD, Mason IJ, Licht JD (2006) Branching morphogenesis of the ureteric epithelium during kidney development is coordinated by the opposing functions of GDNF and Sprouty1. Dev Biol 299(2):466–477
16. Batourina E, Choi C, Paragas N, Bello N, Hensle T, Costantini FD, Schuchardt A, Bacallao RL, Mendelsohn CL (2002) Distal ureter morphogenesis depends on epithelial cell remodeling mediated by vitamin A and Ret. Nat Genet 32(1):109–115
17. Batourina E, Tsai S, Lambert S, Sprenkle P, Viana R, Dutta S, Hensle T, Wang F, Niederreither K, McMahon AP, Carroll TJ, Mendelsohn CL (2005) Apoptosis induced by vitamin A signaling is crucial for connecting the ureters to the bladder. Nat Genet 37(10):1082–1089
18. Battin M, Albersheim S, Newman D (1995) Congenital genitourinary tract abnormalities following cocaine exposure in utero. Am J Perinatol 12(6): 425–428
19. Bergmann C, von Bothmer J, Ortiz Bruchle N, Venghaus A, Frank V, Fehrenbach H, Hampel T, Pape L, Buske A, Jonsson J, Sarioglu N, Santos A, Ferreira JC, Becker JU, Cremer R, Hoefele J, Benz MR, Weber LT, Buettner R, Zerres K (2011) Mutations in multiple PKD genes may explain early and severe polycystic kidney disease. J Am Soc Nephrol 22(11):2047–2056
20. Bingham C, Bulman MP, Ellard S, Allen LI, Lipkin GW, Hoff WG, Woolf AS, Rizzoni G, Novelli G, Nicholls AJ, Hattersley AT (2001) Mutations in the

hepatocyte nuclear factor-1beta gene are associated with familial hypoplastic glomerulocystic kidney disease. Am J Hum Genet 68(1):219–224
21. Bingham C, Ellard S, Allen L, Bulman M, Shepherd M, Frayling T, Berry PJ, Clark PM, Lindner T, Bell GI, Ryffel GU, Nicholls AJ, Hattersley AT (2000) Abnormal nephron development associated with a frameshift mutation in the transcription factor hepatocyte nuclear factor-1 beta. Kidney Int 57(3): 898–907
22. Blomqvist SR, Vidarsson H, Fitzgerald S, Johansson BR, Ollerstam A, Brown R, Persson AE, Bergstrom GG, Enerback S (2004) Distal renal tubular acidosis in mice that lack the forkhead transcription factor Foxi1. J Clin Invest 113(11):1560–1570
23. Bok G, Drews U (1983) The role of the Wolffian ducts in the formation of the sinus vagina: an organ culture study. J Embryol Exp Morphol 73: 275–295
24. Bort R, Signore M, Tremblay K, Martinez Barbera JP, Zaret KS (2006) Hex homeobox gene controls the transition of the endoderm to a pseudostratified, cell emergent epithelium for liver bud development. Dev Biol 290(1):44–56
25. Boualia SK, Gaitan Y, Murawski I, Nadon R, Gupta IR, Bouchard M (2011) Vesicoureteral reflux and other urinary tract malformations in mice compound heterozygous for Pax2 and Emx2. PLoS One 6(6):e21529
26. Bouchard M, Souabni A, Mandler M, Neubuser A, Busslinger M (2002) Nephric lineage specification by Pax2 and Pax8. Genes Dev 16(22):2958–2970
27. Boyle S, de Caestecker M (2006) Role of transcriptional networks in coordinating early events during kidney development. Am J Physiol Renal Physiol 291(1):F1–F8
28. Boyle S, Misfeldt A, Chandler KJ, Deal KK, Southard-Smith EM, Mortlock DP, Baldwin HS, de Caestecker M (2008) Fate mapping using Cited1-CreERT2 mice demonstrates that the cap mesenchyme contains self-renewing progenitor cells and gives rise exclusively to nephronic epithelia. Dev Biol 313(1):234–245
29. Brenner-Anantharam A, Cebrian C, Guillaume R, Hurtado R, Sun TT, Herzlinger D (2007) Tailbud-derived mesenchyme promotes urinary tract segmentation via BMP4 signaling. Development 134(10):1967–1975
30. Brenner BM, Anderson S (1992) The interrelationships among filtration surface area, blood pressure, and chronic renal disease. J Cardiovas Pharmacol 19(Suppl 6):S1–S7
31. Brenner BM, Garcia DL, Anderson S (1988) Glomeruli and blood pressure. Less of one, more the other? Am J Hypertens 1(4 Pt 1):335–347
32. Bridgewater D, Cox B, Cain J, Lau A, Athaide V, Gill PS, Kuure S, Sainio K, Rosenblum ND (2008) Canonical WNT/beta-catenin signaling is required for ureteric branching. Dev Biol 317(1):83–94
33. Brodbeck S, Englert C (2004) Genetic determination of nephrogenesis: the Pax/Eya/Six gene network. Pediatr Nephrol 19(3):249–255
34. Brophy PD, Ostrom L, Lang KM, Dressler GR (2001) Regulation of ureteric bud outgrowth by Pax2-dependent activation of the glial derived neurotrophic factor gene. Development 128:4747–4756
35. Brunskill EW, Aronow BJ, Georgas K, Rumballe B, Valerius MT, Aronow J, Kaimal V, Jegga AG, Yu J, Grimmond S, McMahon AP, Patterson LT, Little MH, Potter SS (2008) Atlas of gene expression in the developing kidney at microanatomic resolution. Dev Cell 15(5):781–791
36. Burn SF, Webb A, Berry RL, Davies JA, Ferrer-Vaquer A, Hadjantonakis AK, Hastie ND, Hohenstein P (2011) Calcium/NFAT signalling promotes early nephrogenesis. Dev Biol 352(2):288–298
37. Bush KT, Sakurai H, Steer DL, Leonard MO, Sampogna RV, Meyer TN, Schwesinger C, Qiao J, Nigam SK (2004) TGF-beta superfamily members modulate growth, branching, shaping, and patterning of the ureteric bud. Dev Biol 266(2):285–298
38. Cacalano G, Farinas I, Wang LC, Hagler K, Forgie A, Moore M, Armanini M, Phillips H, Ryan AM, Reichardt LF, Hynes M, Davies A, Rosenthal A (1998) GFRalpha1 is an essential receptor component for GDNF in the developing nervous system and kidney. Neuron 21:53–62
39. Cain JE, Hartwig S, Bertram JF, Rosenblum ND (2008) Bone morphogenetic protein signaling in the developing kidney: present and future. Differentiation 76(8):831–842
40. Cain JE, Islam E, Haxho F, Blake J, Rosenblum ND (2011) GLI3 repressor controls functional development of the mouse ureter. J Clin Invest 121(3): 1199–1206
41. Cain JE, Islam E, Haxho F, Chen L, Bridgewater D, Nieuwenhuis E, Hui CC, Rosenblum ND (2009) GLI3 repressor controls nephron number via regulation of Wnt11 and Ret in ureteric tip cells. PLoS One 4(10):e7313
42. Cain JE, Nion T, Jeulin D, Bertram JF (2005) Exogenous BMP-4 amplifies asymmetric ureteric branching in the developing mouse kidney in vitro. Kidney Int 67(2):420–431
43. Cancilla B, Davies A, Cauchi JA, Risbridger GP, Bertram JF (2001) Fibroblast growth factor receptors and their ligands in the adult rat kidney. Kidney Int 60(1):147–155
44. Cano-Gauci DF, Song H, Yang H, McKerlie C, Choo B, Shi W, Pullano R, Piscione TD, Grisaru S, Soon S, Sedlackova L, Tanswell AK, Mak TW, Yeger H, Rosenblum ND, Filmus J (1999) Glypican-3-deficient mice exhibit developmental overgrowth and some of the renal abnormalities typical of Simpson-Golabi-Behmel syndrome. J Cell Biol 146:255–264
45. Cantley LG, Barros EJG, Gandhi M, Rauchman M, Nigam SK (1994) Regulation of mitogenesis, motogenesis, and tubulogenesis by hepatocyte growth

factor in renal collecting duct cells. Am J Physiol 267:F271–F280

46. Cao M, Liu B, Cunha G, Baskin L (2008) Urothelium patterns bladder smooth muscle location. Pediatr Res 64(4):352–357
47. Cao M, Tasian G, Wang MH, Liu B, Cunha G, Baskin L (2010) Urothelium-derived Sonic hedgehog promotes mesenchymal proliferation and induces bladder smooth muscle differentiation. Differentiation 79(4–5):244–250
48. Carroll TJ, Park JS, Hayashi S, Majumdar A, McMahon AP (2005) Wnt9b plays a central role in the regulation of mesenchymal to epithelial transitions underlying organogenesis of the mammalian urogenital system. Dev Cell 9(2):283–292
49. Caruana G, Cullen-McEwen L, Nelson AL, Kostoulias X, Woods K, Gardiner B, Davis MJ, Taylor DF, Teasdale RD, Grimmond SM, Little MH, Bertram JF (2006) Spatial gene expression in the T-stage mouse metanephros. Gene Expr Patterns 6(8):807–825
50. Caubit X, Lye CM, Martin E, Core N, Long DA, Vola C, Jenkins D, Garratt AN, Skaer H, Woolf AS, Fasano L (2008) Teashirt 3 is necessary for ureteral smooth muscle differentiation downstream of SHH and BMP4. Development 135(19):3301–3310
51. Cebrian C, Borodo K, Charles N, Herzlinger DA (2004) Morphometric index of the developing murine kidney. Dev Dyn 231(3):601–608
52. Challen G, Gardiner B, Caruana G, Kostoulias X, Martinez G, Crowe M, Taylor DF, Bertram J, Little M, Grimmond SM (2005) Temporal and spatial transcriptional programs in murine kidney development. Physiol Genom 23(2):159–171
53. Chatterjee R, Ramos E, Hoffman M, Vanwinkle J, Martin DR, Davis TK, Hoshi M, Hmiel SP, Beck A, Hruska K, Coplen D, Liapis H, Mitra R, Druley T, Austin P, Jain S (2012) Traditional and targeted exome sequencing reveals common, rare and novel functional deleterious variants in RET-signaling complex in a cohort of living US patients with urinary tract malformations. Human Genet 131(11):1725–1738
54. Chen L, Al-Awqati Q (2005) Segmental expression of Notch and Hairy genes in nephrogenesis. Am J Physiol Renal Physiol 288(5):F939–F952
55. Cheng HT, Kim M, Valerius MT, Surendran K, Schuster-Gossler K, Gossler A, McMahon AP, Kopan R (2007) Notch2, but not Notch1, is required for proximal fate acquisition in the mammalian nephron. Development 134(4):801–811
56. Cheng W, Yeung CK, Ng YK, Zhang JR, Hui CC, Kim PC (2008) Sonic Hedgehog mediator Gli2 regulates bladder mesenchymal patterning. J Urol 180(4):1543–1550
57. Chertin B, Puri P (2003) Familial vesicoureteral reflux. J Urol 169(5):1804–1808
58. Chi L, Saarela U, Railo A, Prunskaite-Hyyrylainen R, Skovorodkin I, Anthony S, Katsu K, Liu Y, Shan J, Salgueiro AM, Belo JA, Davies J, Yokouchi Y, Vainio SJ (2011) A secreted BMP antagonist, Cer1, fine tunes the spatial organization of the ureteric bud tree during mouse kidney development. PLoS One 6(11):e27676
59. Chi L, Zhang S, Lin Y, Prunskaite-Hyyrylainen R, Vuolteenaho R, Itaranta P, Vainio S (2004) Sprouty proteins regulate ureteric branching by coordinating reciprocal epithelial Wnt11, mesenchymal Gdnf and stromal Fgf7 signalling during kidney development. Development 131(14):3345–3356
60. Chi X, Michos O, Shakya R, Riccio P, Enomoto H, Licht JD, Asai N, Takahashi M, Ohgami N, Kato M, Mendelsohn C, Costantini F (2009) Ret-dependent cell rearrangements in the Wolffian duct epithelium initiate ureteric bud morphogenesis. Dev Cell 17(2):199–209
61. Chia I, Grote D, Marcotte M, Batourina E, Mendelsohn C, Bouchard M (2011) Nephric duct insertion is a crucial step in urinary tract maturation that is regulated by a Gata3-Raldh2-Ret molecular network in mice. Development 138(10):2089–2097
62. Chiba S (2006) Notch signaling in stem cell systems. Stem Cells (Dayton, Ohio) 24(11):2437–2447
63. Clarren SK (1994) Chapter 27: Malformations of the renal system. In: Holliday MA, Barratt TM, Avner ED (eds) Pediatric nephrology, 3rd edn. Williams & Wilkins, Baltimore
64. Clark AT, Young RJ, Bertram JF (2001) In vitro studies on the roles of transforming growth factor-beta 1 in rat metanephric development. Kidney Int 59:1641–1653
65. Clarke JC, Patel SR, Raymond RM Jr, Andrew S, Robinson BG, Dressler GR, Brophy PD (2006) Regulation of c-Ret in the developing kidney is responsive to Pax2 gene dosage. Hum Mol Genet 15(23):3420–3428
66. Constantinou CE (1978) Contractility of the pyeloureteral pacemaker system. Urol Int 33(6):399–416
67. Coppes MJ, Liefers GJ, Higuchi M, Zinn AB, Balfe JW, Williams BR (1992) Inherited WT1 mutation in Denys-Drash syndrome. Cancer Res 52(21):6125–6128
68. Costantini F (2010) GDNF/Ret signaling and renal branching morphogenesis: from mesenchymal signals to epithelial cell behaviors. Organogenesis 6(4):252–262
69. Cui S, Schwartz L, Quaggin SE (2003) Pod1 is required in stromal cells for glomerulogenesis. Dev Dyn 226(3):512–522
70. David SG, Cebrian C, Vaughan ED Jr, Herzlinger D (2005) c-kit and ureteral peristalsis. J Urol 173(1):292–295
71. Deschamps J, van Nes J (2005) Developmental regulation of the Hox genes during axial morphogenesis in the mouse. Development 132(13):2931–2942
72. Dewulf N, Verschueren K, Lonnoy O, Morén A, Grimsby S, Vande Spiegle K, Miyazono K, Huylebroeck D, Ten Dijke P (1995) Distinct spatial and temporal expression patterns of two type 1 receptors

for bone morphogenetic proteins during mouse embryogenesis. Endocrinology 136:2652–2663
73. Donovan MJ, Natoli TA, Sainio K, Amstutz A, Jaenisch R, Sariola H, Kreidberg JA (1999) Initial differentiation of the metanephric mesenchyme is independent of WT1 and the ureteric bud. Dev Genet 24:252–262
74. Douglas-Denton R, Moritz KM, Bertram JF, Wintour EM (2002) Compensatory renal growth after unilateral nephrectomy in the ovine fetus. J Am Soc Nephrol 13(2):406–410
75. Dressler GR (2006) The cellular basis of kidney development. Annu Rev Cell Dev Biol 22:509–529
76. Dressler GR (2009) Advances in early kidney specification, development and patterning. Development 136(23):3863–3874
77. Drews U, Sulak O, Schenck PA (2002) Androgens and the development of the vagina. Biol Reprod 67(4):1353–1359
78. Dreyer SD, Zhou G, Baldini A, Winterpacht A, Zabel B, Cole W, Johnson RL, Lee B (1998) Mutations in LMX1B cause abnormal skeletal patterning and renal dysplasia in nail patella syndrome. Nat Genet 19:47–50
79. Dudley AT, Lyons KM, Robertson EJ (1995) A requirement for bone morphogenetic protein-7 during development of the mammalian kidney and eye. Genes Dev 9:2795–2807
80. Dudley AT, Robertson EJ (1997) Overlapping expression domains of bone morphogenetic protein family members potentially account for limited tissue defects in BMP7 deficient embryos. Dev Dyn 208:349–362
81. Dunn NR, Winnier GE, Hargett LK, Schrick JJ, Fogo AB, Hogan BLM (1997) Haploinsufficient phenotypes in Bmp4 heterozygous null mice and modification by mutations in Gli3 and Alx4. Dev Biol 188:235–247
82. Durbec P, Marcos-Gutierrez CV, Kilkenny C, Grigoriou M, Wartiowaara K, Suvanto P, Smith D, Ponder B, Costantini F, Saarma M, Sariola H, Pachnis V (1996) GDNF signalling through the Ret receptor tyrosine kinase. Nature 381:789–792
83. Edery P, Lyonnet S, Mulligan LM, Pelet A, Dow E, Abel L, Holder S, Nihoul-Fekete C, Ponder BAJ, Munnich A (1994) Mutations of the *RET* proto-oncogene in Hirschprung's disease. Nature 367:378–380
84. Edwin F, Anderson K, Ying C, Patel TB (2009) Intermolecular interactions of Sprouty proteins and their implications in development and disease. Mol Pharmacol 76(4):679–691
85. El-Dahr SS, Harrison-Bernard LM, Dipp S, Yosipiv IV, Meleg-Smith S (2000) Bradykinin B2 null mice are prone to renal dysplasia: gene-environment interactions in kidney development. Physiol Genom 3(3):121–131
86. Ellisen LW, Bird J, West DC, Soreng AL, Reynolds TC, Smith SD, Sklar J (1991) TAN-1, the human homolog of the Drosophila notch gene, is broken by chromosomal translocations in T lymphoblastic neoplasms. Cell 66(4):649–661
87. Emerick KM, Rand EB, Goldmuntz E, Krantz ID, Spinner NB, Piccoli DA (1999) Features of Alagille syndrome in 92 patients: frequency and relation to prognosis. Hepatology 29(3):822–829
88. Enomoto H, Araki T, Jackman A, Heuckeroth RO, Snider WD, Johnson EMJ, Milbrandt J (1998) GFRa 1-deficient mice have deficits in the enteric nervous system and kidneys. Neuron 21:317–324
89. Eremina V, Cui S, Gerber H, Ferrara N, Haigh J, Nagy A, Ema M, Rossant J, Jothy S, Miner JH, Quaggin SE (2006) Vascular endothelial growth factor a signaling in the podocyte-endothelial compartment is required for mesangial cell migration and survival. J Am Soc Nephrol 17(3):724–735
90. Eremina V, Sood M, Haigh J, Nagy A, Lajoie G, Ferrara N, Gerber HP, Kikkawa Y, Miner JH, Quaggin SE (2003) Glomerular-specific alterations of VEGF-A expression lead to distinct congenital and acquired renal diseases. J Clin Invest 111(5):707–716
91. Erkner A, Gallet A, Angelats C, Fasano L, Kerridge S (1999) The role of Teashirt in proximal leg development in Drosophila: ectopic Teashirt expression reveals different cell behaviours in ventral and dorsal domains. Dev Biol 215(2):221–232
92. Evan AP, Gattone VH II, Schwartz GJ (1983) Development of solute transport in rabbit proximal tubule. II. Morphologic segmentation. Am J Physiol 245(3):F391–F407
93. Fagman H, Andersson L, Nilsson M (2006) The developing mouse thyroid: embryonic vessel contacts and parenchymal growth pattern during specification, budding, migration, and lobulation. Dev Dyn 235(2):444–455
94. Fasano L, Roder L, Core N, Alexandre E, Vola C, Jacq B, Kerridge S (1991) The gene teashirt is required for the development of Drosophila embryonic trunk segments and encodes a protein with widely spaced zinc finger motifs. Cell 64(1):63–79
95. Favor J, Sandulache R, Neuhauser-Klaus A, Pretsch W, Chaterjee B, Senft E, Wurst W, Blanquet V, Grimes P, Sporle R, Schughart K (1996) The mouse Pax (1Neu) mutation is identical to a human PAX2 mutation in a family with renal-coloboma syndrome and results in developmental defects of the brain, ear, eye and kidney. Proc Natl Acad Sci U S A 93:13870–13875
96. Fenske S, Mader R, Scharr A, Paparizos C, Cao-Ehlker X, Michalakis S, Shaltiel L, Weidinger M, Stieber J, Feil S, Feil R, Hofmann F, Wahl-Schott C, Biel M (2011) HCN3 contributes to the ventricular action potential waveform in the murine heart. Circ Res 109(9):1015–1023
97. Fetterman GH, Shuplock NA, Philipp FJ, Gregg HS (1965) The growth and maturation of human glomeruli and proximal convolutions from term to adulthood: studies by microdissection. Pediatrics 35:601–619

98. Fischer E, Legue E, Doyen A, Nato F, Nicolas JF, Torres V, Yaniv M, Pontoglio M (2006) Defective planar cell polarity in polycystic kidney disease. Nat Genet 38(1):21–23
99. Gao F, Maiti S, Sun G, Ordonez NG, Udtha M, Deng JM, Behringer RR, Huff V (2004) The Wt1+/R394W mouse displays glomerulosclerosis and early-onset renal failure characteristic of human Denys-Drash syndrome. Mol Cell Biol 24(22):9899–9910
100. Garrod DR, Fleming S (1990) Early expression of desmosomal components during kidney tubule morphogenesis in human and murine embryos. Development 108(2):313–321
101. Georgas K, Rumballe B, Valerius MT, Chiu HS, Thiagarajan RD, Lesieur E, Aronow BJ, Brunskill EW, Combes AN, Tang D, Taylor D, Grimmond SM, Potter SS, McMahon AP, Little MH (2009) Analysis of early nephron patterning reveals a role for distal RV proliferation in fusion to the ureteric tip via a cap mesenchyme-derived connecting segment. Dev Biol 332(2):273–286
102. Gilpin SA, Gosling JA (1983) Smooth muscle in the wall of the developing human urinary bladder and urethra. J Anat 137(Pt 3):503–512
103. Godin RE, Robertson EJ, Dudley AT (1999) Role of BMP family members during kidney development. Int J Dev Biol 43:405–411
104. Godin RE, Takaesu NT, Robertson EJ, Dudley AT (1998) Regulation of BMP7 expression during kidney development. Development 125:3473–3482
105. Gong KQ, Yallowitz AR, Sun H, Dressler GR, Wellik DM (2007) A Hox-Eya-Pax complex regulates early kidney developmental gene expression. Mol Cell Biol 27(21):7661–7668
106. Grieshammer U, Cebrian C, Ilagan R, Meyers E, Herzlinger D, Martin GR (2005) FGF8 is required for cell survival at distinct stages of nephrogenesis and for regulation of gene expression in nascent nephrons. Development 132(17):3847–3857
107. Grieshammer U, Le M, Plump AS, Wang F, Tessier-Lavigne M, Martin GR (2004) SLIT2-mediated ROBO2 signaling restricts kidney induction to a single site. Dev Cell 6(5):709–717
108. Grote D, Boualia SK, Souabni A, Merkel C, Chi X, Costantini F, Carroll T, Bouchard M (2008) Gata3 acts downstream of beta-catenin signaling to prevent ectopic metanephric kidney induction. PLoS Genet 4(12):e1000316
109. Grote D, Souabni A, Busslinger M, Bouchard M (2006) Pax 2/8-regulated Gata 3 expression is necessary for morphogenesis and guidance of the nephric duct in the developing kidney. Development 133(1):53–61
110. Guillaume R, Bressan M, Herzlinger D (2009) Paraxial mesoderm contributes stromal cells to the developing kidney. Dev Biol 329(2):169–175
111. Guo G, Morrison DJ, Licht JD, Quaggin SE (2004) WT1 activates a glomerular-specific enhancer identified from the human nephrin gene. J Am Soc Nephrol 15(11):2851–2856
112. Guo JK, Menke AL, Gubler MC, Clarke AR, Harrison D, Hammes A, Hastie ND, Schedl A (2002) WT1 is a key regulator of podocyte function: reduced expression levels cause crescentic glomerulonephritis and mesangial sclerosis. Hum Mol Genet 11(6):651–659
113. Hall JG, Pallister PD, Clarren SK, Beckwith JB, Wiglesworth FW, Fraser FC, Cho S, Benke PJ, Reed SD (1980) Congenital hypothalamic hamartoblastoma, hypopituitarism, imperforate anus and postaxial polydactyly–a new syndrome? Part I: Clinical, causal, and pathogenetic considerations. Am J Med Genet 7(1):47–74
114. Hammes A, Guo JK, Lutsch G, Leheste JR, Landrock D, Ziegler U, Gubler MC, Schedl A (2001) Two splice variants of the Wilms' tumor 1 gene have distinct functions during sex determination and nephron formation. Cell 106(3):319–329
115. Hanson J, Gorman J, Reese J, Fraizer G (2007) Regulation of vascular endothelial growth factor, VEGF, gene promoter by the tumor suppressor, WT1. Front Biosci: J Virtual Libr 12: 2279–2290
116. Haraguchi R, Mo R, Hui C, Motoyama J, Makino S, Shiroishi T, Gaffield W, Yamada G (2001) Unique functions of Sonic hedgehog signaling during external genitalia development. Development 128(21): 4241–4250
117. Harding SD, Armit C, Armstrong J, Brennan J, Cheng Y, Haggarty B, Houghton D, Lloyd-MacGilp S, Pi X, Roochun Y, Sharghi M, Tindal C, McMahon AP, Gottesman B, Little MH, Georgas K, Aronow BJ, Potter SS, Brunskill EW, Southard-Smith EM, Mendelsohn C, Baldock RA, Davies JA, Davidson D (2011) The GUDMAP database–an online resource for genitourinary research. Development 138(13):2845–2853
118. Harrison MR, Golbus MS, Filly RA, Nakayama DK, Callen PW, de Lorimier AA, Hricak H (1982) Management of the fetus with congenital hydronephrosis. J Pediatr Surg 17(6):728–742
119. Hartwig S, Bridgewater D, Di Giovanni V, Cain J, Mishina Y, Rosenblum ND (2008) BMP receptor ALK3 controls collecting system development. J Am Soc Nephrol 19(1):117–124
120. Hartwig S, Ho J, Pandey P, Macisaac K, Taglienti M, Xiang M, Alterovitz G, Ramoni M, Fraenkel E, Kreidberg JA (2010) Genomic characterization of Wilms' tumor suppressor 1 targets in nephron progenitor cells during kidney development. Development 137(7):1189–1203
121. Hartwig S, Hu MC, Cella C, Piscione T, Filmus J, Rosenblum ND (2005) Glypican-3 modulates inhibitory Bmp2-Smad signaling to control renal development in vivo. Mech Dev 122(7–8):928–938
122. Hatini V, Huh SO, Herzlinger D, Soares VC, Lai E (1996) Essential role of stromal mesenchyme in kidney morphogenesis revealed by targeted disruption of Winged Helix transcription factor *BF-2*. Genes Dev 10:1467–1478

123. Hendry C, Rumballe B, Moritz K, Little MH (2011) Defining and redefining the nephron progenitor population. Pediatr Nephrol 26(9):1395–1406
124. Higgins JP, Wang L, Kambham N, Montgomery K, Mason V, Vogelmann SU, Lemley KV, Brown PO, Brooks JD, van de Rijn M (2004) Gene expression in the normal adult human kidney assessed by complementary DNA microarray. Mol Biol Cell 15(2):649–656
125. Hinchliffe SA, Lynch MR, Sargent PH, Howard CV, Van Velzen D (1992) The effect of intrauterine growth retardation on the development of renal nephrons. Br J Obstet Gynaecol 99(4):296–301
126. Hinchliffe SA, Sargent PH, Howard CV, Chan YF, van Velzen D (1991) Human intrauterine renal growth expressed in absolute number of glomeruli assessed by the disector method and Cavalieri principle. Lab Invest 64(6):777–784
127. Hoppe CC, Evans RG, Bertram JF, Moritz KM (2007) Effects of dietary protein restriction on nephron number in the mouse. Am J Physiol Regul Integr Comp Physiol 292(5):R1768–R1774
128. Hoskins BE, Cramer CH 2nd, Tasic V, Kehinde EO, Ashraf S, Bogdanovic R, Hoefele J, Pohl M, Hildebrandt F (2008) Missense mutations in EYA1 and TCF2 are a rare cause of urinary tract malformations. Nephrol Dial Transplant 23(2):777–779
129. Hoy WE, Bertram JF, Denton RD, Zimanyi M, Samuel T, Hughson MD (2008) Nephron number, glomerular volume, renal disease and hypertension. Curr Opin Nephrol Hypertens 17(3):258–265
130. Hu MC, Rosenblum ND (2003) Genetic regulation of branching morphogenesis: lessons learned from loss-of-function phenotypes. Pediatr Res 54(4):433–438
131. Hughson M, Farris AB 3rd, Douglas-Denton R, Hoy WE, Bertram JF (2003) Glomerular number and size in autopsy kidneys: the relationship to birth weight. Kidney Int 63(6):2113–2122
132. Hui CC, Angers S (2011) Gli proteins in development and disease. Annu Rev Cell Dev Biol 27:513–537
133. Hurtado R, Bub G, Herzlinger D (2010) The pelvis-kidney junction contains HCN3, a hyperpolarization-activated cation channel that triggers ureter peristalsis. Kidney Int 77(6):500–508
134. Hyink DP, Tucker DC, St John PL, Leardkamolkarn V, Accavitti MA, Abrass CK, Abrahamson DR (1996) Endogenous origin of glomerular endothelial and mesangial cells in grafts of embryonic kidneys. Am J Physiol 270(5 Pt 2):F886–F899
135. Hynes PJ, Fraher JP (2004) The development of the male genitourinary system. I. The origin of the urorectal septum and the formation of the perineum. Br J Plast Surg 57(1):27–36
136. Iafolla K, Fratkin JD, Spiegel PK, Cohen MM Jr, Graham JM Jr (1989) Case report and delineation of the congenital hypothalamic hamartoblastoma syndrome (Pallister-Hall syndrome). Am J Med Genet 33(4):489–499
137. Iglesias DM, Hueber PA, Chu L, Campbell R, Patenaude AM, Dziarmaga AJ, Quinlan J, Mohamed O, Dufort D, Goodyer PR (2007) Canonical WNT signaling during kidney development. Am J Physiol Renal Physiol 293(2):F494–F500
138. Ishibe S, Karihaloo A, Ma H, Zhang J, Marlier A, Mitobe M, Togawa A, Schmitt R, Czyczk J, Kashgarian M, Geller DS, Thorgeirsson SS, Cantley LG (2009) Met and the epidermal growth factor receptor act cooperatively to regulate final nephron number and maintain collecting duct morphology. Development 136(2):337–345
139. Hutson J (2008) Development of the urogenital system. In: Standring S (ed) Gray's anatomy. 40th edn. Churchill Livingstone Elsevier, Edinburgh/New York, pp 1305–1325
140. Jackson SM, Nakato H, Sugiura M, Jannuzi A, Oakes R, Kaluza V, Golden C, Selleck SB (1997) dally, a drosophila glypican, controls cellular responses to the TGF-ß-related morphogen, Dpp. Development 124:4113–4120
141. James RG, Kamei CN, Wang Q, Jiang R, Schultheiss TM (2006) Odd-skipped related 1 is required for development of the metanephric kidney and regulates formation and differentiation of kidney precursor cells. Development 133(15):2995–3004
142. James RG, Schultheiss TM (2003) Patterning of the avian intermediate mesoderm by lateral plate and axial tissues. Dev Biol 253(1):109–124
143. James RG, Schultheiss TM (2005) Bmp signaling promotes intermediate mesoderm gene expression in a dose-dependent, cell-autonomous and translation-dependent manner. Dev Biol 288(1):113–125
144. Jeanpierre C, Denamur E, Henry I, Cabanis MO, Luce S, Cecille A, Elion J, Peuchmaur M, Loirat C, Niaudet P, Gubler MC, Junien C (1998) Identification of constitutional WT1 mutations, in patients with isolated diffuse mesangial sclerosis, and analysis of genotype/phenotype correlations by use of a computerized mutation database. Am J Hum Genet 62(4):824–833
145. Jeanpierre C, Mace G, Parisot M, Moriniere V, Pawtowsky A, Benabou M, Martinovic J, Amiel J, Attie-Bitach T, Delezoide AL, Loget P, Blanchet P, Gaillard D, Gonzales M, Carpentier W, Nitschke P, Tores F, Heidet L, Antignac C, Salomon R (2011) RET and GDNF mutations are rare in fetuses with renal agenesis or other severe kidney development defects. J Med Genet 48(7):497–504
146. Jenkins D, Bitner-Glindzicz M, Malcolm S, Hu CC, Allison J, Winyard PJ, Gullett AM, Thomas DF, Belk RA, Feather SA, Sun TT, Woolf AS (2005) De novo Uroplakin IIIa heterozygous mutations cause human renal adysplasia leading to severe kidney failure. J Am Soc Nephrol 16(7):2141–2149
147. Jeong HW, Jeon US, Koo BK, Kim WY, Im SK, Shin J, Cho Y, Kim J, Kong YY (2009) Inactivation of Notch signaling in the renal collecting duct causes nephrogenic diabetes insipidus in mice. J Clin Invest 119(11):3290–3300

148. Kang S, Graham JM Jr, Olney AH, Biesecker LG (1997) GLI3 frameshift mutations cause autosomal dominant Pallister-Hall syndrome. Nat Genet 15(3):266–268
149. Karihaloo A, O'Rourke DA, Nickel C, Spokes K, Cantley LG (2001) Differential MAPK pathways utilized for HGF- and EGF-dependent renal epithelial morphogenesis. J Biol Chem 276(12):9166–9173
150. Karner CM, Chirumamilla R, Aoki S, Igarashi P, Wallingford JB, Carroll TJ (2009) Wnt9b signaling regulates planar cell polarity and kidney tubule morphogenesis. Nat Genet 41(7):793–799
151. Kispert A, Vainio S, McMahon AP (1998) Wnt-4 is a mesenchymal signal for epithelial transformation of metanephric mesenchyme in the developing kidney. Development 125:4225–4234
152. Kispert A, Vainio S, Shen L, Rowitch DH, McMahon AP (1996) Proteoglycans are required for maintenance of *Wnt-11* expression in the ureter tips. Development 122:3627–3637
153. Kitamoto Y, Tokunaga H, Tomita K (1997) Vascular endothelial growth factor is an essential molecule for mouse kidney development: glomerulogenesis and nephrogenesis. J Clin Invest 99(10):2351–2357
154. Klamt B, Koziell A, Poulat F, Wieacker P, Scambler P, Berta P, Gessler M (1998) Frasier syndrome is caused by defective alternative splicing of WT1 leading to an altered ratio of WT1+/-KTS splice isoforms. Hum Mol Genet 7:709–714
155. Klein G, Langegger M, Goridis C, Ekblom P (1988) Neural cell adhesion molecules during embryonic induction and development of the kidney. Development 102(4):749–761
156. Kleinman LI, Lubbe RJ (1972) Factors affecting the maturation of glomerular filtration rate and renal plasma flow in the new-born dog. J Physiol 223(2): 395–409
157. Kobayashi A, Kwan KM, Carroll TJ, McMahon AP, Mendelsohn CL, Behringer RR (2005) Distinct and sequential tissue-specific activities of the LIM-class homeobox gene Lim1 for tubular morphogenesis during kidney development. Development 132(12): 2809–2823
158. Kobayashi A, Valerius MT, Mugford JW, Carroll TJ, Self M, Oliver G, McMahon AP (2008) Six2 defines and regulates a multipotent self-renewing nephron progenitor population throughout mammalian kidney development. Cell Stem Cell 3(2):169–181
159. Kohan DE (2008) Progress in gene targeting: using mutant mice to study renal function and disease. Kidney Int 74(4):427–437
160. Kohlhase J, Wischermann A, Reichenbach H, Froster U, Engel W (1998) Mutations in the SALL1 putative transcription factor gene cause Townes-Brocks syndrome. Nat Genet 18:81–83
161. Koleda P, Apoznanski W, Wozniak Z, Rusiecki L, Szydelko T, Pilecki W, Polok M, Kalka D, Pupka A (2012) Changes in interstitial cell of Cajal-like cells density in congenital ureteropelvic junction obstruction. Int Urol Nephrol 44(1):7–12
162. Kong XT, Deng FM, Hu P, Liang FX, Zhou G, Auerbach AB, Genieser N, Nelson PK, Robbins ES, Shapiro E, Kachar B, Sun TT (2004) Roles of uroplakins in plaque formation, umbrella cell enlargement, and urinary tract diseases. J Cell Biol 167(6):1195–1204
163. Korostylev A, Worzfeld T, Deng S, Friedel RH, Swiercz JM, Vodrazka P, Maier V, Hirschberg A, Ohoka Y, Inagaki S, Offermanns S, Kuner R (2008) A functional role for semaphorin 4D/plexin B1 interactions in epithelial branching morphogenesis during organogenesis. Development 135(20): 3333–3343
164. Kreidberg JA (2003) Podocyte differentiation and glomerulogenesis. J Am Soc Nephrol 14(3): 806–814
165. Kreidberg JA, Sariola H, Loring JM, Maeda M, Pelletier J, Housman D, Jaenisch R (1993) WT-1 is required for early kidney development. Cell 74:679–691
166. Kume T, Deng K, Hogan BL (2000) Murine forkhead/winged helix genes Foxc1 (Mf1) and Foxc2 (Mfh1) are required for the early organogenesis of the kidney and urinary tract. Development 127:1387–1395
167. Langley-Evans SC, Welham SJ, Jackson AA (1999) Fetal exposure to a maternal low protein diet impairs nephrogenesis and promotes hypertension in the rat. Life Sci 64(11):965–974
168. Leveen P, Pekny M, Gebre-Medhin S, Swolin B, Larsson E, Betsholtz C (1994) Mice deficient for PDGF B show renal, cardiovascular, and hematological abnormalities. Genes Dev 8:1875–1887
169. Levinson RS, Batourina E, Choi C, Vorontchikhina M, Kitajewski J, Mendelsohn CL (2005) Foxd1-dependent signals control cellularity in the renal capsule, a structure required for normal renal development. Development 132(3):529–539
170. Levitt MA, Pena A (2007) Anorectal malformations. Orphanet J Rare Dis 2
171. Liang FX, Bosland MC, Huang H, Romih R, Baptiste S, Deng FM, Wu XR, Shapiro E, Sun TT (2005) Cellular basis of urothelial squamous metaplasia: roles of lineage heterogeneity and cell replacement. J Cell Biol 171(5):835–844
172. Lien SC, Usami S, Chien S, Chiu JJ (2006) Phosphatidylinositol 3-kinase/Akt pathway is involved in transforming growth factor-beta1-induced phenotypic modulation of 10T1/2 cells to smooth muscle cells. Cellular Signalling 18:1270–1278
173. Limwongse C, Clarren SK, Cassidy SB (1999) Syndromes and malformations of the urinary tract. In: Barratt TM, Avner ED, Harmon WE (eds) Pediatric nephrology, 3rd edn. Williams & Wilkins, Baltimore, pp 427–452
174. Lin Y, Zhang S, Tuukkanen J, Peltoketo H, Pihlajaniemi T, Vainio S (2003) Patterning parameters associated with the branching of the ureteric bud regulated by epithelial-mesenchymal interactions. Int J Dev Biol 47(1):3–13

175. Lindahl P, Hellström M, Kalén M, Karlsson L, Pekny M, Pekna M, Soriano P, Betsholtz C (1998) Paracrine PDGF-B/PDGF-Rß signaling controls mesangial cell development in kidney glomeruli. Development 125:3313–3322
176. Little M, Georgas K, Pennisi D, Wilkinson L (2010) Kidney development: two tales of tubulogenesis. Curr Top Dev Biol 90:193–229
177. Little MH, Williamson KA, Mannens M, Kelsey A, Gosden C, Hastie ND, van Heyningen V (1993) Evidence that WT1 mutations in Denys-Drash syndrome patients may act in a dominant-negative fashion. Hum Mol Genet 2(3):259–264
178. Liu W, Li Y, Cunha S, Hayward G, Baskin L (2000) Diffusable growth factors induce bladder smooth muscle differentiation. In Vitro Cell Dev Biol 36(7):476–484
179. Lu BC, Cebrian C, Chi X, Kuure S, Kuo R, Bates CM, Arber S, Hassell J, MacNeil L, Hoshi M, Jain S, Asai N, Takahashi M, Schmidt-Ott KM, Barasch J, D'Agati V, Costantini F (2009) Etv4 and Etv5 are required downstream of GDNF and Ret for kidney branching morphogenesis. Nat Genet 41(12):1295–1302
180. Lu W, van Eerde AM, Fan X, Quintero-Rivera F, Kulkarni S, Ferguson H, Kim HG, Fan Y, Xi Q, Li QG, Sanlaville D, Andrews W, Sundaresan V, Bi W, Yan J, Giltay JC, Wijmenga C, de Jong TP, Feather SA, Woolf AS, Rao Y, Lupski JR, Eccles MR, Quade BJ, Gusella JF, Morton CC, Maas RL (2007) Disruption of ROBO2 is associated with urinary tract anomalies and confers risk of vesicoureteral reflux. Am J Hum Genet 80(4):616–632
181. Luyckx VA, Brenner BM (2010) The clinical importance of nephron mass. J Am Soc Nephrol 21(6):898–910
182. Lye CM, Fasano L, Woolf AS (2010) Ureter myogenesis: putting Teashirt into context. J Am Soc Nephrol 21(1):24–30
183. Mackenzie HS, Lawler EV, Brenner BM (1996) Congenital oligonephropathy: the fetal flaw in essential hypertension? Kidney Int 55:S30–S34
184. Mackie GG, Stephens FD (1975) Duplex kidneys: a correlation of renal dysplasia with position of the ureteral orifice. J Urol 114:274–280
185. Maeshima A, Sakurai H, Choi Y, Kitamura S, Vaughn DA, Tee JB, Nigam SK (2007) Glial cell-derived neurotrophic factor independent ureteric bud outgrowth from the Wolffian duct. J Am Soc Nephrol 18(12):3147–3155
186. Majumdar A, Vainio S, Kispert A, McMahon J, McMahon AP (2003) Wnt11 and Ret/Gdnf pathways cooperate in regulating ureteric branching during metanephric kidney development. Development 130(14):3175–3185
187. Manalich R, Reyes L, Herrera M, Melendi C, Fundora I (2000) Relationship between weight at birth and the number and size of renal glomeruli in humans: a histomorphometric study. Kidney Int 58(2):770–773
188. Marose TD, Merkel CE, McMahon AP, Carroll TJ (2008) Beta-catenin is necessary to keep cells of ureteric bud/Wolffian duct epithelium in a precursor state. Dev Biol 314(1):112–126
189. Matsuno T, Tokunaka S, Koyanagi T (1984) Muscular development in the urinary tract. J Urol 132(1):148–152
190. Mauch TJ, Yang G, Wright M, Smith D, Schoenwolf GC (2000) Signals from trunk paraxial mesoderm induce pronephros formation in chick intermediate mesoderm. Dev Biol 220(1):62–75
191. McCright B, Gao X, Shen L, Lozier J, Lan Y, Maguire M, Herzlinger D, Weinmaster G, Jiang R, Gridley T (2001) Defects in development of the kidney, heart and eye vasculature in mice homozygous for a hypomorphic Notch2 mutation. Development 128:491–502
192. McCright B, Lozier J, Gridley T (2002) A mouse model of Alagille syndrome: Notch2 as a genetic modifier of Jag1 haploinsufficiency. Development 129:1075–1082
193. McDill BW, Li SZ, Kovach PA, Ding L, Chen F (2006) Congenital progressive hydronephrosis (cph) is caused by an S256L mutation in aquaporin-2 that affects its phosphorylation and apical membrane accumulation. Proc Natl Acad Sci U S A 103(18): 6952–6957
194. McPherson E, Carey J, Kramer A, Hall JG, Pauli RM, Schimke RN, Tasin MH (1987) Dominantly inherited renal adysplasia. Am J Med Genet 26(4): 863–872
195. Michael L, Davies JA (2004) Pattern and regulation of cell proliferation during murine ureteric bud development. J Anat 204(4):241–255
196. Michos O (2009) Kidney development: from ureteric bud formation to branching morphogenesis. Curr Opin Genet Dev 19(5):484–490
197. Michos O, Cebrian C, Hyink D, Grieshammer U, Williams L, D'Agati V, Licht JD, Martin GR, Costantini F (2010) Kidney development in the absence of Gdnf and Spry1 requires Fgf10. PLoS Genet 6(1):e1000809
198. Michos O, Goncalves A, Lopez-Rios J, Tiecke E, Naillat F, Beier K, Galli A, Vainio S, Zeller R (2007) Reduction of BMP4 activity by gremlin 1 enables ureteric bud outgrowth and GDNF/WNT11 feedback signalling during kidney branching morphogenesis. Development 134(13):2397–2405
199. Michos O, Panman L, Vintersten K, Beier K, Zeller R, Zuniga A (2004) Gremlin-mediated BMP antagonism induces the epithelial-mesenchymal feedback signaling controlling metanephric kidney and limb organogenesis. Development 131(14):3401–3410
200. Miner JH, Li C (2000) Defective glomerulogenesis in the absence of laminin alpha5 demonstrates a developmental role for the kidney glomerular basement membrane. Dev Biol 217(2):278–289
201. Miner JH, Morello R, Andrews KL, Li C, Antignac C, Shaw AS, Lee B (2002) Transcriptional induction of slit diaphragm genes by Lmx1b is required in podocyte differentiation. J Clin Invest 109(8): 1065–1072

202. Miner JH, Sanes JR (1994) Collagen IV alpha 3, alpha 4, and alpha 5 chains in rodent basal laminae: sequence, distribution, association with laminins, and developmental switches. J Cell Biol 127(3): 879–891
203. Miner JH, Sanes JR (1996) Molecular and functional defects in kidneys of mice lacking collagen alpha 3(IV): implications for Alport syndrome. J Cell Biol 135(5):1403–1413
204. Miyamoto N, Yoshida M, Kuratani S, Matuso I, Aizawa S (1997) Defects of urogenital development in mice lacking *Emx2*. Development 124: 1653–1664
205. Miyazaki Y, Ichikawa I (2003) Ontogeny of congenital anomalies of the kidney and urinary tract, CAKUT. Pediatr Int: Official J Jpn Pediatr Soc 45(5):598–604
206. Miyazaki Y, Oshima K, Fogo A, Hogan BLM, Ichikawa I (2000) Bone morphogenetic protein 4 regulates the budding site and elongation of the mouse ureter. J Clin Invest 105:863–873
207. Miyazaki Y, Oshima K, Fogo A, Ichikawa I (2003) Evidence that bone morphogenetic protein 4 has multiple biological functions during kidney and urinary tract development. Kidney Int 63(3):835–844
208. Miyazaki Y, Tsuchida S, Nishimura H, Pope JC IV, Harris RC, McKanna JM, Inagami T, Hogan BLM, Fogo A, Ichikawa I (1998) Angiotensin induces the urinary peristaltic machinery during the perinatal period. J Clin Invest 102:1489–1497
209. Montesano R, Soriano JV, Pepper MS, Orci L (1997) Induction of epithelial branching tubulogenesis in vitro. J Cell Physiol 173:152–161
210. Moore MW, Klein RD, Farinas I, Sauer H, Armanini M, Phillips H, Reichardt LF, Ryan AM, Carver-Moore K, Rosenthal A (1996) Renal and neuronal abnormalities in mice lacking GDNF. Nature 382:76–79
211. Moritz KM, Mazzuca MQ, Siebel AL, Mibus A, Arena D, Tare M, Owens JA, Wlodek ME (2009) Uteroplacental insufficiency causes a nephron deficit, modest renal insufficiency but no hypertension with ageing in female rats. J Physiol 587(Pt 11):2635–2646
212. Mugford JW, Sipila P, Kobayashi A, Behringer RR, McMahon AP (2008) Hoxd11 specifies a program of metanephric kidney development within the intermediate mesoderm of the mouse embryo. Dev Biol 319(2):396–405
213. Mugford JW, Sipila P, McMahon JA, McMahon AP (2008) Osr1 expression demarcates a multi-potent population of intermediate mesoderm that undergoes progressive restriction to an Osr1-dependent nephron progenitor compartment within the mammalian kidney. Dev Biol 324(1):88–98
214. Mugford JW, Yu J, Kobayashi A, McMahon AP (2009) High-resolution gene expression analysis of the developing mouse kidney defines novel cellular compartments within the nephron progenitor population. Dev Biol 333(2):312–323
215. Murawski IJ, Gupta IR (2006) Vesicoureteric reflux and renal malformations: a developmental problem. Clin Genet 69(2):105–117
216. Murawski IJ, Maina RW, Malo D, Guay-Woodford LM, Gros P, Fujiwara M, Morgan K, Gupta IR (2010) The C3H/HeJ inbred mouse is a model of vesico-ureteric reflux with a susceptibility locus on chromosome 12. Kidney Int 78(3):269–278
217. Murawski IJ, Watt CL, Gupta IR (2011) Vesico-ureteric reflux: using mouse models to understand a common congenital urinary tract defect. Pediatr Nephrol 26(9):1513–1522
218. Murnaghan GF (1958) The dynamics of the renal pelvis and ureter with reference to congenital hydronephrosis. Br J Urol 30(3):321–329
219. Nagata M, Nakayama K, Terada Y, Hoshi S, Watanabe T (1998) Cell cycle regulation and differentiation in the human podocyte lineage. Am J Pathol 153(5):1511–1520
220. Naiche LA, Harrelson Z, Kelly RG, Papaioannou VE (2005) T-box genes in vertebrate development. Annu Rev Genet 39:219–239
221. Nakai S, Sugitani Y, Sato H, Ito S, Miura Y, Ogawa M, Nishi M, Jishage K, Minowa O, Noda T (2003) Crucial roles of Brn1 in distal tubule formation and function in mouse kidney. Development 130(19):4751–4759
222. Nakayama M, Nozu K, Goto Y, Kamei K, Ito S, Sato H, Emi M, Nakanishi K, Tsuchiya S, Iijima K (2010) HNF1B alterations associated with congenital anomalies of the kidney and urinary tract. Pediatr Nephrol 25(6):1073–1079
223. Neiss WF (1982) Histogenesis of the loop of Henle in the rat kidney. Anat Embryol (Berl) 164(3): 315–330
224. Neiss WF, Klehn KL (1981) The postnatal development of the rat kidney, with special reference to the chemodifferentiation of the proximal tubule. Histochemistry 73(2):251–268
225. Nelson RG, Morgenstern H, Bennett PH (1998) Intrauterine diabetes exposure and the risk of renal disease in diabetic Pima Indians. Diabetes 47(9): 1489–1493
226. Netter FH, Cochard LR (2002) Netter's Atlas of human embryology. Icon Learning Systems, Teterboro
227. Newman J, Antonakopoulos GN (1989) The fine structure of the human fetal urinary bladder. Development and maturation. A light, transmission and scanning electron microscopic study. J Anat 166:135–150
228. Nie X, Xu J, El-Hashash A, Xu PX (2011) Six1 regulates Grem1 expression in the metanephric mesenchyme to initiate branching morphogenesis. Dev Biol 352(1):141–151
229. Nievelstein RA, van der Werff JF, Verbeek FJ, Valk J, Vermeij-Keers C (1998) Normal and abnormal embryonic development of the anorectum in human embryos. Teratology 57(2):70–78
230. Niimura F, Labostky PA, Kakuchi J, Okubo S, Yoshida H, Oikawa T, Ichiki T, Naftilan AJ, Fogo A,

Inagami T et al (1995) Gene targeting in mice reveals a requirement for angiotensin in the development and maintenance of kidney morphology and growth factor regulation. J Clin Invest 96:2947–2954
231. Nishimura H, Yerkes E, Hohenfellner K, Miyazaki Y, Ma J, Hunley TE, Yoshida H, Ichiki T, Threadgill D, Phillips JA, Hogan BML, Fogo A, Brock JW, Inagami T, Ichikawa I (1999) Role of the angiotensin type 2 receptor gene in congenital anomalies of the kidney and urinary tract, CAKUT, of mice and men. Mol Cell 3:1–10
232. Nishinakamura R, Matsumoto Y, Nakao K, Nakamura K, Sato A, Copeland NG, Gilbert DJ, Jenkins NA, Scully S, Lacey DL, Katsuki M, Asashima M, Yokota T (2001) Murine homolog of SALL1 is essential for ureteric bud invasion in kidney development. Development 128:3105–3115
233. Noakes PG, Miner JH, Gautam M, Cunningham JM, Sanes JR, Merlie JP (1995) The renal glomerulus of mice lacking s-laminin/laminin ß2: nephrosis despite molecular compensation by laminin ß1. Nat Genet 10:400–406
234. Nyengaard JR, Bendtsen TF (1992) Glomerular number and size in relation to age, kidney weight, and body surface in normal man. Anat Rec 232:194–201
235. O'Brien LL, Grimaldi M, Kostun Z, Wingert RA, Selleck R, Davidson AJ (2011) Wt1a, Foxc1a, and the Notch mediator Rbpj physically interact and regulate the formation of podocytes in zebrafish. Dev Biol 358(2):318–330
236. Obara-Ishihara T, Kuhlman J, Niswander L, Herzlinger D (1999) The surface ectoderm is essential for nephric duct formation in intermediate mesoderm. Development 126:1103–1108
237. Oh S, Shin S, Janknecht R (2012) ETV1, 4 and 5: an oncogenic subfamily of ETS transcription factors. Biochim Biophys Acta 1826(1):1–12
238. Olatunbosun ST, Bella AF (2000) Relationship between height, glucose intolerance, and hypertension in an urban African black adult population: a case for the "thrifty phenotype" hypothesis? J Natl Med Assoc 92(6):265–268
239. Osafune K, Takasato M, Kispert A, Asashima M, Nishinakamura R (2006) Identification of multipotent progenitors in the embryonic mouse kidney by a novel colony-forming assay. Development 133(1):151–161
240. Osathanondh V, Potter EL (1963) Development of human kidney as shown by microdissection. II. Renal pelvis, calyces, and papillae. Arch Pathol 76:277–289
241. Osathanondh V, Potter EL (1963) Development of human kidney as shown by microdissection.III. Formation and interrelationship of collecting tubules and nephrons. Arch Pathol 76:66–78
242. Osathanondh V, Potter EL (1966) Development of human kidney as shown by microdissection. Arch Pathol 82:391–402
243. Palmer RE, Kotsianti A, Cadman B, Boyd T, Gerald W, Haber DA (2001) WT1 regulates the expression of the major glomerular podocyte membrane protein Podocalyxin. Curr Biol 11(22):1815–1809
244. Park JS, Valerius MT, McMahon AP (2007) Wnt/beta-catenin signaling regulates nephron induction during mouse kidney development. Development 134(13):2533–2539
245. Patek CE, Little MH, Fleming S, Miles C, Charlieu JP, Clarke AR, Miyagawa K, Christie S, Doig J, Harrison DJ, Porteous DJ, Brookes AJ, Hooper ML, Hastie ND (1999) A zinc finger truncation of murine WT1 results in the characteristic urogenital abnormalities of Denys-Drash syndrome. Proc Natl Acad Sci U S A 96(6):2931–2936
246. Pavenstadt H, Kriz W, Kretzler M (2003) Cell biology of the glomerular podocyte. Physiol Rev 83(1): 253–307
247. Pedersen A, Skjong C, Shawlot W (2005) Lim 1 is required for nephric duct extension and ureteric bud morphogenesis. Dev Biol 288(2):571–581
248. Pelletier J, Schalling M, Buckler AJ, Rogers A, Haber DA, Housman D (1991) Expression of the Wilms' tumor gene WT1 in the murine urogenital system. Genes Dev 5:1345–1356
249. Pena A, Levitt MA, Hong A, Midulla P (2004) Surgical management of cloacal malformations: a review of 339 patients. J Pediatr Surg 39(3):470–479, discussion 470-479
250. Pepicelli CV, Kispert A, Rowitch D, McMahon AP (1997) GDNF induces branching and increased cell proliferation in the ureter of the mouse. Dev Biol 192:193–198
251. Perantoni AO, Timofeeva O, Naillat F, Richman C, Pajni-Underwood S, Wilson C, Vainio S, Dove LF, Lewandoski M (2005) Inactivation of FGF8 in early mesoderm reveals an essential role in kidney development. Development 132(17):3859–3871
252. Perriton CL, Powles N, Chiang C, Maconochie MK, Cohn MJ (2002) Sonic hedgehog signaling from the urethral epithelium controls external genital development. Dev Biol 247(1):26–46
253. Pichel JG, Shen L, Sheng HZ, Granholm A-C, Drago J, Grinberg A, Lee EJ, Huang SP, Saarmas M, Hoffer BJ, Sariola H, Westphal H (1996) Defects in enteric innervation and kidney development in mice lacking GDNF. Nature 382:73–76
254. Pini Prato A, Musso M, Ceccherini I, Mattioli G, Giunta C, Ghiggeri GM, Jasonni V (2009) Hirschsprung disease and congenital anomalies of the kidney and urinary tract (CAKUT): a novel syndromic association. Medicine 88(2):83–90
255. Piscione TD, Phan T, Rosenblum ND (2001) BMP7 controls collecting tubule cell proliferation and apoptosis via Smad1-dependent and -independent pathways. Am J Physiol 280:F19–F33
256. Piscione TD, Rosenblum ND (1999) The malformed kidney: disruption of glomerular and tubular development. Clin Genet 56(5):343–358
257. Piscione TD, Waters AM (2008) Structural and functional development of the kidney. In: Geary DF, Schaefer F (eds) Comprehensive pediatric

nephrology, 1st edn. Mosby, Inc., Philadelphia, pp 91–130
258. Piscione TD, Wu MY, Quaggin SE (2004) Expression of hairy/enhancer of split genes, Hes1 and Hes5, during murine nephron morphogenesis. Gene Expr Patterns 4(6):707–711
259. Piscione TD, Yager TD, Gupta IR, Grinfeld B, Pei Y, Attisano L, Wrana JL, Rosenblum ND (1997) BMP-2 and OP-1 exert direct and opposite effects on renal branching morphogenesis. Am J Physiol 273:F961–F975
260. Poladia DP, Kish K, Kutay B, Hains D, Kegg H, Zhao H, Bates CM (2006) Role of fibroblast growth factor receptors 1 and 2 in the metanephric mesenchyme. Dev Biol 291(2):325–339
261. Potter EL (1972) Normal and abnormal development of the kidney. Year Book Medical Publishers Inc, Chicago
262. Povey S, Lovering R, Bruford E, Wright M, Lush M, Wain H (2001) The HUGO Gene Nomenclature Committee (HGNC). Human Genet 109(6):678–680
263. Preger-Ben Noon E, Barak H, Guttmann-Raviv N, Reshef R (2009) Interplay between activin and Hox genes determines the formation of the kidney morphogenetic field. Development 136(12):1995–2004
264. Price KL, Long DA, Jina N, Liapis H, Hubank M, Woolf AS, Winyard PJ (2007) Microarray interrogation of human metanephric mesenchymal cells highlights potentially important molecules in vivo. Physiol Genom 28(2):193–202
265. Pulido R, Krueger NX, Serra-Pages C, Saito H, Streuli M (1995) Molecular characterization of the human transmembrane protein-tyrosine phosphatase delta. Evidence for tissue-specific expression of alternative human transmembrane protein-tyrosine phosphatase delta isoforms. J Biol Chem 270(12):6722–6728
266. Qazi Q, Masakawa A, Milman D, McGann B, Chua A, Haller J (1979) Renal anomalies in fetal alcohol syndrome. Pediatrics 63(6):886–889
267. Qi BQ, Beasley SW, Frizelle FA (2002) Clarification of the processes that lead to anorectal malformations in the ETU-induced rat model of imperforate anus. J Pediatr Surg 37(9):1305–1312
268. Qiao J, Bush KT, Steer DL, Stuart RO, Sakurai H, Wachsman W, Nigam SK (2001) Multiple fibroblast growth factors support growth of the ureteric bud but have different effects on branching morphogenesis. Mech Dev 109(2):123–135
269. Qiao J, Sakurai H, Nigam SK (1999) Branching morphogenesis independent of mesenchymal-epithelial contact in the developing kidney. Proc Natl Acad Sci U S A 96:7330–7335
270. Qiao J, Uzzo R, Obara-Ishihara T, Degenstein L, Fuchs E, Herzlinger D (1999) FGF-7 modulates ureteric bud growth and nephron number in the developing kidney. Development 126:547–554
271. Qiao S, Iwashita T, Furukawa T, Yamamoto M, Sobue G, Takahashi M (2001) Differential effects of leukocyte common antigen-related protein on biochemical and biological activities of RET-MEN2A and RET-MEN2B mutant proteins. J Biol Chem 276(12):9460–9467
272. Quaggin SE, Schwartz L, Cui S, Igarashi P, Deimling J, Post M, Rossant J (1999) The basic-helix-loop-helix protein pod1 is critically important for kidney and lung organogenesis. Development 126: 5771–5783
273. Queisser-Luft A, Stolz G, Wiesel A, Schlaefer K, Spranger J (2002) Malformations in newborn: results based on 30,940 infants and fetuses from the Mainz congenital birth defect monitoring system (1990–1998). Arch Gynecol Obstetr 266(3):163–167
274. Raatikainen-Ahokas A, Hytonen M, Tenhunen A, Sainio K, Sariola H (2000) Bmp-4 affects the differentiation of metanephric mesenchyme and reveals an early anterior-posterior axis of the embryonic kidney. Dev Dyn 217:146–158
275. Ricono JM, Xu YC, Arar M, Jin DC, Barnes JL, Abboud HE (2003) Morphological insights into the origin of glomerular endothelial and mesangial cells and their precursors. J Histochem Cytochem 51(2): 141–150
276. Robboy SJ, Taguchi O, Cunha GR (1982) Normal development of the human female reproductive tract and alterations resulting from experimental exposure to diethylstilbestrol. Human Pathol 13(3):190–198
277. Robert B, St John PL, Hyink DP, Abrahamson DR (1996) Evidence that embryonic kidney cells expressing flk-1 are intrinsic, vasculogenic angioblasts. Am J Physiol 271(3 Pt 2):F744–F753
278. Rodriguez MM, Gomez AH, Abitbol CL, Chandar JJ, Duara S, Zilleruelo GE (2004) Histomorphometric analysis of postnatal glomerulogenesis in extremely preterm infants. Pediatr Dev Pathol 7(1):17–25
279. Rogers SA, Ryan G, Purchio AF, Hammerman MR (1993) Metanephric transforming growth factor-b1 regulates nephrogenesis in vitro. Am J Physiol 264: F996–F1002
280. Roodhooft AM, Birnholz JC, Holmes LB (1984) Familial nature of congenital absence and severe dysgenesis of both kidneys. N Engl J Med 310(21): 1341–1345
281. Ruano-Gil D, Coca-Payeras A, Tejedo-Mateu A (1975) Obstruction and normal recanalization of the ureter in the human embryo. Its relation to congenital ureteric obstruction. Eur Urol 1(6):287–293
282. Rudolph AM, Heymann MA (1970) Circulatory changes during growth in the fetal lamb. Circ Res 26(3):289–299
283. Rumballe BA, Georgas KM, Combes AN, Ju AL, Gilbert T, Little MH (2011) Nephron formation adopts a novel spatial topology at cessation of nephrogenesis. Dev Biol 360(1):110–122
284. Saburi S, Hester I, Fischer E, Pontoglio M, Eremina V, Gessler M, Quaggin SE, Harrison R, Mount R, McNeill H (2008) Loss of Fat4 disrupts PCP signaling and oriented cell division and leads to cystic kidney disease. Nat Genet 40(8):1010–1015
285. Sadl V, Jin F, Yu J, Cui S, Holmyard D, Quaggin S, Barsh G, Cordes S (2002) The mouse Kreisler

(Krml1/MafB) segmentation gene is required for differentiation of glomerular visceral epithelial cells. Dev Biol 249(1):16–29
286. Sainio K, Hellstedt P, Kreidberg JA, Saxen L, Sariola H (1997) Differential regulation of two sets of mesonephric tubules by WT-1. Development 124: 1293–1299
287. Sainio K, Nonclercq D, Saarma M, Palgi J, Saxen L, Sariola H (1994) Neuronal characteristics in embryonic renal stroma. Int J Dev Biol 38(1):77–84
288. Sainio K, Suvanto P, Davies J, Wartiovaara J, Wartiovaara K, Saarma M, Arumäe U, Meng X, Lindahl M, Pachnis V, Sariola H (1997) Glial-cell-line-derived neurotrophic factor is required for bud initiation from ureteric epithelium. Development 124:4077–4087
289. Saisawat P, Tasic V, Vega-Warner V, Kehinde EO, Gunther B, Airik R, Innis JW, Hoskins BE, Hoefele J, Otto EA, Hildebrandt F (2012) Identification of two novel CAKUT-causing genes by massively parallel exon resequencing of candidate genes in patients with unilateral renal agenesis. Kidney Int 81(2):196–200
290. Sakurai H, Barros EJ, Tsukamoto T, Barasch J, Nigam SK (1997) An in vitro tubulogenesis system using cell lines derived from the embryonic kidney shows dependence on multiple soluble growth factors. Proc Natl Acad Sci U S A 94:6279–6284
291. Sakurai H, Nigam S (1997) Transforming growth factor-beta selectively inhibits branching morphogenesis but not tubulogenesis. Am J Physiol 272(1 Pt 2):F139–F146
292. Salerno A, Kohlhase J, Kaplan BS (2000) Townes-Brocks syndrome and renal dysplasia: a novel mutation in the SALL1 gene. Pediatr Nephrol 14(1):25–28
293. Sanchez MP, Silos-Santiago I, Frisen J, He B, Lira SA, Barbacid M (1996) Renal agenesis and the absence of enteric neurons in mice lacking GDNF. Nature 382:70–73
294. Sanders KM, Koh SD, Ward SM (2006) Interstitial cells of Cajal as pacemakers in the gastrointestinal tract. Annu Rev Physiol 68:307–343
295. Sanyanusin P, Schimmenti LA, McNoe LA, Ward TA, Pierpont ME, Sullivan MJ, Dobyns WB, Eccles MR (1995) Mutation of the PAX2 gene in a family with optic nerve colobomas, renal anomalies and vesicoureteral reflux. Nat Genet 9(4):358–364
296. Sariola H, Ekblom P, Lehtonen E, Saxen L (1983) Differentiation and vascularization of the metanephric kidney grafted on the chorioallantoic membrane. Dev Biol 96(2):427–435
297. Sariola H, Holm K, Henke-Fahle S (1988) Early innervation of the metanephric kidney. Development 104(4):589–599
298. Saxen L (1987) Organogenesis of the kidney. Cambridge University Press, Cambridge
299. Schimmenti LA, Pierpont ME, Carpenter BL, Kashtan CE, Johnson MR, Dobyns WB (1995) Autosomal dominant optic nerve colobomas, vesicoureteral reflux, and renal anomalies. Am J Med Genet 59(2):204–208
300. Schmidt-Ott KM, Yang J, Chen X, Wang H, Paragas N, Mori K, Li JY, Lu B, Costantini F, Schiffer M, Bottinger E, Barasch J (2005) Novel regulators of kidney development from the tips of the ureteric bud. J Am Soc Nephrol 16(7):1993–2002
301. Schmidt IM, Damgaard IN, Boisen KA, Mau C, Chellakooty M, Olgaard K, Main KM (2004) Increased kidney growth in formula-fed versus breast-fed healthy infants. Pediatr Nephrol 19(10): 1137–1144
302. Schonfelder EM, Knuppel T, Tasic V, Miljkovic P, Konrad M, Wuhl E, Antignac C, Bakkaloglu A, Schaefer F, Weber S (2006) Mutations in Uroplakin IIIA are a rare cause of renal hypodysplasia in humans. Am J Kidney Dis 47(6):1004–1012
303. Schuchardt A, D'Agati V, Larsson-Blomberg L, Costantini F, Pachnis V (1994) Defects in the kidney and enteric nervous system of mice lacking the tyrosine kinase receptor Ret. Nature 367:380–383
304. Schuchardt A, D'Agati V, Pachnis V, Costantini F (1996) Renal agenesis and hypodysplasia in *ret-k⁻* mutant mice result from defects in ureteric bud development. Development 122:1919–1929
305. Schwab K, Patterson LT, Aronow BJ, Luckas R, Liang HC, Potter SS (2003) A catalogue of gene expression in the developing kidney. Kidney Int 64(5):1588–1604
306. Seifert AW, Bouldin CM, Choi KS, Harfe BD, Cohn MJ (2009) Multiphasic and tissue-specific roles of sonic hedgehog in cloacal septation and external genitalia development. Development 136(23):3949–3957
307. Seikaly MG, Ho PL, Emmett L, Fine RN, Tejani A (2003) Chronic renal insufficiency in children: the 2001 annual report of the NAPRTCS. Pediatr Nephrol 18(8):796–804
308. Self M, Lagutin OV, Bowling B, Hendrix J, Cai Y, Dressler GR, Oliver G (2006) Six2 is required for suppression of nephrogenesis and progenitor renewal in the developing kidney. EMBO J 25(21): 5214–5228
309. Shakya R, Jho EH, Kotka P, Wu Z, Kholodilov N, Burke R, D'Agati V, Costantini F (2005) The role of GDNF in patterning the excretory system. Dev Biol 283(1):70–84
310. Shakya R, Watanabe T, Costantini F (2005) The role of GDNF/Ret signaling in ureteric bud cell fate and branching morphogenesis. Dev Cell 8(1):65–74
311. Shawlot W, Behringer RR (1995) Requirement for *Lim1* in head-organizer function. Nature 374:425–430
312. Shimizu K, Chiba S, Hosoya N, Kumano K, Saito T, Kurokawa M, Kanda Y, Hamada Y, Hirai H (2000) Binding of Delta1, Jagged1, and Jagged2 to Notch2 rapidly induces cleavage, nuclear translocation, and hyperphosphorylation of Notch2. Mol Cell Biol 20(18):6913–6922
313. Shimizu K, Chiba S, Kumano K, Hosoya N, Takahashi T, Kanda Y, Hamada Y, Yazaki Y, Hirai H

(1999) Mouse jagged1 physically interacts with notch2 and other notch receptors. Assessment by quantitative methods. J Biol Chem 274(46):32961–32969
314. Shiroyanagi Y, Liu B, Cao M, Agras K, Li J, Hsieh MH, Willingham EJ, Baskin LS (2007) Urothelial sonic hedgehog signaling plays an important role in bladder smooth muscle formation. Differentiation 75(10):968–977
315. Sichieri R, Siqueira KS, Pereira RA, Ascherio A (2000) Short stature and hypertension in the city of Rio de Janeiro, Brazil. Public Health Nutr 3(1):77–82
316. Sims-Lucas S, Argyropoulos C, Kish K, McHugh K, Bertram JF, Quigley R, Bates CM (2009) Three-dimensional imaging reveals ureteric and mesenchymal defects in Fgfr2-mutant kidneys. J Am Soc Nephrol 20(12):2525–2533
317. Skibo LK, Lyons EA, Levi CS (1992) First-trimester umbilical cord cysts. Radiology 182(3):719–722
318. Skinner MA, Safford SD, Reeves JG, Jackson ME, Freemerman AJ (2008) Renal aplasia in humans is associated with RET mutations. Am J Hum Genet 82(2):344–351
319. Solari V, Piotrowska AP, Puri P (2003) Altered expression of interstitial cells of Cajal in congenital ureteropelvic junction obstruction. J Urol 170(6 Pt 1):2420–2422
320. Soriano P (1994) Abnormal kidney development and hematological disorders in PDGF ß-receptor mutant mice. Genes Dev 8:1888–1896
321. Spencer J, Wang Z, Hoy W (2001) Low birth weight and reduced renal volume in Aboriginal children. Am J Kidney Dis 37(5):915–920
322. Spitzer A, Brandis M (1974) Functional and morphologic maturation of the superficial nephrons. Relationship to total kidney function. J Clin Invest 53(1):279–287
323. Stark K, Vainio S, Vassileva G, McMahon AP (1994) Epithelial transformation of metanephric mesenchyme in the developing kidney regulated by *Wnt-4*. Nature 372:679–683
324. Surendran K, Selassie M, Liapis H, Krigman H, Kopan R (2010) Reduced Notch signaling leads to renal cysts and papillary microadenomas. J Am Soc Nephrol 21(5):819–832
325. Tacciuoli M, Lotti T, de Matteis A, Laurenti C (1975) Development of the smooth muscle of the ureter and vesical trigone: histological investigation in human fetus. Eur Urol 1(6):282–286
326. Takemoto M, He L, Norlin J, Patrakka J, Xiao Z, Petrova T, Bondjers C, Asp J, Wallgard E, Sun Y, Samuelsson T, Mostad P, Lundin S, Miura N, Sado Y, Alitalo K, Quaggin SE, Tryggvason K, Betsholtz C (2006) Large-scale identification of genes implicated in kidney glomerulus development and function. EMBO J 25(5):1160–1174
327. Tanagho EA, Meyers FH, Smith DR (1968) The trigone: anatomical and physiological considerations. I. In relation to the ureterovesical junction. J Urol 100(5):623–632
328. Tang MJ, Cai Y, Tsai SJ, Wang YK, Dressler GR (2002) Ureteric bud outgrowth in response to RET activation is mediated by phosphatidylinositol 3-kinase. Dev Biol 243(1):128–136
329. Tang MJ, Worley D, Sanicola M, Dressler GR (1998) The RET-glial cell-derived neurotrophic factor (GDNF) pathway stimulates migration and chemoattraction of epithelial cells. J Cell Biol 142(5):1337–1345
330. Tanigawa S, Wang H, Yang Y, Sharma N, Tarasova N, Ajima R, Yamaguchi TP, Rodriguez LG, Perantoni AO (2011) Wnt4 induces nephronic tubules in metanephric mesenchyme by a non-canonical mechanism. Dev Biol 352(1):58–69
331. Tasian G, Cunha G, Baskin L (2010) Smooth muscle differentiation and patterning in the urinary bladder. Differentiation 80(2–3):106–117
332. Thomas R, Sanna-Cherchi S, Warady BA, Furth SL, Kaskel FJ, Gharavi AG (2011) HNF1B and PAX2 mutations are a common cause of renal hypodysplasia in the CKiD cohort. Pediatr Nephrol 26(6):897–903
333. Torban E, Dziarmaga A, Iglesias D, Chu LL, Vassilieva T, Little M, Eccles M, Discenza M, Pelletier J, Goodyer P (2006) PAX2 activates WNT4 expression during mammalian kidney development. J Biol Chem 281(18):12705–12712
334. Torihashi S, Ward SM, Nishikawa S, Nishi K, Kobayashi S, Sanders KM (1995) c-kit-dependent development of interstitial cells and electrical activity in the murine gastrointestinal tract. Cell Tissue Res 280(1):97–111
335. Torres M, Gomez-Pardo E, Dressler GR, Gruss P (1995) Pax-2 controls multiple steps of urogenital development. Development 121(12):4057–4065
336. Tsang TE, Shawlot W, Kinder SJ, Kobayashi A, Kwan KM, Schughart K, Kania A, Jessell TM, Behringer RR, Tam PP (2000) Lim1 activity is required for intermediate mesoderm differentiation in the mouse embryo. Dev Biol 223(1):77–90
337. Tufro A, Norwood VF, Carey RM, Gomez RA (1999) Vascular endothelial growth factor induces nephrogenesis and vasculogenesis. J Am Soc Nephrol 10(10):2125–2134
338. Tufro A, Teichman J, Woda C, Villegas G (2008) Semaphorin3a inhibits ureteric bud branching morphogenesis. Mech Dev 125(5–6):558–568
339. Uetani N, Bertozzi K, Chagnon MJ, Hendriks W, Tremblay ML, Bouchard M (2009) Maturation of ureter-bladder connection in mice is controlled by LAR family receptor protein tyrosine phosphatases. J Clin Invest 119(4):924–935
340. Uetani N, Bouchard M (2009) Plumbing in the embryo: developmental defects of the urinary tracts. Clin Genet 75(4):307–317
341. van der Putte SC (2005) The development of the perineum in the human. A comprehensive histological study with a special reference to the role of the stromal components. Adv Anat Embryol Cell Biol 177:1–131

342. Van Esch H, Groenen P, Nesbit MA, Schuffenhauer S, Lichtner P, Vanderlinden G, Harding B, Beetz R, Bilous RW, Holdaway I, Shaw NJ, Fryns JP, Van de Ven W, Thakker RV, Devriendt K (2000) GATA3 haplo-insufficiency causes human HDR syndrome. Nature 406(6794):419–422
343. Vega QC, Worby CA, Lechner MS, Dixon JE, Dressler GR (1996) Glial cell line-derived neurotrophic factor activates the receptor tyrosine kinase RET and promotes kidney morphogenesis. Proc Natl Acad Sci U S A 93(20):10657–10661
344. Veille JC, McNeil S, Hanson R, Smith N (1998) Renal hemodynamics: longitudinal study from the late fetal life to one year of age. J Matern Fetal Investig 8(1):6–10
345. Verschueren K, Dewulf N, Goumans MJ, Lonnoy O, Feijen A, Grimsby S, Vande Spiegle K, ten Dijke P, Moren A, Vanscheeuwijck P, Heldin C-H, Miyazono K, Mummery C, Van Den Eijnden-Van Raaij J, Huylebroeck D (1995) Expression of type I and type IB receptors for activin in midgestation mouse embryos suggests distinct functions in organogenesis. Mech Dev 52:109–123
346. Viana R, Batourina E, Huang H, Dressler GR, Kobayashi A, Behringer RR, Shapiro E, Hensle T, Lambert S, Mendelsohn C (2007) The development of the bladder trigone, the center of the anti-reflux mechanism. Development 134(20):3763–3769
347. Wagner CA, Devuyst O, Bourgeois S, Mohebbi N (2009) Regulated acid-base transport in the collecting duct. Pflugers Arch 458(1):137–156
348. Wagner KD, Wagner N, Schedl A (2003) The complex life of WT1. J Cell Sci 116(Pt 9):1653–1658
349. Wagner N, Wagner KD, Xing Y, Scholz H, Schedl A (2004) The major podocyte protein nephrin is transcriptionally activated by the Wilms' tumor suppressor WT1. J Am Soc Nephrol 15(12): 3044–3051
350. Wang GJ, Brenner-Anantharam A, Vaughan ED, Herzlinger D (2009) Antagonism of BMP4 signaling disrupts smooth muscle investment of the ureter and ureteropelvic junction. J Urol 181(1):401–407
351. Watanabe T, Costantini F (2004) Real-time analysis of ureteric bud branching morphogenesis in vitro. Dev Biol 271(1):98–108
352. Weber S (2012) Novel genetic aspects of congenital anomalies of kidney and urinary tract. Curr Opin Pediatr 24(2):212–218
353. Weber S, Landwehr C, Renkert M, Hoischen A, Wuhl E, Denecke J, Radlwimmer B, Haffner D, Schaefer F, Weber RG (2011) Mapping candidate regions and genes for congenital anomalies of the kidneys and urinary tract (CAKUT) by array-based comparative genomic hybridization. Nephrol Dial Transplant 26(1):136–143
354. Weber S, Moriniere V, Knuppel T, Charbit M, Dusek J, Ghiggeri GM, Jankauskiene A, Mir S, Montini G, Peco-Antic A, Wuhl E, Zurowska AM, Mehls O, Antignac C, Schaefer F, Salomon R (2006) Prevalence of mutations in renal developmental genes in children with renal hypodysplasia: results of the ESCAPE study. J Am Soc Nephrol 17(10):2864–2870
355. Weiss JP (1988) Embryogenesis of ureteral anomalies: a unifying theory. Aust N Z J Surg 58(8): 631–638
356. Wellik DM, Hawkes PJ, Capecchi MR (2002) Hox11 paralogous genes are essential for metanephric kidney induction. Genes Dev 16(11):1423–1432
357. Wesson MB (1925) Anatomical, embryological, and physiological studies of the trigone and bladder neck. J Urol 4:280–306
358. White JT, Zhang B, Cerqueira DM, Tran U, Wessely O (2010) Notch signaling, wt1 and foxc2 are key regulators of the podocyte gene regulatory network in Xenopus. Development 137(11): 1863–1873
359. Wiesel A, Queisser-Luft A, Clementi M, Bianca S, Stoll C (2005) Prenatal detection of congenital renal malformations by fetal ultrasonographic examination: an analysis of 709,030 births in 12 European countries. Eur J Med Genet 48(2):131–144
360. Winnier G, Blessing M, Labosky PA, Hogan BLM (1995) Bone morphogenetic protein-4 is required for mesoderm formation and patterning in the mouse. Genes Dev 9:2105–2116
361. Woodburne RT (1965) The ureter, ureterovesical junction, and vesical trigone. Anat Rec 151: 243–249
362. Woods LL, Weeks DA, Rasch R (2004) Programming of adult blood pressure by maternal protein restriction: role of nephrogenesis. Kidney Int 65(4): 1339–1348
363. Woolf AS, Kolatsi-Joannou M, Hardman P, Andermarcher E, Moorby C, Fine LG, Jat PS, Noble MD, Gherardi E (1995) Roles of hepatocyte growth factor/scatter factor and the met receptor in the early development of the metanephros. J Cell Biol 128(1–2):171–184
364. Woolf AS, Winyard P, Hermanns MH, Welham SJ (2003) 21. Maldevelopment of the human kidney and lower urinary tract: an overview. In: Vize PD, Woolf AS, Bard JB (eds) The kidney: from normal development to congenital disease, 1st edn. Elsevier Science, San Diego, pp 377–393
365. Xiao J, Nguyen TV, Ngui K, Strijbos PJ, Selmer IS, Neylon CB, Furness JB (2004) Molecular and functional analysis of hyperpolarisation-activated nucleotide-gated (HCN) channels in the enteric nervous system. Neuroscience 129(3):603–614
366. Xu P-X, Adams J, Peters H, Brown MC, Heaney S, Maas R (1999) Eya1-deficient mice lack ears and kidneys and show abnormal apoptosis of organ primordia. Nat Genet 23:113–117
367. Xu PX, Zheng W, Huang L, Maire P, Laclef C, Silvius D (2003) Six1 is required for the early organogenesis of mammalian kidney. Development 130(14):3085–3094
368. Yamaguchi OA, Constantinou CE (1989) Renal calyceal and pelvic contraction rhythms. Am J Physiol 257(4 Pt 2):R788–R795

369. Yang Y, Jeanpierre C, Dressler GR, Lacoste M, Niaudet P, Gubler MC (1999) WT1 and PAX-2 podocyte expression in Denys-Drash syndrome and isolated diffuse mesangial sclerosis. Am J Pathol 154(1):181–192
370. Yeger H, Forget D, Alami J, Williams BR (1996) Analysis of WT1 gene expression during mouse nephrogenesis in organ culture. In Vitro Cell Dev Biol 32:496–504
371. Yi SE, Daluiski A, Pederson R, Rosen V, Lyons KM (2000) The type I BMP receptor BMPRIB is required for chondrogenesis in the mouse limb. Development 127:621–630
372. Yosypiv IV (2009) Renin-angiotensin system-growth factor cross-talk: a novel mechanism for ureteric bud morphogenesis. Pediatr Nephrol 24(6):1113–1120
373. Yosypiv IV, Boh MK, Spera MA, El-Dahr SS (2008) Downregulation of Spry-1, an inhibitor of GDNF/Ret, causes angiotensin II-induced ureteric bud branching. Kidney Int 74(10):1287–1293
374. Yu J, Carroll TJ, McMahon AP (2002) Sonic hedgehog regulates proliferation and differentiation of mesenchymal cells in the mouse metanephric kidney. Development 129(22):5301–5312
375. Yu J, Carroll TJ, Rajagopal J, Kobayashi A, Ren Q, McMahon AP (2009) A Wnt7b-dependent pathway regulates the orientation of epithelial cell division and establishes the cortico-medullary axis of the mammalian kidney. Development 136(1):161–171
376. Zhang H, Bradley A (1996) Mice deficient for BMP2 are nonviable and have defects in amnion/chorion and cardiac development. Development 122:2977–2986
377. Zhang S, Lin Y, Itaranta P, Yagi A, Vainio S (2001) Expression of Sprouty genes 1, 2 and 4 during mouse organogenesis. Mech Dev 109(2):367–370
378. Zhang Z, Quinlan J, Hoy W, Hughson MD, Lemire M, Hudson T, Hueber PA, Benjamin A, Roy A, Pascuet E, Goodyer M, Raju C, Houghton F, Bertram J, Goodyer P (2008) A common RET variant is associated with reduced newborn kidney size and function. J Am Soc Nephrol 19(10):2027–2034
379. Zhao H, Kegg H, Grady S, Truong HT, Robinson ML, Baum M, Bates CM (2004) Role of fibroblast growth factor receptors 1 and 2 in the ureteric bud. Dev Biol 276(2):403–415
380. Zimanyi MA, Bertram JF, Black MJ (2002) Nephron number and blood pressure in rat offspring with maternal high-protein diet. Pediatr Nephrol 17(12):1000–1004

2 Development of Renal Function in the Fetus and Newborn

Lyndsay A. Harshman and Patrick D. Brophy

Fetal renal function is inherently related to fetal development, and management of preterm infants requires knowledge of renal developmental stage in conjunction with gestational age and/or post-menstrual age. A variety of factors, including maternal health and gestational medication use, may result in renal dysfunction even in term infants. Optimal prenatal and postnatal care in cases of suspected renal dysfunction is required to decrease the likelihood of long-term renal disease into adulthood.

2.1 Developmental Regulation of Renal Structure

Renal development is marked by a series of transitional developmental structures prior to the generation of a final mature kidney with key processes broadly defined as nephrogenesis and branching morphogenesis. Early renal structures and tubular function begin to appear at 9–12 weeks' gestation in humans with a full complement of new nephrons formed through the 36th week gestation; thus, in the preterm infant, nephrogenesis continues after birth leading to 36 weeks post-menstrual age [1]. Early regionalization within the primitive kidney requires a series of molecular interactions key for formation of the metanephros (mature kidney), of which developmental understanding continues to evolve. A stepwise series of both spatial and temporally regulated gene expression is required to provide proteins needed for key transcription factors, growth factors, receptors, and extracellular matrix components in renal development [2]. An in-depth review of these processes can be found by Dressler [3].

The developing kidney arises from intermediate mesoderm with demarcation of this territory noted by expression of two paired-box, or *PAX*, genes – *PAX-2* and *PAX-8* [4]. The earliest renal precursor in mammals, the nephric duct, arises from intermediate mesoderm [5]. The nephric duct extends caudally in the fetus with primitive renal tubular development demonstrated at approximately gestational week three with appearance of nonfunctional organs called the pronephric tubules. These primitive tubules subsequently involute with resultant formation of the mesonephric tubules – 20 pairs of thick walled tubules and corresponding glomeruli. The mesonephros is capable of urine formation by week 5 gestation. The mesonephros subsequently develops an outgrowth, called the ureteric bud, from the caudal end of the former nephric duct itself.

Appearance of the ureteric bud corresponds with degeneration of the mesonephros at weeks 11–12 gestation. At this time, there is growth of the ureteric bud toward the nephrogenic blastema,

L.A. Harshman (✉) • P.D. Brophy
Division of Nephrology, University of Iowa Children's Hospital, University of Iowa Carve College of Medicine, 200 Hawkins Drive, 2400 Colloton Pavilion, Iowa City, Iowa 52242, IA, USA

A.S. Chishti et al. (eds.), *Kidney and Urinary Tract Diseases in the Newborn*,
DOI 10.1007/978-3-642-39988-6_2, © Springer-Verlag Berlin Heidelberg 2014

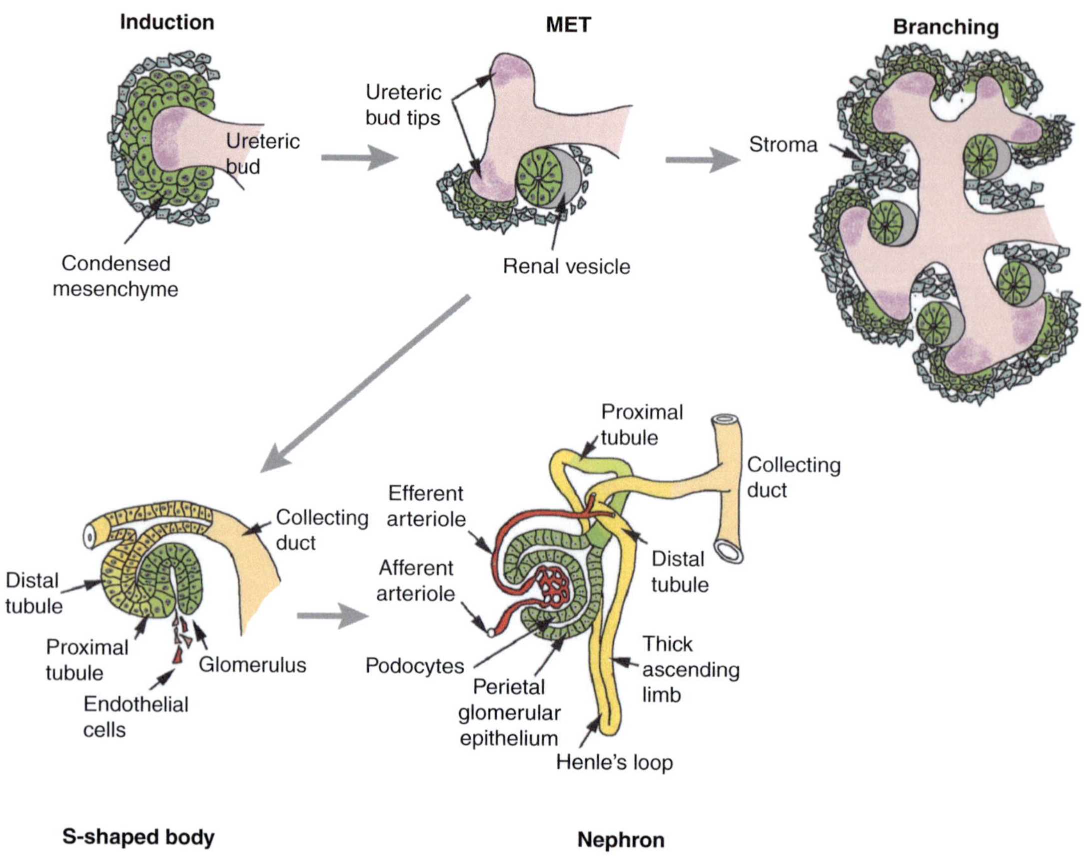

Fig. 2.1 Sequential steps of nephrogenesis. Induction of the metanephric mesenchyme by the ureteric bud promotes aggregation of the condensed mesenchyme around the bud tips. These aggregates become polarized as they undergo mesenchyme-to-epithelial (*MET*) conversion to generate the renal vesicle. Meanwhile, the ureteric bud continues to branch and induce new aggregates at the bud tips [5]

an undifferentiated mesenchymal cell mass within the metanephric mesenchyme. Conversion of the metanephric mesenchyme and ureteric bud into the metanephros requires both spatial and temporal regulation of gene expression (as well as gene repression). This conversion is mediated by reciprocal inductive signaling between the ureteric bud and metanephric mesenchyme, leading to development of the metanephros. Reciprocal induction between the ureteric bud and mesenchyme requires both secretion of glial-derived neurotrophic growth factor (GDNF) from the metanephric mesenchyme and intact expression of the GDNF receptor, *c-ret*, within the ureteric bud [6]. This inductive signaling event catalyzes what is known as the mesenchyme-to-epithelial transition (see Fig. 2.1). As part of this transition, outgrowth from the ureteric bud forms a renal vesicle, which subsequently involutes to form a second structure called a comma-shaped body. The comma-shaped body involutes a second time to form the s-shaped body. In conjunction, new epithelial cells within the s-shaped body come into contact with nearby invading endothelial cells to form an early glomerular basement membrane. This repetitive process is termed branching morphogenesis and results in formation of the renal collecting system. Recruitment and growth of nearby endothelial cells and mesangial precursors yields glomerular capillary tufts as nephrons continue to develop from the innermost aspect of the fetal kidney toward the young renal cortex.

Proper nephrogenesis requires several genetic factors be present to allow for full final nephron complement. In the developing mammalian kidney, the expression pattern of the transcription factor *PAX-2* plays an important functional role in the differentiation of the renal epithelium [7]. Although *PAX* expression is noted very early in development within the intermediate mesoderm, *PAX-2* gene activation requires induction via the ureteric bud and is not an inherent property of the metanephric mesenchyme. During a well-defined sequence of morphogenic events, *PAX-2* expression is observed in the ureteric bud, comma-shaped bodies, nuclei of condensing mesenchyme, and early collecting tubule [8]. Expression persists in the collecting ducts, comma-shaped body, and in the distal two-thirds of the s-shaped body; however, *PAX-2* downregulation is noted in the proximal segment of the s-shaped body where podocyte precursors originate. Overexpression of *PAX-2* within these initial structures, as well as mature tubules, has been demonstrated to lead to atrophic glomeruli and microcystic tubular dilation [9].

The Wilms' tumor suppressor gene *WT1* is an early marker of metanephric mesenchyme and is essential in the survival of the metanephric mesenchyme, for regulation of GDNF expression, and the promotion of survival of uninduced cells [10]. WT1 expression is temporally and spatially regulated, and in later stages of development, *WT1* is expressed at high levels in the newly formed podocyte cells of the glomerulus as well as the s-shaped body. The *WT1* gene is associated with developmental abnormalities in the developing human genitourinary system, and *WT1* knockout mice demonstrate an absence of renal and genital development [11].

Literature demonstrates genes such as *PAX-2* and *WT1*, as well as the proto-oncogenes *c*-myc and *n*-myc, are involved in the development of specialized renal epithelial cells and may also impact development of other renal cell lineages. *C*-myc is found widely within uninduced mesenchyme as well as early epithelial structures [12]. The proto-oncogene *n*-myc, in contrast, is not noted within uninduced mesenchyme but rather is upregulated in early epithelial differentiation [13]. Failure of *c*-myc expression to downregulate is associated with tubular hyperplasia and cyst formation [14].

Multiple growth factors work synergistically with transcription factors such as *PAX-2* and *WT1* in renal cell differentiation [15, 16]. One key growth factor has been previously mentioned—GDNF. This factor is required for proper ureteric bud outgrowth and also provides the ligand and signal to the *c-ret* oncogene receptor within the ureteric bud [7]. Other important growth factors known to influence renal organogenesis include transforming growth factor-α (TGF-α) and TGF-β, as well as platelet-derived growth factor [17–20]. TGF-β has been shown to stimulate extracellular matrix deposition and antibodies to TGF-α are noted to block cell growth and differentiation [18, 21]. Platelet-derived growth factor is key in development of the glomerular vascular stock [22].

Regulation of fluid and electrolyte balance in the developed kidney is dependent on both a spatial and temporal relationship of gene expression within the developing fetus. The aforementioned epithelial-mesenchymal interactions and subsequent branching morphogenesis are essential for mature renal functions in order that renal hemodynamics are well controlled and glomerular function established to allow for fluid and electrolyte balance after birth.

2.2 Fetal Regulation of Renal Hemodynamics

2.2.1 Renal Blood Flow

Sheep models have provided a large amount of the primary experimental work to date regarding renal blood flow and hemodynamics. A high state of renal vascular resistance and low filtration fraction contribute to the difference in renal blood flow between the fetus and neonate, with the newborn receiving approximately 15 % of cardiac output compared to ~3 % in utero [23, 24]. At the time of birth in lambs, there are both a redistribution of blood flow from the inner to outer superficial renal cortex and an immediate, overall increase in renal blood flow [24, 25]. The increase in renal blood flow is linear in nature and associated with a rise in arterial blood pressure and corresponding decrease in renal vascular resistance; however, multiple other factors contribute significantly to postnatal changes in renal hemodynamics, including the renin-angiotensin system, renal neurovascular adaptations, and small molecule influences such as adenosine, atrial natriuretic factor (ANF), and prostaglandins [26–28].

The ability to autoregulate blood flow despite alterations in perfusion pressure becomes increasingly more evident after birth. The fetal kidney appears to have a moderate degree of autoregulation capability despite low perfusion pressures in the fetus of 40–60 mmHg. The adult kidney's ability to maintain blood flow with alterations in perfusion pressure between 80 and 150 mmHg is likely due to the neurovascular bundle in moderating flow, whereas fetal adaptation may be more under the influence of small molecules such as arginine vasopressin (AVP) [29, 30].

2.2.2 Renin-Angiotensin System

Several studies have demonstrated the ability of the renin-angiotensin system in the regulation of fetal blood pressure and renal blood flow. Additionally, angiotensin II (AII) has both important properties as a growth factor and is also required for normal nephrogenesis. Impairment of the perinatal renin-angiotensin system, present from the developing mesonephros, has been demonstrated to impair nephrogenesis as well as lead to a reduced perinatal mass and hypertension in adults [31–35]. The fetus is able to release renin into fetal circulation with generally higher fetal than maternal levels of renin noted [32–35]. Physiologically, AII serves to increase glomerular efferent tone in the fetus. Additionally, the fetus is able to self-generate AII with stimulation of renin release [32, 34]. AII administered intravenously to the fetus leads to increases in arterial blood pressure. In contrast, despite decreases in renal blood flow with administration of AII in fetal sheep, the fetal glomerular filtration rate (GFR) remains constant [36]. Administration of losartan, an AII receptor blocker, as well as the angiotensin-converting enzyme inhibitor, captopril, in the third trimester of fetal sheep development results in decreased fetal blood pressure, a decrease in fetal vascular resistance, and increase in renal blood flow which all contribute to a decrease in GFR [37]. Histologically, manifestations of AII receptor blocker usage may be seen as severely disturbed renal architecture including tubular dysgenesis associated with underdeveloped vasa recta (see Fig. 2.2) [38].

The development and actions of the renin-angiotensin system in the fetus have significant ramifications for long-term postnatal morbidity with abnormalities in the renin-angiotensin system leading to abnormal glomeruli and tubular abnormalities. Maternal low-protein diets have been noted to have an impact on AII actions in utero, leading to a decrease in renal mass and adult hypertension [39]. Salient observations persist regarding the use of both losartan and captopril in pregnant women with harmful fetal effects including fetal hypotension, renal tubular dysplasia, pulmonary hypoplasia, growth retardation, patent ductus arteriosus, as well as increased fetal and neonatal mortality [40, 41]. Additionally, the renin-angiotensin system plays a key role in fetal cardiovascular and renal responses to blood loss with a substantial rise in renin and angiotensin levels in response to rapid reduction in fetal blood volume [42–45].

2.2.3 Renal Sympathetic Nervous System

Studies have suggested that circulating catecholamines and the sympathetic nervous system play a role in the hemodynamics of the developing renal system [30, 46–48]. The renal sympathetic nervous system (SNS) increases renal vascular tone in both the afferent and efferent arterioles and plays a vital role in fetal adaption to

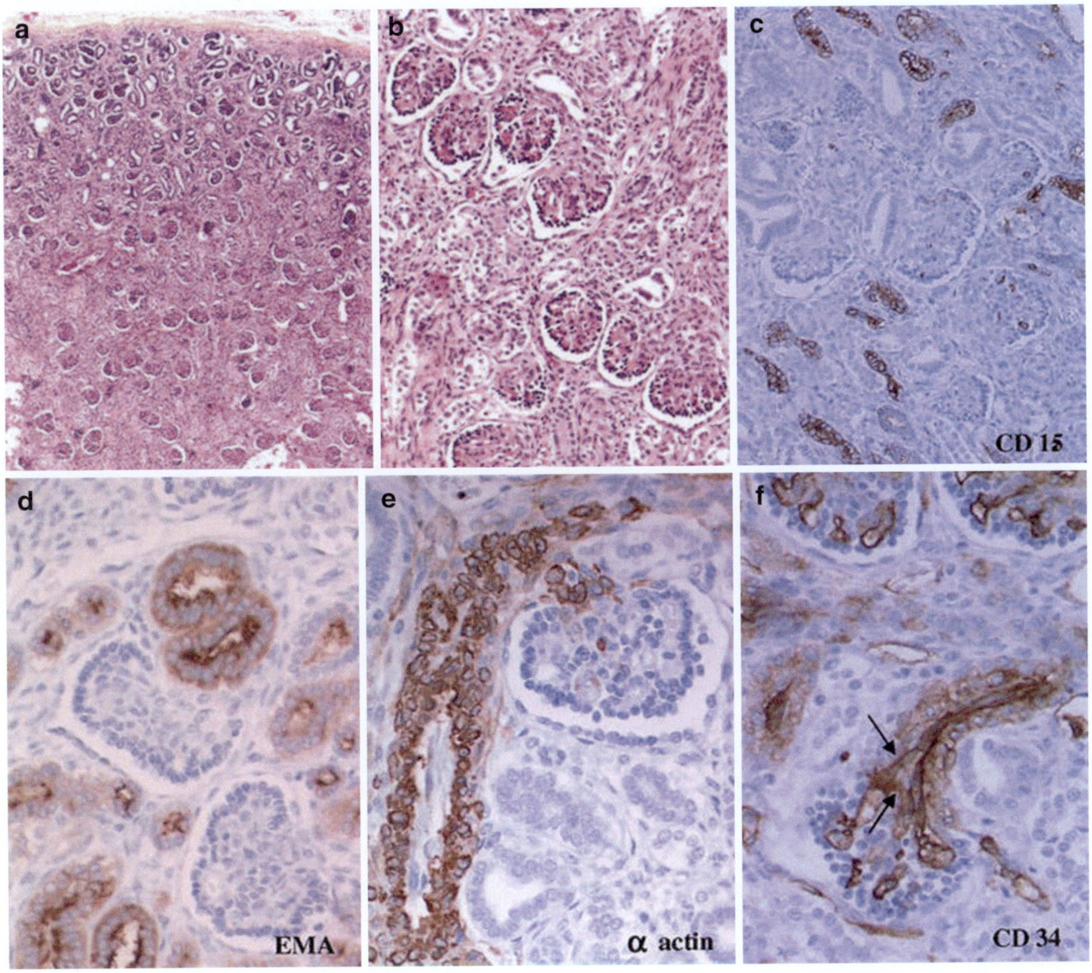

Fig. 2.2 (**a**) Kidney section showing cortical disarray, absent medullary rays, and increased number of glomeruli (hematoxylin and eosin). (**b**) High magnification of the same section showing ischemic glomeruli with retracted tuft in glomerular chamber, decreased numbers of tubules, poorly differentiated, and abundant Mesenchymal tissue. (**c**) Immunoperoxidase staining (CD 15 antibody) showed decreased numbers of proximal tubules, very poorly differentiated. (**d**) Immunoperoxidase staining (*EMA* antibody) showed decreased numbers of distal tubules, poorly differentiated. (**e**) Immunoperoxidase staining (α – smooth muscle actin antibody) showed hypertrophy of the arterial and arteriolar media cells. (**f**) Immunoperoxidase staining (CD 34 antibody) showed hypertrophied endothelial cells of the arterioles (With kind permission from Springer: Daikha-Dahmane et al. [38])

challenges such as fetal asphyxia. SNS responses develop significantly in the third trimester, with a general consensus suggesting that the overall function of the sympathetic state appears to be increased renal vascular tone. Studies in fetal lambs have corroborated this with the demonstration that fetal renal vasculature seems to be more sensitive to α1-adrenoceptor stimulation than in either newborns or adult sheep [49, 50]. These data are supported by the observation that low-level renal nerve stimulation can produce a greater fall in renal blood flow and a subsequent larger rise in renal vascular resistance in fetal versus newborn lambs [48]. Stimulation of the renal sympathetic system at higher levels is associated with greater renal vasoconstriction in newborn lambs than fetuses. Furthermore, the renal vasculature appears to be less responsive to renal nerve stimulation in newborn piglets than it is in adult comparisons [48, 51]. With maturation of the renal system, and consistent with other vascular beds in the developing body, upregulation of α2-adrenoceptors is associated with concomitant downregulation of the ß2-adrenoceptors in the renal vessels.

2.2.4 Small Molecule Mediators of Renal Blood Flow In Utero

2.2.4.1 Prostaglandins

With the advent of selected cyclooxygenase-2 inhibitors and a better understanding of the prostaglandin synthetic pathway, it has become apparent that prostaglandins are inherently important in the regulation of renal function [52–54]. Past investigators demonstrated and suggested that prostaglandins, specifically prostaglandins E2 and I2, produced within the fetal kidney and placenta were involved in renal hemodynamic regulation and function through promoting systemic and renal vasodilation as well as diuresis [53, 54]. Clinical support for these hypotheses is present, with the relatively consistently recognized decreased in renal output after prostaglandin inhibitors, such as indomethacin, in preterm and term infants with patent ductus arteriosus. Studies in fetal sheep have demonstrated that inhibition of prostaglandin synthesis during fetal life can produce a significant decrease in blood flow with a subsequent rise in renal vascular resistance and arterial blood pressure [54, 55]. The use of medications such as indomethacin to stop preterm labor has been associated with oligohydramnios and neonatal oliguria [56], and this effect is likely secondary to a decrease in fetal urinary output resulting from decreased renal fetal blood flow [54]. Further research has demonstrated that prolonged indomethacin therapy, such as for patent ductus arteriosus, can transiently reduce renal blood flow in the very low birth weight infant with symptomatic patent ductus arteriosus [57]. Therefore, in the newborn period, a reduction in renal blood flow does appear to be a direct effect of indomethacin. In general, it appears that the high circulating plasma levels of vasodilatory prostaglandins counteract with highly activated vasoconstricted state of the neonatal microcirculation [57]. Thus, the renal vasoconstrictor effect by prostaglandin synthesis inhibitors can certainly be detrimental, especially in the immature kidney.

2.2.4.2 Kallikrein-Kinin System

Bradykinin is a vasodilator and diuretic peptide produced by the kallikrein enzymes in the collecting tubules of the kidney and thought to play a role in renal morphogenesis. Renal expression of kallikrein is initially low at birth but rapidly rises in the postnatal period. The excretion of bradykinin in fetal urine also correlates with a rise in renal blood flow. In the adult, the intrarenal kinins apparently act in a paracrine fashion and influence renal hemodynamics, along with sodium and water excretion in the kidney. In the developing rat kidney, kallikrein immunoreactivity is localized to the intracortical nephrons within the distal tubules [58]. The kallikrein expression follows a central fugal pattern of nephron maturation. This finding suggests that the kinins may contribute to a preferential distribution of blood flow toward the inner cortex during early development. Findings in fetal sheep as well as in rats and humans all support the apparent increase in activity of the kallikrein system after birth [58–60].

2.2.4.3 Nitric Oxide

The overall relevance of nitric oxide and its role in different kidney function have not been fully elucidated [61–64]. Certainly, it appears that nitric oxide is involved in vasodilation and the regulation of proximal reabsorption of fluid, salt, and phosphorus; however, its underlying specific functions and role under basal conditions are still unclear [65]. Nitric oxide definitely plays a role in regulating the renal vascular endothelium during development [61, 62]. Nitric oxide does play an extensive role in normal renal function; whereby, when nitric oxide is inhibited in the third trimester of fetal sheep, there is an increase in renal vascular resistance, a decrease in GFR, and a decline in urinary excretion of sodium [61].

2.2.4.4 Atrial Natriuretic Factor (ANF)

Atrial natriuretic factor (ANF) has potent diuretic, natriuretic, and vasodilatory effects. ANF is secreted by cardiac myocytes and can increase GFR, inhibit renin and aldosterone release, as well as relax and increase vascular permeability [66–69]. Evidence further suggests that ANF plays a role in the physiologic adaptation of the fetus and neonate to a changing fluid environment via regulation of blood pressure, fluid volume, and natriuresis [70]. Plasma ANF concentrations in the human are elevated in the first days of life and decrease as maturation progresses, suggestive of a primary role in the natriuresis and diuresis that occur postnatally [70]. After this initial diuresis, the neonate develops a stage of positive sodium balance, which is required for proper somatic growth.

Various stimuli have been observed to increase ANF levels in the fetus. Circulating ANF levels are detectable by mid-gestation in fetal sheep and are normally greater in fetal versus maternal circulation [46, 67, 71–74]. Additionally, preterm infants have been noted to have higher ANF levels than full-term neonates [66]. Certain stimuli are known to increase fetal plasma ANF levels, including acute volume expansion and blood transfusion in the human fetus [70]. The renal effects of infused ANF are blunted in the fetus compared with the adult.

Overall, the effects of ANF in the fetus are similar to those in the adult in that ANF decreases arterial pressure and blood volume in both [75]. There is also an increase in fetal urinary flow and electrolyte excretion, as well as a notable vasodilation in the renal splanchnic bed [46, 66, 75–77]. The effects of ANF in the renal vasculature in the fetus appeared to be mediated by high-affinity binding sites for a membrane-bound guanylate cyclase with subsequent increased production of cyclic guanosine 3′, 5′-monophosphate [78]. ANF not only binds guanylate cyclase receptor, but it also binds to an even greater number of receptors that are not coupled to the guanylate cyclase system. These have been classified as clearance receptors and are believed to contribute to the regulation of plasma ANF by removal of this hormone from the plasma [70].

2.2.4.5 Endothelin

Endothelin is a potent vasoconstrictor active within the fetal circulation. There are three known indigenous isoforms of endothelin in humans, designated ETI to ETIII [79]. The actions of these isoforms are mediated by two known-receptor subtypes, ETA and ETB. In humans, ETA receptors are present mainly on vascular smooth muscle cells and are chiefly responsible for muscle contraction. Endothelin infusions in adults increase blood pressure and decrease cardiac output. In addition to these phenomena, endothelin stimulation may enhance the release of nitric oxide and/or prostaglandins [79].

In addition to its vasoconstrictor effects, endothelin is known to increase fetal blood pressure and may induce hypoxemia and acidemia consistent with noted effects on the umbilical blood vessels [80]. Endothelin has been found in maternal blood, amniotic fluid, and fetal circulation [81–84]. In contrast to adults, endothelin increases urinary flow rates and urinary electrolyte excretion in the fetus [80, 85]. This finding suggests that fetal endothelin has minimal vasoconstrictive effects on renal afferent arterioles, in contrast to its known hemodynamic effects on the adult [85]. Once again, there may be a blunted effect in the fetus overall [79].

2.3 Glomerular and Tubular Function In Utero

The maturation of GFR during fetal life is a result of the combination of all the events that occur during the change from fetal to extrauterine life. Many of the potential stressors that the neonate faces during adaptation to extrauterine life can have a detrimental effect on renal output [86]. Certainly, neonatal adversity (such as hypoxemia) may change the overall renal status and alter the transition to extrauterine life. In general, multiple factors oppose and promote filtration in tandem, including changes in renal vascular resistance, increasing nephron mass, and modification of the forces involved in the process of ultrafiltration with subsequent development of concentration gradients through proper sodium and urea deposition. There is a gradual increase in GFR in the first week of life [71, 87, 88]. The rapidity of the GFR rise is indicative of a functional rather than a morphologic change occurring within the kidney. Current opinion is that there is enhanced glomerular perfusion, resulting in the recruitment of the more superficial cortical nephrons that make up the nephron masses [25, 26]. To complicate matters, the fetus is exposed to various medications in the clinical environment that can be inhibit or alter the vasoactive forces at work in the subsequent development of GFR.

The adaptation of the fetus to the postnatal environment requires a preprogrammed change in the GFR of the kidneys. The GFR is known to be low during fetal life due to placental maintenance of fluid and electrolyte balance and clearance of metabolic wastes; thus, GFR is low, but it increases progressively with gestational age [89–92]. The GFR, especially in preterm neonates, is as low as one-third to one-fourth of values in the neonatal period [89–92]. Glomerular filtration rate values depend on gestational age, with a direct correlation between the GFR and the gestational age of newborn infants delivered between 27 and 43 weeks' gestation [93, 94]. After the 1st month of life, GFR increases progressively and reaches adult levels between 1 and 2 years of life.

Although the sequence of development of renal tubules is becoming better understood, the sentinel events that allow differentiation and specification of the proximal versus the other portions of the tubules remain elusive. The role of the kidney in fluid and electrolyte homeostasis is especially dependent on tubular maturation. In utero, the placenta assumes the task of fetal fluid and electrolyte balance while renal tubules mature. Prior to 20 weeks' gestation, fetal urine is nearly isotonic with plasma due to immature tubular function and during later increasing gestation fetal urine becomes increasingly hypotonic [95].

2.3.1 Factors Influencing Renal Tubular Function

Although the fetal kidney's hemodynamic status and vasculature are affected by endocrine factors such as AVP, aldosterone, renin, AII, prostaglandins, and ANF, these hormones also have a graded effect on tubular function in the developing fetus.

2.3.1.1 Aldosterone

Aldosterone is a salt-retaining steroid hormone that is produced in the adrenal cortex. It has been demonstrated to cross the placenta easily from the maternal circulation into the fetus [96, 97]. Accordingly, the fetal component of aldosterone accounts for approximately 60 % of the total noted in fetal circulation in guinea pigs and approximately 80 % in fetal sheep [98, 99]. Additionally, there is a correlation between fetal plasma aldosterone levels and both plasma renin activity and potassium level. Renal aldosterone levels also correlate with the ratio of urinary sodium to urinary potassium; the ratio decreases during fetal maturation as the plasma aldosterone level rises [100]. The responsiveness of the fetus to aldosterone occurs in the same order of magnitude as it does in the adult and is also known to decrease plasma renin activity [101–103]. Some evidence suggests that aldosterone-mediated tubular sodium reabsorption and potassium secretion are not coupled during development. Contrary to the antinatriuretic effect of aldosterone on the fetal kidney, there is no noted increase in potassium excretion [101]. These findings have also been extended to the newborn animal. Further evidence that the fetal kidney is less responsive to aldosterone infusion is the observation that the fractional excretion of sodium is greater than 1 % during either long-term or short-term aldosterone infusion in the fetus when compared with the adult [104]. At this point, it is unclear whether this is a receptor-mediated effect of aldosterone in the tubules or whether other factors may interfere with aldosterone action on the fetal renal tubule.

2.3.1.2 Renin-Angiotensin System

With respect to its tubular function, the renin-angiotensin system appears to have a similar effect on fetal and adult kidneys. As expected, there is an inverse correlation between plasma renin activity and urinary sodium excretion [105]. Furosemide administration in fetal sheep causes both water and salt loss, stimulates renin release, and promotes a subsequent decrease in sodium reabsorption [106]. The factors that could be responsible for this result include a direct effect of the renin-angiotensin system on the renal tubular sodium absorption and the establishment of tubular feedback mechanisms from the macula densa on reabsorption of sodium in the kidney.

2.3.1.3 Prostaglandins

There may be a role for prostaglandins in modulating fetal and neonatal sodium homeostasis. It is known that urinary excretion of prostaglandins is increased during fetal life and subsequently decreases in the neonatal period [54, 107]. Prostaglandins E2 and I2 are known to be natriuretic in adult animals. As mentioned prior, cyclooxygenase inhibitors such as indomethacin decrease sodium excretion in the adult but are conversely noted to cause increased sodium and chloride loss when administered to fetal sheep, despite a noted decrease in renal blood flow [54]. Because of the complex nature of other vasoactive peptides and hormones activated at the time of fetal development, it is difficult to delineate the specific role of prostaglandins in this process, and further investigation is required.

2.3.1.4 Atrial Natriuretic Factor

It has been demonstrated that the renal responsiveness to ANF changes with advancing fetal age. Toward the end of the third trimester of gestation, the fetal kidney exhibits a minimal or modest natriuretic response to ANF infusion without changes in urine volume or GFR [108]. However, other data suggest that ANF may be involved in regulation of fetal urinary sodium excretion and urinary flow rates. These data also indicate that ANF is involved in the maintenance of arterial pressure in near-term fetal sheep [108]. Younger fetuses in mid-third trimester exhibit greater diuresis and natriuresis in response to ANF infusions, associated with a significant increase in GFR [77, 109]. The seemingly contradictory results may indicate that these responses are not necessarily caused by lower levels of ANF but rather that they may depend on an increased proportion of ANF clearance receptors in older fetuses, thus providing a feedback control mechanism for this renal response [67].

2.3.2 Tubular Regulation of Fluid and Electrolyte Balance

2.3.2.1 Sodium

The fetal excretion of sodium is greater in fetal life than later in either a newborn or an adult. This pattern has also been observed in premature infants, with sodium reabsorption ranging between 85 and 95 %, and increases with gestational age. In the adult, more than 99 % of the filtered sodium load is reabsorbed in the renal tubules, and thus the fractional excretion of sodium is relatively low compared with the fetal and neonatal periods [89–91]. Various factors have been thought to contribute to the high rate of sodium excretion by the immature kidney including the presence of circulating natriuretic factors, the relative insensitivity to tubular reabsorption of sodium, the large extracellular fluid volume, and the relative renal tubular immaturity in the fetus and neonate [100, 110–114]. In addition, mechanisms that are not clearly understood may play a role in a differential sodium reabsorption between a proximal and distal portion of the nephron [115], and, for example, in the fetal sheep, a significantly greater fraction of filtered sodium load is reabsorbed in the distal portion of the nephron than the proximal portion; this is the opposite of that which occurs in the adult kidney (Fig. 2.3).

As the renal tubular cells differentiate into their respective portions of the nephron, associated maturation and obligatory changes occur in the function and abundance of many membrane proteins responsible for ion transport and nutrients transport in the nephron. The obligatory changes are based on the requirements of that particular portion of the tubule. Although it may have less of an impact in the fetus, the proximal tubule still retains the ability to absorb the greatest amount of sodium in the fetus and neonate. The sodium/hydrogen exchanger (NHE) likely plays the most important regulatory role in this process by mediating the electroneutral exchange of one

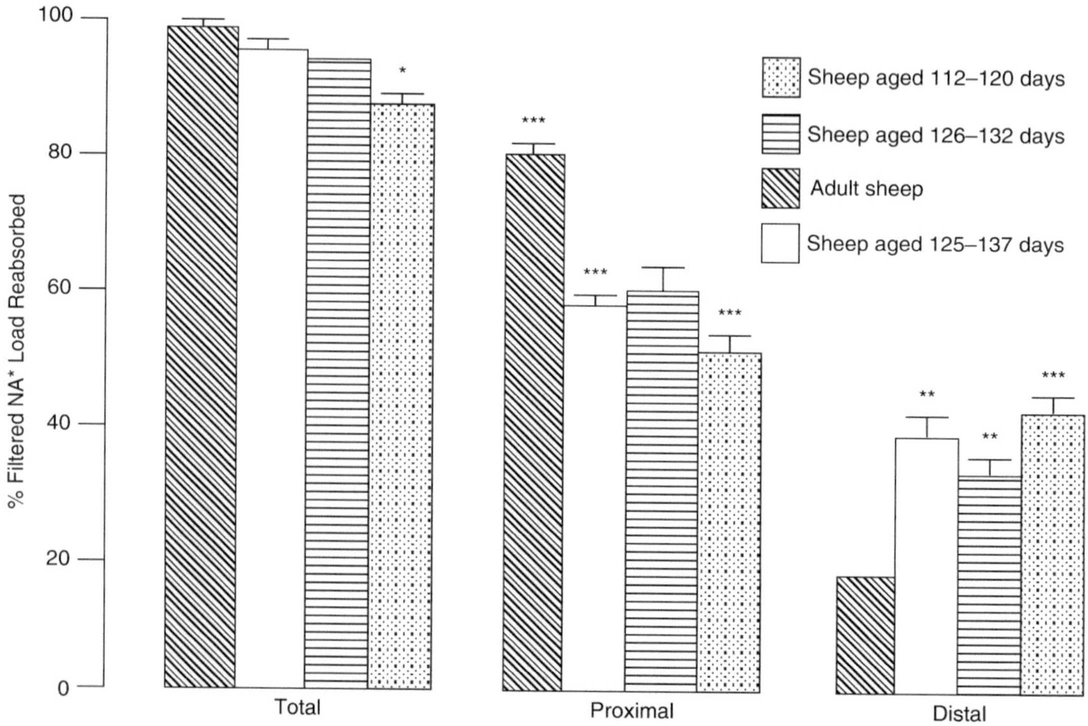

Fig. 2.3 Total fractional sodium reabsorption (Total) and fractional reabsorption of sodium by the proximal tubules (Proximal) and by the distal tubules (Distal) of fetal sheep aged 112–120 days ▒ and 126–132 days ☰ and adult sheep ▧ in which proximal tubular sodium reabsorption was determined from the fractional reabsorption of lithium and a group of fetal sheep aged 125–137 days □ in which it was measured by blocking distal tubular sodium reabsorption with ethacrynic acid and amiloride. *$p<0.05$; **$p<0.01$; ***$p<0.001$, fetal compared with adult values (From Lumbers et al. [115]. © 2008 Canadian Science Publishing or its licensors. Reproduced with permission)

sodium for one hydrogen, and thereby playing a role in the acidification of urine [116]. At least four different isoforms (NHE1-4) have been isolated [117–119]. NHE3 is thought to be the isoform present at the apical (luminal) membrane in the kidney and is therefore likely responsible for the bulk of transepithelial sodium reabsorption. NHE1 has been localized along the lateral plasma membrane of multiple nephron segments and does not appear to contribute to the transepithelial sodium transport [119]. The function of this particular transporter seems to be more consistent with cell volume regulation, growth, and pH defense [120]. NHE4 is mainly found in the collecting tubules of the kidney, suggesting that it may play a specialized role in rectifying cell volume in response to extreme osmotic fluctuations that occur in this area of the kidney [121].

The interdependence of various sodium channels has become partially clarified with the understanding of how NHE transporters may affect the sodium, potassium-adenosine triphosphatase (Na+,K+-ATPase) channels. These enzymes are responsible for active sodium transport in eukaryotic cells. In the mature kidney, they are located in the basolateral membrane of renal tubular cells. The interdependence of Na+,K+-ATPase and NHE channels may be related to the increase in sodium filtrate associated with renal maturation. The increase in sodium filtrate may be an important factor in influencing the postnatal rise in Na+,K+-ATPase activity. Studies in rats have demonstrated that an increase or decrease in NHE activity can stimulate or inhibit Na+,K+-ATPase activity, respectively [122].

2.3.2.2 Potassium

Potassium secretion by the kidney is low early in gestation and increases toward term, leading toward a positive potassium balance in the fetus [115]. Data suggest that the secretory pathways for potassium appear to mature during late fetal life [100, 105, 111]. In general, it appears that potassium balance in the fetus is impacted by capability for tubular reabsorption, secretion after filtration across the glomerular membrane, and relative fetal parathyroid insufficiency. It has been thought that the increase in potassium secretion as the fetus approaches term results from a larger tubular surface area available for potassium secretion. In addition, there may also be a contribution from an increase in Na+,K+-ATPase activity or an increase in the sensitivity of fetal nephron to aldosterone that enhances potassium excretion [100, 105, 111]. Furthermore, as urinary flow increases through the fetal kidneys, an increased gradient may allow for removal of more potassium in the urine. As such, from a clinical standpoint, it is not uncommon to have high potassium levels in the immediate neonatal period, especially in preterm infants.

Glucose

Interest in the effect of maternal hypoglycemia on multiple organ systems has grown substantially since the early 1990s. In general, the reabsorption capacity for glucose is quite high in the fetus as demonstrated with work done in guinea pigs, fetal sheep, and newborn puppies [123–125]. In fetal sheep, compared with adult sheep, investigators noted that the corrected maximal tubule excretory capacity of the kidneys for glucose is greater in the fetus than in adult sheep. This is also true on the renal plasma threshold for glucose, which is greater during fetal life and increases with gestational age [124]. The sodium-dependent glucose transport system in fetal rabbit proximal tubules, late in gestation, is stereospecific, electrogenic, cation specific, and pH sensitive [126].

2.3.2.3 Acid–Base Homeostasis

The ability for the fetal and neonatal kidney to handle organic acids and bases is limited. Secretion of the organic acid *p*-aminohippurate is quite low in both fetal and neonatal periods [127, 128]. There is some evidence to suggest that the fetal kidney can secrete organic bases but to a significantly lesser degree than adults. It is thought that these findings reflect immature tubular secretory pathways present during development. These phenomena may also be explained by the finding that the juxtamedullary circulation shunts blood through the vasa recta, thereby decreasing the peritubular circulation perfusing the secretory cells. As the kidney matures, blood flow changes and allows for improved secretory capability of the kidney itself.

Without the presence of an appropriately functioning kidney in the adult, acid-base balance is unattainable. The kidney itself is responsible for reabsorption of the entire filtered bicarbonate load in proximal portions of the nephron and is also responsible for secretion of hydrogen ions and the generation of new bicarbonate through the urinary buffering systems of titratable acid and ammonium. Without the presence of these homeostatic mechanisms, the other metabolic processes of life, including growth and development are severely restricted. Urinary pH is always less than the plasma titratable acid and ammonium associated with the rise in acid excretion [92, 129]. It has been demonstrated that 80–100 % of filtered bicarbonate load is reabsorbed by the fetal sheep [92, 130, 131]. This bicarbonate absorption provides the driving force for chloride reabsorption in the mature proximal tubule and also requires the presence of adequate carbonic anhydrase activity in these same segments. Both bicarbonate and chloride reabsorption have been noted to increase with age in the ovine fetus. This finding may reflect increasing carbonic anhydrase activity, because inhibition with acetazolamide produces significant increase in bicarbonate excretion and also an increase in urinary pH [130]. Corroborating this hypothesis is the observation that carbonic anhydrase is present in human fetal kidney in the late gestational phase [132]. Although there is a blunted renal response in the fetus to metabolic acidosis compared with the adult, the qualitative response of increased hydrogen ion excretion is similar to that found in the adult animal [133, 134]. In the presence of fetal hyperglycemia, the resulting metabolic acidosis has not been noted to cause a change in the excretion rate of urinary buffers or urinary pH in the fetus, a finding suggesting that the placental regulation of fetal acid–base balance is sufficient and contributes a portion of the buffering capabilities and capacity required by the fetus [135].

2.3.2.4 Phosphate

Fetal plasma is noted to contain a greater concentration of inorganic phosphate when compared with maternal plasma. This is inversely related to gestational age. The importance of phosphorus to the fetus is validated by the observation that it is transported across the placenta from the mother to the fetus against a concentration gradient [136]. There appears to be a unique sodium-phosphorus cotransporter in kidneys of growing animals that differs from the sodium-inorganic phosphorus-2 transporter, which is known to be modulated by dietary phosphorus intake. This cotransporter is thought to contribute to the high rate of renal phosphorus reabsorption during renal development [137]. In fetal sheep, between 60 and 100 % of phosphorus is reabsorbed; the concentration of inorganic phosphorus in fetal urine is quite low [131]. The fetal kidney responds to parathyroid hormone with an increase of urinary excretion of calcium and cyclic adenosine monophosphate [138]. There is a blunted and limited effect of parathyroid hormone on the urinary excretion rate of phosphorus during fetal life. Thus, hyperphosphatemia may result in the presence of relative parathyroid insufficiency during fetal life and may compound the already low fetal renal clearance of phosphorus.

2.3.3 Concentration Capacity in the Developing Kidney

During the last trimester of gestation, the fetal sheep has a urinary flow rate of approximately 1,500 mL/day or urine, which is 0.5–1 mL/min [27, 90, 139, 140]. The urinary flow rate in human fetuses increases ten-fold from 0.1 mL/min at 20 weeks to 1 mL/min at 40 weeks with a subsequent reduction to 0.1 mL/min in the neonate [141].

Fetal urine is usually hypotonic with respect to fetal plasma due to a variety of factors including low collecting duct sensitivity to AVP, structural immaturity of the loop of Henle, as well as an immature concentration gradient in the fetal renal medulla due to limited protein intake (i.e., a urea deficit). The range of osmolality is 100–250 mOsm/kg H_2O. However, the fetal kidney can adapt to its environment. The fetal kidney is able to produce diluted or concentrated urine, depending on the state of hydration of the mother as well as the fetus. One sees a fall in urinary flow rate and a decrease in free water clearance when mannitol is administered to pregnant ewes or when the mother has been deprived of water [142–145]. Direct infusion of AVP into the fetus also appears to cause a decrease in fetal free water clearance [146, 147]. Free water clearance has been directly correlated with the transfer of fluid across the placenta. Therefore, decreases in net fluid transfer across the placenta from the mother to the fetus result in decreased fetal urine production and may account for increased osmolality and decreased urine flow in utero in response to fetal stress [148, 149]. Although this may partially explain the decrease in urine flow rates in conditions of stress, other neuroendocrine pathways may also play a role. The kidney is not able to concentrate urine to adult levels until well after birth. Various factors are thought to contribute to the inability of the fetal kidney to concentrate urine [150]. A decrease in sensitivity of the collecting ducts to the circulating AVP appears to be one such factor. Thus, the actions of vasopressin are hindered, and the fetus has an obligatory water loss. There are also limitations in the movement of urea and the reabsorption of sodium and chloride along the ascending limb of Henle, owing to structural immaturity and a preferential distribution of blood flow through the inner cortex. These factors result in a high flow through the vasa recta and prevent generation of a medullary concentration gradient. In addition, the fetus, generally speaking, has not had a sufficiently high protein intake to generate significant amounts of urea for the initial production of a concentration gradient in the medulla. Although the fetal kidney has a decreased ability to concentrate urine (because of what appears to be decreased responsiveness to AVP), the fetus has the ability to synthesize and/or secrete AVP [151]. Both synthesis and secretion of AVP occur during the last trimester of gestation [151]. In fetal sheep during the last trimester of gestation, both the volume and osmolality receptors controls for AVP secretion are fully functional [152]. In fact, AVP levels increase in fetal circulation after hemorrhage, hypoxemia, diuretic administration, or osmotic stimulus. An AVP challenge administered to fetal animals demonstrates the increased sensitivity to AVP when compared with the adult nephron [97, 153, 154]. Under these conditions, the urinary osmolality is approximately one-third of what an adult animal would obtain for the same plasma AVP concentration [29]. Previous studies have demonstrated that when the V2 receptor for AVP is activated, fetal water reabsorption can increase early in gestation [155]. Expression and activation of collecting duct-specific water channels influences the ability of the active V2 receptor to increase water reabsorption. Membrane water channels called aquaporins (AQP) are also important in renal water absorption. Within the kidney, AQP-2, the collecting duct AQP, has been demonstrated to be the AVP-regulated water channel [156, 157]. This channel has been localized to the apical membrane of collecting duct cells, and its expression is regulated directly by the V2 receptor [158]. AQP-2 is expressed in the medulla of the rat embryo as early as day 18, and by the time of birth, the overall distribution of AQP-2 in the newborn kidney is similar to that observed in the adult kidney [159]. These data provide support for studies that have demonstrated a role for AVP in the regulation of water balance in the fetus.

References

1. Kumar KU, Pillay VV (1996) Estimation of fetal age by histological study of kidney. Med Sci Law 36(3):226–230
2. Igarashi P (1994) Transcription factors and apoptosis in kidney development. Curr Opin Nephrol Hypertens 3(3):308–317
3. Dressler GR (2002) Development of the excretory system. In: Rossant J, Patrick T (eds) Mouse development, patterning, morphogenesis, and organogenesis. Academic, New York, pp 395–420
4. Bouchard M, Souabni A, Mandler M, Neubuser A, Busslinger M (2002) Nephric lineage specification by Pax2 and Pax8. Genes Dev 16(22):2958–2970
5. Dressler GR (2006) The cellular basis of kidney development. Annu Rev Cell Dev Biol 22:509–529
6. Costantini F, Shakya R (2006) GDNF/Ret signaling and the development of the kidney. Bioessays 28(2):117–127
7. Brophy PD, Ostrom L, Lang KM, Dressler GR (2001) Regulation of ureteric bud outgrowth by Pax2-dependent activation of the glial derived neurotrophic factor gene. Development 128(23):4747–4756
8. Dressler GR, Douglass EC (1992) Pax-2 is a DNA-binding protein expressed in embryonic kidney and Wilms tumor. Proc Natl Acad Sci U S A 89(4):1179–1183
9. Dressler GR, Wilkinson JE, Rothenpieler UW, Patterson LT, Williams-Simons L, Westphal H (1993) Deregulation of Pax-2 expression in transgenic mice generates severe kidney abnormalities. Nature 362(6415):65–67
10. Kreidberg JA, Sariola H, Loring JM et al (1993) WT-1 is required for early kidney development. Cell 74(4):679–691
11. Rauscher FJ 3rd (1993) The WT1 Wilms tumor gene product: a developmentally regulated transcription factor in the kidney that functions as a tumor suppressor. FASEB J 7(10):896–903
12. Mugrauer G, Ekblom P (1991) Contrasting expression patterns of three members of the myc family of protooncogenes in the developing and adult mouse kidney. J Cell Biol 112(1):13–25
13. Mugrauer G, Alt FW, Ekblom P (1988) N-myc protooncogene expression during organogenesis in the developing mouse as revealed by in situ hybridization. J Cell Biol 107(4):1325–1335
14. Trudel M, D'Agati V, Costantini F (1991) C-myc as an inducer of polycystic kidney disease in transgenic mice. Kidney Int 39(4):665–671
15. Bacallao R, Fine LG (1989) Molecular events in the organization of renal tubular epithelium: from nephrogenesis to regeneration. Am J Physiol 257(6 Pt 2):F913–F924
16. Hammerman MR, Rogers SA, Ryan G (1992) Growth factors and metanephrogenesis. Am J Physiol 262(4 Pt 2):F523–F532
17. Toback FG, Walsh-Reitz MM, Mendley SR, Kartha S (1990) Kidney epithelial cells release growth factors in response to extracellular signals. Pediatr Nephrol 4(4):363–371
18. Avner ED, Sweeney WE Jr (1990) Polypeptide growth factors in metanephric growth and segmental nephron differentiation. Pediatr Nephrol 4(4):372–377
19. Sariola H, Ekblom P, Lehtonen E, Saxen L (1983) Differentiation and vascularization of the metanephric kidney grafted on the chorioallantoic membrane. Dev Biol 96(2):427–435

20. Sariola H, Saarma M, Sainio K et al (1991) Dependence of kidney morphogenesis on the expression of nerve growth factor receptor. Science 254(5031):571–573
21. Rogers SA, Ryan G, Hammerman MR (1992) Metanephric transforming growth factor-alpha is required for renal organogenesis in vitro. Am J Physiol 262(4 Pt 2):F533–F539
22. Alpers CE, Seifert RA, Hudkins KL, Johnson RJ, Bowen-Pope DF (1992) Developmental patterns of PDGF B-chain, PDGF-receptor, and alpha-actin expression in human glomerulogenesis. Kidney Int 42(2):390–399
23. Rudolph AM, Heymann MA (1973) Control of the fetal circulation. In: Hafez ES (ed) The mammalian fetus: comparative biology and methodology. Charles C Thomas, Springfield, pp 5–19
24. Paton JB, Fisher DE, Peterson EN, DeLannoy CW, Behrman RE (1973) Cardiac output and organ blood flows in the baboon fetus. Biology Neonat 22(1):50–57
25. Aperia A, Broberger O, Herin P, Joelsson I (1977) Renal hemodynamics in the perinatal period. A study in lambs. Acta Physiol Scand 99(3):261–269
26. Robillard JE, Weismann DN, Herin P (1981) Ontogeny of single glomerular perfusion rate in fetal and newborn lambs. Pediatr Res 15(9):1248–1255
27. Gruskin AB, Edelmann CM Jr, Yuan S (1970) Maturational changes in renal blood flow in piglets. Pediatr Res 4(1):7–13
28. Jose PA, Logan AG, Slotkoff LM, Lilienfield LS, Calcagno PL, Eisner GM (1971) Intrarenal blood flow distribution in canine puppies. Pediatr Res 5(8):335–344
29. Robillard JE, Weitzman RE (1980) Developmental aspects of the fetal renal response to exogenous arginine vasopressin. Am J Physiol 238(5):F407–F414
30. Robillard JE, Segar JL, Smith FG, Jose PA (1992) Regulation of sodium metabolism and extracellular fluid volume during development. Clin Perinatol 19(1):15–31
31. Ingelfinger JR, Woods LL (2002) Perinatal programming, renal development, and adult renal function. Am J Hypertens 15(2 Pt 2):46S–49S
32. Broughton Pipkin F, Kirkpatrick SM, Lumbers ER, Mott JC (1974) Renin and angiotensin-like levels in foetal, new-born and adult sheep. J Physiol 241(3):575–588
33. Broughton Pipkin F, Lumbers ER, Mott JC (1974) Factors influencing plasma renin and angiotensin II in the conscious pregnant ewe and its foetus. J Physiol 243(3):619–636
34. Smith FG Jr, Lupu AN, Barajas L, Bauer R, Bashore RA (1974) The renin-angiotensin system in the fetal lamb. Pediatr Res 8(6):611–620
35. Stevens AD, Lumbers ER (1986) Effect on maternal and fetal renal function and plasma renin activity of a high salt intake by the ewe. J Dev Physiol 8(4): 267–275
36. Robillard JE, Gomez RA, VanOrden D, Smith FG Jr (1982) Comparison of the adrenal and renal responses to angiotensin II fetal lambs and adult sheep. Circ Res 50(1):140–147
37. Stevenson KM, Gibson KJ, Lumbers ER (1996) Effects of losartan on the cardiovascular system, renal haemodynamics and function and lung liquid flow in fetal sheep. Clin Exp Pharmacol Physiol 23(2): 125–133
38. Daikha-Dahmane F, Levy-Beff E, Jugie M, Lenclen R (2006) Foetal kidney maldevelopment in maternal use of angiotensin II type I receptor antagonists. Pediatr Nephrol 21(5):729–732
39. Woods LL, Ingelfinger JR, Nyengaard JR, Rasch R (2001) Maternal protein restriction suppresses the newborn renin-angiotensin system and programs adult hypertension in rats. Pediatr Res 49(4):460–467
40. Pryde PG, Sedman AB, Nugent CE, Barr M Jr (1993) Angiotensin-converting enzyme inhibitor fetopathy. J Am Soc Nephrol 3(9):1575–1582
41. Rosa FW, Bosco LA, Graham CF, Milstien JB, Dreis M, Creamer J (1989) Neonatal anuria with maternal angiotensin-converting enzyme inhibition. Obstet Gynecol 74(3 Pt 1):371–374
42. Iwamoto HS, Rudolph AM (1981) Role of renin-angiotensin system in response to hemorrhage in fetal sheep. Am J Physiol 240(6):H848–H854
43. Gomez RA, Meernik JG, Kuehl WD, Robillard JE (1984) Developmental aspects of the renal response to hemorrhage during fetal life. Pediatr Res 18(1):40–46
44. Robillard JE, Weitzman RE, Fisher DA, Smith FG Jr (1979) The dynamics of vasopressin release and blood volume regulation during fetal hemorrhage in the lamb fetus. Pediatr Res 13(5 Pt 1):606–610
45. Brace RA, Cheung CY (1986) Fetal cardiovascular and endocrine responses to prolonged fetal hemorrhage. Am J Physiol 251(2 Pt 2):R417–R424
46. Robillard JE, Nakamura KT, Varille VA, Andresen AA, Matherne GP, VanOrden DE (1988) Ontogeny of the renal response to natriuretic peptide in sheep. Am J Physiol 254(5 Pt 2):F634–F641
47. Robillard JE, Nakamura KT, DiBona GF (1986) Effects of renal denervation on renal responses to hypoxemia in fetal lambs. Am J Physiol 250(2 Pt 2):F294–F301
48. Robillard JE, Nakamura KT, Wilkin MK, McWeeny OJ, DiBona GF (1987) Ontogeny of renal hemodynamic response to renal nerve stimulation in sheep. Am J Physiol 252(4 Pt 2):F605–F612
49. Guillery EN, Karniski LP, Mathews MS, Robillard JE (1994) Maturation of proximal tubule Na+/H+ antiporter activity in sheep during transition from fetus to newborn. Am J Physiol 267(4 Pt 2):F537–F545
50. Matherne GP, Nakamura KT, Robillard JE (1988) Ontogeny of alpha-adrenoceptor responses in renal vascular bed of sheep. Am J Physiol 254(2 Pt 2):R277–R283
51. Buckley NM, Brazeau P, Gootman PM, Frasier ID (1979) Renal circulatory effects of adrenergic stimuli in anesthetized piglets and mature swine. Am J Physiol 237(6):H690–H695

52. Pace-Asciak CR (1977) Prostaglandin biosynthesis and catabolism in the developing fetal sheep kidney. Prostaglandins 13(4):661–668
53. Terragno NA, Terragno A, Early JA, Roberts MA, McGiff JC (1978) Endogenous prostaglandin synthesis inhibitor in the renal cortex. Effects on production of prostacyclin by renal blood vessels. Clin Sci Mol Med Suppl 4:199s–202s
54. Matson JR, Stokes JB, Robillard JE (1981) Effects of inhibition of prostaglandin synthesis on fetal renal function. Kidney Int 20(5):621–627
55. Kirshon B, Mari G, Moise KJ Jr (1990) Indomethacin therapy in the treatment of symptomatic polyhydramnios. Obstet Gynecol 75(2):202–205
56. Hendricks SK, Smith JR, Moore DE, Brown ZA (1990) Oligohydramnios associated with prostaglandin synthetase inhibitors in preterm labour. Br J Obstet Gynaecol 97(4):312–316
57. Seyberth HW, Rascher W, Hackenthal R, Wille L (1983) Effect of prolonged indomethacin therapy on renal function and selected vasoactive hormones in very-low-birth-weight infants with symptomatic patent ductus arteriosus. J Pediatr 103(6):979–984
58. el-Dahr SS, Yosipiv I (1993) Developmentally regulated kallikrein enzymatic activity and gene transcription rate in maturing rat kidneys. Am J Physiol 265(1 Pt 2):F146–F150
59. Robillard JE, Lawton WJ, Weismann DN, Sessions C (1982) Developmental aspects of the renal kallikrein-like activity in fetal and newborn lambs. Kidney Int 22(6):594–601
60. Vio CP, Olavarria F, Krause S, Herrmann F, Grob K (1987) Kallikrein excretion: relationship with maturation and renal function in human neonates at different gestational ages. Biol Neonat 52(3):121–126
61. Bogaert GA, Kogan BA, Mevorach RA (1993) Effects of endothelium-derived nitric oxide on renal hemodynamics and function in the sheep fetus. Pediatr Res 34(6):755–761
62. Solhaug MJ, Wallace MR, Granger JP (1993) Endothelium-derived nitric oxide modulates renal hemodynamics in the developing piglet. Pediatr Res 34(6):750–754
63. Furchgott RF, Zawadzki JV (1980) The obligatory role of endothelial cells in the relaxation of arterial smooth muscle by acetylcholine. Nature 288(5789):373–376
64. Bastron RD, Kaloyanides GJ (1972) Effect of sodium nitroprusside on function in the isolated and intact dog kidney. J Pharmacol Exp Ther 181(2):244–249
65. Persson PB (2002) Nitric oxide in the kidney. Am J Physiol Regul Integr Comp Physiol 283(5):R1005–R1007
66. Cheung CY (1991) Role of endogenous atrial natriuretic factor in the regulation of fetal cardiovascular and renal function. Am J Obstet Gynecol 165(5 Pt 1):1558–1567
67. Dodd A, Kullama LK, Ervin MG, Leake RD, Ross MG (1994) Ontogeny of ovine fetal renal atrial natriuretic factor receptors. Life Sci 54(15):1101–1107
68. Cheung CY, Roberts VJ (1993) Developmental changes in atrial natriuretic factor content and localization of its messenger ribonucleic acid in ovine fetal heart. Am J Obstet Gynecol 169(5):1345–1351
69. Kikuchi K, Nakao K, Hayashi K et al (1987) Ontogeny of atrial natriuretic polypeptide in the human heart. Acta Endocrinol 115(2):211–217
70. Walsh P (2002) Hormonal control of renal function during development. In: Walsh P (ed) Campbell's textbook of urology. Elsevier Science, Philadelphia, pp 1772–1774
71. Smith FG, Lumbers ER (1989) Comparison of renal function in term fetal sheep and newborn lambs. Biol Neonat 55(4–5):309–316
72. Cheung CY, Gibbs DM, Brace RA (1987) Atrial natriuretic factor in maternal and fetal sheep. Am J Physiol 252(2 Pt 1):E279–E282
73. Ervin MG, Ross MG, Castro R et al (1988) Ovine fetal and adult atrial natriuretic factor metabolism. Am J Physiol 254(1 Pt 2):R40–R46
74. Tulassay T, Rascher W, Seyberth HW, Lang RE, Toth M, Sulyok E (1986) Role of atrial natriuretic peptide in sodium homeostasis in premature infants. J Pediatr 109(6):1023–1027
75. Brace RA, Cheung CY (1987) Cardiovascular and fluid responses to atrial natriuretic factor in sheep fetus. Am J Physiol 253(4 Pt 2):R561–R567
76. Varille VA, Nakamura KT, McWeeny OJ, Matherne GP, Smith FG, Robillard JE (1989) Renal hemodynamic response to atrial natriuretic factor in fetal and newborn sheep. Pediatr Res 25(3):291–294
77. Shine P, McDougall JG, Towstoless MK, Wintour EM (1987) Action of atrial natriuretic peptide in the immature ovine kidney. Pediatr Res 22(1):11–15
78. Fujino Y, Ross MG, Ervin MG, Castro R, Leake RD, Fisher DA (1992) Ovine maternal and fetal glomerular atrial natriuretic factor receptors: response to dehydration. Biol Neonat 62(2–3):120–126
79. Davenport AP, Battistini B (2002) Classification of endothelin receptors and antagonists in clinical development. Clin Sci (Lond) 103(Suppl 48):1S–3S
80. Cheung CY (1994) Regulation of atrial natriuretic factor release by endothelin in ovine fetuses. Am J Physiol 267(2 Pt 2):R380–R386
81. Usuki S, Saitoh T, Sawamura T et al (1990) Increased maternal plasma concentration of endothelin-1 during labor pain or on delivery and the existence of a large amount of endothelin-1 in amniotic fluid. Gynecol Endocrinol 4(2):85–97
82. Nisell H, Hemsen A, Lunell NO, Wolff K, Lundberg MJ (1990) Maternal and fetal levels of a novel polypeptide, endothelin: evidence for release during pregnancy and delivery. Gynecol Obstet Invest 30(3):129–132
83. Nakamura T, Kasai K, Konuma S et al (1990) Immunoreactive endothelin concentrations in maternal and fetal blood. Life Sci 46(15):1045–1050

84. Haegerstrand A, Hemsen A, Gillis C, Larsson O, Lundberg JM (1989) Endothelin: presence in human umbilical vessels, high levels in fetal blood and potent constrictor effect. Acta Physiol Scand 137(4):541–542
85. Han SP, Trapani AJ, Fok KF, Westfall TC, Knuepfer MM (1989) Effects of endothelin on regional hemodynamics in conscious rats. Eur J Pharmacol 159(3):303–305
86. Toth-Heyn P, Drukker A, Guignard JP (2000) The stressed neonatal kidney: from pathophysiology to clinical management of neonatal vasomotor nephropathy. Pediatr Nephrol 14(3):227–239
87. Nakamura KT, Matherne GP, McWeeny OJ, Smith BA, Robillard JE (1987) Renal hemodynamics and functional changes during the transition from fetal to newborn life in sheep. Pediatr Res 21(3):229–234
88. Smith FG, Lumbers ER (1988) Changes in renal function following delivery of the lamb by caesarean section. J Dev Physiol 10(2):145–148
89. Rankin JH, Gresham EL, Battaglia FC, Makowski EL, Meschia G (1972) Measurement of fetal renal inulin clearance in a chronic sheep preparation. J Appl Physiol 32(1):129–133
90. Robillard JE, Sessions C, Kennedey RL, Hamel-Robillard L, Smith FG Jr (1977) Interrelationship between glomerular filtration rate and renal transport of sodium and chloride during fetal life. Am J Obstet Gynecol 128(7):727–734
91. Robillard JE, Kulvinskas C, Sessions C, Burmeister L, Smith FG Jr (1975) Maturational changes in the fetal glomerular filtration rate. Am J Obstet Gynecol 122(5):601–606
92. Kesby GJ, Lumbers ER (1986) Factors affecting renal handling of sodium, hydrogen ions, and bicarbonate by the fetus. Am J Physiol 251(2 Pt 2):F226–F231
93. Leake RD, Trygstad CW, Oh W (1976) Inulin clearance in the newborn infant: relationship to gestational and postnatal age. Pediatr Res 10(8):759–762
94. Guignard JP, Torrado A, Da Cunha O, Gautier E (1975) Glomerular filtration rate in the first three weeks of life. J Pediatr 87(2):268–272
95. Nicolini U, Spelzini F (2001) Invasive assessment of fetal renal abnormalities: urinalysis, fetal blood sampling and biopsy. Prenat Diagn 21(11):964–969
96. Bayard F, Ances IG, Tapper AJ, Weldon VV, Kowarski A, Migeon CJ (1970) Transplacental passage and fetal secretion of aldosterone. J Clin Invest 49(7):1389–1393
97. Siegel SR, Leake RD, Weitzman RE, Fisher DA (1980) Effects of furosemide and acute salt loading on vasopressin and renin secretion in the fetal lamb. Pediatr Res 14(7):869–871
98. Giry J, Delost P (1979) Placental transfer of aldosterone in the guinea-pig during late pregnancy. J Steroid Biochem 10(5):541–547
99. Wintour EM, Coghlan JP, Hardy KJ, Lingwood BE, Rayner M, Scoggins BA (1980) Placental transfer of aldosterone in the sheep. J Endocrinol 86(2):305–310
100. Robillard JE, Ramberg E, Sessions C et al (1980) Role of aldosterone on renal sodium and potassium excretion during fetal life and newborn period. Dev Pharmacol Ther 1(4):201–216
101. Robillard JE, Nakamura KT, Lawton WJ (1985) Effects of aldosterone on urinary kallikrein and sodium excretion during fetal life. Pediatr Res 19(10):1048–1052
102. Lingwood B, Hardy KJ, Coghlan JP, Wintour EM (1978) Effect of aldosterone on urine composition in the chronically cannulated ovine foetus. J Endocrinol 76(3):553–554
103. Ganong WF, Mulrow PJ (1958) Rate of change in sodium and potassium excretion after injection of aldosterone into the aorta and renal artery of the dog. Am J Physiol 195(2):337–342
104. Horisberger JD, Diezi J (1983) Effects of mineralocorticoids on Na+ and K+ excretion in the adrenalectomized rat. Am J Physiol 245(1):F89–F99
105. Stevens AD, Lumbers ER (1981) The relationship between plasma renin activity and renal electrolyte excretion in the fetal sheep. J Dev Physiol 3(2):101–110
106. Lumbers ER, Stevens AD (1987) The effects of frusemide, saralasin and hypotension on fetal plasma renin activity and on fetal renal function. J Physiol 393:479–490
107. Walker DW, Mitchell MD (1978) Prostaglandins in urine of foetal lambs. Nature 271(5641):161–162
108. Brace RA, Bayer LA, Cheung CY (1989) Fetal cardiovascular, endocrine, and fluid responses to atrial natriuretic factor infusion. Am J Physiol 257(3 Pt 2):R580–R587
109. Castro R, Ervin MG, Leake RD, Ross MG, Sherman DJ, Fisher DA (1991) Fetal renal response to atrial natriuretic factor decreases with maturation. Am J Physiol 260(2 Pt 2):R346–R352
110. Kleinman LI (1982) Developmental renal physiology. Physiologist 25(2):104–110
111. Lumbers ER (1984) A brief review of fetal renal function. J Dev Physiol 6(1):1–10
112. Siegel SR, Oh W (1976) Renal function as a marker of human fetal maturation. Acta Paediatr Scand 65(4):481–485
113. Aperia A, Broberger O, Herin P, Zetterstrom R (1979) Sodium excretion in relation to sodium intake and aldosterone excretion in newborn pre-term and full-term infants. Acta Paediatr Scand 68(6):813–817
114. Spitzer A (1982) The role of the kidney in sodium homeostasis during maturation. Kidney Int 21(4):539–545
115. Lumbers ER, Hill KJ, Bennett VJ (1988) Proximal and distal tubular activity in chronically catheterized fetal sheep compared with the adult. Can J Physiol Pharmacol 66(6):697–702
116. Bianchini L, Pouyssegur J (1995) Na+/H+ exchangers: structure, function and regulation. In: Schlondorff D, Bonventre J (eds) Molecular biology of the kidney in health and disease. Marcel Dekker, New York

117. Orlowski J, Lingrel JB (1988) Tissue-specific and developmental regulation of rat Na, K-ATPase catalytic alpha isoform and beta subunit mRNAs. J Biol Chem 263(21):10436–10442
118. Tse CM, Levine SA, Yun CH et al (1993) Cloning and expression of a rabbit cDNA encoding a serum-activated ethylisopropylamiloride-resistant epithelial Na+/H+ exchanger isoform (NHE-2). J Biol Chem 268(16):11917–11924
119. Tse CM, Brant SR, Walker MS, Pouyssegur J, Donowitz M (1992) Cloning and sequencing of a rabbit cDNA encoding an intestinal and kidney-specific Na+/H+ exchanger isoform (NHE-3). J Biol Chem 267(13):9340–9346
120. Sardet C, Franchi A, Pouyssegur J (1989) Molecular cloning, primary structure, and expression of the human growth factor-activatable Na+/H+ antiporter. Cell 56(2):271–280
121. Bookstein C, Musch MW, DePaoli A et al (1994) A unique sodium-hydrogen exchange isoform (NHE-4) of the inner medulla of the rat kidney is induced by hyperosmolarity. J Biol Chem 269(47):29704–29709
122. Larsson SH, Aperia A (1991) Renal growth in infancy and childhood–experimental studies of regulatory mechanisms. Pediatr Nephrol 5(4):439–442
123. Merlet-Benichou C, Pegorier M, Muffat-Joly M, Augeron C (1981) Functional and morphologic patterns of renal maturation in the developing guinea pig. Am J Physiol 241(6):F618–F624
124. Robillard JE, Sessions C, Kennedy RL, Smith FG Jr (1978) Maturation of the glucose transport process by the fetal kidney. Pediatr Res 12(5):680–684
125. Arant BS Jr, Edelmann CM Jr, Nash MA (1974) The renal reabsorption of glucose in the developing canine kidney: a study of glomerulotubular balance. Pediatr Res 8(6):638–646
126. Beck JC, Lipkowitz MS, Abramson RG (1988) Characterization of the fetal glucose transporter in rabbit kidney. Comparison with the adult brush border electrogenic Na+-glucose symporter. J Clin Invest 82(2):379–387
127. Alexander DP, Nixon DA (1962) Plasma clearance of p-aminohippuric acid by the kidneys of foetal, neonatal and adult sheep. Nature 194:483–484
128. Buddingh F, Parker HR, Ishizaki G, Tyler WS (1971) Long-term studies of the functional development of the fetal kidney in sheep. Am J Vet Res 32(12):1993–1998
129. Robillard JE, Sessions C, Burmeister L, Smith FG Jr (1977) Influence of fetal extracellular volume contraction on renal reabsorption of bicarbonate in fetal lambs. Pediatr Res 11(5):649–655
130. Robillard JE, Sessions C, Smith FG Jr (1978) In vivo demonstration of renal carbonic anhydrase activity in the fetal lamb. Biol Neonat 34(5–6):253–258
131. Hill KJ, Lumbers ER (1988) Renal function in adult and fetal sheep. J Dev Physiol 10(2):149–159
132. Lonnerholm G, Wistrand PJ (1983) Carbonic anhydrase in the human fetal kidney. Pediatr Res 17(5):390–397
133. Smith FG Jr, Schwartz A (1970) Response of the intact lamb fetus to acidosis. Am J Obstet Gynecol 106(1):52–58
134. Kesby GJ, Lumbers ER (1988) The effects of metabolic acidosis on renal function of fetal sheep. J Physiol 396:65–74
135. Smith FG, Lumbers ER (1988) Effects of maternal hyperglycemia on fetal renal function in sheep. Am J Physiol 255(1 Pt 2):F11–F14
136. Economou-Mavrou C, Mc CR (1958) Calcium, magnesium and phosphorus in foetal tissues. Biochem J 68(4):573–580
137. Smith FG Jr, Alexander DP, Buckle RM, Britton HG, Nixon DA (1972) Parathyroid hormone in foetal and adult sheep: the effect of hypocalcaemia. J Endocrinol 53(3):339–348
138. Davicco MJ, Coxam V, Lefaivre J, Barlet JP (1992) Parathyroid hormone-related peptide increases urinary phosphate excretion in fetal lambs. Exp Physiol 77(2):377–383
139. Robillard JE, Nakamura KT (1988) Neurohormonal regulation of renal function during development. Am J Physiol 254(6 Pt 2):F771–F779
140. Brace RA, Moore TR (1991) Diurnal rhythms in fetal urine flow, vascular pressures, and heart rate in sheep. Am J Physiol 261(4 Pt 2):R1015–R1021
141. Rabinowitz R, Peters MT, Vyas S, Campbell S, Nicolaides KH (1989) Measurement of fetal urine production in normal pregnancy by real-time ultrasonography. Am J Obstet Gynecol 161(5):1264–1266
142. Lumbers ER, Stevens AD (1983) Changes in fetal renal function in response to infusions of a hyperosmotic solution of mannitol to the ewe. J Physiol 343:439–446
143. Bell RJ, Congiu M, Hardy KJ, Wintour EM (1984) Gestation-dependent aspects of the response of the ovine fetus to the osmotic stress induced by maternal water deprivation. Q J Exp Physiol 69(1):187–195
144. Ross MG, Sherman DJ, Ervin MG, Castro R, Humme J (1988) Maternal dehydration-rehydration: fetal plasma and urinary responses. Am J Physiol 255(5 Pt 1):E674–E679
145. Stevens AD, Lumbers ER (1985) The effect of maternal fluid intake on the volume and composition of fetal urine. J Dev Physiol 7(3):161–166
146. Woods LL, Cheung CY, Power GG, Brace RA (1986) Role of arginine vasopressin in fetal renal response to hypertonicity. Am J Physiol 251(1 Pt 2):F156–F163
147. Lingwood B, Hardy KJ, Horacek I, McPhee ML, Scoggins BA, Wintour EM (1978) The effects of antidiuretic hormone on urine flow and composition in the chronically-cannulated ovine fetus. Q J Exp Physiol Cogn Med Sci 63(4):315–330
148. Lumbers ER, Smith FG, Stevens AD (1985) Measurement of net transplacental transfer of fluid to the fetal sheep. J Physiol 364:289–299
149. Wintour EM, Bell RJ, Congui M, MacIsaac RJ, Wang X (1985) The value of urine osmolality as an index of stress in the ovine fetus. J Dev Physiol 7(5):347–354

150. Rees L, Brook CG, Forsling ML (1983) Continuous urine collection in the study of vasopressin in the newborn. Horm Res 17(3):134–140
151. Levina SE (1968) Endocrine features in development of human hypothalamus, hypophysis, and placenta. Gen Comp Endocrinol 11(1):151–159
152. Leake RD, Weitzman RE, Effros RM, Siegel SR, Fisher DA (1979) Maternal fetal osmolar homeostasis: fetal posterior pituitary autonomy. Pediatr Res 13(7):841–844
153. Weitzman RE, Fisher DA, Robillard J, Erenberg A, Kennedy R, Smith F (1978) Arginine vasopressin response to an osmotic stimulus in the fetal sheep. Pediatr Res 12(1):35–38
154. Rurak DW (1979) Plasma vasopressin levels during haemorrhage in mature and immature fetal sheep. J Dev Physiol 1(1):91–101
155. Ervin MG, Terry KA, Calvario GC et al (1994) Vascular effects alter early-gestation fetal renal responses to vasopressin. Am J Physiol 266(3 Pt 2):R722–R729
156. Fushimi K, Uchida S, Hara Y, Hirata Y, Marumo F, Sasaki S (1993) Cloning and expression of apical membrane water channel of rat kidney collecting tubule. Nature 361(6412):549–552
157. Sasaki S, Fushimi K, Saito H et al (1994) Cloning, characterization, and chromosomal mapping of human aquaporin of collecting duct. J Clin Invest 93(3):1250–1256
158. Hayashi M, Sasaki S, Tsuganezawa H et al (1994) Expression and distribution of aquaporin of collecting duct are regulated by vasopressin V2 receptor in rat kidney. J Clin Invest 94(5): 1778–1783
159. Baum M, Quigley R (1993) Glucocorticoids stimulate rabbit proximal convoluted tubule acidification. J Clin Invest 91(1):110–114

3 Fluid and Electrolyte Physiology in the Fetus and Neonate

Isa F. Ashoor, Nilka de Jesús-González, and Michael J.G. Somers

Core Messages

1. During both fetal and neonatal development, total body water and its distribution into extracellular and intracellular compartments vary. With maturation, total body water as a proportion of body weight decreases, and there is increasing distribution of water into the intracellular compartment.
2. Neonates can produce dilute urine but they have reduced urinary concentrating ability due to anatomic, biochemical, and hormonal factors affecting the kidney. These factors change with maturation, allowing increased water reabsorption in the nephron and an improved ability to maintain water balance and volume homeostasis across a broad spectrum of clinical conditions.
3. Positive sodium balance is important for growth of the fetus and neonate. Sodium balance also significantly affects extracellular fluid volume and effective circulating volume. Accordingly, multiple mechanisms that vary according to developmental needs and nephron segment differentiation are coordinated to regulate sodium homeostasis.
4. Positive potassium balance is also necessary for fetal and neonatal growth. Active transport mechanisms across the placenta from the mother insure adequate delivery of potassium to the fetus. After birth, maturational changes occur in all nephron segments to enhance potassium handling and allow for its reabsorption or excretion as clinically indicated.
5. Calcium, magnesium, and phosphorus are the major divalent ions that factor significantly in fetal and neonatal growth and development. Their renal handling is often linked to homeostatic mechanisms that involve bone accretion and turn over as well as the gastrointestinal tract.

Case Vignette

A 19-year-old primigravida woman was admitted after premature rupture of membranes at 35 weeks' gestation. Antenatal history was unremarkable except for mildly reduced amniotic fluid volume noted on an initial 18-week gestation ultrasound that resolved on follow-up imaging. She delivered a 3,200 g boy vaginally who did well

I.F. Ashoor • N. de Jesús-González
M.J.G. Somers, MD (✉)
Division of Nephrology, Harvard Medical School, Boston Children's Hospital, 300 Longwood Avenue, Boston, MA 02115, USA
e-mail: michael.somers@childrens.harvard.edu

A.S. Chishti et al. (eds.), *Kidney and Urinary Tract Diseases in the Newborn*, DOI 10.1007/978-3-642-39988-6_3, © Springer-Verlag Berlin Heidelberg 2014

in the newborn nursery with only routine care. The infant was discharged home with the breastfeeding mother after 48 h with a weight of 3,000 g.

At 1 week of age, the baby was brought to the pediatrician's office for routine care. The mother reports that he is a "good" baby who seems to be generally quiet and sleepy. In response to questions from the pediatrician, his mother reported poor latching when he breastfeeds and slow feeding. She thinks her milk supply is just now becoming better established. She also reports perhaps fewer wet diapers in the day prior to this visit. On exam, the infant was arousable but the mucus membranes were dry and the anterior fontanel was depressed. Vital signs demonstrated no fever, a pulse of 150, and a respiratory rate of 40. Blood pressure was not performed, but capillary refill was thought adequate. Weight was decreased to 2,500 g.

Given the 20 % weight loss from birth and the clinical circumstances, the infant was admitted for further evaluation, hydration, and observation. As part of a diagnostic evaluation on admission, an electrolyte panel, BUN, and creatinine were obtained, revealing a sodium of 146 mmol/L, potassium of 5.9 mmol/L, chloride 110 mmol/L, carbon dioxide 19 mmol/L, blood urea nitrogen 25 mg/dL, and serum creatinine of 0.5 mg/dL. After an initial bolus of 40 mL of 0.9 % NaCl, the baby was offered formula and avidly drank nearly an ounce, and no further intravenous hydration was provided. A lactation consultant arrived and observed the mother nursing the baby. She worked closely with the mother to optimize breastfeeding technique. Over the course of the next 2 days, the infant demonstrated weight gains of nearly 30 g daily and the mother and the nursing staff were both satisfied with the technical aspects of breastfeeding. Following discharge, the baby continued to thrive, weighing 4 kg at the 1-month well-child visit.

3.1 Introduction

Body fluid distribution and composition in the fetus and neonate differ from what is found in older children and adults. In fact, during intrauterine and perinatal life and persisting into the early postnatal period, high water content characterizes body composition, with significant and dynamic changes then occurring in its distribution as the child ages and grows. Maintaining the appropriate body fluid balance at different developmental stages is critical for cell growth and differentiation and for organ formation and function. Accordingly, a host of unique regulatory mechanisms determine the distribution and composition of body fluids in the fetus and newborn and contribute to ongoing volume and biochemical homeostasis in early childhood. In the following chapter, the main aspects of fluid and electrolyte physiology in the fetus and neonate are reviewed, with particular emphasis on mechanisms regulating water, sodium, potassium, and the divalent ions.

3.2 Body Fluid

3.2.1 Body Fluid Distribution

Water, the most abundant substance in the body, is distributed into two main body compartments—the intracellular fluid (ICF) and the extracellular fluid (ECF)—separated by the cell membrane. The ECF compartment is further subdivided into the intravascular space (plasma) and the extravascular space (interstitium), anatomically separated by the capillary wall.

During development, the proportion of total body water (TBW) as well as its distribution between ECF and ICF compartments varies (Fig. 3.1). Fetal composition is characterized by an extremely high proportion of TBW and, as gestation progresses, TBW decreases. In early pregnancy, TBW accounts for up to 95 % of the body's weight, decreasing to 80 % at 26 weeks' gestation and 75 % at term. Similar to TBW, ECF volume also decreases throughout gestation. Two-thirds of TBW is distributed into the ECF

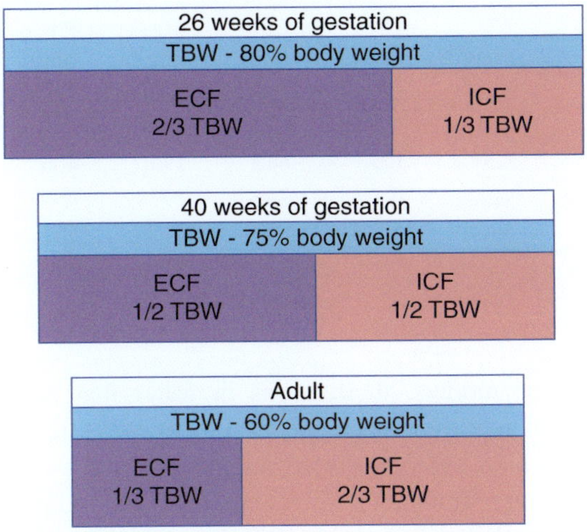

Fig. 3.1 Proportion of total body water (*TBW*) relative to body weight and distribution of TBW in body fluid compartments at different ages. During development, TBW relative to body weight decreases. The proportion of extracellular fluid (*ECF*) relative to TBW decreases during development, while the proportion of intracellular fluid (*ICF*) to TBW increases

compartment by 20 weeks of gestation, decreasing to about half by 37–40 weeks. Of note, plasma volume does not change, remaining constant at 4–5 % of body weight, with interstitial fluid volumes shifting more. As a result, the ICF volume actually increases during fetal development. In early gestation, only one-third of TBW is distributed to the ICF but this increases to one-half of TBW at term [52]. These changes seem to reflect increases in cell density, body mass accretion, and fat deposition [54].

In the perinatal period, changes in the intravascular volume also take place. First, the relative intrapartum hypoxia increases fetal capillary permeability leading to redistribution of the intravascular fluid to the interstitium [19]. Postnatally, with good oxygenation, capillary integrity is restored, and the interstitial fluid redistributes back to the intravascular space [19]. Second, vasoactive hormones such as vasopressin, norepinephrine, and cortisol seem to play a role in reducing the intravascular volume. In animal models, infusion of these hormones into the fetal circulation reduced circulating blood volume and plasma volume [20, 144, 160]. Interestingly, elevated levels of these hormones have been reported in human neonates following vaginal delivery. Third, animal studies suggest that fetal arterial blood pressure increases in the days just prior to delivery and this could serve to drive fluid out of the intravascular compartment via transcapillary redistribution [32]. Fourth, the timing of cord clamping after delivery affects intravascular volume in the newborn during the first days of life. If the cord is clamped immediately, blood volume remains stable. If the cord is clamped late, however, or the newborn is positioned at or above placental level, blood will flow from the neonate back into the placenta, leading to a decrease in intravascular blood volume [84].

At birth, further TBW and weight loss ensue. Full-term neonates lose about 5–10 % of body weight during the first week of life, while very low birth weight preterm infants may have weight losses as high as 15 % [30, 131]. It is largely accepted that neonatal weight loss is mainly associated with ECF contraction, although the mechanisms mediating this process are not completely understood [9, 68, 131]. One hypothesis proposes that as pulmonary vascular resistance decreases and left atrial venous return increases after birth, atria overstretch stimulates the release of atrial natriuretic peptide (ANP) from myocardial cells [149]. Once released, ANP enters the circulation and enhances renal Na^+ and water excretion [120]. In contrast, others propose that the fluid lost is mainly intracellular as a result of Na^+ translocation out of the cellular milieu mediated by the effect of prolactin, though this requires there to be some ECF loss that then happens for actual weight loss [34].

3.2.2 Body Fluid Composition

The ICF and ECF solute composition are very different. In the ICF, the major cations are potassium (K^+) and magnesium (Mg^{2+}), while the major anions are organic phosphates and proteins. In contrast, in the ECF, sodium (Na^+) is the major cation, while chloride (Cl^-) and bicarbonate (HCO_3^-) are the major anions. This asymmetric distribution of cations (especially Na^+ and K^+) across plasma membranes is maintained by the

Table 3.1 Changes in body ion content throughout gestation[a]

Gestational age (weeks)	Na^+ (meq)[b]	K^+ (meq)[b]	Cl^- (meq)[b]	Ca++ (mg)[b]	Mg++ (mg)[b]	Ph (mg)[b]
24	9.9	4	7	621	17.8	387
28	9.4	4.2	6.9	610	17.4	385
32	9.1	4.3	6.6	640	17.8	406
36	8.8	4.5	6.1	726	19	460
40	8.7	4.6	5.7	882	21.1	551

[a]Adapted from Ziegler et al. [164]
[b]These values are referenced per 100 g fat-free weight

activity of Na^+/K^+ ATPase, which uses cellular energy to pump $3Na^+$ out of the cell in exchange for $2K^+$ moving intracellularly. Changes in the ECF osmolality drive the net movement of water [90]. Thus, a tight control of the ECF osmolality is required to maintain the ECF volume and, notably, the circulatory system, as well as to control the size and osmolality of the ICF. In the ECF, the capillary wall separating the intravascular from the extravascular compartments is freely permeable to ions but not proteins. Thus, the interstitial fluid and plasma are similar in ionic composition, but protein concentration is significantly higher in the plasma. This difference provides the oncotic pressure required to maintain fluids in the intravascular space.

The total body distribution of ions does vary as the fetus develops (Table 3.1). For example, during early gestation, the fetal body has high Na^+ content and low K^+ content. As gestation progresses, Na^+ content decreases and K^+ content increases [164]. Similarly, there are gestational increases in calcium, magnesium, and phosphorus.

3.3 Water Balance in the Fetus and the Newborn

3.3.1 Water Balance in the Fetus

Fetal water acquisition primarily occurs across the placenta through complex processes whose regulation is poorly understood. Water flux may occur through both paracellular and transcellular routes and may potentially be driven by hydrostatic and osmotic pressure differences or active transport mechanisms. In guinea pigs and sheep models, fluctuations in water flux have been reported when the perfusion pressure on the fetal side is altered suggesting that water transfer across the placenta may be a flow-dependent process [21, 127]. Interestingly, studies in human placentas suggest that hydrostatic pressures are lower in the intervillous space (maternal side) than the umbilical vein (fetal side) [78] suggesting water movement from the fetus to the mother that argues against hydrostatic pressure as a mechanism explaining fetal water acquisition. From the osmotic pressure perspective, fetal plasma osmolality is equal to or slightly greater than maternal plasma osmolality [42], and this would, in theory, potentially drive water from the mother to the fetus. The principal plasma solutes contributing to plasma osmolality are Na^+ and Cl^-, however, and these are both permeable across the placenta and should not contribute to any actual osmotic force [38]. An active transport of Na^+ across the placenta, creating local osmotic difference and influencing local water flux, has been proposed and such a mechanism has actually been described in rats [142]. Whether hydrostatic or osmotic pressure or some combination of both serves as the main determinants of net water flux during fetal development is uncertain and requires further research.

There is evidence supporting transcellular solute-free water flow through water channels or aquaporins (AQPs) in the placenta. AQPs are membrane proteins that form hydrophilic pores. In the placenta, four different AQPs have been identified (AQPs 1, 3, 8, and 9). AQP 3 is expressed in the apical membranes of the syncytiotrophoblasts [37] and its expression changes throughout gestation [10]. In mouse models, AQP 3 expression increases early in fetal life and then decreases with advancing gestation [10], a pattern that is also seen in studies evaluating placental permeability to water [75]. These findings suggest that AQP 3 expression may be an important factor regulating placental water flux.

On the other hand, AQP 1 is located in the fetal chorioamnion [95] and seems to be involved in the movement of water between the fetus and amniotic fluid. In fact, alterations in AQP 1 expression appear to affect amniotic fluid volume, leading to pathologic conditions such as polyhydramnios. This is supported by evidence showing that the amniotic fluid volumes in AQP 1 knockout mice are significantly altered [94]. Moreover, the expression of AQP 1 in the placenta of patients with elevated amniotic fluid volumes is increased [93]. Similar to AQP 3, AQP 1 expression varies with gestation, being the highest early in gestation, decreasing thereafter, and rising again near term [85]. Finally, although AQP 8 and 9 have been identified in human placentas, their roles in water flux remain to be elucidated [37, 154].

3.3.2 Water Balance in the Newborn

In the early neonatal period, the infant's body composition is characterized by a TBW excess and this water load can generally be excreted over the first few days [119]. In fact, neonates can dilute their urine as well as older children and adults, though their ability to excrete a water load is limited by their initial low GFR. On the other hand, during the early neonatal period, urinary concentrating ability remains immature. In the typical early postpartum neonate, there is no need for maximal urinary concentrating ability, however, given the TBW excess. As a neonate matures and volume balance needs better regulation, urinary concentrating ability increases [110]. The reduced urinary concentrating ability is due to an anatomically shorter loop of Henle, a relatively low interstitial NaCl and urea concentration, and decreased responsiveness to ADH by principal cells in the distal tubule. These factors are more pronounced in premature neonates [16, 47].

ADH increases water permeability across the collecting duct (Fig. 3.2). ADH is produced in the paraventricular and supraoptic nuclei of the anterior hypothalamus and stored in the posterior hypothalamus. Its secretion is stimulated by an increase in serum osmolality (>285 mOsm/kg) sensed by hypothalamic osmoreceptors or a decrease in volume sensed by carotid baroreceptors. Once in the circulation, ADH binds to the vasopressin receptor (V2R) on the basolateral membrane of the principal cell and activates the adenylate cyclase second messenger system [62, 121]. This increases intracellular cAMP and activates a downstream protein, protein kinase A (PKA), which then phosphorylates the cytoplasmic carboxyterminal end of AQP 2, resulting in the incorporation of this water channel into the apical membrane of the cell [55, 56, 103]. Water flux will then ensue, entering the cell via apical AQP 2 and leaving through AQP 3 and 4 located in the basolateral membrane [86].

In the neonate, low responsiveness to ADH is likely secondary to an immature intracellular second messenger system rather than low secretion of ADH or inadequate number of VR2. This is supported by data showing that the generation of adenylcyclase, stimulated by ADH as well as the cAMP response, are both markedly reduced in the neonatal period [16–18, 114]. Moreover, cAMP degradation is increased, along with an increase in phosphodiesterase IV and subsequent inhibition of cAMP production by prostaglandin E2 [113]. ADH levels are actually elevated at birth [65], and no major changes are observed in the first weeks of life [116]. Likewise, based on data in rodents, V2R expression is thought to be present in early gestation [105], and the number of V2R does not change during the first weeks of life [1].

To enhance water reabsorption, a hypertonic medullary interstitium is needed so that water will move down a concentration gradient from the tubular lumen [80]. The neonatal interstitium has a low tonicity secondary to limited concentrations of both NaCl and urea [49]. This is due

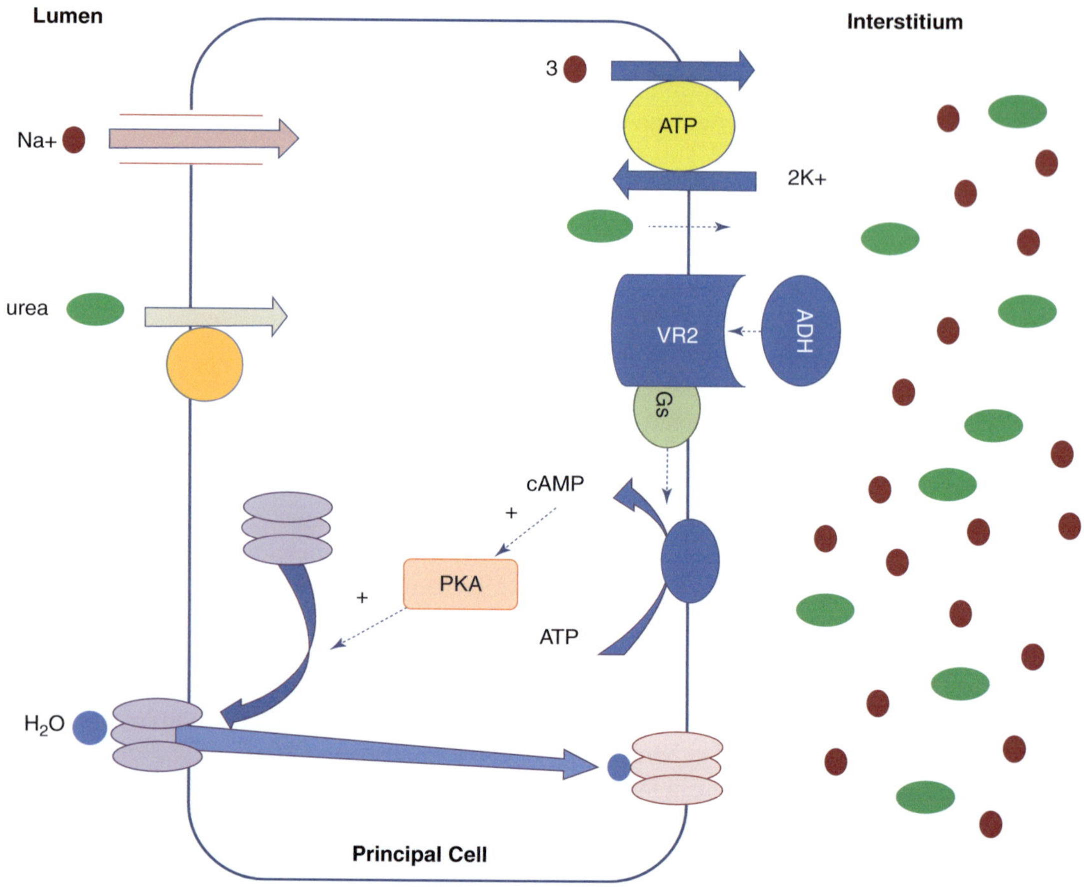

Fig. 3.2 Water transport across principal cell in the distal tubule and collecting duct [16]. Antidiuretic hormone (ADH) secretion from the hypothalamus is stimulated by an increase in serum osmolality sensed by hypothalamic osmoreceptors or a decrease in volume sensed by carotid baroreceptors. Once in the circulation, ADH binds to the vasopressin receptor (V2R) on the basolateral membrane of the principal cell and activates the adenylate cyclase (AC) second messenger system. This increases intracellular cAMP and activates a downstream protein, protein kinase A (PKA), which then phosphorylates the cytoplasmic carboxyterminal end of aquaporin (AQP) 2 resulting in the incorporation of this water channel into the apical membrane of the cell. Water flux will then ensue, entering the cell via apical AQP 2 and leaving through AQP 3 and 4 located in the basolateral membrane. A hypertonic medullary interstitium is also needed for water to get reabsorbed from the tubular lumen. During the first weeks of life, an increased number of urea transporters (UT-A) take place which in turn increases the interstitial urea concentration. This mechanism also contributes to water transport across principal cells

to low Na^+ transport across the thick ascending loop of Henle [71], low expression of urea transporters [79], and a short loop of Henle [29, 87]. With maturation and enhancing Na^+/K^+ ATPase activity, Na^+ transport across the thick ascending loop of Henle increases [165]. Likewise, the loop of Henle physically elongates and penetrates the medulla, forming tubulovascular units [137]. Also, animal studies have reported an increased number of urea transporters during the first 2 weeks of life to increase interstitial urea concentration [49, 79]. Temporally, all these changes parallel the increasing concentrating ability observed in the maturing neonate, suggesting that these mechanisms do indeed contribute to the increasing interstitial tonicity.

3.4 Sodium Balance in the Fetus and Neonate

Na^+ is the main extracellular cation. In fact, more than 95 % of total body Na^+ is in the extracellular compartment, with concentrations ranging from 135 to 145 mmol/L. Conversely, the intracellular fluid contains a relatively low Na^+ concentration of ~10 mmol/L. This significant electrochemical Na^+ gradient across the cell membrane provides the driving force for the cotransport of other substances, either along with or in exchange for Na^+. The Na^+ balance is an essential determinant of the ECF volume which, in turn, is crucial to sustaining the circulatory system and delivery of oxygen and nutrients to cells. Given this important role, multiple mechanisms are coordinated to regulate Na^+ concentration, varying according to specific developmental stages.

3.4.1 Sodium Physiology in the Fetus

During fetal life, appropriate Na^+ provision is required for growth. Mathematical models estimate that normal human fetal growth requires approximately 1.8 mmol of Na^+/kg/day. This Na^+ balance is primarily regulated by the placenta, with the fetal kidneys having a minimal role. Na^+ is thought to be passively and bidirectionally transported, via paracellular diffusion across the placenta between the mother and the fetus. Fetal plasma concentration of Na^+ remains similar to or slightly lower than maternal concentration between 18 and 40 weeks of gestation [61], supporting a passive bidirectional transport of Na^+ (Fig. 3.1). Moreover, gross Na^+ transfer from mother to fetus is 10–100 times higher than the Na^+ actually retained by the fetus [48], again suggesting bidirectional passive transport.

Given such passive Na^+ flux, active transport of Na^+ to the fetus does not seem to be necessarily required for the fetus to maintain Na^+ balance. Evidence exists, however, that there are active Na^+ transport systems in the placental syncytiotrophoblast, including Na^+/H^+ exchangers [7], Na^+/Pi exchangers [82], and Na-amino acid cotransporters [99] on the maternal side and Na^+/K^+ ATPase [155] on the fetal side (Fig. 3.3). Interestingly, some of these Na^+ transporters undergo changes in expression and activity during gestation. For example, the activity of the Na^+/H^+ exchanger increases as gestation progresses [73, 91]. At the same time, pathologic characteristics in the fetal milieu seem to have an effect on the activity of these transporters. For instance, the activity of the Na^+/H^+ exchanger and Na^+/K^+ ATPase is reduced in newborns with intrauterine growth retardation [76, 107]. These findings suggest that the active transport mechanisms across the placenta do indeed factor in some aspects of fetal solute homeostasis although, at this point, their specific physiological relevance remains unclear.

3.4.2 Sodium Physiology in the Neonate

During infancy, a positive Na^+ balance is required longitudinally for adequate growth [67]. Since neonatal Na^+ intake is limited due to the low Na^+ content in breast milk or formula, the kidneys play a major role in allowing Na^+ balance to be attained, and there seem to be specific maturational changes in the nephron during the neonatal period that permit such a positive Na^+ balance.

Although eventually a positive Na^+ balance prevails throughout infancy, in the immediate period after birth, neonates actually manifest a negative Na^+ balance associated with increased urinary Na^+ excretion and high fractional excretion of Na^+ (FeNa). Notably, urinary excretion of Na^+ is inversely related to gestational age. Premature neonates <30 weeks of gestation have a FeNa near 5 % [133], whereas full-term neonates have a FeNa closer to 3 % [156]. With advancing gestational and postnatal age, FeNa can decrease and renal Na^+ conservation can improve [118]. With most full-term babies, FeNa falls to values less than 1 % within days, whereas in premature neonates FeNa reaches these levels within 2 weeks [150].

This high initial perinatal FeNa results, in part, from a physiologic natriuresis that occurs

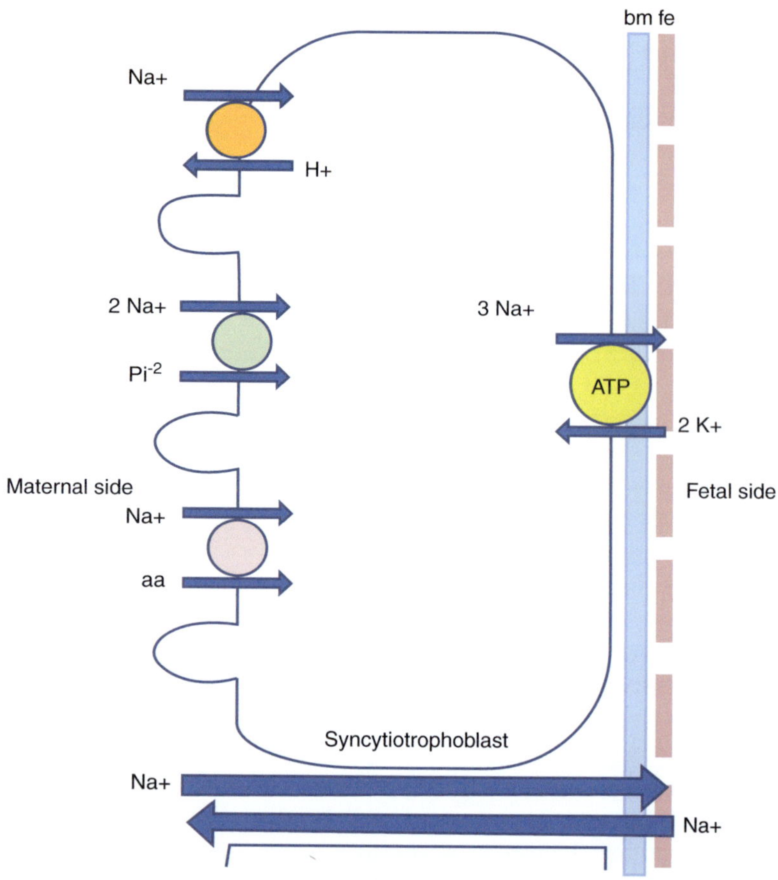

Fig. 3.3 Na^+ transfer mechanisms across the placenta. A passive bidirectional transport via paracellular diffusion accomplishes Na^+ transport across the human placenta. Although active transport mechanisms are also present in human placenta, their physiological significance is not clear. *Pi* inorganic phosphorus, *aa* amino acids, *bm* basement membrane, and *fe* fetal endothelium

as an adaptation to extrauterine life, presumably to eliminate excess ECW and Na^+. In preterm infants, this process is proportionately greater than in term infants [53], and in all infants, atrial natriuretic peptide (ANP) release has been thought to mediate this perinatal physiologic natriuresis [149]. Specifically, pulmonary vascular resistance decreases and left atrial venous return increases after birth; the atria overstretch and stimulate the release of ANP from myocardial cells [60]. Once released, ANP enters the circulation, binds to its receptor in the basolateral membrane of the collecting duct principal cells, activates guanylate cyclase thereby increasing intracellular levels of cGMP, and inhibits Na^+ reabsorption by closing the amiloride-sensitive Na^+ channels (ENaC) [31]. ANP release has also been implicated in other actions that may promote natriuresis including an increase in GFR, vasodilation, and inhibition of the renin-angiotensin-aldosterone [60]. As a neonate matures, ANP levels tend to decrease [14].

In addition to the decrease in circulating levels of ANP, maturational changes in the renal Na^+ transport systems also affect FeNa in the neonate (Table 3.2). At birth, Na^+ transporters in the kidney are relatively low in both distribution and activity. As maturation progresses, they increase in number and also acquire maximal enzymatic potential, resulting in an increased Na^+ transporting capacity along the renal tubule [138].

Of particular importance is the Na^+/K^+ ATPase located in the basolateral membrane of renal tubular cells [44]. As previously noted, the Na^+/K^+ ATPase actively exchanges $3Na^+$ ions out of the cell for $2K^+$ ions that enter into the cell, resulting in an intracellular Na^+

Table 3.2 Summary of developmental changes in Na^+ transport mechanisms

	Maturational changes in Na^+ transport systems		
Nephron segment	Transporter	Activity of transporter as gestation progresses	Mechanism regulating developmental changes
Proximal tubule	Na^+/H^+ exchanger 3	Increases	Induced by glucocorticoids, and angiotensin II
	Na^+/Pi	Decreases	Induced by growth hormone and IGF; inhibited by PTH
	Na^+ glucose (or aa)	Increases	?
	Na^+/K^+ ATPase	Increases	Induced by glucocorticoids and thyroid hormones; inhibited by dopamine
Loop of Henle	$Na^+/2Cl^-/K^+$	Increases	?
	Na^+/K^+ ATPase	Increases; its activity is greater in this segment than in other segments	Induced by glucocorticoids and thyroid hormones; inhibited by dopamine
Early distal tubule	Na^+/Cl^-	Increases	?
	Na^+/K^+ ATPase	Increases	Induced by glucocorticoids and thyroid hormones; inhibited by dopamine
Late distal tubule and collecting duct	ENaC	Increases	?; endogenous glucocorticoids do not induce ENaC developmental changes
	Na^+/K^+ ATPase	Increases	Induced by glucocorticoids and thyroid hormones; inhibited by dopamine

concentration one-tenth that of plasma and a −60 mV potential difference across the plasma membrane. Na^+/K^+ ATPase activity undergoes developmental changes in the fetus and neonate. In neonates born before 35 weeks of gestation, red blood cells Na^+/K^+ ATPase activity is lower than that in neonates of more advanced gestation [15]. Likewise, in renal epithelial cells, animal studies have shown increases in Na^+/K^+ ATPase activity paralleling the increased Na^+ reabsorption observed during kidney maturation [2, 125, 128]. By 2 weeks of life, Na^+/K^+ ATPase activity is similar in all neonates irrespective of gestational age [15]. Glucocorticoids have been posited to play an important role regulating these developmental changes. This is supported by evidence in rats showing that exposure to betamethasone during development increases Na^+/K^+ ATPase activity [3]. Thyroid hormone surge at birth may also enhance Na^+/K^+ ATPase [98]. In contrast to glucocorticoids and thyroid hormone, dopamine seems to inhibit Na^+/K^+ ATPase activity, with animal studies suggesting that during development, the natriuretic response to dopamine is decreased, in part due to a reduced inhibitory effect on Na^+/K^+ ATPase activity [12].

3.4.3 Sodium Handling Sequentially in the Renal Tubule

The sequential tubular segments of the nephron—proximal convoluted tubule (early and late segments), loop of Henle, distal tubule (early and late segments), and collecting ducts (cortical and medullary)—each play an important role in maintaining Na^+ balance (Fig. 3.4). How they accomplish this homeostasis is a reflection on their differing Na^+ transport systems.

3.4.3.1 Proximal Convoluted Tubule

The bulk of Na^+ reabsorption takes place in the proximal tubule (~65 % of filtered Na^+). These multiple Na^+ transporter systems are mainly driven by the electrochemical gradient generated by the Na^+/K^+ ATPase. In the early segment of the proximal tubule, several cotransporters reabsorb Na^+ mostly with organic solutes and HCO_3^-, whereas in the late segment Na^+ is primarily reabsorbed with Cl^-. During the neonatal period, the reabsorption of Na^+ in the proximal segment increases three- to fourfold along with the increased activity in Na^+/K^+ ATPase, sodium-proton (Na^+/H^+) exchanger, sodium-dependent

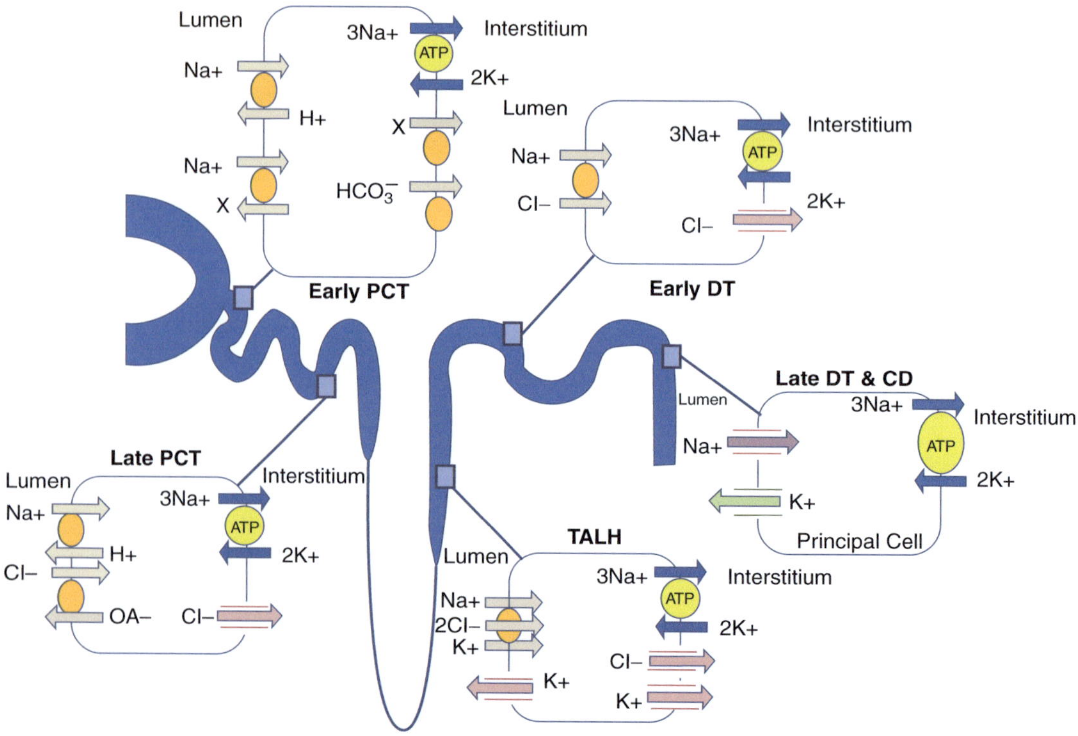

Fig. 3.4 Sodium and potassium transport along the entire renal tubule. *PT* proximal tubule, *TALH* thick ascending loop of Henle, *DT* distal tubule, *CD* collecting duct, *X* solutes (i.e., glucose, amino acids), *OA* organic acids

phosphate (Na^+/Pi) cotransporter, Na^+/glucose cotransporter, and Na^+/amino acid cotransporter [28].

The electroneutral Na^+/H^+ exchanger is the principal mediator of Na^+ reabsorption in the proximal tubule [35, 36]. Of note, multiple Na^+/H^+ exchanger isoforms are present in the kidney, and the Na^+/H^+ exchanger 3, located on the apical side of proximal tubule epithelial cells, carries Na^+ into the cell in exchange for H^+ secretion [13, 22]. The net product of this exchange is reabsorption of $NaHCO_3$ by mechanisms that will be discussed in a later chapter. Na^+/H^+ exchangers 1 and 4 are isoforms found on the basolateral side of the proximal tubule cell [13, 22, 78]. Na^+/H^+ exchanger activity as well as mRNA expression of some of the Na^+/H^+ exchangers may undergo maturational changes [132]. The postnatal maturation seems to be enhanced by glucocorticoids stimulation, as demonstrated by animal studies showing increased Na^+/H^+ activity and mRNA/protein expression in fetuses exposed to glucocorticoids [11, 64]. In addition to glucocorticoids, rodent models also suggest that angiotensin II may also be contributing to postnatal maturation and stimulation of the Na^+/H^+ exchanger [112], although these findings were not observed in young sheep [64].

In the early proximal tubule, Na^+ also enters the epithelial cell via the Na^+/Pi cotransporters. Various isoforms of Na^+/Pi cotransporters have been identified in the proximal tubular cell (Na^+/Pi 1–3), and Na^+/Pi 2 isoform is specific to the brush border and seems to play a major role in Na^+ dependent Pi reabsorption in this segment [24, 157]. In contrast to the Na^+/H^+ exchanger, the Na^+/Pi cotransporters in newborns demonstrate higher transport rates than that in adults, presumably associated with a poor ability of the neonate to adapt to changes in dietary Pi intake [139]. Contrary to other Na^+ transporters, Na^+/Pi cotransporter does not seem to be regulated by glucocorticoids. Instead, growth hormone and insulin-like growth factor have been implicated as stimulators of Na^+/Pi uptake [8, 66], whereas PTH has been found to inhibit proximal Na^+/Pi cotransport [66].

Na^+/amino acid and Na^+/glucose cotransporters also contribute to net Na^+ reabsorption in the early proximal tubule. Similar to the Na^+/H^+ exchanger and Na^+/K^+ ATPase, the activity of these transporters is low at birth and increases with maturation. This in part explains the glucosuria and aminoaciduria frequently seen during the first weeks of life [70]. The mechanisms regulating developmental changes in these transporters are poorly understood.

In the late segment of the proximal tubule, Na^+ is primarily reabsorbed with Cl^- as other solutes (glucose, HCO_3^-, and amino acids) have already preferentially been reabsorbed. NaCl is reabsorbed by both cellular and paracellular pathways. The cellular pathway involves coupled function of both the Na^+/H^+ exchanger and the Cl^-/formate (or oxalate) anion exchanger and leads to the net reabsorption of NaCl. Once inside the cell, Na^+ moves into the blood by the Na^+/K^+ ATPase, and Cl^- diffuses out via Cl^- channels [5]. Whether these mechanisms undergo developmental changes remains a question.

3.4.3.2 Loop of Henle

Approximately 20–25 % of the filtered Na^+ load is reabsorbed in the loop of Henle. It is composed of three segments: thin descending limb, thin ascending limb, and thick ascending limb. Na^+ is passively reabsorbed in the thin segments, while in the thick segment Na^+ is absorbed primarily by active transport via a specific $Na^+/K^+/2Cl^-$ cotransporter [111]. The $Na^+/K^+/2Cl^-$ cotransporter is the site of action of loop diuretics such as furosemide. In vitro studies have shown variable expression of this transporter during nephrogenesis [126], although the physiological significance of these fetal changes remains to be elucidated. Postnatally, although Na^+/K^+ ATPase activity increases in all tubular segments, studies in rats and rabbits demonstrate that its activity is greater in the loop of Henle than other tubular segments [115].

3.4.3.3 Distal Tubule and Collecting Duct

The early distal tubule reabsorbs ~5 % of filtered Na^+. In this segment, Na^+ is reabsorbed via the electroneutral Na^+/Cl^- cotransporter, the site of action of the thiazide diuretics. In the fully mature distal tubule, the Na^+/Cl^- cotransporter is expressed along the entire distal tubule [104]. During nephrogenesis, Na^+/Cl^- cotransporter mRNA expression in the early distal tubule is detected before $Na^+/K^+/2Cl^-$ mRNA expression in the loop of Henle. As development advances, the Na^+/Cl^- cotransporter localizes into the post-macula segment [126], although again, the physiological significance or evolutionary advantage of this variable expression is poorly understood.

The late distal tubule and the collecting duct, anatomically and functionally similar, come to reabsorb only 1–3 % of filtered Na^+. These segments play an important role, however, in determining the final Na^+ concentration in the urine, essentially fine-tuning overall Na^+ balance. Unlike other nephron segments in which coupled transport mechanisms mediate Na^+ reabsorption, in these segments, Na^+ is reabsorbed down its electrochemical gradient via the amiloride-sensitive Na^+ channel (ENaC) located in the luminal membrane of principal cells [45]. ENaC is composed of an alpha subunit that forms a transmembranous channel as well as beta and gamma subunits that stabilize this channel and allow for its appropriate insertion into the membrane [26]. Aldosterone directly upregulates ENaC expression and alters its assembly, trafficking, and degradation, ultimately resulting in enhanced Na^+ reabsorption [46].

The sodium transporting capacity of these segments also undergoes maturational changes. First, in early gestation, ENaC is located along the medullary collecting duct and then redistributes to the cortical collecting duct as the fetal kidney undergoes further maturation. Second, studies in animals have shown that early in life, the Na^+ transport in this segment is limited by high passive permeability, low active transport of Na^+, aldosterone unresponsiveness, and low density and activity of ENaC [151]. During the first weeks of life, the passive Na^+ permeability decreases, followed by an increase in both Na^+ active transport capacity and mineralocorticoid responsiveness [151]. Although these developmental changes have been described, the mechanisms regulating them are not well understood. Prenatal exposure to exogenous glucocorticoids does enhance the expression of the ENaC alpha subunit. Evidence in mice shows, however, that there is no difference in ENaC subunit expression in corticotropin-releasing hormone knockout mice compared to wild type, suggesting that endogenous glucocorticoids do not have a major role on perinatal maturation [101]. Inactivation of endogenous but not exogenous glucocorticoids by 11-beta hydrogenase type 2 has been proposed, given evidence demonstrating an increased expression of this enzyme in embryonic murine kidneys [25].

3.5 Potassium

Approximately 98 % of total body potassium (K^+) stores are intracellular, and potassium (K^+) is the major intracellular cation with a concentration of 100–150 mmol/L. This is in contrast to the extracellular K^+ fluid concentration that ranges from 3.5 to 5 mmol/L in older children and adults and up to 6.7 mmol/L in neonates [88]. This steep K^+ gradient across cell membranes is important to maintain the resting membrane potential that determines nerve and muscle excitability. As a result, K^+ homeostasis is tightly regulated by a host of mechanisms that undergo maturational changes during fetal and neonatal life.

3.5.1 Potassium Physiology in the Fetus

Similar to what is seen with Na^+, a positive K^+ balance is necessary for fetal and neonatal growth. This is different from the healthy adult where the goal is to remain in an even K^+ balance between intake and excretion [162]. During fetal life, K^+ is actively transported across the placenta from the mother to the fetus. This helps to explain the significantly higher plasma K^+ concentrations in the umbilical cord blood of newborn infants than in their mothers [96]. This active transport mechanism also likely explains the observation in several animal models of stable fetal K^+ concentration even when the pregnant female is fed a K^+ deficient diet and develops low plasma K^+ concentration [39, 130]. In contrast, both urea and creatinine freely diffuse across the placenta, resulting in the highly correlated levels between the mother and neonate seen immediately after birth.

3.5.2 Potassium Physiology in the Neonate

A sequence of maturational changes in the neonatal nephron allows for the net positive K^+ balance required for postnatal growth (Table 3.3). Total body K^+ content subsequently increases, with the majority attributed to increased intracellular K^+ concentration in myocytes as muscle mass is gained [43].

Rapid regulation of the ECF K^+ concentration is accomplished by modulating the activity of the basolateral Na^+-K^+-ATPase pump. As detailed earlier in this chapter, this cellular pump actively transports Na^+ out and K^+ into cells, against concentration gradients in a 3:2 ratio. Diminished activity of this pump in very premature infants up to 30–32 weeks' gestation is believed to account for the commonly elevated plasma K^+ levels in the first 24–72 h after birth [63, 89, 123, 140]. In the absence of exogenous K^+ intake and renal failure, this elevation of plasma K^+, often to levels >6.5 mmol/L, is referred to as non-oliguric hyperkalemia. Correction of this condition in the premature infant is hampered by a further limited capacity to excrete K^+ due to low GFR and limited distal nephron K^+ secretion [162]. Both insulin and B_2-adrenergic stimulants such as albuterol, by virtue of stimulating the Na^+-K^+-ATPase pump, drive K^+ intracellularly from the ECF compartment and can be employed to acutely lower the plasma K^+ concentration [92, 136] until physiologic diuresis occurs around 48 h of life [89].

Table 3.3 Summary of developmental changes in K^+ handling

Nephron segment	Postnatal maturational changes in potassium handling
Glomerulus	K^+ is freely filtered. The filtered load increases in proportion to the GFR which doubles by 2 weeks and reaches about 50–60 mL/min/1.73 m^2 by 4 weeks in term infants
Proximal convoluted tubule	Up to 65 % of K^+ is reabsorbed by solvent drag in association with water and Na^+ reabsorption
Thick ascending limb of the loop of Henle	K^+ reabsorption is mediated by apical NKCC2 channels. Up to an additional 25 % of filtered K^+ load is reabsorbed in this segment by the end of the neonatal period
Cortical collecting duct	Principal cells:
	K^+ secretion via apical ROMK channels (basal conditions) and Maxi-K^+ channels (high tubular flow)
	ROMK and Maxi-K^+ mRNA transcripts and protein expression first detectable towards the end of second and fourth postnatal weeks, respectively
	Functional hypoaldosteronism in the neonatal period
	Intercalated cells:
	K^+ reabsorption coupled to active H^+ secretion via H^+-K^+-ATPase
	Enhanced activity detected in the neonatal period likely contributes to net K^+ retention

Long-term control of total body K^+ stores in the neonate is a balance between intake and output, with the kidney being the major excretory organ responsible for regulation of external K^+ balance. K^+ is freely filtered at the glomerulus and the majority (~65 %) is reabsorbed in the proximal tubule. No specific K^+ channels have been identified in this segment, and the reabsorption process is accomplished by solvent drag in association with water and Na^+ reabsorption. K^+ reabsorption in the thick ascending limb loop of Henle (TALH) is mediated by the sodium-potassium-chloride (NKCC2) cotransporter. This membrane protein, which shuttles sodium, potassium, and two chloride ions from the tubular lumen into the cells, is expressed on the apical surface of TALH and is encoded by the SLC12A1 gene [134]. Loss of function genetic mutations affecting NKCC2 activity results in an inherited salt-losing tubulopathy (antenatal Bartter syndrome) characterized by polyhydramnios, significant salt wasting, and hypokalemia [108]. Micropuncture studies in newborn rats have shown that up to 35 % of the filtered K^+ load can traverse the TALH and reach the distal nephron [83]. This is significantly higher than the 10 % filtered K^+ load that reaches the adult distal nephron, suggesting a maturational increase in the reabsorptive capacity of TALH [162].

The final determination of net renal K^+ excretion is then determined by the balance of K^+ secretion and reabsorption in the late distal tubule and cortical collecting duct (CCD), accomplished by both the principal and intercalated cells that exist only in this segment. Maturational changes that occur during the neonatal period facilitate the net positive K^+ balance required for somatic growth in this early period.

As discussed in an earlier section, Na^+ reabsorption in the principal cells occurs via the amiloride-sensitive epithelial Na^+ channel (ENaC). As Na^+ is reabsorbed, K^+ is secreted through renal outer medullary K^+ (ROMK) channels under basal conditions [58, 106, 163] and flow-stimulated Maxi-K^+ channels under conditions of high tubular fluid rate [158, 159]. Animal micropuncture studies of the CCD have shown no significant net K^+ secretion until after the third week of postnatal life under basal physiological flow rates [122]. This is believed to be secondary to low expression of ROMK channel protein on principal cells in early infancy as these mRNA transcripts and proteins were not detected until the second postnatal week in rodents [166]. Similarly, when rabbit CCDs were microperfused in vitro at high physiological flow rates, net K^+ secretion only increased in the adult animals, while no significant change was noted in the first month of postnatal life [162]. Maxi-K^+ channel mRNA transcription and protein expression mirrored this finding and were only detectable after the fourth week of life [159]. Loss of function genetic mutations involving the KCNJ1 gene encoding ROMK channels explains the initial transient hyperkalemia noted in a subset of patients with antenatal Bartter syndrome, which later normalizes and trends towards hypokalemia when salt wasting and increased tubular fluid rate activates K^+ secretion through Maxi-K^+ channels beyond the neonatal period [108].

Principal cells also form the primary target for hormonal control by aldosterone, mediated by intracellular mineralocorticoid receptors (MR). In the fully mature distal tubule, aldosterone stimulates Na^+ absorption through ENaC channels, and K^+ secretion through ROMK channels follows as a result of the generated negative lumen potential. Aldosterone levels were found to be higher in umbilical cord blood of healthy newborns compared to their mothers [96]. Yet, the transtubular potassium gradient (TTKG) is low in the neonatal period, particularly in premature infants despite the high aldosterone levels, suggesting a state of functional hypoaldosteronism [117]. In agreement with this observation, molecular studies on mouse kidneys detected MR at day 16 postcoitum, peaking at day 18, and then reaching very low levels at birth followed by a progressive rise afterwards [97]. Studies on fetal, neonatal, and infantile kidney specimens detected a similar pattern of MR expression, first detectable between 15 and 24 weeks' gestation and then disappearing below any threshold of detection from 30 weeks' gestation until 10 months of age [97].

The intercalated cells primarily function in maintaining acid–base balance by actively secreting hydrogen (H^+) ions into the tubular lumen via the apical H^+-K^+-ATPase pump. For every H^+ ion secreted, a K^+ ion is reabsorbed from the tubular lumen. It is believed that upregulation of this pump's activity is particularly important for K^+ retention under conditions of chronic K^+ depletion. In neonates, significant activity of the apical H^+-K^+-ATPase pump in intercalated cells is identified by fluorescent functional assays, suggesting that the CCD has the capacity for K^+ retention [33]. Table 3.3 summarizes the maturational changes observed in the various nephron segments that influence K^+ physiology during the neonatal period.

3.6 Divalent Ions

Calcium, magnesium, and phosphorus make up the three major divalent ions in the body and are primarily stored in bone. In plasma, they can be found in protein-bound forms, complexed with other ions, or as free ions. The free non-protein-bound fraction undergoes glomerular filtration. Renal handling contributes to regulation of the serum concentration of divalent ions in concert with other homeostatic mechanisms, particularly bone turnover and absorption from the gastrointestinal tract.

3.6.1 Divalent Ion Physiology in the Fetus

The growing fetal skeleton requires significant calcium and phosphorus delivery [40, 100]. Ultimately at term gestation, a total of 30 g of calcium is accumulated in the fetus, with up to 80 % occurring during the third trimester [102]. This is in contrast to the transplacental transfer of magnesium, which occurs throughout pregnancy, and especially during the first trimester [4].

The placenta actively transports calcium from the maternal to the fetal compartment against a concentration gradient [27, 141]. Extrusion of calcium from the trophoblast into the fetal blood is mediated by an ATP-dependent Ca^{2+} pump on the trophoblast basal membrane [141]. The total calcium concentration in cord plasma increases with gestational age, and the term fetus is hypercalcemic relative to the mother [72, 81, 109, 124]. This suppresses PTH release during fetal life [81].

Phosphorus and magnesium are also transferred actively across the placenta. The uptake of phosphorus by human trophoblasts is highly dependent on Na^+, while the efflux from the placenta to the fetus is presumably passive [141]. Based on animal models, it is believed that a Mg^{2+}–Na^+ exchanger is the principal mechanism of transfer across the trophoblast plasma membrane [141].

3.6.2 Divalent Ion Physiology in the Neonate

3.6.2.1 Calcium

Calcium homeostasis in the postnatal period involves a complex interaction between the parathyroid glands, the kidneys, the bone compartment, and the gastrointestinal tract to keep the ionized serum calcium concentration within a tight range. The following discussion will focus specifically on the renal contribution to homeostatic calcium regulation.

Immediately after birth, the infant's serum calcium levels fall with the abrupt termination of active placental transport of calcium [145]. This drop in serum calcium stimulates PTH release, mobilizing calcium from bone and stimulating the synthesis of 1,25 $(OH)_2$ vitamin D by renal tubular cells, which in turn enhances calcium absorption from the gastrointestinal tract. In term infants, normal serum calcium concentrations will typically be reached by the second week of life [153]. The decline in serum calcium levels seen immediately postpartum is exaggerated in premature infants and is believed to be related to a state of functional hypoparathyroidism and end organ unresponsiveness to PTH [40, 145, 147]. Similar mechanisms are thought to account for the hypocalcemia noted in infants of diabetic mothers [146].

As is true for other divalent ions, only the non-protein-bound plasma calcium fraction (about 50 % of total calcium) is freely filtered at the glomerulus and then reabsorbed along the tubular segments. Approximately 70 % of filtered Ca^{2+} is reabsorbed in the proximal tubule and 20 % in the TALH. This process is primarily passive and paracellular, driven by sodium reabsorption in those segments and a positive lumen potential. The final 5–10 % of filtered Ca^{2+} can be reabsorbed in the distal tubule in an active transcellular fashion. The process is mediated by the Ca^{2+}-selective TRPV5 channel activated by PTH. The transcellular calcium movement then is mediated by calbindins, calcium-binding proteins whose expression is upregulated by vitamin D. Calcium then gets extruded from the tubular cells into the blood compartment by two proteins on the basolateral membrane: the plasma membrane Ca^{2+}-ATPase (PMCA1b) and the $3Na^+$–Ca^{2+} exchanger [51, 59]. The PMCA1b activity is stimulated by both PTH and vitamin D [50]. The final amount of calcium excreted in normal neonates is therefore determined by the balance of homeostatic mechanisms acting on the distal tubule.

Several extrinsic factors such as medications can also increase calcium excretion in preterm and term neonates. Loop diuretics such as furosemide, often used in preterm infants with lung disease or older babies with bronchopulmonary dysplasia or cardiac issues, are associated with increased urinary calcium excretion [6]. Infants provided loop diuretics are at increased risk of developing nephrocalcinosis. Also, the aminoglycoside gentamicin, typically used for the treatment of neonatal sepsis, is associated with a post infusion increase in the urinary calcium excretion. The significance of these early alterations on long-term calcium handling as the kidney develops further remains to be seen. The acute transient calcium losses may, however, be detrimental, especially in premature neonates who have even lower calcium stores and blood calcium levels than term neonates [57].

3.6.2.2 Phosphorus

Phosphate in the major divalent anion in the body and is particularly important during periods of rapid growth. Neonates and children have higher phosphate concentration than adults [23]. Free phosphate in the plasma exists in the forms HPO_4^{2-} and $H_2PO_4^-$ which act as a buffer pair. This non-protein-bound phosphate fraction is freely filtered at the glomerulus and then reabsorbed by the tubule. Phosphate reabsorption kinetics follows a transport maximum (Tm_{Pi}) model so that filtered phosphate in excess of the reabsorption threshold is excreted. The majority

(80 %) of tubular phosphate reabsorption occurs in the proximal tubule by a transcellular process mediated by sodium-phosphate cotransporters on the apical brush border surface of tubular cells. The tubular reabsorption of phosphate (TRP) in older children and adults is around 80–85 % of the filtered load but can be as high as 90–99 % in neonates in the first week of life [69]. Those differences are mirrored by the expression of different sodium-phosphate transporter isoforms in the proximal tubule during kidney development. The most important isoforms for inorganic phosphate reabsorption are two members of the type 2 family: the $2Na^+$-Pi IIa and the $2Na^+$-Pi IIc cotransporters. Human studies suggest the $2Na^+$-Pi IIc isoform is the most relevant in phosphate reabsorption [152]. This isoform has been found to be expressed at higher levels in weaning animals and has reduced function in adults, potentially explaining the developmental changes in TRP values seen in humans [129]. Additionally, the response to parathyroid hormone (PTH) is less pronounced in the first few weeks of life [74]. PTH acts as a phosphaturic hormone promoting phosphate excretion by accelerating the endocytosis of the cotransporters from the brush border membrane to the subapical compartment. FGF-23 acts as a phosphaturic hormone in a similar fashion, in addition to accelerating cotransporter degradation in lysosomes [143].

3.6.2.3 Magnesium

Only 1 % of total body magnesium is found in the extracellular fluid, while the majority is stored in bone and soft tissues. Total plasma magnesium relates inversely to postconceptional age in premature and full-term neonates [77, 148]. Plasma values of the diffusible fraction of plasma magnesium (UFMg), which is not protein bound and is freely filtered, were found to be constant at different gestational ages, despite variation in total plasma magnesium [4].

More than 95 % of filtered magnesium is reabsorbed along the nephron. This process is highly efficient and not affected by postconceptional age in infancy, as demonstrated by a similar fractional excretion of magnesium in both preterm and term neonates [4]. In infants, approximately 70 % of the filtered magnesium load is reabsorbed in the proximal tubule of the developing kidney by paracellular transport. This is in contrast to older children and adults where two-thirds of the filtered load is reabsorbed in the thick ascending limb of the loop of Henle, while the proximal tubule only reabsorbs about 20 % of the filtered load [41]. Absorption at these sites is mediated by passive paracellular transport and involves paracellin-1, which is important in tight junction formation. Maturational changes in tight junction permeability contribute to the changing reabsorption pattern in the proximal tubule and TALH [135]. The remainder (~5 %) of the filtered magnesium load is actively reabsorbed in the distal convoluted tubule through an apical magnesium channel (TRPM6). The autosomal recessive condition termed hypomagnesemia with secondary hypocalcemia is caused by mutations in the TRPM6 channel and presents with severe hypomagnesemia in infancy [161].

References

1. Ammar A, Roseau S, Butlen D (1992) Postnatal ontogenesis of vasopressin receptors in the rat collecting duct. Mol Cell Endocrinol 86(3):193–203
2. Aperia A, Larsson L (1984) Induced development of proximal tubular NaKATPase, basolateral cell membranes and fluid reabsorption. Acta Physiol Scand 121(2):133–141
3. Aperia A, Larsson L, Zetterstrom R (1981) Hormonal induction of Na-K-ATPase in developing proximal tubular cells. Am J Physiol 241(4):F356–F360
4. Ariceta G, Rodriguez-Soriano J, Vallo A (1995) Magnesium homeostasis in premature and full-term neonates. Pediatr Nephrol 9(4):423–427
5. Aronson PS (2006) Ion exchangers mediating Na+, HCO_3 – and Cl– transport in the renal proximal tubule. J Nephrol 19(Suppl 9):S3–S10
6. Atkinson SA, Shah JK, McGee C, Steele BT (1988) Mineral excretion in premature infants receiving various diuretic therapies. J Pediatr 113(3):540–545
7. Balkovetz DF, Leibach FH, Mahesh VB, Devoe LD, Cragoe EJ Jr, Ganapathy V (1986) Na+-H+ exchanger of human placental brush-border membrane: identification and characterization. Am J Physiol 251(6 Pt 1): C852–C860
8. Barac-Nieto M, Corey H, Liu SM, Spitzer A (1993) Role of intracellular phosphate in the regulation of

renal phosphate transport during development. Pediatr Nephrol 7(6):819–822
9. Bauer K, Bovermann G, Roithmaier A, Gotz M, Proiss A, Versmold HT (1991) Body composition, nutrition, and fluid balance during the first two weeks of life in preterm neonates weighing less than 1500 grams. J Pediatr 118(4 Pt 1):615–620
10. Beall MH, Wang S, Yang B, Chaudhri N, Amidi F, Ross MG (2007) Placental and membrane aquaporin water channels: correlation with amniotic fluid volume and composition. Placenta 28(5–6):421–428. doi:10.1016/j.placenta.2006.06.005
11. Beck JC, Lipkowitz MS, Abramson RG (1991) Ontogeny of Na/H antiporter activity in rabbit renal brush border membrane vesicles. J Clin Invest 87(6):2067–2076. doi:10.1172/JCI115237
12. Bertorello AM, Hopfield JF, Aperia A, Greengard P (1990) Inhibition by dopamine of (Na(+) + K+) ATPase activity in neostriatal neurons through D1 and D2 dopamine receptor synergism. Nature 347(6291):386–388. doi:10.1038/347386a0
13. Biemesderfer D, Rutherford PA, Nagy T, Pizzonia JH, Abu-Alfa AK, Aronson PS (1997) Monoclonal antibodies for high-resolution localization of NHE3 in adult and neonatal rat kidney. Am J Physiol 273(2 Pt 2):F289–F299
14. Bierd TM, Kattwinkel J, Chevalier RL, Rheuban KS, Smith DJ, Teague WG, Carey RM, Linden J (1990) Interrelationship of atrial natriuretic peptide, atrial volume, and renal function in premature infants. J Pediatr 116(5):753–759
15. Bistritzer T, Berkovitch M, Rappoport MJ, Evans S, Arieli S, Goldberg M, Tavori I, Aladjem M (1999) Sodium potassium adenosine triphosphatase activity in preterm and term infants and its possible role in sodium homeostasis during maturation. Arch Dis Child Fetal Neonatal Ed 81(3):F184–F187
16. Bonilla-Felix M (2004) Development of water transport in the collecting duct. Am J Physiol Renal Physiol 287(6):F1093–F1101. doi:10.1152/ajprenal.00119.2004
17. Bonilla-Felix M, John-Phillip C (1994) Prostaglandins mediate the defect in AVP-stimulated cAMP generation in immature collecting duct. Am J Physiol 267(1 Pt 2):F44–F48
18. Bonilla-Felix M, Vehaskari VM, Hamm LL (1999) Water transport in the immature rabbit collecting duct. Pediatr Nephrol 13(2):103–107
19. Brace RA (1987) Fetal blood volume responses to fetal haemorrhage: autonomic nervous contribution. J Dev Physiol 9(2):97–103
20. Brace RA, Cheung CY (1987) Role of catecholamines in mediating fetal blood volume decrease during acute hypoxia. Am J Physiol 253(4 Pt 2):H927–H932
21. Brace RA, Moore TR (1991) Transplacental, amniotic, urinary, and fetal fluid dynamics during very-large-volume fetal intravenous infusions. Am J Obstet Gynecol 164(3):907–916
22. Brant SR, Bernstein M, Wasmuth JJ, Taylor EW, McPherson JD, Li X, Walker S, Pouyssegur J, Donowitz M, Tse CM et al (1993) Physical and genetic mapping of a human apical epithelial Na+/H+ exchanger (NHE3) isoform to chromosome 5p15.3. Genomics 15(3):668–672
23. Brodehl J, Gellissen K, Weber HP (1982) Postnatal development of tubular phosphate reabsorption. Clin Nephrol 17(4):163–171
24. Brooks HL, Sorensen AM, Terris J, Schultheis PJ, Lorenz JN, Shull GE, Knepper MA (2001) Profiling of renal tubule Na+ transporter abundances in NHE3 and NCC null mice using targeted proteomics. J Physiol 530(Pt 3):359–366
25. Brown RW, Diaz R, Robson AC, Kotelevtsev YV, Mullins JJ, Kaufman MH, Seckl JR (1996) The ontogeny of 11 beta-hydroxysteroid dehydrogenase type 2 and mineralocorticoid receptor gene expression reveal intricate control of glucocorticoid action in development. Endocrinology 137(2):794–797
26. Canessa CM, Schild L, Buell G, Thorens B, Gautschi I, Horisberger JD, Rossier BC (1994) Amiloride-sensitive epithelial Na+ channel is made of three homologous subunits. Nature 367(6462):463–467. doi:10.1038/367463a0
27. Care AD (1991) The placental transfer of calcium. J Dev Physiol 15(5):253–257
28. Celsi G, Larsson L, Aperia A (1986) Proximal tubular reabsorption and Na-K-ATPase activity in remnant kidney of young rats. Am J Physiol 251(4 Pt 2):F588–F593
29. Cha JH, Kim YH, Jung JY, Han KH, Madsen KM, Kim J (2001) Cell proliferation in the loop of henle in the developing rat kidney. J Am Soc Nephrol 12(7):1410–1421
30. Cheek DB, Wishart J, MacLennan AH, Haslam R (1984) Cell hydration in the normally grown, the premature and the low weight for gestational age infant. Early Hum Dev 10(1–2):75–84
31. Chevalier RL (1993) Atrial natriuretic peptide in renal development. Pediatr Nephrol 7(5):652–656
32. Comline RS, Silver M (1972) The composition of foetal and maternal blood during parturition in the ewe. J Physiol 222(1):233–256
33. Constantinescu A, Silver RB, Satlin LM (1997) H-K-ATPase activity in PNA-binding intercalated cells of newborn rabbit cortical collecting duct. Am J Physiol 272(2 Pt 2):F167–F177
34. Coulter DM (1984) Differing effects of prolactin on the water content of individual tissues in the rabbit pup at 72 h of age. Biol Neonate 46(3):131–138
35. Counillon L, Pouyssegur J (2000) The expanding family of eucaryotic Na(+)/H(+) exchangers. J Biol Chem 275(1):1–4
36. Counillon L, Touret N, Bidet M, Peterson-Yantorno K, Coca-Prados M, Stuart-Tilley A, Wilhelm S, Alper SL, Civan MM (2000) Na+/H+ and CI-/HCO3-antiporters of bovine pigmented ciliary epithelial cells. Pflug Arch 440(5):667–678
37. Damiano A, Zotta E, Goldstein J, Reisin I, Ibarra C (2001) Water channel proteins AQP3 and AQP9 are present in syncytiotrophoblast of human term

placenta. Placenta 22(8–9):776–781. doi:10.1053/plac.2001.0717
38. Dancis J, Kammerman S, Jansen V, Schneider H, Levitz M (1981) Transfer of urea, sodium, and chloride across the perfused human placenta. Am J Obstet Gynecol 141(6):677–681
39. Dancis J, Springer D (1970) Fetal homeostasis in maternal malnutrition: potassium and sodium deficiency in rats. Pediatr Res 4(4):345–351. doi:10.1203/00006450-197007000-00005
40. David L, Anast CS (1974) Calcium metabolism in newborn infants. The interrelationship of parathyroid function and calcium, magnesium, and phosphorus metabolism in normal, "sick," and hypocalcemic newborns. J Clin Invest 54(2):287–296. doi:10.1172/JCI107764
41. de Rouffignac C, Quamme G (1994) Renal magnesium handling and its hormonal control. Physiol Rev 74(2):305–322
42. Delivoria-Papadopoulos M, Battaglia FC, Meschia G (1969) A comparison of fetal versus maternal plasma colloidal osmotic pressure im man. Proc Soc Exp Biol Med 131(1):84–87
43. Dickerson JW, Widdowson EM (1960) Chemical changes in skeletal muscle during development. Biochem J 74:247–257
44. Doucet A (1988) Function and control of Na-K-ATPase in single nephron segments of the mammalian kidney. Kidney Int 34(6):749–760
45. Duc C, Farman N, Canessa CM, Bonvalet JP, Rossier BC (1994) Cell-specific expression of epithelial sodium channel alpha, beta, and gamma subunits in aldosterone-responsive epithelia from the rat: localization by in situ hybridization and immunocytochemistry. J Cell Biol 127(6 Pt 2):1907–1921
46. Eaton DC, Malik B, Saxena NC, Al-Khalili OK, Yue G (2001) Mechanisms of aldosterone's action on epithelial Na+ transport. J Membr Biol 184(3):313–319. doi:10.1007/s00232-001-0098-x
47. Edelmann CM, Barnett HL, Troupkou V (1960) Renal concentrating mechanisms in newborn infants. Effect of dietary protein and water content, role of urea, and responsiveness to antidiuretic hormone. J Clin Invest 39:1062–1069. doi:10.1172/JCI104121
48. Flexner LB, Cowie DB et al (1948) The permeability of the human placenta to sodium in normal and abnormal pregnancies and the supply of sodium to the human fetus as determined with radioactive sodium. Am J Obstet Gynecol 55(3):469–480
49. Forrest JN Jr, Stanier MW (1966) Kidney composition and renal concentration ability in young rabbits. J Physiol 187(1):1–4
50. Friedlander G, Amiel C (1994) Cellular mode of action of parathyroid hormone. Adv Nephrol Necker Hosp 23:265–279
51. Friedman PA (2000) Mechanisms of renal calcium transport. Exp Nephrol 8(6):343–350. doi:20688 [pii]
52. Friis-Hansen B (1961) Body water compartments in children: changes during growth and related changes in body composition. Pediatrics 28:169–181
53. Friis-Hansen B (1971) Body composition during growth. In vivo measurements and biochemical data correlated to differential anatomical growth. Pediatrics 47(1):Suppl 2:264+
54. Friis-Hansen B (1983) Water distribution in the foetus and newborn infant. Acta Paediatr Scand Suppl 305:7–11
55. Fushimi K, Sasaki S, Marumo F (1997) Phosphorylation of serine 256 is required for cAMP-dependent regulatory exocytosis of the aquaporin-2 water channel. J Biol Chem 272(23):14800–14804
56. Fushimi K, Uchida S, Hara Y, Hirata Y, Marumo F, Sasaki S (1993) Cloning and expression of apical membrane water channel of rat kidney collecting tubule. Nature 361(6412):549–552. doi:10.1038/361549a0
57. Giapros VI, Cholevas VI, Andronikou SK (2004) Acute effects of gentamicin on urinary electrolyte excretion in neonates. Pediatr Nephrol 19(3):322–325. doi:10.1007/s00467-003-1381-0
58. Giebisch G (1998) Renal potassium transport: mechanisms and regulation. Am J Physiol 274(5 Pt 2): F817–F833
59. Gkika D, Hsu YJ, van der Kemp AW, Christakos S, Bindels RJ, Hoenderop JG (2006) Critical role of the epithelial Ca2+ channel TRPV5 in active Ca2+ reabsorption as revealed by TRPV5/calbindin-D28K knockout mice. J Am Soc Nephrol 17(11):3020–3027. ASN.2006060676 [pii], doi:10.1681/ASN.2006060676
60. Goetz KL (1988) Physiology and pathophysiology of atrial peptides. Am J Physiol 254(1 Pt 1):E1–E15
61. Gozzo ML, Noia G, Barbaresi G, Colacicco L, Serraino MA, De Santis M, Lippa S, Calla C, Caruso A, Mancuso S, Giardina B (1998) Reference intervals for 18 clinical chemistry analytes in fetal plasma samples between 18 and 40 weeks of pregnancy. Clin Chem 44(3):683–685
62. Grantham JJ, Burg MB (1966) Effect of vasopressin and cyclic AMP on permeability of isolated collecting tubules. Am J Physiol 211(1):255–259
63. Gruskay J, Costarino AT, Polin RA, Baumgart S (1988) Nonoliguric hyperkalemia in the premature infant weighing less than 1000 grams. J Pediatr 113(2):381–386
64. Guillery EN, Karniski LP, Mathews MS, Robillard JE (1994) Maturation of proximal tubule Na+/H+ antiporter activity in sheep during transition from fetus to newborn. Am J Physiol 267(4 Pt 2):F537–F545
65. Hadeed AJ, Leake RD, Weitzman RE, Fisher DA (1979) Possible mechanisms of high blood levels of vasopressin during the neonatal period. J Pediatr 94(5):805–808
66. Hammerman MR, Karl IE, Hruska KA (1980) Regulation of canine renal vesicle Pi transport by growth hormone and parathyroid hormone. Biochim Biophys Acta 603(2):322–335
67. Haycock GB (1993) The influence of sodium on growth in infancy. Pediatr Nephrol 7(6):871–875
68. Heimler R, Doumas BT, Jendrzejczak BM, Nemeth PB, Hoffman RG, Nelin LD (1993) Relationship

between nutrition, weight change, and fluid compartments in preterm infants during the first week of life. J Pediatr 122(1):110–114
69. Hohenauer L, Rosenberg TF, Oh W (1970) Calcium and phosphorus homeostasis on the first day of life. Biol Neonate 15(12):49–56
70. Holtback U, Aperia AC (2003) Molecular determinants of sodium and water balance during early human development. Semin Neonatol 8(4):291–299. doi:10.1016/S1084-2756(03)00042-3
71. Horster M (1978) Loop of Henle functional differentiation: in vitro perfusion of the isolated thick ascending segment. Pflug Arch 378(1):15–24
72. Hsu SC, Levine MA (2004) Perinatal calcium metabolism: physiology and pathophysiology. Semin Neonatol 9(1):23–36. doi:10.1016/j.siny.2003.10.002, S1084275603001593 [pii]
73. Hughes JL, Doughty IM, Glazier JD, Powell TL, Jansson T, D'Souza SW, Sibley CP (2000) Activity and expression of the Na(+)/H(+) exchanger in the microvillous plasma membrane of the syncytiotrophoblast in relation to gestation and small for gestational age birth. Pediatr Res 48(5):652–659. doi:10.1203/00006450-200011000-00017
74. Imbert-Teboul M, Chabardes D, Clique A, Montegut M, Morel F (1984) Ontogenesis of hormone-dependent adenylate cyclase in isolated rat nephron segments. Am J Physiol 247(2 Pt 2):F316–F325
75. Jansson T, Powell TL, Illsley NP (1999) Gestational development of water and non-electrolyte permeability of human syncytiotrophoblast plasma membranes. Placenta 20(2–3):155–160. doi:10.1053/plac.1998.0371
76. Johansson M, Glazier JD, Sibley CP, Jansson T, Powell TL (2002) Activity and protein expression of the Na+/H+ exchanger is reduced in syncytiotrophoblast microvillous plasma membranes isolated from preterm intrauterine growth restriction pregnancies. J Clin Endocrinol Metab 87(12):5686–5694
77. Jukarainen E (1971) Plasma magnesium levels during the first five days of life. Acta Paediatr Scand Suppl 222:1–58
78. Karimu AL, Burton GJ (1994) The effects of maternal vascular pressure on the dimensions of the placental capillaries. Br J Obstet Gynaecol 101(1):57–63
79. Kim YH, Kim DU, Han KH, Jung JY, Sands JM, Knepper MA, Madsen KM, Kim J (2002) Expression of urea transporters in the developing rat kidney. Am J Physiol Renal Physiol 282(3):F530–F540. doi:10.1152/ajprenal.00246.2001
80. Knepper MA, Nielsen S, Chou CL, DiGiovanni SR (1994) Mechanism of vasopressin action in the renal collecting duct. Semin Nephrol 14(4):302–321
81. Kovacs CS, Kronenberg HM (1997) Maternal-fetal calcium and bone metabolism during pregnancy, puerperium, and lactation. Endocr Rev 18(6):832–872
82. Lajeunesse D, Brunette MG (1988) Sodium gradient-dependent phosphate transport in placental brush border membrane vesicles. Placenta 9(2):117–128
83. Lelievre-Pegorier M, Merlet-Benichou C, Roinel N, de Rouffignac C (1983) Developmental pattern of water and electrolyte transport in rat superficial nephrons. Am J Physiol 245(1):F15–F21
84. Linderkamp O (1982) Placental transfusion: determinants and effects. Clin Perinatol 9(3):559–592
85. Liu H, Koukoulas I, Ross MC, Wang S, Wintour EM (2004) Quantitative comparison of placental expression of three aquaporin genes. Placenta 25(6):475–478. doi:10.1016/j.placenta.2003.10.008
86. Liu H, Wintour EM (2005) Aquaporins in development – a review. Reprod Biol Endocrinol 3:18. doi:10.1186/1477-7827-3-18
87. Liu W, Morimoto T, Kondo Y, Iinuma K, Uchida S, Imai M (2001) "Avian-type" renal medullary tubule organization causes immaturity of urine-concentrating ability in neonates. Kidney Int 60(2):680–693. doi:10.1046/j.1523-1755.2001.060002680.x
88. Lorenz JM (1997) Assessing fluid and electrolyte status in the newborn. Natl Acad Clin Biochem Clin Chem 43(1):205–210
89. Lorenz JM, Kleinman LI, Markarian K (1997) Potassium metabolism in extremely low birth weight infants in the first week of life. J Pediatr 131(1 Pt 1):81–86. doi:S002234769700262X [pii]
90. Macknight AD, Leaf A (1977) Regulation of cellular volume. Physiol Rev 57(3):510–573
91. Mahendran D, Byrne S, Donnai P, D'Souza SW, Glazier JD, Jones CJ, Sibley CP (1994) Na+ transport, H+ concentration gradient dissipation, and system A amino acid transporter activity in purified microvillous plasma membrane isolated from first-trimester human placenta: comparison with the term microvillous membrane. Am J Obstet Gynecol 171(6):1534–1540
92. Malone TA (1991) Glucose and insulin versus cation-exchange resin for the treatment of hyperkalemia in very low birth weight infants. J Pediatr 118(1):121–123
93. Mann SE, Dvorak N, Gilbert H, Taylor RN (2006) Steady-state levels of aquaporin 1 mRNA expression are increased in idiopathic polyhydramnios. Am J Obstet Gynecol 194(3):884–887. doi:10.1016/j.ajog.2005.07.004
94. Mann SE, Ricke EA, Torres EA, Taylor RN (2005) A novel model of polyhydramnios: amniotic fluid volume is increased in aquaporin 1 knockout mice. Am J Obstet Gynecol 192(6):2041–2044; discussion 2044–2046. doi:10.1016/j.ajog.2005.02.046
95. Mann SE, Ricke EA, Yang BA, Verkman AS, Taylor RN (2002) Expression and localization of aquaporin 1 and 3 in human fetal membranes. Am J Obstet Gynecol 187(4):902–907
96. Martinerie L, Pussard E, Foix-L'Helias L, Petit F, Cosson C, Boileau P, Lombes M (2009) Physiological partial aldosterone resistance in human newborns. Pediatr Res 66(3):323–328. doi:10.1203/PDR.0b013e3181b1bbec
97. Martinerie L, Viengchareun S, Delezoide AL, Jaubert F, Sinico M, Prevot S, Boileau P, Meduri G, Lombes M (2009) Low renal mineralocorticoid receptor expression at birth contributes to partial aldosterone resistance in neonates. Endocrinology 150(9):4414–4424. en.2008-1498 [pii], doi:10.1210/en.2008-1498

98. McDonough AA, Brown TA, Horowitz B, Chiu R, Schlotterbeck J, Bowen J, Schmitt CA (1988) Thyroid hormone coordinately regulates Na+-K+-ATPase alpha- and beta-subunit mRNA levels in kidney. Am J Physiol 254(2 Pt 1):C323–C329
99. Moe AJ, Smith CH (1989) Anionic amino acid uptake by microvillous membrane vesicles from human placenta. Am J Physiol 257(5 Pt 1):C1005–C1011
100. Moniz CF, Nicolaides KH, Tzannatos C, Rodeck CH (1986) Calcium homeostasis in second trimester fetuses. J Clin Pathol 39(8):838–841
101. Nakamura K, Stokes JB, McCray PB Jr (2002) Endogenous and exogenous glucocorticoid regulation of ENaC mRNA expression in developing kidney and lung. Am J Physiol Cell Physiol 283(3):C762–C772. doi:10.1152/ajpcell.00029.2002
102. Namgung R, Tsang RC (2003) Bone in the pregnant mother and newborn at birth. Clin Chim Acta 333(1):1–11. doi:S0009898102000256 [pii]
103. Nielsen S, Chou CL, Marples D, Christensen EI, Kishore BK, Knepper MA (1995) Vasopressin increases water permeability of kidney collecting duct by inducing translocation of aquaporin-CD water channels to plasma membrane. Proc Natl Acad Sci U S A 92(4):1013–1017
104. Obermuller N, Bernstein P, Velazquez H, Reilly R, Moser D, Ellison DH, Bachmann S (1995) Expression of the thiazide-sensitive Na-Cl cotransporter in rat and human kidney. Am J Physiol 269(6 Pt 2):F900–F910
105. Ostrowski NL, Young WS 3rd, Knepper MA, Lolait SJ (1993) Expression of vasopressin V1a and V2 receptor messenger ribonucleic acid in the liver and kidney of embryonic, developing, and adult rats. Endocrinology 133(4):1849–1859
106. Palmer LG (1999) Potassium secretion and the regulation of distal nephron K channels. Am J Physiol 277(6 Pt 2):F821–F825
107. Persson A, Johansson M, Jansson T, Powell TL (2002) Na(+)/K(+)-ATPase activity and expression in syncytiotrophoblast plasma membranes in pregnancies complicated by diabetes. Placenta 23(5):386–391. doi:10.1053/plac.2002.0807
108. Peters M, Jeck N, Reinalter S, Leonhardt A, Tonshoff B, Klaus GG, Konrad M, Seyberth HW (2002) Clinical presentation of genetically defined patients with hypokalemic salt-losing tubulopathies. Am J Med 112(3):183–190. doi:S0002934301010865 [pii]
109. Pitkin RM (1985) Calcium metabolism in pregnancy and the perinatal period: a review. Am J Obstet Gynecol 151(1):99–109. doi:0002-9378(85)90434-X [pii]
110. Polacek E, Vocel J, Neugebauerova L, Sebkova M, Vechetova E (1965) The osmotic concentrating ability in healthy infants and children. Arch Dis Child 40:291–295
111. Quaggin SE, Payne JA, Forbush B 3rd, Igarashi P (1995) Localization of the renal Na-K-Cl cotransporter gene (Slc12a1) on mouse chromosome 2. Mamm Genome Off J Int Mamm Genome Soc 6(8):557–558
112. Quan A, Baum M (1998) Endogenous angiotensin II modulates rat proximal tubule transport with acute changes in extracellular volume. Am J Physiol 275(1 Pt 2):F74–F78
113. Quigley R, Chakravarty S, Baum M (2004) Antidiuretic hormone resistance in the neonatal cortical collecting tubule is mediated in part by elevated phosphodiesterase activity. Am J Physiol Renal Physiol 286(2):F317–F322. doi:10.1152/ajprenal.00122.2003
114. Rajerison RM, Butlen D, Jard S (1976) Ontogenic development of antidiuretic hormone receptors in rat kidney: comparison of hormonal binding and adenylate cyclase activation. Mol Cell Endocrinol 4(4):271–285
115. Rane S, Aperia A (1985) Ontogeny of Na-K-ATPase activity in thick ascending limb and of concentrating capacity. Am J Physiol 249(5 Pt 2):F723–F728
116. Rees L, Forsling ML, Brook CG (1980) Vasopressin concentrations in the neonatal period. Clin Endocrinol 12(4):357–362
117. Rodriguez-Soriano J, Ubetagoyena M, Vallo A (1990) Transtubular potassium concentration gradient: a useful test to estimate renal aldosterone bio-activity in infants and children. Pediatr Nephrol 4(2):105–110
118. Rodriguez-Soriano J, Vallo A, Oliveros R, Castillo G (1983) Renal handling of sodium in premature and full-term neonates: a study using clearance methods during water diuresis. Pediatr Res 17(12):1013–1016
119. Rodriguez G, Ventura P, Samper MP, Moreno L, Sarria A, Perez-Gonzalez JM (2000) Changes in body composition during the initial hours of life in breast-fed healthy term newborns. Biol Neonate 77(1):12–16
120. Sagnella GA, MacGregor GA (1984) Physiology: cardiac peptides and the control of sodium excretion. Nature 309(5970):666–667
121. Sands JM, Nonoguchi H, Knepper MA (1987) Vasopressin effects on urea and H_2O transport in inner medullary collecting duct subsegments. Am J Physiol 253(5 Pt 2):F823–F832
122. Satlin LM (1994) Postnatal maturation of potassium transport in rabbit cortical collecting duct. Am J Physiol 266(1 Pt 2):F57–F65
123. Sato K, Kondo T, Iwao H, Honda S, Ueda K (1995) Internal potassium shift in premature infants: cause of nonoliguric hyperkalemia. J Pediatr 126(1):109–113. doi:S0022-3476(95)70511-2 [pii]
124. Schauberger CW, Pitkin RM (1979) Maternal-perinatal calcium relationships. Obstet Gynecol 53(1):74–76
125. Schmidt U, Horster M (1977) Na-K-activated ATPase: activity maturation in rabbit nephron segments dissected in vitro. Am J Physiol 233(1): F55–F60
126. Schmitt R, Ellison DH, Farman N, Rossier BC, Reilly RF, Reeves WB, Oberbaumer I, Tapp R, Bachmann S (1999) Developmental expression of sodium entry pathways in rat nephron. Am J Physiol 276(3 Pt 2):F367–F381

127. Schroder H, Leichtweiss HP (1977) Perfusion rates and the transfer of water across isolated guinea pig placenta. Am J Physiol 232(6):H666–H670
128. Schwartz GJ, Evan AP (1984) Development of solute transport in rabbit proximal tubule. III. Na-K-ATPase activity. Am J Physiol 246(6 Pt 2): F845–F852
129. Segawa H, Kaneko I, Takahashi A, Kuwahata M, Ito M, Ohkido I, Tatsumi S, Miyamoto K (2002) Growth-related renal type II Na/Pi cotransporter. J Biol Chem 277(22):19665–19672. doi:10.1074/jbc.M200943200, M200943200 [pii]
130. Serrano CV, Talbert LM, Welt LG (1964) Potassium deficiency in the pregnant dog. J Clin Invest 43:27–31. doi:10.1172/JCI104890
131. Shaffer SG, Quimiro CL, Anderson JV, Hall RT (1987) Postnatal weight changes in low birth weight infants. Pediatrics 79(5):702–705
132. Shah M, Gupta N, Dwarakanath V, Moe OW, Baum M (2000) Ontogeny of Na+/H+ antiporter activity in rat proximal convoluted tubules. Pediatr Res 48(2):206–210. doi:10.1203/00006450-200008000-00014
133. Simon DB, Karet FE, Hamdan JM, DiPietro A, Sanjad SA, Lifton RP (1996) Bartter's syndrome, hypokalaemic alkalosis with hypercalciuria, is caused by mutations in the Na-K-2Cl cotransporter NKCC2. Nat Genet 13(2):183–188. doi:10.1038/ng0696-183
134. Simon DB, Lu Y, Choate KA, Velazquez H, Al-Sabban E, Praga M, Casari G, Bettinelli A, Colussi G, Rodriguez-Soriano J, McCredie D, Milford D, Sanjad S, Lifton RP (1999) Paracellin-1, a renal tight junction protein required for paracellular Mg2+ resorption. Science 285(5424):103–106. doi:7616 [pii]
135. Singh BS, Sadiq HF, Noguchi A, Keenan WJ (2002) Efficacy of albuterol inhalation in treatment of hyperkalemia in premature neonates. J Pediatr 141(1):-16–20. S0022-3476(02)00032-X [pii], doi:10.1067/mpd.2002.125229
136. Speller AM, Moffat DB (1977) Tubulo-vascular relationships in the developing kidney. J Anat 123(Pt 2):487–500
137. Spitzer A (1982) The role of the kidney in sodium homeostasis during maturation. Kidney Int 21(4): 539–545
138. Spitzer A, Barac-Nieto M (2001) Ontogeny of renal phosphate transport and the process of growth. Pediatr Nephrol 16(9):763–771. doi:10.1007/s004670100763
139. Stefano JL, Norman ME, Morales MC, Goplerud JM, Mishra OP, Delivoria-Papadopoulos M (1993) Decreased erythrocyte Na+, K(+)-ATPase activity associated with cellular potassium loss in extremely low birth weight infants with nonoliguric hyperkalemia. J Pediatr 122(2):276–284
140. Stulc J (1997) Placental transfer of inorganic ions and water. Physiol Rev 77(3):805–836
141. Stulc J, Stulcova B, Sibley CP (1993) Evidence for active maternal-fetal transport of Na+ across the placenta of the anaesthetized rat. J Physiol 470:637–649
142. Tiosano D, Hochberg Z (2009) Hypophosphatemia: the common denominator of all rickets. J Bone Miner Metab 27(4):392–401. doi:10.1007/s00774-009-0079-1
143. Tomita H, Brace RA, Cheung CY, Longo LD (1985) Vasopressin dose–response effects on fetal vascular pressures, heart rate, and blood volume. Am J Physiol 249(5 Pt 2):H974–H980
144. Tsang RC, Chen IW, Friedman MA, Chen I (1973) Neonatal parathyroid function: role of gestational age and postnatal age. J Pediatr 83(5):728–738
145. Tsang RC, Kleinman LI, Sutherland JM, Light IJ (1972) Hypocalcemia in infants of diabetic mothers. Studies in calcium, phosphorus, and magnesium metabolism and parathormone responsiveness. J Pediatr 80(3):384–395
146. Tsang RC, Light IJ, Sutherland JM, Kleinman LI (1973) Possible pathogenetic factors in neonatal hypocalcemia of prematurity. The role of gestation, hyperphosphatemia, hypomagnesemia, urinary calcium loss, and parathormone responsiveness. J Pediatr 82(3):423–429
147. Tsang RC, Oh W (1970) Serum magnesium levels in low birth weight infants. Am J Dis Child 120(1):44–48
148. Tulassay T, Seri I, Rascher W (1987) Atrial natriuretic peptide and extracellular volume contraction after birth. Acta Paediatr Scand 76(3):444–446
149. Vanpee M, Herin P, Zetterstrom R, Aperia A (1988) Postnatal development of renal function in very low birthweight infants. Acta Paediatr Scand 77(2):191–197
150. Vehaskari VM (1994) Ontogeny of cortical collecting duct sodium transport. Am J Physiol 267(1 Pt 2):F49–F54
151. Wagner CA, Biber J, Murer H (2008) Of men and mice: who is in control of renal phosphate reabsorption? J Am Soc Nephrol 19(9):1625–1626. ASN.2008060611 [pii], doi:10.1681/ASN.2008060611
152. Wandrup J, Kroner J, Pryds O, Kastrup KW (1988) Age-related reference values for ionized calcium in the first week of life in premature and full-term neonates. Scand J Clin Lab Invest 48(3):255–260
153. Wang S, Kallichanda N, Song W, Ramirez BA, Ross MG (2001) Expression of aquaporin-8 in human placenta and chorioamniotic membranes: evidence of molecular mechanism for intramembranous amniotic fluid resorption. Am J Obstet Gynecol 185(5):1226–1231. doi:10.1067/mob.2001.117971
154. Whitsett JA, Wallick ET (1980) [3H]ouabain binding and Na+-K+-ATPase activity in human placenta. Am J Physiol 238(1):E38–E45
155. Wilkinson AW (1973) Some aspects of renal function in the newly born. J Pediatr Surg 8(2):103–116
156. Woda C, Mulroney SE, Halaihel N, Sun L, Wilson PV, Levi M, Haramati A (2001) Renal tubular sites of increased phosphate transport and NaPi-2 expression in the juvenile rat. Am J Physiol Regul Integr Comp Physiol 280(5):R1524–R1533

157. Woda CB, Bragin A, Kleyman TR, Satlin LM (2001) Flow-dependent K+ secretion in the cortical collecting duct is mediated by a maxi-K channel. Am J Physiol Renal Physiol 280(5):F786–F793
158. Woda CB, Miyawaki N, Ramalakshmi S, Ramkumar M, Rojas R, Zavilowitz B, Kleyman TR, Satlin LM (2003) Ontogeny of flow-stimulated potassium secretion in rabbit cortical collecting duct: functional and molecular aspects. Am J Physiol Renal Physiol 285(4):F629–F639. doi:10.1152/ajprenal.00191.2003, 00191.2003 [pii]
159. Wood CE, Cheung CY, Brace RA (1987) Fetal heart rate, arterial pressure, and blood volume responses to cortisol infusion. Am J Physiol 253(6 Pt 2):R904–R909
160. Xi Q, Hoenderop JG, Bindels RJ (2009) Regulation of magnesium reabsorption in DCT. Pflug Arch 458(1):89–98. doi:10.1007/s00424-008-0601-7
161. Zhou H, Satlin LM (2004) Renal potassium handling in healthy and sick newborns. Semin Perinatol 28(2):103–111
162. Zhou H, Tate SS, Palmer LG (1994) Primary structure and functional properties of an epithelial K channel. Am J Physiol 266(3 Pt 1):C809–C824
163. Ziegler EE, O'Donnell AM, Nelson SE, Fomon SJ (1976) Body composition of the reference fetus. Growth 40(4):329–341
164. Zink H, Horster M (1977) Maturation of diluting capacity in loop of Henle of rat superficial nephrons. Am J Physiol 233(6):F519–F524
165. Zolotnitskaya A, Satlin LM (1999) Developmental expression of ROMK in rat kidney. Am J Physiol 276(6 Pt 2):F825–F836

4 Electrolyte Disorders in the Newborn

Michael L. Moritz

4.1 Hyponatremia

> **Core Messages**
> - Hyponatremia typically results from a combination of arginine vasopressin excess plus free water intake.
> - 3 % sodium chloride is the most effective therapy for treating hyponatremic encephalopathy.

> **Case Vignette**
> A 4-kg 2-week-old child is admitted to the hospital for severe bronchiolitis with hypoxia and tachypnea. The child is placed on parenteral fluids with 0.225 % sodium chloride (39 mEq/L) in 5 % dextrose in water at a rate of 16 mL/h. Twenty-four hours following admission, the child suffers a generalized tonic-clonic seizure. Biochemistries reveal serum sodium 122 mEq/L, potassium 4 mEq/L, blood urea nitrogen 2 mg/dL, creatinine 0.2 mg/dL, osmolality 238 mOsm/kg H_2O, urine osmolality 400 mOsm/kg H_2O, and urine sodium plus potassium concentration 90 mEq/L.

M.L. Moritz, MD
Division of Nephrology, Children's Hospital of Pittsburgh of UPMC, 4401 Penn Ave, Pittsburgh, PA 15224, USA
e-mail: moritzml@upmc.edu

4.1.1 Introduction

Hyponatremia is defined as a serum sodium level <135 mEq/L [1]. It is one of the most common electrolyte disorders encountered in the newborn in both the outpatient and inpatient setting. The cause is usually easily identified by history, but in many cases, it can be elusive. Hyponatremia has typically been viewed as relatively benign condition, but there is increasing evidence in both children and adults suggesting that hyponatremia is a serious condition [2]. Numerous studies in adults have revealed that even mild and asymptomatic hyponatremia is an independent predictor of mortality [3]. Studies in neonates have revealed that hyponatremia is an independent predictor of poor neuromotor outcome and has been associated with impaired neonatal growth and development, sensorineural hearing loss, cerebral palsy, and intracranial hemorrhages [4, 5]. The most serious complication of hyponatremia is that of hyponatremic encephalopathy. Increasing evidence has revealed that the majority of hyponatremic encephalopathy in children is iatrogenic and related to errors in parenteral fluid therapy [6].

4.1.2 Pathogenesis of Hyponatremia

Under normal circumstances, the human body can maintain plasma sodium levels within the normal range (135–145 mEq/L [135–145 mmol/L]), despite wide fluctuations in fluid intake. The

A.S. Chishti et al. (eds.), *Kidney and Urinary Tract Diseases in the Newborn*,
DOI 10.1007/978-3-642-39988-6_4, © Springer-Verlag Berlin Heidelberg 2014

Table 4.1 Causes of hyponatremia in the newborn

1. Water intoxication: improperly mixed infant formula
2. Gastrointestinal losses (a) Diarrheal dehydration, congenital chloride diarrhea, intestinal fistulas (b) Vomiting, pyloric stenosis, nasogastric suction
3. Skin losses: cystic fibrosis
4. Renal losses (a) Salt-wasting nephropathy (i) Bartter syndrome/Gitelman syndrome (ii) Renal tubular acidosis/Fanconi syndrome (iii) Nephronophthisis diuretics (b) Mineralocorticoid deficiency (i) Congenital adrenal hyperplasia (ii) Bilateral adrenal hemorrhage (c) Mineralocorticoid resistance (i) Pseudohypoaldosteronism type 1 (ii) Obstructive uropathy (iii) Pyelonephritis (d) Diuretics (e) Cerebral salt wasting (f) Hyponatremic hypertensive syndrome (g) Polyuric phase of acute kidney injury
5. Edematous states (a) Heart failure (b) Cirrhosis (c) Nephrotic syndrome
6. Decrease peripheral vascular resistance (a) Sepsis (b) Hypothyroidism
7. Renal failure (a) Acute (b) Chronic
8. Non-hypovolemic states of ADH excess (a) SIADH (Table 4.2) (b) Postoperative state (c) Nausea, vomiting (d) Pain, stress (e) Glucocorticoid deficiency
9. Nephrogenic syndrome of inappropriate antidiuresis (NSIAD)

body's primary defense against developing hyponatremia is the kidney's ability to generate dilute urine and excrete free water. The primary reasons that children develop hyponatremia encompass underlying conditions that impair the kidney's ability to excrete free water (Table 4.1). Hyponatremia usually occurs in the setting of excess water intake, with or without sodium losses, in the presence of impaired free water excretion. The most common reason for impaired free water excretion is due to arginine vasopressin (AVP) excess. There are numerous hemodynamic and non-hemodynamic stimuli for AVP excess that place virtually all hospitalized patients at risk for developing hyponatremia. Common causes of AVP production are volume depletion, pain, stress, nausea, vomiting, pulmonary disorders, the postoperative state, central nervous system (CNS) disorders, edematous states, and narcotic use. Only under the most extreme circumstances can excess water intake or sodium loss alone lead to hyponatremia in the absence of impaired free water excretion.

4.1.3 Diagnostic Approach

Before embarking on an aggressive therapeutic regimen, it is vital to confirm that hyponatremia is in fact associated with hypoosmolality. Hyponatremia can be associated with either a normal or an elevated serum osmolality (Fig. 4.1). The most common reasons for this are hyperglycemia, severe hyperproteinemia, or hyperlipidemia [7]. Hyperglycemia results in hyperosmolality with a translocation of fluid from the intracellular space to the extracellular space, resulting in a 1.6 mEq/L fall in the serum sodium for every 100 mg/dL elevation in the serum glucose concentration above normal. Severe hyperlipidemia, hypercholesterolemia, hyperproteinemia, or radiocontrast can cause a displacement of plasma water, which will result in a decreased sodium concentration (pseudohyponatremia) with a normal serum osmolality. Serum sodiums are currently measured by either direct or indirect-reading ion-selective electrode potentiometry. The direct method will not result in pseudohyponatremia, as it measures the activity of sodium in the aqueous phase of serum only. The indirect method, on the other hand, can result in pseudohyponatremia as the specimen is diluted with a reagent prior to measurement. The indirect method is currently performed in approximately 60 % of chemistry labs in the United States; therefore,

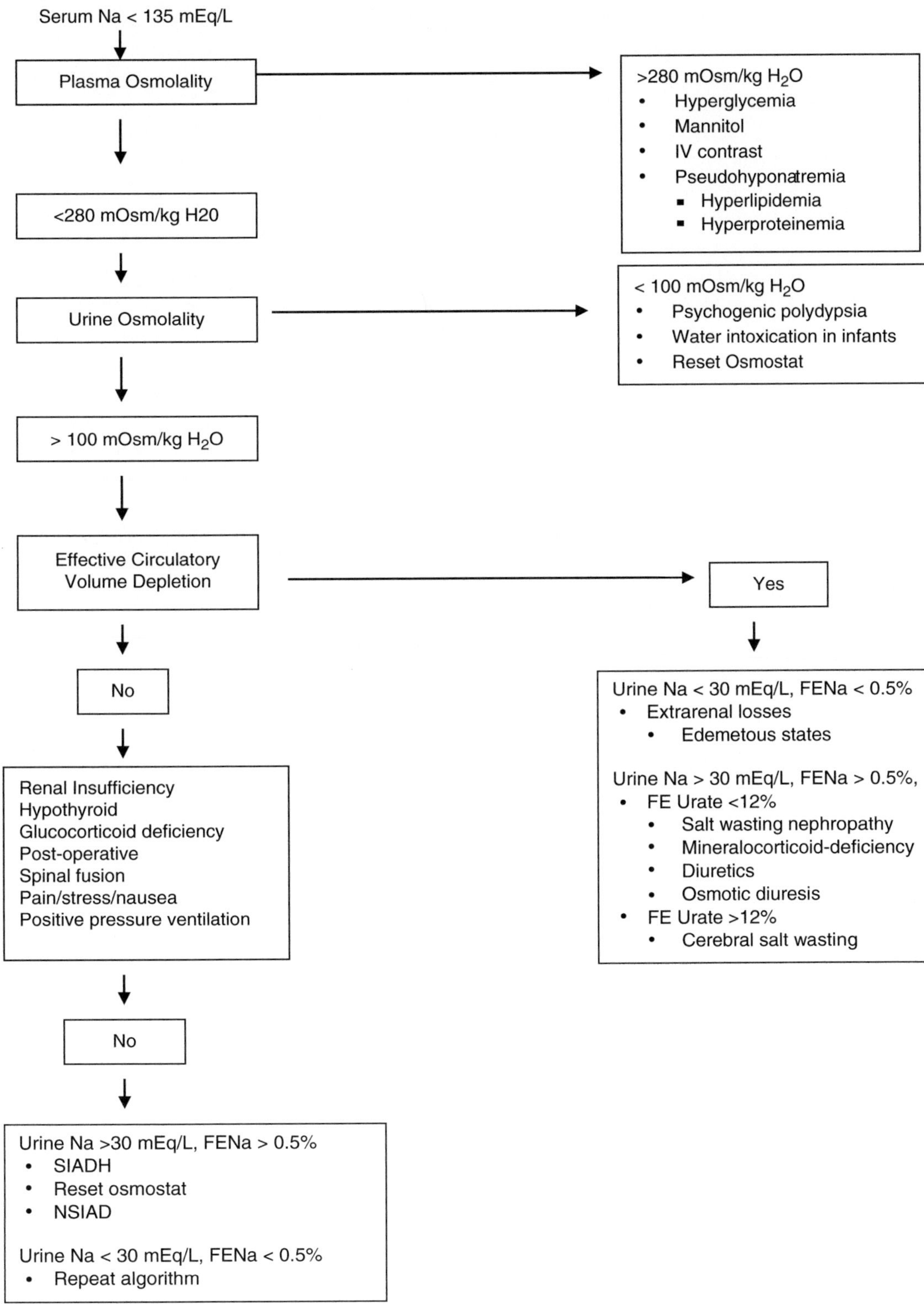

Fig. 4.1 Evaluation of hyponatremia

pseudohyponatremia remains an entity that clinicians need to be aware of. If hyponatremia is associated with hypoosmolality (true hyponatremia) and the history does not suggest an obvious cause, the next step is to measure the urinary osmolality to determine if there is an impaired ability to excrete free water (urine Osm > 100 mOsm/kg).

The information that is most useful in arriving at a correct diagnosis of hyponatremia is a detailed history of fluid balance, weight changes, medications (especially diuretics), and underlying medical illnesses. Hyponatremia is usually a multifactorial disorder, and a detailed history will identify sources of salt and water losses, free water ingestion, and underlying illnesses that cause a nonosmotic stimulus for vasopressin production. An assessment of the volume status on physical examination and the urinary electrolytes can be extremely helpful, but both can be misleading. In patients in whom hyponatremia is due to salt losses, such as diuretics, signs of volume depletion may be absent on physical examination, as the volume deficit may be nearly corrected due to oral intake of hypotonic fluids if the thirst mechanism is intact.

In general, a urinary sodium concentration <30 mEq/L and a fractional excretion of sodium (FENa) <0.5 % in adults are consistent with effective circulating volume depletion, while a urine sodium >30 mEq/L or a FENa >0.5 % is consistent with renal tubular dysfunction, use of diuretics, adrenal insufficiency, the syndrome of inappropriate antidiuretic hormone secretion (SIADH), or cerebral salt wasting [8]. The plasma uric acid and fraction excretion of urate (FE urate) can be helpful in distinguishing SIADH from other hyponatremic states associated with urinary sodium loss [9, 10]. SIADH virtually always associates with increase urate clearance with hypourecemia (serum uric acid <4 mg/dL) and an elevated FE urate (>12 %). There have been no studies to validating if these adult parameters for urine chemistries can be applied to the newborn with hyponatremia. Numerous factors can affect the urine chemistries, making interpretation difficult; therefore, the timing of the urinary measurements in relation to dosages of diuretics, intravenous fluid boluses, or fluid and sodium restriction is also important.

4.1.4 Prevention of Hospital-Acquired Hyponatremia

Hospital-acquired hyponatremia is of particular concern in the newborn as the standard of care in pediatrics has been to administer hypotonic fluids containing 0.2 % sodium chloride (34 mEq/L) as maintenance fluids [11]. The safety of this approach has never been established, and there have been numerous reports of death and permanent neurologic injury from hospital-acquired hyponatremic encephalopathy in children receiving hypotonic fluids [12]. Hospitalized children have numerous nonosmotic stimuli for vasopressin production that place them at risk for developing hyponatremia. Hyponatremia is especially dangerous in children with underlying CNS injury such as encephalitis, with mild hyponatremia (sodium >130 mEq/L) resulting in cerebral edema and even herniation [13, 14]. The most important measure that can be taken to prevent hyponatremia is to avoid using hypotonic fluids in children who have clear risks for nonosmotic AVP secretion and to initially administer isotonic saline, 0.9 % sodium chloride, unless otherwise clinically indicated [12, 15]. The serum sodium should be measured daily in any patient receiving continuous parenteral fluid and adjustments to the composition of intravenous fluids be made accordingly.

4.1.5 Syndrome of Inappropriate Antidiuretic Hormone Production (SIADH)

SIADH is one of the most common causes of hyponatremia in the hospital setting and frequently leads to severe hyponatremia (plasma Na <120 mEq/L). It is caused by elevated AVP secretion in the absence of an osmotic or hypovolemic stimulus. SIADH can occur due to a variety of illnesses but most often occurs due to central nervous system disorders, pulmonary disorders, and

Table 4.2 Common causes of SIADH in the newborn

Central nervous system disorders	*Malignancies*
Infection: meningitis, encephalitis	Neuroblastoma
Neoplasms	Lymphomas
Vascular abnormalities	*Medications*
Hydrocephalus	Vincristine
Brain surgery	Intravenous Cytoxan
Head trauma	Carbamazepine
Intracranial hemorrhage or thrombosis	Oxcarbazepine
Pulmonary disorders	Narcotics
Pneumonia	Nonsteroidal anti-inflammatory drugs
Bronchiolitis	
Asthma	
Cystic fibrosis	
Positive-pressure ventilation	
Pneumothorax	

medications (Table 4.2) [16, 17]. Among the latter, the chemotherapeutic drugs vincristine and Cytoxan and the antiepileptic drug carbamazepine are especially common. SIADH is essentially a diagnosis of exclusion as can be seen from Fig. 4.1. Before SIADH can be diagnosed, diseases causing decreased effective circulating volume, renal impairment, adrenal insufficiency, and hypothyroidism must be excluded. Adrenal insufficiency can be difficult to rule out; therefore, cortisol level should be checked in a patient considered to have SIADH. The hallmarks of SIADH are as follows: mild volume expansion with low to normal plasma concentrations of creatinine, urea, uric acid, and potassium; impaired free water excretion with normal sodium excretion which reflects sodium intake; and hyponatremia which is relatively unresponsive to sodium administration in the absence of fluid restriction.

SIADH is usually of short duration and resolves with treatment of the underlying disorder and discontinuation of the offending medication. Fluid restriction is the cornerstone to therapy. However, fluid restriction results in slow correction of hyponatremia and is frequently impractical in infants who receive most of their nutrition as liquids. All intravenous fluids should be of a tonicity of at least normal saline, and if this does not correct the plasma sodium, 3 % sodium chloride may be given as needed. If a more rapid correction of hyponatremia is needed, the addition of a loop diuretic in combination with hypertonic saline is useful. Vasopressin 2 antagonists are new medications that are now FDA approved for the treatment SIADH in adults [18]. These drugs may have a role for treatment of SIADH in children.

4.1.6 Oral Water Intoxication in Infants

Water intoxication is one of the most common causes of symptomatic hyponatremia in healthy infants; 70 % of infants younger than 6 months of age who develop seizures that have no apparent cause are found to have hyponatremia due to water intoxication [19]. Most of these infants are living in poverty and develop water intoxication when caregivers either dilute formula inappropriately or supplement feedings with water [20]. Because an infant's caloric intake depends almost entirely on a liquid diet, hunger will drive the infant to accept a low-solute formula to the point of water intoxication. Infants typically present with generalized tonic-clonic seizures, respiratory insufficiency, and hypothermia. Affected infants may be managed with rapid and partial correction of hyponatremia via administration of hypertonic or normal saline [21]. The hyponatremia corrects rapidly due to a free water diuresis, and it corrects spontaneously in many infants after they resume normal feeding. With appropriate treatment, the prognosis generally is good without long-term neurologic sequelae.

4.1.7 Diuretics

Diuretics are a relatively common cause of hyponatremia in hospitalized children, with the potential for causing severe and symptomatic hyponatremia [22]. Hyponatremia is primarily seen with thiazide diuretics [23]. Thiazide diuretics can cause both acute and chronic hyponatremia, but typically hyponatremia develops in the first few weeks following the initiation of therapy [24]. Thiazide diuretics frequently are employed to manage chronic lung disease or edema-forming states, and the effects of the diuretic are synergistic with other underlying disorders that cause hyponatremia. Excess water intake also is a major contributing factor to the development of hyponatremia among those receiving diuretics.

4.1.8 Hyponatremic Encephalopathy

A major consequence of hyponatremia is the influx of water into the intracellular space resulting in cellular swelling, which can lead to cerebral edema and encephalopathy [25]. The clinical manifestations of hyponatremia are primarily neurologic and related to cerebral edema caused by hypoosmolality. The symptoms of hyponatremic encephalopathy are quite variable between individuals with the only consistent symptoms being headache, nausea, vomiting, emesis, and weakness. As the cerebral edema worsens, patients then develop behavioral changes, and impaired response to verbal and tactile stimuli. Advanced symptoms are signs of cerebral herniation, with seizures, respiratory arrest, dilated pupils, and decorticate posturing. Headache, nausea, and vomiting are the most consistent symptoms of hyponatremic encephalopathy.

Newborns are at particularly high risk for developing hyponatremic encephalopathy due to their relatively larger brain to intracranial volume ratio as compared to adults [26]. A child's brain reaches adult size by 6 years of age, whereas the skull does not reach adult size until 16 years of age. Consequently, children have less room available in their rigid skulls for brain expansion and are likely to develop brain herniation from hyponatremia at higher serum sodium concentrations than adults. Other risks factors for developing hyponatremic encephalopathy are hypoxia and underlying central nervous system (CNS) disease [27]. Hypoxia impairs brain-cell-volume regulation and decreases cerebral perfusion [28]. Patient with underlying CNS disease are already at risk for intracranial hypertension and fall in serum sodium will exacerbate this.

4.1.8.1 Treatment of Hyponatremic Encephalopathy

Hyponatremic encephalopathy is a medical emergency that requires early recognition and treatment. The definitive therapy for treating hyponatremic encephalopathy is the administration of hypertonic saline (3 % NaCl, 513 mEq/L) [29]. Fluid restriction alone has no role in the management of symptomatic hyponatremia; 0.9 % NaCl is also inappropriate for the treatment of hyponatremic encephalopathy as it is not sufficiently hypertonic to induce the necessary reduction in cerebral edema central to the management of this condition. Once signs of encephalopathy are identified, prompt treatment is required in a monitored setting before imaging studies are performed. Endotracheal intubation and mechanical ventilation may be necessary to ensure appropriate gas exchange.

Children with suspected hyponatremic encephalopathy with either mild or advanced symptoms should receive 2 mL/kg of 3 % NaCl as a bolus over 10 min in order to rapidly reverse brain edema (Table 4.3). A single bolus of 3 % NaCl will result in at most a 2-mEq/L acute rise

Table 4.3 Treatment of symptomatic hyponatremia in the newborn

1. 2 cc/kg bolus of 3 % NaCl over 10 min
2. Repeat bolus 1–2 times as needed until symptoms improve Goal: 5–6 mEq/L increase in serum sodium in first 1–2 h
3. Recheck serum sodium following second bolus or Q 2 h
4. Hyponatremic encephalopathy is unlikely if no clinical improvement following an acute rise in serum sodium of 5–6 mEq/L
5. Stop further therapy with 3 % NaCl boluses when patient is either: (a) Symptom-free: awake, alert, responding to commands, resolution of headache and nausea (b) Acute rise in sodium of 10 mEq/L in if first 5 h
6. Correction in first 48 h should: (a) Not exceed 15–20 mEq/L (b) Avoid normo- or hypernatremia

in serum sodium. This dose might need to be repeated once or twice until symptoms subside, with the goal of correction being 5–6 mEq/L in the first 1–2 h. Children who have not had some neurologic response to three boluses of 3 % NaCl most likely do not have hyponatremic encephalopathy. To prevent complications arising from excessive therapy, 3 % NaCl should be discontinued when symptoms subside. The rate of correction should not exceed 20 mmol/L in the first 48 h, and correction should be to mildly hyponatremic values, avoiding normonatremia and hypernatremia in the first 48 h.

4.1.9 Risk Factors for Developing Cerebral Demyelination

Cerebral demyelination is a rare condition that has been primarily reported in adults with severe chronic hyponatremia (Na <115 mEq/L, >48 h) who have additional risk factors such as liver disease, severe malnutrition, hypokalemia, hypoxia, and a correction of serum sodium >25 mEq/L in the first 24–48 h of therapy [2]. In these high-risk patients, it is not clear that cerebral demyelination can be prevented even with careful correction of hyponatremia. Cerebral demyelination has not been reported in children with acute hospital-acquired hyponatremia, nor have neurologic complications been associated with the use of 3 % NaCl to treat children with hyponatremic encephalopathy. Cerebral demyelination is rarely reported in newborns as a newborn brain is not fully myelinated.

When symptomatic cerebral demyelination does follow the correction of hyponatremia, it typically follows a biphasic pattern. There is initially clinical improvement of the hyponatremic encephalopathy associated with correction of the serum sodium, which is followed by neurologic deterioration 2–7 days later. Cerebral demyelination can be both pontine and extrapontine. Classic features of pontine demyelination include mutism, dysarthria, spastic quadriplegia, pseudobulbar palsy, a pseudocoma with a "locked-in stare," and ataxia. The clinical features of extrapontine lesions are more varied, including behavior changes and movement disorders. Radiographic features of cerebral demyelination typically lag behind the clinical symptoms. Cerebral demyelination is best diagnosed on MRI approximately 14 days following correction. The classic radiographic findings on MRI are symmetrical lesions that are hypointense on T1-weighted images and hyperintense on T2-weighted images. Some data suggest that cerebral demyelination can be detected earlier on MRI with diffusion-weighted imaging.

4.2 Hypernatremia

Core Messages

- The primary cause of hypernatremia is insufficient free water intake.
- Volume expansion with 0.9 % sodium chloride should precede the correction of hypernatremia if volume depletion is present.

Case Vignette

A 7-day-old female infant weighting 2.8 kg presents to the emergency department with a fever and lethargy. The child was born full term via a spontaneously vaginal delivery weighting 3.2 kg to a 22-year-old first-time mother who was exclusively breastfeeding the child. The postnatal course was complicated by neonatal jaundice which required 2 days of home phototherapy. The child is described as being a slow feeder, spending over 30 min on each breast. The child has been sleepy and fussy with a high-pitched cry. She has had two to three bowel movements a day and one diaper appeared to have pink urine. Biochemistries revealed a serum sodium 156 mEq/L, potassium 5.6 mEq/L, total carbon dioxide 12 mEq/L, blood urea nitrogen 40 mg/dL, and creatinine 0.8 mg/dL. Urine biochemistries reveal sodium <5 mEq/L, potassium 20 mEq/L, and osmolality 900 mOsm/kg/H_2O.

4.2.1 Introduction

Hypernatremia is defined as a serum sodium concentration >145 mEq/L. In both children and adults, hypernatremia is seen primarily in hospitals and occurs in individuals who have restricted access to water for a variety of reasons. Typically, affected patients are either debilitated by an acute or chronic illness, have neurologic impairment, or are at the extremes of age. Infants, especially those born preterm, are at particularly high risk for the development of hypernatremia because of their relatively small mass-to-surface area ratio and their dependency on a caretaker to administer fluids. Hypernatremia is particularly dangerous in the newborn as it can result in vascular complication. Diarrheal dehydration is an important cause of hypernatremia in the outpatient setting but is much less common than previously reported, presumably due to the advent of low-solute infant formulas and the increased use and availability of oral rehydration solutions.

A group at high risk for developing hypernatremia in the outpatient setting is that of the breastfed infant [30]. Breastfeeding-associated hypernatremia is on the rise. Over 15 % of mother-infant diads have difficulty establishing successful lactation during the first week postpartum. This is of particular concern for the primiparous infant. Reasons for lactation failure are multifactorial, including physiological factors which require 3–5 days for optimal breast milk production and mechanical factors resulting in a poor latch or insufficient time on the breast to stimulate optimal milk production. Hypernatremic dehydration results from a combination of insufficient lactation and increased breast milk sodium concentration. Hypernatremic dehydration can be difficult to diagnose as hypernatremic infants will have a better preserved extracellular volume.

4.2.2 Pathogenesis of Hypernatremia

The body has two defenses to protect against developing hypernatremia: the ability to produce a concentrated urine and a powerful thirst mechanism. AVP release occurs when the plasma osmolality exceeds 275–280 mOsm/kg and results in a maximally concentrated urine when the plasma osmolality exceeds 290–295 mOsm/kg. Thirst is the body's second line of defense but provides the ultimate protection against hypernatremia. If the thirst mechanism is intact and there is unrestricted access to free water, it is rare for someone to develop sustained hypernatremia from either excess sodium ingestion or a renal concentrating defect.

4.2.3 Diagnosis

Hypernatremia is usually multifactorial and a systematic approach is required to determine the contributing factors (Fig. 4.2) [1]. A serum sodium, glucose, and osmolality must be evaluated. An elevated serum sodium is always associated with hyperosmolality and should be considered abnormal. In cases of significant hyperglycemia, the serum sodium will be depressed due to the associated translocation of fluids from the intracellular to extracellular space. Once the diagnosis of hypernatremia is established, a detailed history and review of fluid intake should be taken to determine if the patient has an intact thirst mechanism, has restricted access to fluids, or is not being provided adequate free water in intravenous fluids. If no apparent cause for hypernatremia is identified, then urine volume should be measured and compared to fluid intake, and the urine osmolality and electrolytes should be determined to assess if the renal concentrating ability is appropriate and to quantify the urinary free water losses. A less than maximally concentrated urine (<800 mOsm/kg) in the face of hypernatremia is a sign of a renal concentrating defect, as hypernatremia is a maximal stimulus for ADH release. In patients with hypernatremia, the following should be evaluated: gastrointestinal losses, urinary output, dermal losses from fever or burns, diet history (including tube feedings and breastfeeding), medication history (including diuretics), and sources of exogenous sodium. Salt poisoning should be suspected whenever the severity of hypernatremia, neurologic

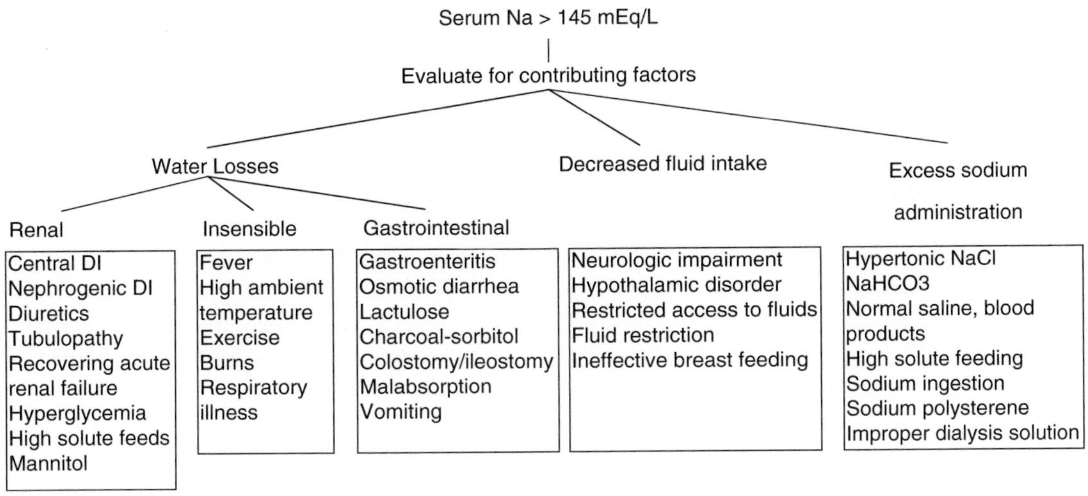

Fig. 4.2 Diagnostic approach to hypernatremia

manifestations, or hospital course does not correlate with the history of present illness. If this is suspected, a gastric sodium sample should be obtained as soon as possible, as a gastric sodium concentration greater than that of plasma is virtually diagnostic of salt poisoning.

4.2.4 Clinical Manifestations of Hypernatremia

Hypernatremia results in an efflux of fluid from the intracellular space to the extracellular space to maintain osmotic equilibrium. This leads to transient cerebral dehydration with cell shrinkage. Brain cell volume can decrease by as much as 10–15 % acutely but then quickly adapts. Within 1 h, the brain significantly increases its intracellular content of sodium and potassium, amino acids, and unmeasured organic substances called idiogenic osmoles. Within 1 week, the brain regains approximately 98 % of its water content [31]. If severe hypernatremia develops acutely, the brain may not be able to increase its intracellular solute sufficiently to preserve its volume, and the resulting cellular shrinkage can cause structural changes. Cerebral dehydration from hypernatremia can result in a physical separation of the brain from the meninges leading to a rupture of the delicate bridging veins and intracranial or intracerebral hemorrhages [32]. Venous sinus thrombosis leading to infarction can also develop. Acute hypernatremia has also been shown to cause cerebral demyelinating lesions in both animals and humans [33]. Patients with hepatic encephalopathy are at the highest risk for developing demyelinating lesions.

Children with hypernatremia are usually agitated and irritable but can progress to lethargy, listlessness, and coma [34]. On neurologic examination, they frequently have increased tone, nuchal rigidity, and brisk reflexes. Myoclonus, asterixis, and chorea can be present; tonic-clonic and absence seizures have been described. Hyperglycemia is a particularly common consequence of hypernatremia in children. Severe hypernatremia can also result in rhabdomyolysis. While earlier reports showed that hypocalcemia was associated with hypernatremia, this has not been found in more recent literature. In adults hypernatremia primarily manifests as central nervous system depression. Adults with hypernatremia are rarely alert, and most have confusion with abnormal speech and obtundation with stupor or coma. The degree of central nervous system depression appears to correlate with the severity of hypernatremia.

4.2.5 Treatment of Hypernatremia

The cornerstone of the management of hypernatremia is providing adequate free water to correct the serum sodium. Hypernatremia is frequently accompanied by volume depletion. Fluid resuscitation with normal saline should be instituted to reestablish distal perfusion prior to any attempt to correct the free water deficit. Following initial volume expansion, the composition of parenteral fluid therapy largely depends on the etiology of the hypernatremia. Patients with sodium overload or a renal concentrating defect will require a more hypotonic fluid than patients with volume depletion and intact renal concentrating ability. Oral hydration should be instituted as soon as it can be safely tolerated. Plasma electrolytes should be checked every 2 h until the patient is neurologically stable.

A simple way of estimating the minimum amount of fluid necessary to correct the serum sodium is by the following equation:

$$\begin{aligned}&Free\,water\,deficit\,(mL)\\&=4\,mL\times lean\,body\,wt\,(kg)\\&\times[desired\ change\ in\ serum\ Na\,mEq\,/\,\mathrm{L}]\end{aligned}$$

Larger amounts of fluid will be required depending on the fluid composition. To correct a 300 mL free water deficit, approximately 400 mL of 0.2 % sodium chloride in water or 600 mL of 0.45 % sodium chloride in water would be required, as they contain approximately 75 and 50 % free water, respectively. The calculated deficit does not account for insensible losses or ongoing urinary or gastrointestinal losses. Maintenance fluids, which include replacement of urine volume with hypotonic fluids, are given in addition to the deficit. Glucose-containing fluids should be limited as they can result in significant hyperglycemia.

The rate of correction of hypernatremia is largely dependent on the severity of the hypernatremia and the etiology. Due to the brain's relative inability to extrude unmeasured organic substances called idiogenic osmoles, rapid correction of hypernatremia can lead to cerebral edema. While there are no definitive studies that document the optimal rate of correction that can be undertaken without developing cerebral edema, empirical data have shown that unless symptoms of hypernatremic encephalopathy are present, a rate of correction not exceeding 1 mEq/h or 15 mEq/24 h is reasonable [35]. In severe hypernatremia (>170 mEq/L), serum sodium should not be corrected to below 150 mEq/L in the first 48–72 h. Seizures occurring during the correction of hypernatremia are not uncommon in children but may be a sign of cerebral edema. Hypotonic fluid infusion should be ceased and hypertonic saline should be administered when signs of cerebral edema occur during the correction of hypernatremia is suspected. Seizures associated with the correction of hyponatremia are usually self-limited and not a sign of long-term neurologic sequelae. Patients with acute hypernatremia, corrected by the oral route, can tolerate a more rapid rate of correction with a much lower incidence of seizures. The type of therapy is largely dependent on the etiology of the hypernatremia and should be tailored to the pathophysiologic events involved in each patient (Table 4.4).

4.2.6 Potassium Homeostasis

Potassium is the most abundant cation in the body, with 98 % of potassium residing intracellular and 2 % extracellular. It is the ratio of intracellular to extracellular potassium concentration that determines the resting membrane

Table 4.4 Management of hypernatremia

Etiology	Treatment[a]
(A) Sodium and water loss Gastroenteritis	0.45 % Sodium chloride in 5 % dextrose in water
(B) Primary water loss Ineffective breastfeeding	0.2–0.45 % Sodium chloride in 5 % dextrose in water
(C) Nephrogenic diabetes insipidus	0.1 % Sodium chloride in 2.5 % dextrose in water (acute management)
(D) Central diabetes insipidus	Desmopressin acetate
(E) Sodium overload	5 % Dextrose in water Diuretics or dialysis may be needed

[a]Avoid 5 % dextrose in water if hyperglycemia is present

potential; therefore, the body must maintain the extracellular potassium concentration in a fairly narrow range of 3.5–5.5 mEq/L to prevent neurologic and conduction disturbances. Potassium can be consumed in large quantities in the diet and is absorbed rapidly in the gastrointestinal tract. The serum potassium is acutely regulated by a transcellular shift of potassium from extracellular to intracellular by the release of insulin and β-adrenergic catecholamines. The long-term regulation of potassium is via urinary excretion which is primarily regulated by aldosterone release. The serum potassium does not reflect the total body potassium content, as disorders in serum potassium may be due to acute intracellular shift or more chronic potassium depletion or overload. Chronic perturbations in serum potassium are better tolerated than acute changes, as the gradient in intracellular to extracellular potassium will be less severe. Chronic states of hyperkalemia generally reflect a disorder in renal function or mineralocorticoid activity, and hypokalemia represents total body potassium depletion.

4.3 Hypokalemia

Core Messages

- Hypokalemia does not cause significant arrhythmias unless there is significant underlying cardiac disease or digoxin use.
- Excessive correction of hypokalemia can result in dangerous hyperkalemia.

Case Vignette

A 3-week-old infant is evaluated for poor weight gain. The child was born at 36 weeks' gestation with a weight of 2.6 kg and a history of maternal polyhydramnios. At approximately 20 days of age, the child developed frequent bowel movements, non-bilious emesis, and abdominal distention. Upon presentation the child weights 2.5 kg. Serum electrolytes reveal a sodium of 132 mEq/L, potassium 2.6 mEq/L, chloride 94 mEq/L, and total carbon dioxide 35 mEq/L.

4.3.1 Clinical Effects of Hypokalemia

Hypokalemia, defined as a serum potassium <3.6 mEq/L, is a common electrolyte abnormality occurring in hospitalized patients [36]. Mild hypokalemia, potassium 3–3.5 mEq/L, is usually asymptomatic. Hypokalemia does not cause significant arrhythmias, other than U waves, unless there is underlying cardiac disease or digoxin use, where even mild hypokalemia can contribute to arrhythmias. Serum potassium <3.0 mEq/L can lead to weakness, myopathy, constipation, and intestinal ileus, while a serum potassium <2.5 mEq/L can cause rhabdomyolysis and ascending paralysis. When hypokalemia develops, the underlying cause should be addressed and corrected as hypokalemia is associated with increased morbidity and mortality in both children and adults.

4.3.2 Causes of Hypokalemia (Table 4.5)

Hypokalemia is not particularly common in the newborn. One of the most common causes of potassium depletion is from the use of loop or thiazide diuretics [37]. Diuretics are frequently used in the neonate with respiratory distress syndrome or bronchopulmonary dysplasia, but there is little evidence to support their use [38]. Loop and thiazide diuretics increase sodium delivery to the collecting duct. This leads to maximal sodium reabsorption in these segments and facilitates potassium excretion. Chronic diuretic use may be associated with effective circulating volume depletion which further stimulates the renin-angiotensin-aldosterone pathway, increasing urinary potassium losses. Hyperchloremic metabolic

Table 4.5 Causes of hypokalemia

1. Inadequate intake
2. Urinary losses
(a) Diuretics
(b) Salt-wasting nephropathy
(i) Fanconi syndrome
(c) Osmotic diuresis
(i) Uncontrolled diabetes
(d) Transport disorder
(i) Bartter and Gitelman syndromes
(e) Mineralocorticoid excess
(f) Magnesium depletion
(i) Amphotericin B
(g) Alkalosis
(h) Non-reabsorbable anions (penicillins)
3. Extrarenal losses
(a) Vomiting
(b) Diarrhea
(c) Malabsorption
(d) Tumors
(e) Dialysis
4. Transcellular shifts
(a) $ß_2$-Adrenergic agents
(b) Insulin
(c) Theophylline
(d) Hyperthyroidism
(e) Hypokalemic periodic paralysis

alkalosis, which is a frequent complication of diuretics, contributes to hypokalemia by impairing chloride-linked sodium reabsorption, thereby increasing distal tubule sodium reabsorption and potassium excretion. Hypomagnesemia, which is a common complication of diuretic therapy, promotes urinary potassium losses by unknown mechanisms. The combination of loop plus thiazide diuretics can lead to profound hypokalemia.

Other disorders leading to hypokalemia are conditions which lead to gastrointestinal losses, transcellular shifts in potassium, or mineralocorticoid excess. Potassium is primarily excreted in the stool by the colonic epithelium; therefore, any process that results in diarrhea can cause large potassium losses. Intestinal losses from an ileostomy or upper gastrointestinal losses from vomiting or nasogastric do not contain significant amounts of potassium. Hyperchloremic alkalosis induced by emesis can cause hypokalemia by increasing urinary potassium losses. $ß_2$-adrenergics, theophylline, and insulin can cause hypokalemia by causing a transcellular shift in potassium. There are numerous medical conditions that are associated with increased mineralocorticoid production or activity that can cause hypokalemia, especially in conjunction with diuretics, such as seen with renovascular hypertension.

4.3.3 Bartter Syndrome

Bartter syndrome is rare but important cause of hypokalemia in the newborn [39]. Bartter syndrome is a heterogenous disorder characterized by defects in distal tubular sodium and chloride reabsorption occurring in the thick ascending limb of the loop of Henle with secondary hyperreninemia and hyperaldosteronism. To date there are five different types of Bartter syndrome. These conditions generally have clinical features similar to that of being on a loop diuretic with hypercalciuria being a prominent feature. A severe form of Bartter syndrome that occurs in the newborn is referred to as antenatal Bartter syndrome or hyperprostaglandin E syndrome. Antenatal Bartter syndrome is associated with maternal polyhydramnios, preterm birth, intrauterine and postnatal polyuria, recurrent vomiting, failure to thrive, growth retardation, and severe bouts of dehydration.

4.3.4 Treatment of Hypokalemia

The treatment of hypokalemia is controversial as excess potassium supplementation, especially via the intravenous route, can cause dangerous hyperkalemia [40]. Hypokalemia is generally asymptomatic, and therapy should aim for a slow correction over a period of days, preferably by the enteral route as potassium chloride in two to three divided doses. In cases of cardiac arrhythmias, severe myopathies, paralysis, or severe hypokalemia (potassium <2 mEq/L), aggressive intravenous administration of potassium is indicated. Potassium should be given as potassium chloride, as there is generally an accompanying chloride deficit. Potassium should not be infused faster than 0.5 mEq/kg/h. The infusion should be stopped every 2–3 h to reassess the serum potassium. A parenteral fluid potassium concentration >60 mEq/L should not be administered through a peripheral intravenous line as it can cause sclerosis of the vein, and potassium infiltration can cause tissue necrosis. Magnesium depletion should be corrected as hypomagnesemia promotes urinary potassium losses. Potassium-sparing diuretics can be helpful to curtail urinary potassium losses.

4.4 Hyperkalemia

Core Messages

- Hyperkalemia can result in fatal cardiac arrhythmias.
- Exchange resins are ineffective and dangerous in the treatment of non-oliguric hyperkalemia of the premature infant.

Case Vignette

A preterm infant is admitted to the neonatal intensive care unit. The child was born at 26 weeks' gestation with a birth weight of 900 g with an Apgar score of 5 at 5 min. The child is intubated and ventilated and is given surfactant. The child did not receive antenatal dexamethasone. The child is placed on intravenous fluids without potassium. At 18 h of life, the child is noted to have peaked T waves on the monitor with a widening QRS. STAT biochemistries reveal a nonhemolyzed potassium of 7.4 mEq/L with a serum sodium of 136 mEq/L, carbon dioxide of 18 mEq/L, and serum creatinine of 0.8 mg/dL. Urine output is normal at 3 mL/kg/h.

Table 4.6 Causes of hyperkalemia

1. Factitious (a) Hemolysis (b) Thrombocytosis (platelets >1,000,000/mm^3) (c) Leukocytosis (white blood cell count >100,000/mm^3) (d) Repeated fist clenching with tourniquet in place
2. Non-oliguric hyperkalemia of the premature infant
3. Impaired potassium excretion (a) Renal insufficiency or failure (b) Mineralocorticoid deficiency (i) Hereditary enzyme deficiencies (ii) Addison's disease (iii) Hyporeninemic hypoaldosteronism (type 4 renal tubular acidosis) (iv) Heparin-induced inhibition of aldosterone synthesis (c) Pseudohypoaldosteronism (i) Hereditary (ii) Pyelonephritis
4. Medications (a) Potassium-sparing diuretics (b) ACE inhibitors (c) Angiotensin receptor blockers (d) NSAIDs (e) Cyclosporine/tacrolimus (f) Trimethoprim (g) Pentamidine
5. Impaired potassium entry into cells (a) Insulin deficiency or resistance (b) Hyperchloremic metabolic acidosis (c) Hypertonicity (uncontrolled diabetes) (d) Massive tissue breakdown (rhabdomyolysis) (e) Familial hyperkalemic periodic paralysis (f) Medications (i) B-blockers (ii) Digoxin (at toxic levels) (iii) Succinylcholine (iv) Arginine (v) Lysine
6. Excess potassium administration (a) Total parenteral nutrition (b) Potassium supplements (c) Diet or enteral feeds (d) RBC transfusion (e) Penicillin G potassium

4.4.1 Newborns at Risk for Hyperkalemia (Table 4.6)

Hyperkalemia is defined as serum potassium >6 mEq/L in newborns and >5 mEq/L in children outside of the newborn period. The preterm neonate is at particularly high risk for developing hyperkalemia. Hyperkalemia is common during the first few days after birth in premature infants with a gestational age <28 weeks. This condition is termed non-oliguric hyperkalemia of the premature infant, which is defined as a serum potassium >7 mEq/L during the first 72 h of life in the presence of normal urinary output >1 mL/kg/h [41]. Neonatal hyperkalemia can result in cardiac arrhythmias and has resulted in sudden death. Non-oliguric hyperkalemia results from a transcellular shift of potassium into the extracellular space and spontaneously resolves after the first few days of life. Hyperkalemia in the older newborn typically results from either excess potassium intake, decreased potassium excretion, or a transcellular shift of potassium from the intracellular to extracellular space. There are usually multiple factors contributing to hyperkalemia; therefore, a detailed evaluation of potassium intake, renal function, and medication history is mandatory.

Pseudohyperkalemia is a common cause of hyperkalemia in the newborn resulting from cell breakdown following venipuncture or capillary sampling [42]. A common setting for serious hyperkalemia in the children is oliguric acute renal failure, such as seen in urinary tract obstruction from posterior urethral valves. Mineralocorticoid deficiency and resistance are also important causes of severe hyperkalemia in the newborn. Severe hyperkalemia can develop in infants with pyelonephritis due to transient pseudohypoaldosteronism with the associated features of hyponatremia, acidosis, and elevated plasma renin activity and aldosterone [43]. A rare but serious form of hyperkalemia in the newborn is that of pseudohypoaldosteronism type 1 (PHA-1) [44]. PHA-1 results from mutations in the mineralocorticoid receptor. It results in severe hyperkalemia in the first week of life with salt loss, acidosis, and elevated aldosterone levels. It requires lifelong sodium supplementation and dietary potassium restriction. Hyperkalemia from acute and chronic kidney disease or from massive tissue breakdown from rhabdomyolysis or tumor lysis syndrome is much less common in newborn than in the older child. Hyperkalemia from hyperchloremic metabolic acidosis is relatively common in children and results from a transcellular shift in potassium. Serum potassium rises on average 0.6 mEq/L (0.24–1.7 mEq/L) for every 0.1 unit fall in pH. An elevated anion gap acidosis has little or no effect on serum potassium.

4.4.2 Clinical Effects of Hyperkalemia

The ratio of intracellular to extracellular potassium is the major determinant of the resting membrane potential [42]. Hyperkalemia decreases resting membrane potential facilitating depolarization and impairing repolarization. The symptoms of mild to moderate hyperkalemia are usually asymptomatic; however, the first presenting symptom may be a fatal cardiac arrhythmia. Clinical manifestations that can result from membrane potential effects in striated muscle include weakness, paresthesias, and ascending paralysis. Ascending paralysis is usually seen in patients with chronic renal insufficiency when the serum potassium exceeds 7.5 mEq/L.

The effects of potassium on cardiac conduction are the most worrisome features (Table 4.7). Hyperkalemia interferes with atrioventricular and intraventricular conduction pathways leading to arrhythmias. The risks of arrhythmias usually correlate with the degree of hyperkalemia,

Table 4.7 Electrographic manifestations of hyperkalemia

Serum potassium level	Expected ECG abnormality
Mild hyperkalemia 5.5–6.5 mEq/L	Tall, tent-shaped ("peaked") T waves with narrow base, best seen in precordial leads (lead II)
Moderate hyperkalemia 6.5–8.0 mEq/L	Peaked T waves
	Prolonged PR interval
	Decreased amplitude of P waves
	Widening of QRS complex
Severe hyperkalemia >8.0 mEq/L	Absence of P wave
	Intraventricular blocks, fascicular blocks, bundle branch blocks, QRS axis shift
	Progressive widening of the QRS complex resulting in bizarre QRS morphology
	Eventual "sine-wave" pattern (sinoventricular rhythm), ventricular fibrillation, asystole

Table 4.8 Emergency management of hyperkalemia

1. Evaluation (a) Confirm that potassium value is venous and nonhemolyzed (b) Place patient on cardiac monitor (lead II) and obtain ECG
2. Conduction abnormalities (a) Calcium gluconate (10 %) 100 mg/kg/dose (1 mL/kg/dose) over 3–5 min. Works immediately with a 15–30-min duration. Can be repeated in 15 min
3. Serum potassium >6.5 mEq/L (a) Move potassium into cells: (i) Regular insulin 0.1 U/kg with 25 % glucose 2 mL/kg over 30 min. Onset is 10–20 min with a duration of 2–3 h (ii) Albuterol nebulization 0.5 % 0.25 mg/kg/dose over 10 min. Onset of action 20–30 min, duration 2–3 h. Can be used in conjunction with insulin and glucose (iii) Sodium bicarbonate 1 mEq/kg, only if hyperchloremic metabolic acidosis, onset of action is 1–3 h (b) Remove potassium from body: (i) Loop diuretic (ii) Hemodialysis or peritoneal dialysis (iii) Fludrocortisone

but arrhythmias are more likely to occur with rapid increases in serum potassium then with gradual increases. The most consistent ECG finding of hyperkalemia is increased T waves followed by widening of the QRS complex. There is no clear cutoff where arrhythmias will develop, but patients with serum potassium >6.0 mEq/L should be considered at risk for arrhythmias, and patients with levels exceeding 6.5 mEq/L or electrocardiographic features should receive immediate treatment.

4.4.3 Treatment of Hyperkalemia

The treatment of hyperkalemia largely depends on both the etiology and severity of hyperkalemia [42]. The presence of ECG changes or serum potassium exceeding 6.5 mEq/L requires immediate therapy (Table 4.8). Calcium can reverse cardiac conduction abnormalities and should be administered if ECG changes or present. Calcium must be administered through a properly function intravenous line as extravasation can cause tissue necrosis. This is of particular concern in the term and preterm infant where reliable vascular access can be difficult to establish. The acute management of hyperkalemia involves shifting potassium intracellularly. The administration of insulin and glucose is the most reliable first-line therapy for the treatment of hyperkalemia. β_2-adrenergic agent such as albuterol has been used successfully both intravenously and nebulized in the treatment of hyperkalemia. These agents both lower serum potassium by 0.6–1 mEq/L within 30 min and have an additive effect when use together. Insulin is effective in all patients but has the disadvantage of potentially causing hypoglycemia and requiring vascular access, which can be difficult to establish in small children. Albuterol's main advantage is that it can be administered quickly and repeatedly without the need for vascular access with minimal side effects. The main disadvantage of albuterol is that it is ineffective in 10–20 % of patients. Both insulin and albuterol lower the serum potassium for 2–3 h, while additional therapies can be instituted to remove potassium from the body. Sodium bicarbonate has recently lost favor in the acute management of hyperkalemia as it is relatively ineffective in the absence of severe acidosis, has a delayed onset of action of 1 h, and can cause fluid overload and hypernatremia.

Following the acute lowering of serum potassium by causing an intracellular shift in potassium, the next objective is to remove potassium from the body via urine, stool, or dialytic therapies. The preferred method of removing potassium from the body is via urinary losses, and measures should be undertaken to improve urinary flow. Prerenal causes of acute renal failure should be promptly treated with volume expansion, obstructive causes should be corrected, and urinary flow should be optimized with diuretics. When potassium removal via urinary losses is not possible, then an exchange transfusion or dialysis may be indicated. Sodium polystyrene (Kayexalate) is an exchange resin which has been used for the treatment of hyperkalemia. Kayexalate removes 0.5–1.0 mEq of potassium in exchange for 2–3 mEq of sodium. The primary site of potassium removal is the colon; therefore, the gastric administration of Kayexalate can take 6 h for potassium removal, while a retention enema can work in hours. Kayexalate is unpalatable, and to quickly deliver any significant volume to a child will likely require nasogastric administration or a retention enema. Kayexalate can have serious intestinal complications, particularly in the preterm infant [45]. There have been multiple reports of bowel necrosis, intestinal perforation, bowel impaction, and intestinal bezoars. Kayexalate has not been found to be effective in the treatment of non-oliguric hyperkalemia and has been associated with a high mortality. Kayexalate should not be used for the treatment of non-oliguric hyperkalemia in the premature infant and is best avoided in the term newborn. Hemodialysis is a rapid and effective means of potassium removal when there is a severe renal impairment and an acutely rising serum potassium.

References

1. Moritz ML, Ayus JC (2002) Disorders of water metabolism in children: hyponatremia and hypernatremia. Pediatr Rev 23:371–380
2. Moritz ML, Ayus JC (2010) New aspects in the pathogenesis, prevention, and treatment of hyponatremic encephalopathy in children. Pediatr Nephrol 25:1225–1238
3. Wald R, Jaber BL, Price LL, Upadhyay A, Madias NE (2010) Impact of hospital-associated hyponatremia on selected outcomes. Arch Intern Med 170:294–302
4. Baraton L, Ancel PY, Flamant C, Orsonneau JL, Darmaun D, Roze JC (2009) Impact of changes in serum sodium levels on 2-year neurologic outcomes for very preterm neonates. Pediatrics 124:e655–e661
5. Moritz ML, Ayus JC (2009) Hyponatremia in preterm neonates: not a benign condition. Pediatrics 124:e1014–e1016
6. Moritz ML, Ayus JC (2011) Prevention of hospital-acquired hyponatremia: do we have the answers? Pediatrics 128(5):980–983
7. Fortgens P, Pillay TS (2011) Pseudohyponatremia revisited: a modern-day pitfall. Arch Pathol Lab Med 135:516–519
8. Decaux G, Musch W (2008) Clinical laboratory evaluation of the syndrome of inappropriate secretion of antidiuretic hormone. Clin J Am Soc Nephrol 3:1175–1184
9. Maesaka JK, Imbriano LJ, Ali NM, Ilamathi E (2009) Is it cerebral or renal salt wasting? Kidney Int 76:934–938
10. Moritz ML (2012) Syndrome of inappropriate antidiuresis and cerebral salt wasting syndrome: are they different and does it matter? Pediatr Nephrol 27(5):689–693
11. Holliday MA, Segar WE (1957) The maintenance need for water in parenteral fluid therapy. Pediatrics 19:823–832
12. Moritz ML, Ayus JC (2005) Preventing neurological complications from dysnatremias in children. Pediatr Nephrol 20:1687–1700
13. McJunkin JE, de los Reyes EC, Irazuzta JE et al (2001) La Crosse encephalitis in children. N Engl J Med 344:801–807
14. Moritz ML, Ayus JC (2001) La Crosse encephalitis in children. N Engl J Med 345:148–149
15. Moritz ML, Ayus JC (2003) Prevention of hospital-acquired hyponatremia: a case for using isotonic saline. Pediatrics 111:227–230
16. Bartter FC, Schwartz WB (1967) The syndrome of inappropriate secretion of antidiuretic hormone. Am J Med 42:790–806
17. Robertson GL (2006) Regulation of arginine vasopressin in the syndrome of inappropriate antidiuresis. Am J Med 119:S36–S42
18. Decaux G, Soupart A, Vassart G (2008) Non-peptide arginine-vasopressin antagonists: the vaptans. Lancet 371:1624–1632
19. Farrar HC, Chande VT, Fitzpatrick DF, Shema SJ (1995) Hyponatremia as the cause of seizures in infants: a retrospective analysis of incidence, severity, and clinical predictors. Ann Emerg Med 26:42–48
20. Keating JP, Schears GJ, Dodge PR (1991) Oral water intoxication in infants. An American epidemic. Am J Dis Child 145:985–990
21. David R, Ellis D, Gartner JC (1981) Water intoxication in normal infants: role of antidiuretic hormone in pathogenesis. Pediatrics 68:349–353
22. Wattad A, Chiang ML, Hill LL (1992) Hyponatremia in hospitalized children. Clin Pediatr (Phila) 31:153–157
23. Sonnenblick M, Friedlander Y, Rosin AJ (1993) Diuretic-induced severe hyponatremia. Review and analysis of 129 reported patients. Chest 103:601–606
24. Glover M, Clayton J (2011) Thiazide-induced hyponatraemia: epidemiology and clues to pathogenesis. Cardiovasc Ther 30(5):e219–e226
25. Moritz ML, Ayus JC (2003) The pathophysiology and treatment of hyponatraemic encephalopathy: an update. Nephrol Dial Transplant 18:2486–2491
26. Arieff AI, Ayus JC, Fraser CL (1992) Hyponatraemia and death or permanent brain damage in healthy children. BMJ 304:1218–1222
27. Moritz ML, Carlos Ayus J (2007) Hospital-acquired hyponatremia–why are hypotonic parenteral fluids still being used? Nat Clin Pract Nephrol 3:374–382
28. Ayus JC, Armstrong D, Arieff AI (2006) Hyponatremia with hypoxia: effects on brain adaptation, perfusion, and histology in rodents. Kidney Int 69:1319–1325

29. Moritz ML, Ayus JC (2010) 100 cc 3% sodium chloride bolus: a novel treatment for hyponatremic encephalopathy. Metab Brain Dis 25:91–96
30. Moritz ML, Manole MD, Bogen DL, Ayus JC (2005) Breastfeeding-associated hypernatremia: are we missing the diagnosis? Pediatrics 116:e343–e347
31. Ayus JC, Armstrong DL, Arieff AI (1996) Effects of hypernatraemia in the central nervous system and its therapy in rats and rabbits. J Physiol 492:243–255
32. Finberg L, Luttrell C, Redd H (1959) Pathogenesis of lesions in the nervous system in hypernatremic states. II. Experimental studies of gross anatomic changes and alterations of chemical composition of the tissues. Pediatrics 23:46–53
33. Brown WD, Caruso JM (1999) Extrapontine myelinolysis with involvement of the hippocampus in three children with severe hypernatremia. J Child Neurol 14:428–433
34. Finberg L (1959) Pathogenesis of lesions in the nervous system in hypernatremic states. I. Clinical observations of infants. Pediatrics 23:40–45
35. Rosenfeld W, deRomana GL, Kleinman R, Finberg L (1977) Improving the clinical management of hypernatremic dehydration. Observations from a study of 67 infants with this disorder. Clin Pediatr (Phila) 16:411–417
36. Gennari FJ (1998) Hypokalemia. N Engl J Med 339:451–458
37. Greger R (1997) Why do loop diuretics cause hypokalaemia? Nephrol Dial Transplant 12:1799–1801
38. Stewart A, Brion LP, Soll R (2011) Diuretics for respiratory distress syndrome in preterm infants. Cochrane Database Syst Rev 2011, CD001454
39. Brochard K, Boyer O, Blanchard A et al (2009) Phenotype-genotype correlation in antenatal and neonatal variants of Bartter syndrome. Nephrol Dial Transplant 24:1455–1464
40. Gennari FJ (2002) Disorders of potassium homeostasis. Hypokalemia and hyperkalemia. Crit Care Clin 18:273–288, vi
41. Yaseen H (2009) Nonoliguric hyperkalemia in neonates: a case-controlled study. Am J Perinatol 26:185–189
42. Masilamani K, van der Voort J (2012) The management of acute hyperkalaemia in neonates and children. Arch Dis Child 97:376–380
43. Gil-Ruiz MA, Alcaraz AJ, Maranon RJ, Navarro N, Huidobro B, Luque A (2012) Electrolyte disturbances in acute pyelonephritis. Pediatr Nephrol 27:429–433
44. Guran T, Degirmenci S, Bulut IK, Say A, Riepe FG, Guran O (2011) Critical points in the management of pseudohypoaldosteronism type 1. J Clin Res Pediatr Endocrinol 3:98–100
45. Mildenberger E, Versmold HT (2002) Pathogenesis and therapy of non-oliguric hyperkalaemia of the premature infant. Eur J Pediatr 161:415–422

Assessment of Renal Function

5

Aftab S. Chishti

5.1 Introduction

Core Messages

(a) Kidney and urinary tract abnormalities are common neonatal and congenital findings that warrant appropriate and timely assessment of structural and functional integrity of the kidneys.
(b) Renal dysfunction is often subtle and asymptomatic requiring reliance on various laboratory tests to identify and manage underlying conditions.
(c) Awareness of antenatal and postnatal laboratory evaluation methods is the key to timely interventions.
(d) Ability to understand the age and gestation-associated variation of certain tests might avoid unnecessary investigations.

Case Vignette

A 6-week-old male neonate, born to a 23-year-old healthy primigravida, was brought to the pediatrician's office with history of reddish discoloration noticed in the diaper for about a week. There was no associated change in urine output. He has been feeding well on breast milk. Physical examination was unremarkable with adequate anthropometric measurements (>75th percentile for weight and height). The pediatrician performed a dipstick urinalysis to asses for a possible urinary tract infection, which was negative for blood; a CBC and renal function panel were normal but a renal sonogram revealed slightly small and mildly echogenic kidneys bilaterally, which can be seen in this age group. The patient was then referred to a nephrologist for further evaluation. At the nephrologist's office, the diagnosis of uric acid crystalluria was considered as the possible cause, and urine was evaluated for urinalysis, microscopy, and urine electrolytes including creatinine. Tubular functions were assessed which were essentially normal including fractional excretion of sodium of 0.5 % {FeNa}, urinary uric acid to GFR ratio of 0.3 (<0.56 mg/dL of GFR), urine calcium to creatinine ratio of

A.S. Chishti, MD, FAAP, CCST
Division of Pediatric Nephrology, Hypertension and Renal Transplantation, Kentucky Children's Hospital, University of Kentucky,
William R Willard Medical Science Building,
800 Rose Street, Lexington, KY 40536-0298, USA
e-mail: aftab.chishti@uky.edu

A.S. Chishti et al. (eds.), *Kidney and Urinary Tract Diseases in the Newborn*,
DOI 10.1007/978-3-642-39988-6_5, © Springer-Verlag Berlin Heidelberg 2014

1 (<0.8), and tubular reabsorption of phosphorus was 96 %. These tests were done to reassure the family of completely normal neonatal renal function.

Renal disease is usually silent; the changes are usually subtle and can only be elicited if precisely sought for. Pediatricians must use the best of the clinical acumen and use the appropriate diagnostic tools, with the knowledge of the differences in the normal ranges at various ages. The diagnostic tools in the assessments of renal function have improved over the last few decades.

5.2 Urine Analysis (UA)

UA is the oldest method of diagnostic urine testing, first used more than 6,000 years ago [20]. Often neglected by the clinicians and poorly performed by laboratories, it is an inexpensive, readily available, and easy to interpret test with or without automated analyzers. It is an excellent indicator of a variety of renal functions, and some people consider it as a medical "poor man's" biopsy of the kidney.

Urinalysis has two components: (1) Dipstick urinalysis gives semiquantitative analysis of chemical and metabolic abnormalities. Most commercially available dipsticks can screen for pH, specific gravity, ketones, glucose, protein, bilirubin, white blood cells, red blood cells, and nitrites. Newer dipsticks can even detect microalbumin as well. (2) Wet urinalysis consists of macroscopic appearances and microscopic analysis of the cellular elements, crystals, and bacteria in the urine. The urine specimen has to preferably be evaluated within an hour of voiding.

Macroscopic assessment of urine is useful and informative. Color, clarity, and odor of urine can give a wealth of information. Depending on concentration, the color of urine varies from clear to dark yellow. Amber to reddish brown urine suggests presence of hemoglobin, myoglobin, and hemosiderin. Bright red color signifies fresh blood, urate crystals (pink diaper syndrome), porphyrins, food coloring, and foods like beets. Brown-black discoloring is seen in alkaptonuria. Urine normally is clear, but the presence of white blood cells, bacteria, amorphous phosphates, and urates can turn it cloudy.

Urine specific gravity is commonly measured by a reagent strip; it ranges from 1.001 to 1.035, and it is indicative of tubular function. High-specific gravity is associated with volume depletion, syndrome of inappropriate antidiuretic hormone, and in glycosuria. It is rather low with diuretic use, in diabetes insipidus, and in impaired renal function [47].

Urinary pH is also assessed by the reagent strips, but it is not very accurate; in circumstances when exact pH is desirable, it should be measured using a pH meter in freshly voided urine. Assessment of urinary pH is useful in assessing acid–base status in a variety of conditions and in the evaluation for renal tubular acidosis as well as mixed respiratory and metabolic disturbances. It is also useful for the monitoring and treatment of nephrolithiasis.

Glucose is usually not present in the urine as it is completely reabsorbed in the proximal tubule after being filtered. It can be seen in significant hyperglycemic states (serum glucose >200 mg/dL), isolated renal glycosuria due to altered SGLT −1 or GLUT 2 transport proteins and in proximal tubular injury due to Fanconi's syndrome. The reagent strips are only sensitive to the presence of glucose, so other reducing sugars have to be tested for independently.

Ketone bodies are the product of fat metabolism and consist of acetoacetic acid, beta hydroxybutyrate, and acetone. Reagents on the dipstick only detect acetoacetic acid so dipstick underestimates the burden of ketone bodies in the system. Ketones are seen in the urine in diabetic ketoacidosis, glycogen storage diseases, starvation, high-fat diets, and in hyperthyroidism.

Urinary nitrites are produced by the conversion of dietary nitrates by the action of bacteria and are indicative of urinary tract infection (UTI) [42], mostly due to gram-negative bacteria. The absence of nitrites does not rule out an infection, as the urine may not have stayed long enough (usually about 4 h) in the bladder for the chemical reaction to be completed. False-negative results could be seen with excess of vitamin C in the urine, patients on vegan diets, and infection by yeast or gram-positive bacteria and especially in neonates in whom frequent emptying of the bladder may not allow the chemical reaction to be completed.

Crystals are seldom seen in freshly voided urine, but their presence can definitely suggest various pathologies like cystinuria and several others. Some are more readily seen in acidic urine like calcium oxalate and uric acid, while calcium phosphates, amorphous phosphates, and magnesium ammonium phosphates are readily visualized in alkaline samples.

White blood cells in the urine are seen with UTI or glomerulonephritides, which are detected by the leukocyte esterase, an enzyme present in the leukocyte granules.

Hematuria is detected by the reagent strip and confirmed by the presence of two-five red blood cells per high power field in the centrifuged urine under the microscope. The shape of RBCs can help determine the origin of these cells, as the red blood cells cross the glomerular filtration barrier, their pliable membrane gets distorted, or some part of it is pinched off giving the classic appearance of acanthocytes, and the red blood cells originating in the lower tract keep their eumorphic appearance. In addition red blood cell casts confirm glomerular etiology of hematuria.

5.3 Assessment of Proteinuria

In normal states, minimal amounts of high molecular weight proteins are filtered through the glomerular filtration; low molecular weight proteins that are filtered are mostly reabsorbed by the proximal tubules. Tamm-Horsfall protein is secreted by the tubules constituting the major component of excreted urinary proteins. In a variety of disease states, proteinuria increases either through the glomerular barrier or secreted by the diseased tubules. Albumin is the marker of glomerular proteinuria, while beta-2 microglobulin, alpha-1 microglobulin, and retinol-binding protein are common markers of tubular proteinuria.

5.3.1 Glomerular Proteinuria

Dipstick reagents are highly sensitive for albuminuria. They can give false-positive results due to prolonged immersion of the dipstick in the urine, a high urinary pH (>8.0), or in the presence of pyuria or bacteriuria. Dipsticks are useful for semiquantitative estimation of protein in the urine based on the color change of the strip (trace to 4+ suggestive of 10 mg/dL up to >500 mg/dL). Standard urine dipsticks are of little to no use for assessment of low molecular weight proteins. For the assessment of tubular proteinuria, sulfosalicylic acid precipitation test can be used but that is only a qualitative assessment, and urine protein electrophoresis will be needed for confirmation and quantification.

Spot urine protein to creatinine ratios are commonly used quick and reliable tests for protein excretion. The normal value varies according to the age and gestation; in general a ratio of <0.2 and under is considered normal, and values >2 suggest nephrotic range proteinuria [23]. In premature babies, this ratio can be as high as 0.6.

A 24-h timed urine collection is the gold standard for estimation of urinary protein loss. It is always necessary to check the total amount of creatinine in the same collection to assess adequacy of the collection. Amounts of 4 mg/m^2/day or less are considered normal protein excretion, while protein of >40 mg/m^2/day is confirmatory of nephrotic range proteinuria [23].

5.3.2 Tubular Proteinuria

Impaired proximal tubular reabsorption of filtered low molecular weight proteins leads to tubular proteinuria. Alpha-1 microglobulin (MW 30 kDa), retinol-binding protein (21.4 kDa), and beta-2 microglobulin (11.8 kDa) are the main markers of tubular injury. These proteins are much higher in diseased preterm babies in comparison to healthy preterm and healthy term babies; in addition all babies show decline in their urinary excretion within a few days in postnatal life suggesting tubular maturity happens rather quickly [2].

5.4 Assessment of Glomerular Function

Knowledge of the glomerular filtration rate (GFR) is critical in the management of newborn, infants, and children, not only to assess the renal function itself but also to help with function-based dosing of various medications that might be necessary in the premature infants and neonates, assessing potential risk of radiocontrast materials and in early detection of acute kidney injury.

Glomerular filtration is the commonly used measure of renal function. GFR changes significantly from early fetal life until 2 years of age when it reaches adult levels (Table 5.1). Neonates at term are born with minimal measureable GFR, but it is sufficient for the metabolic needs of the neonate. Glomerular filtration starts between 10 and 12 weeks of gestation; after birth, the GFR in term infants doubles by 2 weeks, triples by 3 months, and quadruples by 6 months of age. In premature babies born at 26 weeks of gestation, average GFR is 6 mL/min/1.732 m^2. A minimal increase in GFR occurs by 34 weeks of gestation (Table 5.1).

GFR increases rather quickly in first few weeks of postnatal life. GFR estimation is done using endogenous substances like creatinine and cystatin C or exogenous markers like inulin and iohexol or radioisotopic agents like DMSA or DTPA.

Table 5.1 Glomerular filtration in infants and children as assessed by the inulin clearance

Age	GFR ± SD mL/min/1.732 m^2
Preterm babies	
1–3 days	14+/−5
1–7 days	18.7+/−5.5
4–8 days	44+/−9.3
3–13 days	47.8+/−10.7
8–14 days	35.4+/−13.4
1.5–4 months	67.4+/−16.6
Term babies	
1–3 days	20.8+/−5
3–4 days	39+/−15.1
4–14 days	36.8+/−7.2
6–14 days	54.6+/−7.6
15–19 days	46.9+/−12.5
1–3 months	60.4+/−17.4
4–6 months	87.4+/−22.3
7–12 months	96.2+/−12.2
1–2 years	105.2+/−17.3

Modified with kind permission Springer: Schwartz and Furth [45]

Table 5.2 Normal serum creatinine levels

Age	Creatinine mg/dL {mmol/L}
<34 weeks of gestation	
<2 weeks old	0.7–1.4 {62–123}
>2 weeks old	0.7–0.9 {62–80}
>34 weeks of gestation	
<2 weeks old	0.4–0.6 {35–53}
>2 weeks old	0.3–0.5 {26–44}
1 month to 2 years	0.2–0.5 {18–44}

Modified from Chan et al. [8]

5.4.1 Creatinine-Based GFR Estimation

Creatinine-based GFR estimation methods are most commonly employed as it correlates well with inulin clearance within normal GFR ranges [45]. Creatinine as a by-product of muscle breakdown, hence it is not an ideal marker of GFR as there is some degree of reabsorption by the renal tubular cells. It is also secreted in the tubules and therefore overestimates the GFR at higher serum creatinine concentrations. Nevertheless it is overall the easiest and most commonly used test to assess GFR (Table 5.2).

The Schwartz formula [46] is quick and easy, utilizing height or length and serum creatinine concentration to calculate GFR; it has been recently modified in 2009, now recommending a fixed K of 0.413:

$$\text{GFR} = 0.413 \times \text{Length or Height}(\text{cm}) / \text{S. Creatinine}(\text{mg/dL})$$

Another commonly used formula is by Counahan [10] for serum creatinine measured in mg/dL or mmol/L, respectively:

$$\text{GFR} = 0.43 \times \text{Length or Height}\ (\text{cm}) / \text{S.Creatinine}(\text{mg/dL})$$

$$\text{GFR} = 0.43 \times \text{Length or Height}\ (\text{cm}) / \text{S.Creatinine}\ (\text{micromol/L})$$

Estimated GFR formulae have an intrinsic limitation, and they cannot be used in cases of severe obesity, malnutrition, and at the extremes of serum creatinine, where the secretory component of the creatinine can result in overestimation of GFR. In addition these cannot be used in critically ill patients with rapidly changing serum creatinine and in acute kidney injury.

Table 5.3 Normal serum cystatin C and creatinine levels

Age	Cystatin C mg/L (range)	Creatinine mmol/L (range)
24–28 weeks GA	1.48 (0.65–3.37)	78 (35–136)
29–36 weeks GA	1.65 (0.62–4.42)	75 (27–175)
0–3 months	1.37 (0.81–2.32)	47 (23–127)
4–11 months	0.98 (0.65–1.49)	42 (32–100)
1–3 years	0.79 (0.5–1.25)	45 (33–60)
1–17 years	0.8 (0.5–1.27)	56 (33–88)

Adapted from Finney et al. [14]. Copyright (2000) with permission from BMJ Publishing Group Ltd.

5.4.2 Cystatin C-Based GFR Estimation

Cystatin C is an endogenous low molecular weight protein (13.4 kD) and a member of cysteine protease inhibitor protein. It is produced by all the nucleated cells at a constant rate, completely filtered by the glomeruli, and almost 100 % metabolized by the renal tubular cells. Cystatin C is not affected much by age (the serum level decreases from birth to age 1 year and remain stable thereafter), gender, body composition, inflammatory conditions, and muscle mass. It can be affected by steroid use, thyroid disorders, and cigarette smoking. Multiple adult studies [18, 48] and a large pediatric study [14] suggest that cystatin C measurements correlate better with measured GFR and are more sensitive to subtle changes in GFR in comparison to creatinine (Table 5.3).

There are multiple cystatin C-based GFR formulae *without* measurement of serum creatinine:

Filler	$91.62 \times \text{Cystatin C}^{-1.123}$	{mL/min/1.732 m²} [13]
Zappitelli	$75.94 \times \text{Cystatin C}^{-1.17}$	{mL/min/1.732 m²} [55]
Grubb	$83.93 \times \text{Cystatin C}^{-1.676}$	{mL/min/1.732 m²} [19]
Larsson	$77.24 \times \text{Cystatin C}^{-1.2623}$	{mL/min} [25]

Some calculations include the serum creatinine:

Zappitelli

$$\frac{\left(507.76 \times e^{0.0003\text{Ht}}\right)}{\text{CystC}^{0.634}\ \ \text{Cr}^{0.547}\ \ 1.165^{\text{Tx}}}$$

$$\{\text{Cr mmol/L and Cystatin C mg/L}\}$$

$$43.82\left[1/\text{CystC}\right]^{0.635}\left[1/\text{Cr}\right]^{0.547}\left[1.35\right]^{\text{Ht}}$$

$$\{\text{Cr mg/dL and Cystatin C mg/L}\}$$

Zappitelli et al. [55].

Bouvet

$$63.2 \times (\text{Cr}/96)^{-0.35} \times (\text{Cyst C}/1.2)^{-0.56} \times (\text{Wt}/45)^{0.3} \times (\text{age}/14)^{0.4}$$

$$\{\text{Cr mmol/L and Cystatin C mg/L}\}$$

Bouvet et al. [7].

$$63.2\left[1.2/\text{CystC}\right]^{0.56}\left[(96/88.4)/\text{S.Cr}\right]^{0.35} \times (\text{Wt}/45)^{0.3} \times (\text{age}/14)^{0.4}$$

$$\{\text{Cr mg/dL and Cystatin C mg/L}\}$$

Schwartz CKiDs

$39.1 \times (\text{HT/S.Cr})^{0.516} \times (1.8/\text{Cyst C})^{0.294} \times (30/\text{BUN})^{0.169} \times (1.099)^{\text{Male}} \times (\text{HT}/1.4)^{0.188}$ (Schwartz et al. [46]).

5.4.3 Exogenous Substrate-Based GFR Estimation

Multiple substrates like inulin [1], iothalmate [37], iohexol [3], ethylenediaminetetraacetic acid {EDTA} [41], and diethylenetriaminepentaacetic acid {DTPA} [41] are used for GFR estimation. Some use radioactivity and others use plasma clearance/disappearance curves. The limitation of inulin, iohexol, and iothalmate is their availability and difficulty in collecting timed urine samples from neonates and infants. Tc-DTPA is a very useful radiotracer as it allows assessment of differential renal function of either kidney, but its limitation is the exposure to radiation. A detailed discussion of these methods is beyond the scope of this chapter.

5.5 Assessment of Tubular Function

Renal tubular cells along all nephron segments are responsible for the processing of glomerular filtrate until it is ready to be excreted as final urine. Tubular cells have a remarkable ability to reabsorb or secrete substances according to the bodily needs; their functions are measured by absolute values of various solutes and proteins excreted along with various determinants like fractional excretion of sodium, fractional excretion of urea nitrogen, trans-tubular potassium gradient, and tubular reabsorption of phosphorus.

5.5.1 Fractional Excretion of Sodium and Urea (FeNa)

It is one of the most sensitive indicators of volume status and tubular integrity.

$$\mathrm{FeNa} = \left\{ \begin{array}{l} \mathrm{Urine\,Na/Plasma\,Na} \times \\ \mathrm{Plasma\,Creatinine/} \\ \mathrm{Urine\,Creatinine} \end{array} \right\} \times 100$$

In older children, the FeNa usually is <1 % in prerenal states and >1 % in acute tubular injury, but in neonates, the threshold raises to 2.5–3.0 % due to inability to concentrate the urine [26, 50]. The value is dependent upon the gestational age as well; at 28 weeks, this could be as high as 12–15 % which gradually drops to 2–5 % by term and continues to fall postnatal even in premature infants [16]. It is also important to note that in face of diuretic use, FeNa cannot be used reliably due to increased sodium excretion caused by the diuretic. Under those circumstances, fractional excretion of urea can be substituted to assess intravascular volume or tubular integrity with a value of <35 % suggesting intravascular volume depletion and >35 % being suggestive of acute tubular injury [12].

$$\mathrm{FeUrea} = \left\{ \begin{array}{l} \mathrm{Urine\,Urea/Plasma\,Urea} \times \\ \mathrm{Plasma\,Creatinine/} \\ \mathrm{Urine\,Creatinine} \end{array} \right\} \times 100$$

5.5.2 Fractional Excretion of Magnesium (FeMg)

Mg is primarily reabsorbed in the proximal tubule and thick ascending limb of the loop of Henle. Mg handling is assessed by FeMg, which is normally 2–4 %.

$$\mathrm{FeMg} = \left\{ \begin{array}{l} \mathrm{Urine\ Mg} \times \mathrm{Plasma\ Creatinine} \times 100/ \\ \mathrm{Plasma\ Mg} \times \mathrm{Urine\ Creatinine} \times 0.7 \end{array} \right\}$$

A factor of 0.7 is used to estimate the free serum Mg concentration, as only the free unbound Mg is available to be filtered by the glomeruli.

5.5.3 Trans-tubular Potassium Gradient (TTKG)

It is an indicator of action of aldosterone on distal tubules and collecting ducts [43]. It is very useful in the differential diagnosis of hypo-/hyperkalemia. Its prerequisite is that the urinary osmolality has to be greater than the serum osmolality, or urinary sodium has to be >25 mmol/L as potassium secretion is markedly reduced in these circumstances.

$$TTKG = \begin{Bmatrix} \text{Urinary Potassium} \times \text{Plasma Osm}/ \\ \text{Plasma Potassium} \times \text{Urine Osm} \end{Bmatrix} \times 100$$

In general, expected values of TTKG are <3–5 in hypokalemic states and 6–10 in hyperkalemia. TTKG in preterm neonates is rather low due to low-potassium excretory capacity of the tubules, but it does increase quickly over the course of the first few weeks of postnatal life [34].

5.5.4 Tubular Reabsorption of Phosphorus (TRP)

Phosphorus excretion is mainly dependent upon tubular handling as 85–95 % of filtered phosphorus is reabsorbed via proximal tubular cells [15]. Tubular reabsorption of phosphorus is significantly lower after 3 months of age [5].

$$TRP = \left\{ 1 - \begin{pmatrix} \text{Urinary Phosphorus} \\ \times \text{Plasma Creatinine} \\ /\text{Plasma Phosphorus} \\ \times \text{Urinary Creatinine} \end{pmatrix} \times 100 \right\}$$

5.5.5 Random Urinary Calcium to Creatinine Ratio (UCa/Cr)

Urinary calcium estimation is useful in the evaluation of a patient with frequency, dysuria, hematuria, nephrocalcinosis, and nephrolithiasis. Random UCa/Cr is dependent on age ranging from 0.2 to 0.8 and the dietary intake of calcium (Table 5.4) [44, 49]. It is also significantly increased with the use of loop diuretics. Confirmation of true calcium excretion is obtained by collecting 24-h urine for calcium (<4 mg/kg/day).

Table 5.4 Norms for spot urinary calcium to creatinine ratio

Age	mg/mg	mmol/mmol
0–6 months	<0.8	<2.24
6–18 months	<0.6	<1.68
2–18 years	<0.2	<0.56

5.5.6 Urinary Uric Acid Estimation

Urinary uric acid excretion is another major indicator of renal tubular function. Newborns and infants tend to excrete a large amount of the filtered uric acid due to tubular immaturity. Adults excrete about 10 % of the filtered load, and this level is achieved at around 1 year of life. Neonates can excrete as much as 30–50 % of the filtered load. Uric acid excretion is related to weight and the gestational age of the newborn [40]. It can be assessed by using the fractional excretion of uric acid (FeUA):FeUA = {Urinary UA (mg/dL)/ Serum UA (mg/dL)/Urinary Creatinine (mg/dL)/ Serum Creatinine (mg/dL)/} × 100

As uric acid excretion also depends on the glomerular filtration, one can assess uric acid excretion per deciliter glomerular filtration, 3.3 mg/dL for children <2 years of age and <0.56 mg/dL for children >2 years of age [51, 52]: UA/GFR = {Urine UA (mg/dL) × Plasma Creatinine (mg/dL)/Urine Creatinine (mg/dL)}

5.6 Assessment of Fetal Renal Function

In the antenatal period, the placenta performs most of the functions that a well-developed and mature kidney performs. Nevertheless, the developing kidney does not stay idle either. Various physiologic mechanisms are underway, which can be assessed by various tests, even though some of these tests are crude and not very sensitive but can predict things to come in the future. Fetal renal function can be assessed by

1. Adequacy of amniotic fluid
2. Fetal urinary biochemical marker
3. Fetal blood sampling
4. Fetal renal biopsy
5. Fetal ultrasonography (see Chap. 8 for details)

Initially amniotic fluid is produced by the placenta but gradually fetal urine becomes the main source by 20 weeks of gestation. Any reduction in the amniotic fluid should alert the perinatologist to potential fetal renal dysfunction which can hamper lung development and maturity especially before 24 weeks of gestation. Similarly

Table 5.5 Predictors of poor neonatal renal function on the basis of fetal urinary markers

Index test	Threshold
Sodium	>100 mmol/L or >95th percentile
Chloride	>90 mmol/L or >95th percentile
Calcium	>1.2 mmol/L or >95th percentile
Osmolality	>200 mOsm/kg
Beta-2 microglobulin	>6 mg/L
Cystatin C	>1 mg/L
Retinol-binding protein	32 mg/L
Alpha-1 microglobulin	47 mg/L

Cobet et al. [9], Morris et al. [30], Muller et al. [31], Vanderheyden et al. [54]

excess of amniotic fluid can be associated with renal anomalies like congenital nephrosis and Bartter syndrome.

Fetal urine has been used to assess renal function for more than quarter century [17]. It is commonly done in cases of obstructive uropathies with dilated urinary tracts. Fetal urine can be assessed for sodium, chloride, calcium, urinary osmolarity, beta-2 microglobulins, and cystatin C. Of those markers, sodium, beta-2 microglobulins, and cystatin C best correlate with postnatal renal tubular function rather than glomerular filtration (Table 5.5).

Fetal urine becomes progressively more dilute with advancing gestational age; it is isotonic by 20 weeks of gestation. Urinary sodium concentrations decrease to <90 mmol/L by 30 weeks of gestation; higher values are indicators of poor renal tubular function. In a meta-analysis of fetal urine studies, it is suggested to use a gestation-specific threshold for urinary Na and beta-2 microglobulins for better diagnostic accuracy.

Cystatin C has evolved into a relatively more sensitive marker of renal function in adults and children. It has also been evaluated in amniotic fluid [33], fetal urine [31, 32], and fetal blood [6] to assess fetal renal function. Cystatin C is a protein (molecular weight 13.8 kD), so it does not cross placental barrier; it is filtered by glomeruli and reabsorbed and metabolized by renal tubules. In normal circumstances, cystatin C is not excreted in urine unless renal tubular cells are injured leading to alterations in tubular cell reabsorption and/or catabolism. Urinary cystatin C has the added advantage of being independent of gestational age.

Fetal blood sampling has become relatively safe with the development of the ultrasound-assisted chordocentesis. Usual clinical markers of renal function like urea, creatinine, and electrolytes pass through the placental barrier, so they are not good markers of renal function in the fetal blood [35]. Various higher molecular weight proteins like alpha-1 microglobulin (30 kD) [9, 36], beta-2 microglobulin (11.8 kD) [4, 11], retinol-binding protein (21 kD), and cystatin C (13.8 kD) [6] are used as markers in fetal blood sample.

Fetal renal biopsies are only in experimental procedure due to its invasiveness and high failure rate.

5.7 Future Developments

5.7.1 Novel Biomarkers and Future Directions

The need to identify novel biomarker to predict AKI has been a major area of research for nephrologists, neonatologists, and cardiologist in the last decade. Among the various promising biomarkers for prediction, stratification, characterizations, and monitoring the course and prognostication of acute kidney injury, four main biomarkers have been studied the most. These are neutrophil gelatinase-associated lipocalin {NGAL}, kidney injury molecule 1 {KIM-1}, and interleukin 18 {IL-18}.

(I) NGAL is a 25 kD, 178 amino acid long protein that has a role in renal tubular cell protection and proliferation. In a prospective study of children undergoing cardiopulmonary bypass, NGAL in the urine and serum samples predicted AKI within 2–6 h, while the creatinine rose 48–72 h later [27]. NGAL has also been found to be a predictor of renal dysfunction and the need for dialysis in renal transplant population [28], hemolytic uremic syndrome [53], contrast nephropathy [22], critically ill children in pediatric ICU setting [56], and chronic kidney disease (CKD) [29]. Unfortunately all these studies were rather small so large multicenter studies are warranted for this promising biomarker.

(II) KIM-1 is a transmembrane protein whose production is upregulated primarily in ischemic tubular injury. It is more specific for ischemic [21] and nephrotoxic AKI [24], then other forms of AKI and CKD. It is detected in high concentration in urine with 6 h of cardiopulmonary bypass in patients who subsequently develop AKI.

(III) IL-18 is an inflammatory mediator, which can be measured in the urine in ischemic AKI [38] but does not rise in nephrotoxic injury, urinary tract infection, or in chronic renal injury. It can also help predict delayed graft function in kidney transplant population [39].

There are other novel biomarkers like proximal renal tubular epithelial antigen, adenosine deaminase-binding protein, N-acetyl-beta-glucosaminidase, and liver fatty acid-binding protein which are being tested to improve our ability to identify renal injury as early as possible and to change the potential course and outcomes. Efforts are also being devoted to use many of these biomarkers either sequentially or as panels to improve their yield and reduce the morbidity and hopefully the mortality.

References

1. Arant BS Jr, Edelmann CM Jr et al (1972) The congruence of creatinine and inulin clearances in children: use of the Technicon AutoAnalyzer. J Pediatr 81(3):559–561
2. Awad H, el-Safty I et al (2002) Evaluation of renal glomerular and tubular functional and structural integrity in neonates. Am J Med Sci 324(5):261–266
3. Back SE, Krutzen E et al (1988) Contrast media as markers for glomerular filtration: a pharmacokinetic comparison of four agents. Scand J Clin Lab Invest 48(3):247–253
4. Berry SM, Lecolier B et al (1995) Predictive value of fetal serum beta 2-microglobulin for neonatal renal function. Lancet 345(8960):1277–1278
5. Bistarakis L, Voskaki I et al (1986) Renal handling of phosphate in the first six months of life. Arch Dis Child 61(7):677–681
6. Bokenkamp A, Dieterich C et al (2001) Fetal serum concentrations of cystatin C and beta2-microglobulin as predictors of postnatal kidney function. Am J Obstet Gynecol 185(2):468–475
7. Bouvet Y, Bouissou F et al (2006) GFR is better estimated by considering both serum cystatin C and creatinine levels. Pediatr Nephrol 21(9):1299–1306
8. Chan JCM, Williams DM et al (2002) Kidney failure in infants and children. Pediatr Rev 23(2):47–60
9. Cobet G, Gummelt T et al (1996) Assessment of serum levels of alpha-1-microglobulin, beta-2-microglobulin, and retinol binding protein in the fetal blood. A method for prenatal evaluation of renal function. Prenat Diagn 16(4):299–305
10. Counahan R, Chantler C et al (1976) Estimation of glomerular filtration rate from plasma creatinine concentration in children. Arch Dis Child 51(11): 875–878
11. Dommergues M, Muller F et al (2000) Fetal serum beta2-microglobulin predicts postnatal renal function in bilateral uropathies. Kidney Int 58(1):312–316
12. Fahimi D, Mohajeri S et al (2009) Comparison between fractional excretions of urea and sodium in children with acute kidney injury. Pediatr Nephrol 24(12):2409–2412
13. Filler G, Lepage N (2003) Should the Schwartz formula for estimation of GFR be replaced by Cystatin C formula? Pediatr Nephrol 18:981–985
14. Finney H, Newman DJ et al (2000) Reference ranges for plasma cystatin C and creatinine measurements in premature infants, neonates, and older children. Arch Dis Child 82(1):71–75
15. Forster IC, Hernando N et al (2006) Proximal tubular handling of phosphate: a molecular perspective. Kidney Int 70(9):1548–1559
16. Gallini F, Maggio L et al (2000) Progression of renal function in preterm neonates with gestational age < or = 32 weeks. Pediatr Nephrol 15(1–2):119–124
17. Glick PL, Harrison MR et al (1985) Management of the fetus with congenital hydronephrosis II: prognostic criteria and selection for treatment. J Pediatr Surg 20(4):376–387
18. Grubb A (1992) Diagnostic value of analysis of cystatin C and protein HC in biological fluids. Clin Nephrol 38(Suppl 1):S20–S27
19. Grubb A, Nyman U et al (2005) Simple cystatin C-based prediction equations for glomerular filtration rate compared with the modification of diet in renal disease prediction equation for adults and the Schwartz and the Counahan-Barratt prediction equations for children. Clin Chem 51(8):1420–1431
20. Haber MH (1988) Pisse prophecy: a brief history of urinalysis. Clin Lab Med 8(3):415–430
21. Han WK, Bailly V et al (2002) Kidney Injury Molecule-1 (KIM-1): a novel biomarker for human renal proximal tubule injury. Kidney Int 62(1): 237–244
22. Hirsch R, Dent C et al (2007) NGAL is an early predictive biomarker of contrast-induced nephropathy in children. Pediatr Nephrol 22(12):2089–2095

23. Hogg RJ, Portman RJ et al (2000) Evaluation and management of proteinuria and nephrotic syndrome in children: recommendations from a pediatric nephrology panel established at the National Kidney Foundation conference on Proteinuria, Albuminuria, Risk, Assessment, Detection, and Elimination (PARADE). Pediatrics 105(6):1242–1249
24. Ichimura T, Hung CC et al (2004) Kidney injury molecule-1: a tissue and urinary biomarker for nephrotoxicant-induced renal injury. Am J Physiol Renal Physiol 286(3):F552–F563
25. Larsson A, Malm J et al (2004) Calculation of glomerular filtration rate expressed in mL/min from plasma cystatin C values in mg/L. Scand J Clin Lab Invest 64(1):25–30
26. Mathew OP, Jones AS et al (1980) Neonatal renal failure: usefulness of diagnostic indices. Pediatrics 65(1):57–60
27. Mishra J, Dent C et al (2005) Neutrophil gelatinase-associated lipocalin (NGAL) as a biomarker for acute renal injury after cardiac surgery. Lancet 365(9466):1231–1238
28. Mishra J, Ma Q et al (2006) Kidney NGAL is a novel early marker of acute injury following transplantation. Pediatr Nephrol 21(6):856–863
29. Mitsnefes MM, Kathman TS et al (2007) Serum neutrophil gelatinase-associated lipocalin as a marker of renal function in children with chronic kidney disease. Pediatr Nephrol 22(1):101–108
30. Morris RK, Quinlan-Jones E et al (2007) Systematic review of accuracy of fetal urine analysis to predict poor postnatal renal function in cases of congenital urinary tract obstruction. Prenat Diagn 27(10):900–911
31. Muller F, Bernard MA et al (1999) Fetal urine cystatin C as a predictor of postnatal renal function in bilateral uropathies. Clin Chem 45(12):2292–2293
32. Muller F, Dommergues M et al (1993) Fetal urinary biochemistry predicts postnatal renal function in children with bilateral obstructive uropathies. Obstet Gynecol 82(5):813–820
33. Mussap M, Fanos V et al (2002) Predictive value of amniotic fluid cystatin C levels for the early identification of fetuses with obstructive uropathies. BJOG 109(7):778–783
34. Nako Y, Ohki Y et al (1999) Transtubular potassium concentration gradient in preterm neonates. Pediatr Nephrol 13(9):880–885
35. Nava S, Bocconi L et al (1996) Aspects of fetal physiology from 18 to 37 weeks' gestation as assessed by blood sampling. Obstet Gynecol 87(6):975–980
36. Nolte S, Mueller B et al (1991) Serum alpha 1-microglobulin and beta 2-microglobulin for the estimation of fetal glomerular renal function. Pediatr Nephrol 5(5):573–577
37. Odlind B, Hallgren R et al (1985) Is 125I iothalamate an ideal marker for glomerular filtration? Kidney Int 27(1):9–16
38. Parikh CR, Abraham E et al (2005) Urine IL-18 is an early diagnostic marker for acute kidney injury and predicts mortality in the intensive care unit. J Am Soc Nephrol 16(10):3046–3052
39. Parikh CR, Jani A et al (2006) Urine NGAL and IL-18 are predictive biomarkers for delayed graft function following kidney transplantation. Am J Transplant 6(7):1639–1645
40. Passwell JH, Modan M et al (1974) Fractional excretion of uric-acid in infancy and childhood – index of tubular maturation. Arch Dis Child 49(11):878–882
41. Rehling M, Moller ML et al (1984) Simultaneous measurement of renal clearance and plasma clearance of 99mTc-labelled diethylenetriaminepenta-acetate, 51Cr-labelled ethylenediaminetetra-acetate and inulin in man. Clin Sci (Lond) 66(5):613–619
42. Roberts KB (2011) Urinary tract infection: clinical practice guideline for the diagnosis and management of the initial UTI in febrile infants and children 2 to 24 months. Pediatrics 128(3):595–610
43. Rodriguez-Soriano J, Vallo A (1988) Renal tubular hyperkalaemia in childhood. Pediatr Nephrol 2(4):498–509
44. Sargent JD, Stukel TA et al (1993) Normal values for random urinary calcium to creatinine ratios in infancy. J Pediatr 123(3):393–397
45. Schwartz GJ, Furth SL (2007) Glomerular filtration rate measurement and estimation in chronic kidney disease. Pediatr Nephrol 22(11):1839–1848
46. Schwartz GJ, Munoz A et al (2009) New equations to estimate GFR in children with CKD. J Am Soc Nephrol 20(3):629–637
47. Simerville JA, Maxted WC et al (2005) Urinalysis: a comprehensive review. Am Fam Physician 71(6):1153–1162
48. Simonsen O, Grubb A et al (1985) The blood serum concentration of cystatin C (gamma-trace) as a measure of the glomerular filtration rate. Scand J Clin Lab Invest 45(2):97–101
49. So NP, Osorio AV et al (2001) Normal urinary calcium/creatinine ratios in African-American and Caucasian children. Pediatr Nephrol 16(2):133–139
50. Stapleton FB, Jones DP et al (1987) Acute renal failure in neonates: incidence, etiology and outcome. Pediatr Nephrol 1(3):314–320
51. Stapleton FB, Linshaw MA et al (1978) Uric acid excretion in normal children. J Pediatr 92(6):911–914
52. Stapleton FB, Nash DA (1983) A screening test for hyperuricosuria. J Pediatr 102(1):88–90
53. Trachtman H, Christen E et al (2006) Urinary neutrophil gelatinase-associated lipocalcin in D+HUS: a novel marker of renal injury. Pediatr Nephrol 21(7):989–994
54. Vanderheyden T, Kumar S et al (2003) Fetal renal impairment. Semin Neonatol 8(4):279–289
55. Zappitelli M, Parvex P et al (2006) Derivation and validation of cystatin C-based prediction equations for GFR in children. Am J Kidney Dis 48(2):221–230
56. Zappitelli M, Washburn KK et al (2007) Urine neutrophil gelatinase-associated lipocalin is an early marker of acute kidney injury in critically ill children: a prospective cohort study. Crit Care 11(4):R84

Nutrition in the Newborn with Renal Disease

6

Sonal Bhatnagar and Steven J. Wassner

Core Messages

- The neonatal period through the first year of life is a critical growth period during which nutritional intake is the prime growth stimulant.
- During infancy, chronic kidney disease is mainly due to renal structural abnormalities. These infants demonstrate significant renal tubular defects including sodium and bicarbonate losses as well as the inability to concentrate urine. Treatment in these infants must be adjusted to repair their excessive electrolyte and water losses.
- Neonatal acute kidney injury is often present as part of a more general picture of neonatal sepsis, congenital heart disease or hypoxic ischemic encephalopathy. Weighing the nutritional requirements for growth against the need to restrict fluid and electrolyte intake requires the collaborative efforts of multiple subspecialists.

Case Vignette

At 28 weeks gestation, a fetal ultrasound reveals that there is a male singleton fetus present but that there is bilateral hydronephrosis and an enlarge bladder. The ultrasound report notes that there is sufficient amniotic fluid present, and lung development is reported to be adequate. The parents ask to speak to you regarding antenatal counseling. You note that the presence of adequate amniotic fluid is a good sign but believe that it is highly likely that their son will be born with posterior urethral valves and will require surgical relief of his urinary obstruction shortly after birth. You stress the importance of delivery at a neonatal center with both pediatric urologic and nephrologic care providers and counsel the parents that their son will likely have some degree of chronic kidney disease but that it is too early to determine the severity of the problem. The infant is born at a regional

S. Bhatnagar, MBBS
Division of Pediatric Nephrology,
Children's Hospital of Philadelphia,
Philadelphia, PA, USA

S.J. Wassner (✉)
Penn State Hershey Children's Hospital,
500 University Drive, Hershey,
PA 17033, USA
e-mail: swassner@hmc.psu.edu

A.S. Chishti et al. (eds.), *Kidney and Urinary Tract Diseases in the Newborn*,
DOI 10.1007/978-3-642-39988-6_6, © Springer-Verlag Berlin Heidelberg 2014

center and is enrolled in a comprehensive chronic kidney disease program. The child goes on to require three hospitalizations within the first 18 months of life for dehydration secondary to infectious diarrhea/emesis but is thereafter stable. At 7 years of age, chronic kidney disease has progressed to **Stage 4** with an estimated creatinine clearance of 22 mL/min/1.73 m^2, and he is referred for renal transplantation. His care to date has required multiple medications and the use of nutritional supplements, but at the time of transplantation, his height and weight are both within −1 standard deviation score of the mean, his head circumference is at the mean for age, and he is developmentally normal.

6.1 Introduction

The role of nutrition is to provide the essential elements necessary for maintenance and growth. This is accomplished through a combination of metabolic adaptations as well as the kidney's exceptional ability to maintain the body's internal milieu. Children born with abnormal renal function are at a significant disadvantage at either conserving or excreting a variety of nutrients and as a result, often suffer nutritional debility during their earliest, most vital growth period. This chapter will attempt to outline both the challenges faced and some of the solutions currently available to achieve optimal growth during the first months of life.

Karlberg [1] proposed a hypothesis that divides growth into three distinct but overlapping phases. The first begins in utero and continues until sometime during the first year. The primary driver in this phase is nutritional not hormonal. The second phase begins later in the first year when nutrition remains important, but the primary stimulant is now growth hormone. The third phase begins at puberty when sex hormone secretion provides an additional stimulant to ongoing growth hormone secretion.

Linear growth rates are highest during the fetal period, averaging approximately 12 cm/month in the third trimester [2]. While growth rates decrease in the neonatal period, they are still higher than those at later periods of life. A normal infant gains about 25 cm in length during the first year of life, which is an increase of almost 50 % over birth length. By the end of the second year of life, a normal infant has completed approximately 30 % of its total growth and has reached 50 % of its final height [3]. At 1 year of age, the standard deviation (SD) for length is approximately 2.5 cm. This means that a growth rate as high as 80 % of normal (20 cm) would still leave them at a height of −2 SD below normal, putting it below the third percentile on the height chart.

During fetal life, it is the placenta that serves as the metabolic filter with the fetal kidney primarily being responsible for the production of amniotic fluid. While the kidney's role is limited, it is vital since infants born with oligohydramnios often die due to pulmonary hypoplasia. For infants born with structural renal disease and decreased renal function, growth failure often begins during the fetal period with newborn length measurements averaging approximately 1 standard deviation score (SDS) below the mean. Growth rates are diminished throughout the first several months of life, and infants with chronic kidney disease (CKD) may lose up to another SDS within the first few months of life [4]. This can account for up to 2/3 of the overall reduction in height SDS occurring over childhood. Data from the Growth Failure in Children with Renal Diseases Study and the North American Pediatric Renal Transplant Collaborative Studies group (NAPRTCS) indicate that the younger a child is at the onset of renal disease, the larger height deficits she/he has [5, 6]. Both height and weight are affected, which explains the classic literature description of infants with CKD as one of small, often cachectic individuals. The importance of this growth failure is magnified by the fact that both in renal disease and in studies in otherwise normal children, growth lost during the first year of life is not fully regained [7, 8].

These findings emphasize the need for early and aggressive intervention to maximize growth. By intervening early, growth velocity can be improved with some degree of catch-up growth obtained. Current studies suggest, however, that for infants with CKD, average height SDS still hover below the mean as opposed to being normally distributed around zero [6, 9].

6.2 Etiology of CKD in Infancy

Approximately 20 % of children diagnosed with CKD each year are under 2 years of age (3/4 of whom are diagnosed in the first year of life). Of these, 70–75 % have a structural abnormality, such as obstructive uropathy, renal aplasia/hypoplasia/dysplasia, or reflux nephropathy, currently grouped together under the acronym CAKUT, which stands for congenital abnormalities of the kidneys or urinary tract. While present, autosomal recessive polycystic kidney disease forms only a small percentage of this group, and the incidence of inflammatory/immunologic disease is quite small [6]. The prevalence of CAKUT is associated with a high incidence of tubular dysfunction, due to both a combination of tubular adaption to hyperfiltration and to the tubular dysfunction present in these infants.

6.3 Conditions with Decreased GFR

6.3.1 Nutritional Intake and Growth

Given that multiple dietary alterations will be required for infants with CKD both as a function of their growth and their changing renal capacity, it is appropriate to consider as a base diet, a low-electrolyte, low-osmolar formula to which substances can be added as necessary. The most efficient infant formula known is human milk, and its use is to be encouraged for nutritional as well as psychological reasons. However, since the infant's volitional intake cannot be counted upon and a variety of additives are likely to be necessary, it is unlikely that the mother will be able to feed her infant at the breast. We have attempted to have mothers express their own milk and feed it to their infants, adding supplements as necessary. Unfortunately, this has rarely been a successful long-term solution, and the majority of mothers switch to one of the low-osmolar, human-milk substitutes. Table 6.1 notes some of the commercial formulas that may be utilized during the first year of life and thereafter, while Table 6.2 lists additional modules utilized to increase energy or protein intakes. The role of the renal dietician is crucial in assisting the mother in the choice of a suitable formula, in monitoring nutritional parameters, and in helping the family with the multiple formula changes required.

Progression to dialysis will affect also the nutritional requirements. Prior to dialysis, remnant kidney function and the requirements associated with solute clearance produce copious amounts of dilute urine. At end stage, urine output decreases and fluid overload becomes a concern. Attention to dietary intake will require marked alteration of fluid and nutrient intake and, where appropriate, will be noted in the sections below.

Infants with CKD do not require higher energy intakes than normal infants. Estimates of total energy requirements for normal infants have been calculated based on average values for breast-fed infants [10]. Since there are variations present within the normal population, it is understandable that infants with CKD would show at least the same variability. The Fluid and Nutrition Board has determined estimated energy requirements (EER) for healthy infants based on estimates of total energy expenditure plus the energy required for growth and tissue deposition. This data can be presented several ways but is most easily seen in Table 6.3 [11]. It should be noted that these calculations assume normal body size/age and were not designed for use in infants who were growth retarded and in whom catch-up growth is desired. It has been suggested that for these children, the appropriate choice for energy intake would be that of an average child of the same height [11]. As can be seen, moving higher on the table automatically increases the energy intake/kilogram body weight. Experimental evidence suggests that intakes of 100–120 % of normal are appropriate and that energy intakes >130 % of normal are unlikely to promote linear growth but may lead to obesity [5, 12, 13].

Table 6.1 Common neonatal and infant formula

Formula name	kcal/oz	kcal/100 mL	Prot (g)[a]	CHO (g)[a]	FAT (g)[a]	Na mEq[a]	K mEq[a]	Ca mg [a]	Ca mEq[a]	P mg[a]	P mmol[a]	Mg mg[a]	Mg mEq[a]	mOsm/kg	RSL mOsm/L[b]
Human milk	21	73	1.1	7.2	4.6	0.8	1.4	33	1.7	15	0.5	3.2	0.3	290	91
Similac® PM 60/40	20	68	1.5	6.9	3.8	0.7	1.4	37.9	1.9	19	0.6	4.1	0.3	280	124
Similac® Advance	20	68	1.4	7.2	3.8	0.7	1.8	53	2.6	28	0.9	4.1	0.3	310	127
Good Start® Gentle Plus	20	67	1.5	7.8	3.4	0.8	1.8	45	2.3	25	0.8	4.7	0.4	250	130
Enfamil® Lipil	20	68	1.4	7.6	3.6	0.8	1.9	53	2.7	29	0.9	5.4	0.4	300	130
Isomil®	20	68	1.7	7.0	3.7	1.3	1.9	71	3.6	51	1.6	51	4.2	200	155
Prosobee®	20	68	1.7	7.2	3.6	1.1	2.1	71	3.6	47	1.5	5.4	0.4	170	156
Pregestimil®	20	68	1.9	6.9	3.8	1.4	1.9	64	3.2	35	1.1	5.4	0.4	320	168
PediaSure®	30	100	2.9	13.9	3.8	1.7	3.4	106	5.3	84	2.7	17	1.4	352	278
Nutren Junior Fibre®	30	100	3.0	11.0	5.0	2.0	3.4	120	6.0	84	2.7	20.0	1.6	350	256

[a]Values per 100 mL of standard dilution formula
[b]Renal solute load

Table 6.2 Modular additions to formulas and diets

Module	Measure	kcal	Prot (g)	CHO (g)	Fat (g)	Na (mEq)	K (mEq)	Ca (mg)	Ca (mEq)	P (mg)	P (mmol)
Similac® Human Milk Fortifier	1 packet (.09 g)	3.5	0.3	0.5	0.09	0.16	0.40	29.3	1.5	16.8	0.5
Enfamil® Human Milk Fortifier	1 vial	7.5	0.55	<0.3	0.58	0.29	0.29	29	1.5	15.8	0.5
Duocal®	1 scoop (5 g)	25	0	3.6	1.12				0.0		0.0
Polycose®	1 teaspoon (2 g)	8		1.9		0.11		0.6	0.0	0.3	0.0
Polycose® Liquid	1 mL	2		0.5		0.03	0.00				
Microlipid®	1 mL	4.5			0.5						
MCT Oil® (medium-chain triglycerides)	1 Tablespoon (15 mL)	116			14						
Beneprotein®	1 scoop (7 g)	25	6			0.7	0.9	<20			

Table 6.3 Average energy requirements during infancy

Age (months)	Average length[a]	Average Wt	EER[b]	EER/kg
1	54.2	4.4	472	107
2	57.8	5.3	567	107
3	60.6	6	572	95
4	63.0	6.7	548	82
5	65.0	7.3	596	82
6	66.7	7.9	645	82
7	68.3	8.4	668	80
8	69.7	8.9	710	80
9	71.1	9.3	746	80
10	72.4	9.7	793	82
11	73.7	10	817	82
12	74.9	10.3	844	82
15	78.3	11.1	908	82
18	81.5	11.7	961	82
21	84.4	12.2	1,006	82
24	87.0	12.7	1,050	83

Adapted from [52]
Total energy expenditure for normal infants of both sexes = 0.89 × body weight (kg) – 100
[a]Average length of male and female infants
[b]EER = estimated energy requirements as the sum of total energy expenditure (TEE) and energy deposition

The institution of hemodialysis does not appear to alter caloric requirements. However, for infants on peritoneal dialysis, it is important to take into account the energy derived from dialysate glucose, which can reach 8–12 kcal/kg/day and make a significant contribution to the total energy intake [14, 15].

6.3.2 Protein

The body's hierarchy places maintenance energy requirements above growth so that when energy requirements are not being met, amino acids will be broken down into their carbon backbones plus nitrogen, with the carbon being converted to energy and the nitrogen to urea. Thus, the first step to ensuring the anabolism necessary for growth is the provision of adequate energy. Again, in the absence of intercurrent illness or surgery, there is no evidence to suggest that infants with CKD have increased protein requirements. On the other hand, provision of excess protein will not lead to improvement in nitrogen balance but rather the formation of excess urea nitrogen and subsequent azotemia. Attempts to delay the progression of renal failure by the institution of low-protein diets to infants and children with CKD have been unsuccessful and may be associated with diminished growth [16, 17]. As renal function declines, however, protein restriction should be enforced and intake limited to currently published standards (Table 6.4).

Table 6.4 Macronutrient intakes for normal infants[a]

Infants	Protein g/kg/day	Sodium g/day	Phosphorous mg/day	Calcium mg/day	Potassium g/day
0–6 month	1.5	0.12	100	210	0.4
7–12 month	1.5[b]	0.37	275	270	0.7

Adapted from [26, 52, 53]
[a]Values are noted as adequate intake (AI), the recommended average daily intake level based on observed or experimentally determined approximations or estimates of nutrient intake by a group (or groups) of apparently healthy people that are assumed to be adequate—used when an DRI cannot be determined
[b]Value listed as the DRI—adequate for 97.5 % of the population [52]

6.3.3 Sodium

Sodium is required for growth, and during the first 6 months, infants must retain approximately 2 mEq/day to account for the increase in total body sodium associated with increased ECF [18]. Breast-fed infants consume about 1 mEq/kg/day and are able to achieve a positive sodium balance due to the ability of normal renal tubules to avidly conserve sodium. In children with CAKUT, tubular damage leads to an increase in the fractional sodium excretion and a negative sodium balance [19–21]. These infants are particularly at risk at times of intercurrent illness when decreased oral intake, emesis, and diarrhea may combine to further increase losses and decrease renal function. The development of dehydration can lead to the rapid development of acidosis, shock, and hyperkalemia, the combination of which can be acutely life threatening. Parents need to be counseled about the importance of maintaining hydration and contacting their physicians at an early stage in their child's illness.

Sodium depletion affects extracellular volume, as well as growth and nitrogen retention [22, 23]. Maintenance of a normal extracellular volume has been shown to be vital for muscle development and bone mineralization.

Standards for normal infant sodium intakes are noted in Table 6.4, but as a rule, infants with neonatal CKD will require additional sodium chloride to be added to their feeds [24, 25]. We begin supplementation with 2–3 mEq sodium/kg/day and aim to keep serum sodium concentrations at or above 140 mEq/L, decreasing sodium intake in the presence of either hypertension or edema formation. Preterm infants may require even larger amounts due to the decreased sodium reabsorptive ability and rapid growth rates. When volume status is still uncertain, serum renin determinations may also be helpful. Early on, the presence of high urinary sodium losses is generally protective against the development of hypertension [26]. As kidney failure progresses and GFR further declines, the amount of sodium intake will have to be adjusted to prevent volume overload.

6.3.4 Potassium

For infants receiving one of the humanized milk formulas, potassium intakes are often acceptable, and normal serum potassium concentrations are maintained through a combination of limited potassium intake and augmented excretion secondary to high urine flow rates, increased urine sodium loss, and hyperaldosteronism. Occasionally, infants with CAKUT develop a form of pseudohypoaldosteronism and may require the small doses of fludrocortisone. More commonly, hyperkalemia presents in the face of intercurrent volume depletion and metabolic acidosis.

When serum potassium concentrations remain elevated in the absence of volume depletion, the use of a sodium-potassium polystyrene resin (Kayexalate®) can be added during preparation of the infant formula. The formula is then decanted and the supernatant fed to the infant [27]. This is effective in lowering potassium intake, but the exchange of potassium for sodium can lead to chronic sodium overload as each gram of resin contains 4 mEq of sodium.

6.3.5 Water

Under normal circumstances, the kidney has enormous capacity to excrete water with up to 10 % of total renal water reabsorption controlled in the collecting duct under the action of antidiuretic hormone. Renal concentrating ability is lost early in infants with CAKUT, while the ability to excrete dilute urine is maintained. Since the amount of urinary osmols to be excreted is related to dietary intake and growth [28], the inability to concentrate urine requires that sufficient free water be presented during feeding. These infants often require as much is 180–200 mL H_2O/kg/day. This can be achieved by diluting infant formula from the standard 20 kcal/oz to approximately 17–18 kcal/oz. Since infants eat to caloric satiety, an average intake of 100 kcal/kg/day will provide sufficient water intake. The ability to dilute urine is preserved until late in the course of CKD so that it is unlikely that fluid intake in this range will lead to volume overload. One area often overlooked is the contribution of formula intake to the production of urinary osmols. This is designated as renal solute load (RSL). A major determinant of RSL is protein content so that appropriate formulas for this group of patients are those with low RSL (see Table 6.1).

6.3.6 Acidosis

Infants with CKD develop acidosis due to both decreased proximal tubular bicarbonate reabsorption and decreased distal hydrogen ion excretion. It has become increasingly clear that acidosis exerts a variety of adverse effects including increased protein degradation, decreased bone mineralization, and possibly even accelerating the rate of GFR decline [29–34].

The need for alkali therapy may be masked by volume contraction. With the use of additional dietary chloride (as the sodium salt) and the use of dilute formulas, intravascular volume is likely to be restored to normal. In this situation, serum bicarbonate concentrations will decrease and the addition of base, either as bicarbonate or citrate, is required.

Acid is produced both from dietary intake and from the calcification of osteoid to bone where the uptake of calcium leads to the release of hydrogen ion. While acid production in adults is generally 1–2 mmol/kg/day, during periods of rapid growth, this may increase to as much as 3–5 mEq/kg/day [26, 35]. There is, therefore, no absolute value for bicarbonate supplementation, but sufficient alkali should be provided to maintain serum bicarbonate concentrations at or above 22 mmol/L. Development of significant metabolic alkalosis in the face of moderate doses of alkali suggests chloride depletion alkalosis. The addition of sodium without chloride generally does not lead to volume overload.

6.3.7 Calcium/Phosphorus

Both calcium and phosphorus are necessary for cellular and bone growth. Human milk provides limited amounts of both of these substances (compared with cow's milk), and adequate renal mass is required to maintain an appropriate balance for both elements. While adequate calcium absorption requires the presence of the activated vitamin D metabolite (1,25-dihydroxcholecalciferol), gastrointestinal phosphate can easily be absorbed in the absence of vitamin D stimulation. Most infant formulas contain excessive quantities of both calcium and phosphate and are inappropriate for infants with CKD. Formulas appropriate for infants with CKD more closely resemble the calcium/phosphate content of human milk with approximately a 2:1 ratio of calcium to phosphorus. It is also true that the development of rickets has been reported in severely premature infants both without evident renal disease. In these infants, however, the etiology is often due to absolute dietary calcium and/or phosphate deficiency in the face of rapid growth rates [36]. While all individuals with CKD will at some point in their progression require the administration of 1,25-dihydroxcholecalciferol, it now appears that there is a role for the maintenance of serum 25-hydroxyvitamin D concentrations as well. While there is still debate as to the minimum requirement, these infants should, at a minimum, receive current recommended daily doses of calciferol or ergocalciferol [37].

6.3.8 Supplemental Feeding

Approximately 40 years ago, Holliday [38] first noted that CKD was associated with decreased caloric intake and that growth could be improved, but not normalized, by caloric supplementation. This has been abundantly confirmed by others [6, 9, 39]. Early attempts to improve intake led to the use of highly concentrated formulas with a high-osmolar load; this approach had the paradoxical effect of increasing renal solute load in the face of decreased tubular concentrating ability. The net effect was the worsening of azotemia, hyperkalemia, and, often, the premature institution of dialysis.

Poor intake may be secondary to poor appetite and/or frequent vomiting, both of which may be clinical manifestations of acidosis or uremia [40]. Symptoms of vomiting, irritability, and discomfort may also be suggestive of gastroesophageal reflux in infants with CKD [41].

When oral intake does not suffice, tube feeding should be initiated to provide adequate nutrition for both predialysis and dialysis-dependent individuals [40]. The use of enteral feeds has allowed physicians to tailor their nutritional therapy and insure more consistent intakes. It also relieves parents of concerns regarding their inability to provide adequate nutrition when their infant will not drink adequate daily volumes. In a large study of infants with CKD who presented at less than 6 months of age, 80 % were tube fed and had a mean height SDS within normal range at 1 year of age [42]. In another study, 12 infants were started on supplemental enteral feeding in association with PD and showed significant improvements in height, weight, and head circumference SDS at 1 year [43].

Nissen fundoplication may be required in severe cases of intractable vomiting and is often performed at the time of gastrostomy tube placement. More recently, the use of gastrojejunal tubes has been suggested as an alternative to fundoplication, but there is little published data on the use of this approach in children with CKD.

Infants who require tube feeds often develop oral feeding dysfunction [44] and require referral to feeding clinics. In our experience, this remains a problem throughout the pretransplant and early transplant period, resolving only after good renal function is established.

For infants and children with advanced renal disease, several formulas have been designed to provide adequate energy and protein intakes with limited fluid and electrolyte content. The use of these formulas implies a significant degree of renal insufficiency and the importance of nephrologic as well as nutritional involvement (Table 6.5).

6.3.9 Growth Hormone

The administration of growth hormone to infants is controversial. If the growth schema noted by Karlberg [1] is correct, then growth hormone is not a major growth stimulant until the later part of the first year. The first 6–9 months of life should therefore be devoted to aggressive attempts to institute and maintain appropriate oral/enteral nutrition and prevent the previously described decline in growth parameters often seen in these children. For those infants in whom growth rates are still not acceptable after adequate nutritional intake is assured and metabolic bone disease has been addressed, the use of recombinant human growth hormone may provide additional improvement in statural growth [45].

6.4 Conditions with Normal GFR

6.4.1 Congenital Nephrotic Syndrome (NS)

Congenital nephrotic syndrome is by definition a condition appearing either at birth or within the first 3 months of life. Unlike CKD, GFR is generally normal early in life, and the main nutritional concerns appear to relate to the provision of a high-energy, high-protein, and low-sodium

Table 6.5 Specialized renal formulas

Formula name	kcal/oz	kcal/100 mL	Prot (g)[a]	CHO (g)[a]	FAT (g)[a]	Na mEq[a]	K mEq[a]	Ca mg[a]	Ca mEq[a]	P mg[a]	P mmol[a]	Mg mg[a]	Mg mEq[a]	mOsm/kg	RSL mOsm/L[b]
Nepro with Carb Steady®[c] Vanilla	54	180	8.1	16.1	9.6	4.6	2.7	106.0	5.3	72.0	2.3	21.0	1.7	745	555
Novasource Renal® (BrikPak)	60	200	9.1	18.3	10.0	4.1	2.4	84.0	4.2	81.9	2.7	19.7	1.6	800	635
Re/Gen HP/HC®[c] Vanilla	58	195	6.8	26.6	9.6	4.4	0.3	8.5	0.4	38.4	1.2	1.7	0.1	225	770
Renalcal®[d]	60	200	3.4	29.0	8.2	0.3	0.2	6.0	0.3	10.0	0.0	2.0	0.0	600	145
Renastart®[e]	30	100	1.5	12.5	4.8	2.1	0.6	22.6	1.1	18.4	0.6	10.6	0.9	225	125
Suplena with Carb Steady®[f] Vanilla	54	180	4.5	19.6	9.6	3.5	2.9	105.5	5.3	71.7	2.3	21.5	1.8	600	344

[a]Values per 100 mL of standard dilution formula
[b]Renal solute load
[c]Intended from individuals on dialysis
[d]Not a nutritionally complete formula
[e]For birth through 10 years of age
[f]Designed for patients with CKD not on dialysis

intake. While the best described form of congenital nephrotic syndrome is the Finnish type, noted for genetic defects in the Nephrin gene, there are a variety of other genetic causes known. In all cases, it is necessary to aggressively limit sodium intake while providing adequate energy and protein intake. These children have traditionally been treated with high-energy formulas, providing up to 130 kcal/kg/day [46]. Human milk or milk formulas may be used, with added glucose polymers to increase the caloric value. Rapeseed, sunflower, or fish oil are generally added to increase the ratio of monounsaturated and polyunsaturated fatty acids. Protein intakes as high as 3–4 g/kg/day are necessary [46, 47] and may be provided in the form of casein-based protein additives. These children may also require intravenous albumin infusions as an adjunct to their enteral feeds to maintain adequate serum albumin concentrations and prevent gross edema necessary [46].

Due to the massive protein loss in the urine, all of these children develop hypothyroidism and require early thyroxine supplementation. Vitamin D supplementation is required, but correction of 25-hydroxyvitamin D concentrations is difficult due to massive urinary losses. During the first several years of life, there is a progressive decline in renal function. These children all develop CKD and will eventually require renal transplantation. The timing of nephrectomy and transplantation is dependent at least to some degree upon the ability to maintain adequate nutrition in the face of nutritional debility [46–48].

6.4.2 Tubular Lesions

Tubular lesions such as renal tubular acidosis, hypophosphatemic states, diabetes insipidus, neonatal Bartter syndrome, or rare cases of the Fanconi syndrome may present within the neonatal period with evidence of volume depletion and electrolyte abnormalities. While specific diagnoses may be delayed, the rapid institution of volume replacement therapies may be lifesaving. In the absence of a family history, the diagnoses of stone-forming diseases such as cystinuria or hyperoxaluria are rarely made within the neonatal period. A full discussion of renal tubular disorders is beyond the scope of this chapter and the reader is referred to Chap. 4 for more complete information.

6.5 Neonatal Acute Kidney Injury (AKI)

6.5.1 Conservative Care

The nutritional care of neonates and infants with AKI is complex, requires the care of multiple services, and should be done only in medical centers with a full complement of pediatric subspecialty care. Children with AKI often present as part of a more general picture of sepsis, congenital heart disease, or hypoxic ischemic encephalopathy. After the initial period of weight/fluid loss, the neonatal period is characterized by a propensity to anabolism, necessary to fuel cellular growth. It is quite difficult to achieve anabolism in any patient with AKI and perhaps even more so in neonates. Often the best that can be achieved is a limitation of tissue catabolism through the provision of a high concentration of energy delivered either enterally or, more often, parenterally. In this instance, the infant's anabolic drive is helpful, and with careful control of energy, protein, and electrolyte intakes, it is possible to avoid dialysis in a significant percentage of infants. Where possible, enteral intake is preferred and formulas can be adapted in a stepwise fashion to provide increasing amounts of energy and protein intake, generally by starting with human milk or a humanized milk formula with the addition of energy in the form of complex carbohydrates or fat, while protein intake can be adjusted upward through the use of protein concentrates (see Table 6.2).

When AKI persists, it is often necessary to institute dialysis in order to achieve adequate nutritional intake. Again, there is no data to suggest that infants with AKI require larger energy or protein intakes than individuals receiving parenteral nutrition for other reasons, and attempts should be made to provide energy and

Table 6.6 Energy and protein intakes for infants requiring dialysis

	Predialysis		Hemodialysis		Peritoneal dialysis	
	Energy[a]	Protein[b]	Energy[a]	Protein[b,c]	Energy[a,d]	Protein[b,e]
0–6 months	100–110	2.2	100–110	2.6	100–110	3
6–12 months	95–105	1.5	95–105	2	95–105	2.4
1–3 years	90	1.1	90	1.6	90	2.0

[a]kcal/kg/day
[b]g/kg/day
[c]Protein intakes increased by approximately 0.4 g/kg/day to account for hemodialysis losses
[d]*Note*: up to 10 % of the total caloric intake (10 kcal/kg/day) can be absorbed as dextrose via the dialysate. Obesity may become a concern for some children and adolescents on peritoneal dialysis
[e]Protein requirements on peritoneal dialysis reflect the significant loss of proteins through the dialysis fluid

protein intakes based on gestational age and size. If possible, the use of indirect calorimetry can be helpful in determining true energy requirements [49, 50].

Current low-solute infant formulas often contain "humanized" concentrations of electrolytes. It is often necessary to modify these formulas to better control calcium, phosphate, alkali, and potassium intake. The addition of calcium will help to decrease phosphate uptake as well as improve serum calcium concentrations. Base can be adjusted by the addition of sodium bicarbonate or citrate. Potassium can also be adjusted, most often decreased by the addition of a sodium-potassium polystyrene resin (Kayexalate®).

6.5.2 Dialysis

Infants with CKD rarely require dialysis in the neonatal period as severe intrauterine renal failure and oliguria will lead to pulmonary hypoplasia and early neonatal demise. The nutritional care of infants requiring dialysis is complex, and adaptations will reflect the type of dialysis therapy used. Given the small size and limited vascular access, peritoneal dialysis is most often utilized for infants with CKD, but the use of hemodialysis and continuous renal replacement therapy (CRRT) all have been reported for this age group. As noted previously, infants on peritoneal dialysis receive a daily transfer of 8–12 kcal/kg via glucose absorbed. Infants on CRRT are often dialyzed using solutions containing glucose. The glucose lost during hemodialysis is not significant. Protein losses can be significant for infants on dialysis, and it has been suggested that protein intakes be increased during both hemo- and peritoneal dialysis (Table 6.6). There is little data on the loss of amino acids for infants on CRRT, but what data is present suggests that children undergo substantial amino acid and protein losses during this procedure [51]. For infants undergoing peritoneal dialysis, it is important to consider the interaction of increased intra-abdominal volume/pressure and rate of nighttime enteral intake, the combination of which may lead to increased filling pressure, worsening gastroesophageal reflux, and consequent decreased food intake.

Conclusion

Normal kidney function gives humans the ability to ingest a wide range of nutritional intakes allowing us to both excrete excess and conserve as conditions demand. During the first year of life, growth rates are high, and infants are primed to conserve electrolytes while excreting the large fluid volumes present in human milk. When renal disease is present during infancy, it becomes more difficult to achieve these goals. Appropriate nutritional care requires the cooperative efforts of physicians and nutritionists working with the family to achieve the optimal growth possible for these infants.

References

1. Karlberg J (1989) On the construction of the infancy-childhood-puberty growth standard. Acta Paediatr Scand 356(Suppl):26–37
2. Tanner JM (1990) Foetus into man: physical growth from conception to maturity, Revised and Enlarged edition. Harvard University, Cambridge, pp 178–221
3. Kuczmarski RJ et al (2000) CDC growth charts: United States. Adv Data 314:1–27
4. Karlberg J et al (1996) Early age-dependent growth impairment in chronic renal failure. Pediatr Nephrol 10(3):283–287
5. Foreman JW et al (1996) Nutritional intake in children with renal insufficiency: a report of the growth failure in children with renal diseases study. J Am Coll Nutr 15(6):579–585
6. North American Pediatric Renal Transplant Collaborative Study (NAPRTCS) 2008 annual report. pp 13–17, 2008. https://web.emmes.com/study/ped/annlrept/Annual%20Report%20-2008.pdf
7. Betts PR, Magrath G (1974) Growth pattern and dietary intake of children with chronic renal insufficiency. Br Med J 2(5912):189–193
8. Satyanarayana K et al (1981) Effect of nutritional deprivation in early childhood on later growth – community study without intervention. Am J Clin Nutr 34:1636–1637
9. Mekahli D et al (2010) Long-term outcome of infants with severe chronic kidney disease. Clin J Am Soc Nephrol 5(1):10–17
10. Wassner SJ et al (1986) Nutritional requirements for infants with renal failure. Am J Kidney Dis 7(4): 300–305
11. KDOQI clinical practice guideline for nutrition in children with CKD: 2008 update. Am J Kidney Dis 2008, 53(3, Suppl 2): S1–S124
12. Wingen AM, Mehls O (2002) Nutrition in children with preterminal chronic renal failure. Myth or important therapeutic aid. Pediatr Nephrol 17:111–120
13. Abitbol CL et al (1990) Linear growth and anthropometric and nutritional measurements in children with mild to moderate renal insufficiency: a report of the growth failure in children with renal diseases study. J Pediatr 116:S46–S47
14. Salusky IB et al (1983) Nutritional status of children undergoing continuous ambulatory peritoneal dialysis. Am J Clin Nutr 38(4):599–611
15. Edefonti A et al (1999) Dietary prescription based on estimated nitrogen balance during peritoneal dialysis. Pediatr Nephrol 13(3):253–258
16. Uauy RD et al (1994) Dietary protein and growth in infants with chronic renal insufficiency: a report from the Southwest Pediatric Nephrology Study Group and the University of California, San Francisco. Pediatr Nephrol 8(1):45–50
17. Wingen AM et al (1997) Randomized multicentre study of a low-protein diet on the progression of chronic renal failure in children. Lancet 349:1117–1123
18. National Academy of Sciences, I.o.M., Food and Nutrition Board (2004) Dietary reference intakes: electrolytes and water, pp 269–423
19. vd Heijden AJ et al (1985) Acute tubular dysfunction in infants with obstructive uropathy. Acta Paediatr Scand 74(4):589–594
20. Kaplan BS et al (1989) Autosomal recessive polycystic kidney disease. Pediatr Nephrol 3(1):43–49
21. Marra G et al (1987) Persistent tubular resistance to aldosterone in infants with congenital hydronephrosis corrected neonatally. J Pediatr 110(6):868–872
22. Wassner SJ, Kulin HE (1990) Diminished linear growth associated with chronic salt depletion. Clin Pediatr 29(12):719–721
23. Wassner SJ (1989) Altered growth and protein turnover in rats fed sodium-deficient diets. Pediatr Res 26(6):608–613
24. Parekh RS et al (2001) Improved growth in young children with severe chronic renal insufficiency who use specified nutritional therapy. J Am Soc Nephrol 12(11):2418–2426
25. Sedman A et al (1996) Nutritional management of the child with mild to moderate chronic renal failure. J Pediatr 129(2):s13–s18
26. Wassner SJ, Baum M (1999) Chronic renal failure: physiology and management. In: Barratt TM, Avner ED, Harmen WE (eds) Pediatric nephrology. Lippincott, Williams &Wilkins, Baltimore, pp 1155–1182
27. Bunchman TE et al (1991) Pretreatment of formula with sodium polystyrene sulfonate to reduce dietary potassium intake. Pediatr Nephrol 5(1):29–32
28. Holliday MA, Segar WE (1957) The maintenance need for water in parenteral fluid therapy. Pediatrics 19(5):823–832
29. Bailey JL et al (1996) The acidosis of chronic renal failure activates muscle proteolysis in rats by augmenting transcription of genes encoding proteins of the ATP-dependent ubiquitin-proteasome pathway. J Clin Invest 97:1447–1453
30. Ballmer PE et al (1995) Chronic metabolic acidosis decreases albumin synthesis and induces negative nitrogen balance in humans. J Clin Investig 95(January):39–45
31. Challa A et al (1993) Metabolic acidosis inhibits growth hormone secretion in rats: mechanism of growth retardation. J Am Physiol Soc 265: E547–E553
32. Hannaford MC et al (1982) Protein wasting due to acidosis of prolonged fasting. Am J Physiol 243: E251–E256
33. Kleinknecht C et al (1996) Acidosis prevents growth hormone-induced growth in experimental uremia. Pediatr Nephrol 10:256–260
34. McSherry E (1978) Acidosis and growth in nonuremic renal disease. Kidney Int 14:349–354
35. McSherry E, Morris RC Jr (1978) Attainment and maintenance of normal stature with alkali therapy in infants and children with classical renal tubular acidosis. J Clin Investig 61:509–527

36. Steichen JJ et al (1981) Elevated serum 1,25 dihydroxyvitamin D concentrations in rickets of very low-birth-weight infants. J Pediatr 99(2):293–298
37. Wagner CL et al (2008) Prevention of rickets and vitamin D deficiency in infants, children, and adolescents. Pediatrics 122(5):1142–1152
38. Chantler C, Holliday M (1973) Growth in children with renal disease with particular reference to the effects of calorie malnutrition: a review. Clin Nephrol 1:230–242
39. Rees L, Mak RH (2011) Nutrition and growth in children with chronic kidney disease. Nat Rev Nephrol 7(11):615–623
40. Haycock GB (2003) Management of acute and chronic renal failure in the newborn. Semin Neonatol 8(4):325–334
41. Ruley EJ et al (1989) Feeding disorders and gastroesophageal reflux in infants with chronic renal failure. Pediatr Nephrol 3(4):424–429
42. Kari JA et al (2000) Outcome and growth of infants with severe chronic renal failure. Kidney Int 57(4):1681–1687
43. Ledermann SE et al (2000) Long-term outcome of peritoneal dialysis in infants. J Pediatr 136(1):24–29
44. Dello Strologo L et al (1997) Feeding dysfunction in infants with severe chronic renal failure after long-term nasogastric tube feeding. Pediatr Nephrol 11(1):84–86
45. Fine R et al (1995) Recombinant human growth hormone in infants and young children with chronic renal insufficiency. Pediatr Nephrol 9:451–457
46. Holmberg C et al (1995) Management of congenital nephrotic syndrome of the Finnish type. Pediatr Nephrol 9(1):87–93
47. Jalanko H, Holmberg C. Congenital nephrotic syndrome. Pediatr Nephrol
48. Mahan J, Mauer S, Sibley R et al (1984) Congenital nephrotic syndrome: evolution of medical management and results of renal transplantation. J Pediatr 105:549–557
49. Briassoulis G, Venkataraman S, Thompson AE (2000) Energy expenditure in critically ill children. Crit Care Med 28(4):1166–1172
50. Vazquez Martinez JL et al (2004) Predicted versus measured energy expenditure by continuous, online indirect calorimetry in ventilated, critically ill children during the early postinjury period [see comment]. Pediatr Crit Care Med 5(1):19–27
51. Maxvold NJ et al (2000) Amino acid loss and nitrogen balance in critically ill children with acute renal failure: a prospective comparison between classic hemofiltration and hemofiltration with dialysis. Crit Care Med 28(4):1161
52. Council NR (2002) Dietary reference intakes for energy, carbohydrate, fiber, fat, fatty acids, cholesterol, protein and amino acids (macronutrients). The National Academies Press, Washington DC
53. Nutritional management of children with renal disease (2008) In: Kleinman R (ed) Pediatric nutrition handbook. 6th ed. American Academy of Pediatrics, Elk Grove Village, pp 905–926

7 Fetal Urology

Amy Hou and Duncan Wilcox

7.1 Introduction

With the advent of prenatal screening, a new population of urological patients has been identified – the fetus. In fact, genitourinary tract anomalies are among the most common congenital anomalies, noted in 1:250–1:1,000 pregnancies. Prenatal ultrasound detects 73–82 % of these anomalies [16, 54]. Many of these patients have transient hydronephrosis that will resolve without medical intervention either during pregnancy or in infancy. Others, such as those with unilateral problems have correctable anomalies that do not warrant intervention during pregnancy as they can be corrected postnatally without any adverse consequences to the child. Consequently, the dilemma following prenatal identification of a urological problem is to identify patients who have a clinical anomaly that is significant enough that prenatal treatment is required and further still in whom the treatment will be beneficial.

Patients with an enlarged bladder, megacystis, are those most concerning as both kidneys can be at risk for renal damage. Despite this, over a half of fetuses detected with megacystis will resolve spontaneously during pregnancy [51], and many that persist will not have evidence of bladder outlet obstruction but may have vesicoureteric reflux or idiopathic causes that do not benefit from early intervention [56].

Lower urinary tract obstruction (LUTO) is seen in 1:5,000–1:8,000 male fetuses, with the most common cause being posterior urethral valves [47]. In girls, urethral atresia accounts for the majority of cases [26]. These two diagnoses, along with prune belly syndrome, comprise the main diagnoses of LUTO that are evaluated for fetal intervention. Lower urinary tract obstruction can result in increased bladder pressure during both the filling and emptying phases. This is known to cause (1) renal dysplasia; (2) pulmonary hypoplasia, as amniotic fluid is crucial to pulmonary development and amniotic fluid volume is decreased with bladder outlet obstruction; and (3) permanent bladder dysfunction in the long run [20].

Complete obstructive uropathy, caused by posterior urethral valves or urethral atresia, may be visualized as early as the first trimester, presenting as first trimester megacystis [48]. Pathologic studies have shown that urethral atresia is more frequently diagnosed at an earlier gestational age, a diagnosis that has historically been considered lethal [27]. Bladder outlet obstruction is a finding that, when combined with oligohydramnios, can be associated with perinatal mortality as high as 95 % [29]. The high mortality rate is attributed to severe pulmonary hypoplasia. This group compares unfavorably with all congenital abnormalities of the kidney and urinary tract (CAKUT) where a recent review found an overall mortality rate of 24 %, ranging from 14.6

A. Hou • D. Wilcox, MD (✉)
The Department of Pediatric Urology, Children's Hospital Colorado, 13123 East 16th Avenue, Box 463, Aurora, CO 80045, USA
e-mail: duncan.wilcox@childrenscolorado.org

A.S. Chishti et al. (eds.), *Kidney and Urinary Tract Diseases in the Newborn*,
DOI 10.1007/978-3-642-39988-6_7, © Springer-Verlag Berlin Heidelberg 2014

to 54 %, highest in the setting of renal agenesis [32]. In addition, almost one third of children under the age of 4 years old with ESRD have obstruction as the underlying cause – 93 % of these patients are male, the majority of which had posterior urethral valves [18].

"Fetal diagnosis prompts the question of fetal surgery" [10]. Currently, the most common treatment of lower urinary tract obstruction is elective termination of the pregnancy [13]. With the majority of LUTO patients being identified prenatally, interest in fetal treatment has increased, to prevent or reverse the sequelae of obstruction. If nothing is done to intervene, the expected outcome for fetuses with severe LUTO and oligohydramnios is that 45 % will die in the first 3 weeks of life and 25 % will have renal failure [37]. With prenatal intervention, the reported neonatal mortality is 38 %. The majority of neonatal deaths are secondary to pulmonary hypoplasia. This chapter aims to identify patients with LUTO whom may benefit from intervention, the types of intervention available, and the outcomes, which currently are not optimistic.

7.1.1 Embryology

The definitive kidney, the metanephros, begins development on day 28 of gestation, when the ureteric bud comes in contact with the metanephric mesenchyme. Through mesenchymal-epithelial interactions, the collecting system is formed from the branching ureteric bud and the nephron from the overlying mesenchyme. Fetal urine production begins as early as week 8 of gestation [40]. By week 12, the collecting system, the ureters, and the bladder are formed. By the 13th week, the smooth muscle and autonomic innervations of the bladder are complete [17]. Nephrogenesis is complete by week 34, with maturation of the existing nephrons continues after birth [28].

By week 16 of gestation, fetal urine maintains the amniotic fluid volume. The canalicular phase of lung development takes place from 16 to 28 weeks. Without adequate amniotic fluid, which is an essential component in fetal lung development, bronchial development does not occur, resulting in pulmonary hypoplasia. Postnatally, death from respiratory failure would be expected. Animal models demonstrated that this process could be reversed by bypassing the obstructed urinary tract, providing normal amniotic fluid levels and allowing for adequate alveolar development [1].

7.2 Investigations

With the advent of prenatal ultrasound screening in the early 1980s, patients were increasingly being identified with hydronephrosis. Currently, in the United States and other countries, it is a normal practice for pregnant mothers to undergo an anomaly scan around 20 weeks of gestation. If this is abnormal then further investigations are arranged. The purposes of these investigations are to:

1. Identify structural anomalies
2. Make an accurate diagnosis where possible
3. Identify patients with associated anomalies
4. Identify patients who are at risk for renal impairment

Structural anomalies are routinely investigated with ultrasonography. However, ultrasound scans are excellent at identifying megacystis but are poor at diagnosing the exact problem. In some studies, up to two thirds of the diagnoses are incorrect [48]. As a result, MRI is now frequently used to further aid in diagnosis. Associated anomalies can also be detected with prenatal ultrasound scans, and maternal and fetal blood sampling has been used to identify fetuses with chromosomal anomalies. Finally fetal urine sampling is being taken in an attempt to identify patients with or who are at risk of renal damage.

7.2.1 Imaging

Definitive diagnosis of underlying etiology for LUTO is not possible with prenatal ultrasound [4]. Prenatal ultrasonography is essential in looking for the presence of other congenital anomalies. In the presence of oligohydramnios or anhydramnios, the ultrasound is limited due

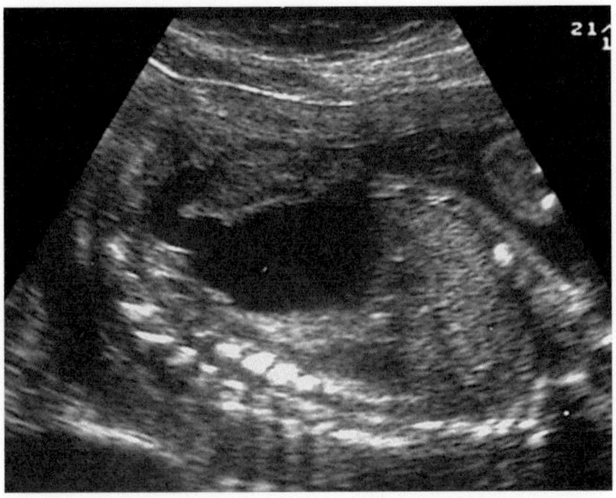

Fig. 7.1 Prenatal ultrasound scan of a male patient with posterior urethral valves. A thick-walled bladder and dilated posterior urethra can be easily identified

to the lack of a fluid window through which the ultrasound transduces. In such cases, amnioinfusion may be necessary to allow for complete fetal survey.

The shape of the bladder can be a clue to the underlying obstruction. Urethral atresia or completely obstructing posterior urethral valves will show a symmetrically thick-walled, distended, and round bladder. In cases of incomplete obstruction, either by incomplete posterior urethral valves, hypoplastic urethras, urethral strictures, or meatal stenosis, a "snowman" bladder may be seen. These bladders will have thickening in the trigone and lower bladder neck region, with minimal thickening at the dome. Dilation of the urethra should also be assessed. A dilated membranous penile urethra can sometimes be traced to the distal end, which has been associated with anterior urethral valves or meatal stenosis [30]. A large series of prenatal ultrasounds found a positive predictive value of 34.6 % of the findings of bilateral hydroureteronephrosis, a dilated bladder and the keyhole sign, with posterior urethral valves (Fig. 7.1) [39].

The presence of cortical cysts or increase in renal echogenicity can be indicative of renal dysplasia. Cortical cysts have been reported to correlate with postnatal findings of renal dysplasia with 100 % specificity and 44 % sensitivity. Increased renal echogenicity correlated with dysplasia, with 73 % sensitivity and 90 % specificity. The presence of cortical cysts or increased echogenicity on ultrasound demonstrated the best predictive accuracy for poor postnatal renal outcome [35].

Fast scanning MRI is a useful supplementary imaging tool in the setting of oligohydramnios. Although, one study looking at MRI as a supplementary imaging modality found that there was no increased information to be gathered regarding fetal anatomy in the setting of normal amniotic fluid [41].

7.2.2 Fetal Urinalysis

Fetal bladder sampling is performed in an attempt to identify patients at risk for current or later renal impairment. Serial fetal bladder sampling is recommended to improve its prognostic value. As the fetal kidneys mature, the urine becomes increasingly hypotonic. In the early second trimester, fetal urine is almost physiologically isotonic, thus making interpretation of fetal urine electrolytes in this time period difficult. Fetal urine sodium and ß-microglobulin decreases during the second half of gestation, whereas urine calcium does not change significantly [38].

Decreased resorption, increased loss of analytes in fetal urine, and hypertonicity has been positively correlated with increased renal impairment and poorer prognosis [46]. A systematic meta-analysis in 2007 [36] reviewing fetal urinalyses found no urine analytes had clinically significant accuracy in predicting poor renal outcome postnatally. The two most accurate parameters were calcium level >95th percentile for gestational age and sodium level >95th percentile for gestational age.

Fetal urine electrolytes play prominently in patient selection, which was confirmed in a consensus of SFU members in 2000. Johnson et al. demonstrated that sequential fetal urine analysis improves the sensitivity and specificity of the test. Good renal function was indicated by urine values falling below the threshold with repeated bladder aspirations. The fetuses with poor outcomes tended to have higher initial values and increasing urine values over time. Urine obtained

Table 7.1 Summary of fetal urine electrolyte levels

	Good prognosis	Poor prognosis
Sodium	<90 mmol/L	>100 mmol/L
Chloride	<80 mmol/L	>90 mmol/L
Osmolality	<180 mOsm/L	>200 mOsm/L
Calcium	<7 mg/dL	>8 mg/dL
Total Protein	<20 mg/dL	>40 mg/dL
β2-Microglobulin	<6 mg/L	>10 mg/L

Reprinted from Mann et al. [30]. Copyright 2010, with permission from Elsevier

on the first bladder aspiration has been present in the bladder for an unknown period of time and is unlikely to accurately reflect urine currently being made by the kidney. The goal is to sample urine shortly after it has been produced by the fetal kidney, to get the most accurate depiction of renal function [24]. A variety of electrolytes have been used, as has beta microglobulin and their respective values are shown in Table 7.1.

The prognostic power of fetal urine electrolytes is debated. Wilkins et al. found no evidence that fetal urine electrolytes facilitate the identification of which fetuses may benefit from intervention [55]. Elders also found a discordance between urinary electrolytes and postnatal renal dysplasia in 50 % of cases [22].

7.2.3 Patient Selection

The screening of appropriate candidates for fetal intervention is important to avoid surgical complications in fetuses that may do well without intervention, as well as to avoid intervention in those fetuses who are unlikely to survive [2].

An algorithm that was proposed by Johnson et al. has been used as a general guideline by many for determining which patients will most benefit from prenatal intervention [23]. A fetal karyotype should be obtained. Then a detailed sonographic evaluation to rule out structural anomalies is performed, as these may impact the fetal prognosis. Fetal intervention would not be recommended if another life-threatening anomaly were found on the fetal survey. Serial fetal urine evaluations were recommended to determine the extent of the underlying renal damage.

Today, an appropriate patient for fetal intervention is a fetus with a normal karyotype, no other structural abnormalities, ultrasound findings consistent with lower urinary tract obstruction, presence of oligohydramnios or anhydramnios, and "favorable" urine electrolytes [42]. Normal-appearing fetal kidneys, in terms of echogenicity and lack of cortical cysts, are also an inclusion criterion for fetal intervention.

In 1986, the International Fetal Surgery Registry summarized the results of fetal intervention on hydronephrosis. They concluded that due to morbidity and mortality, in addition to errors of diagnosis, in utero intervention may improve survival and decrease morbidity, at least in the setting of posterior urethral valves [31]. The goal of fetal intervention in LUTO is to restore amniotic fluid to prevent pulmonary hypoplasia and to decompress the urinary system, to prevent renal impairment.

7.3 Fetal Intervention

Starting in the 1980s Harrison and colleagues in San Francisco have pioneered our approaches to fetal intervention. The aim of intervention is to restore amniotic fluid in time to allow normal pulmonary development and by draining the bladder to decompress the upper renal tracts and to allow more normal renal development so as to minimize renal impairment in childhood. Initially fetal vesicostomies were performed, but today vesicoamniotic shunts and fetal cystoscopy are preferred.

7.3.1 Open Fetal Surgery

Open fetal vesicostomy or ureterostomy has previously been performed for the treatment of LUTO. Crombleholme et al. published a series of five patients who underwent open fetal surgery for oligohydramnios and LUTO. Their group had extensive preparation on fetal animal models, sheep and then primate, prior to performing the operations on human fetuses, which they recommended to others who are considering performing open fetal surgery. The preparation with animal models allowed them to establish a protocol of anesthesia, tocolytics, and surgical technique that greatly aided in minimizing complications during the surgeries on human fetuses. Extrauterine time was 10–12 min when documented. Three patients were live-born. On follow-up, 1 had died at 9 months from septicemia related to bowel disease, 1 was awaiting renal transplantation, and 1 had normal renal function. None of them required pulmonary support after birth. Two patients died as neonates and were found to have pulmonary hypoplasia and bilateral renal dysplasia at autopsy [9].

Open fetal surgery may become preferable over percutaneous fetal shunting when catheter decompression is required for longer periods of time to achieve lung maturity. A vesicostomy achieves a more reliable long-term decompression of the urinary system, without the risks of shunt clogging and repeat procedures to replace the shunt [9].

Postoperative rupture of membrane and preterm labor remain the Achilles' heel of open fetal surgery [10]. Consequently this open procedure is not commonly performed expect in institutions involved in ongoing open fatel studies.

7.3.2 Vesicoamniotic Shunt

The most common method of relieving fetal LUTO is ultrasound-guided vesicoamniotic shunting. Successful use of percutaneous vesicoamniotic shunts in animal models revived an interest in fetal intervention for LUTO. The first clinical case of vesicoamniotic shunt performed in a human fetus was in 1982, at the University of California San Francisco [19].

With the aid of ultrasound, the fetal bladder is visualized. Color Doppler is used to avoid entering into vascular structures. Amniotic infusion may be required in the setting of oligohydramnios or anhydramnios to create a window for ultrasound and also to create a space for the distal end of the shunt to deploy. A trochar and cannula is placed through the maternal abdominal wall and the uterine wall, into the fetal bladder.

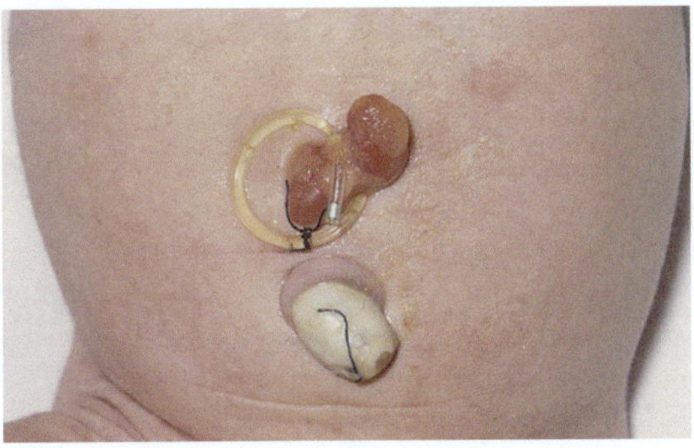

Fig. 7.2 Fetal vesicoamniotic shunt in place

Percutaneous access of the fetal bladder is obtained, and the shunt is deployed into the fetal bladder and the amniotic cavity. Care is taken to place the shunt low in the fetal bladder, to avoid dislodgement of the shunt when the bladder is decompressed (Fig. 7.2). The trochar is carefully manipulated within the amniotic cavity to avoid misplacing the shunt into the maternal uterine wall or the fetal abdomen. The trochar can also be used to gently move the fetus away from the maternal uterine wall, if necessary [49].

A long-term outcomes study following 20 male patients after fetal vesicoamniotic shunting by Biard et al. found a first year survival of 91 %. Their database had 31 patients who underwent prenatal shunting, with 23 confirmed live-born. No evidence of chorioamnionitis was found at the time of delivery. 18 families responded to the long-term follow-up information requests. Diagnoses for the 18 patients were: 7 posterior urethral valves, 7 prune belly syndrome, and 4 urethral atresia. The mean age at follow-up was 5 years (range 1–14 years). In this group, growth abnormalities, with height or weight below the 25th percentile, were seen in 50 % of patient [5]. The Fetal Surgery Registry, in 1984, had reported that 50 % of children were below the fifth percentile for height and 35 % for weight [15]. The decreased severity of growth delays is attributed to increased nutritional support. 61 % (11/18) were spontaneously voiding, 16.5 % (3/18) did a combination of spontaneous voiding and catheterization, 16.5 % (3/18) were dependent on catheterization, and 6 % (1/18) had a vesicostomy. Fifty-five percent (10/18) had normal pulmonary function, with the remainder having asthma, restricted physical activity, recurrent pulmonary infections, and sleep apnea. Importantly, the self-perceived quality of life of the survivor was comparable to normals.

In one series, mortality was found to be 100 % in those patients who did not have restoration of amniotic fluid [45]. In analysis of outcomes based on prognosis determined by urine biochemistry [8, 14], a prediction of poor renal function was confirmed in 88 % (14/16 patients). In the good prognosis group, 85 % of survivors had normal renal function. If amniotic fluid was restored, there was no postnatal pulmonary compromise. A systematic review by Clark et al. found that drainage of the fetal bladder had increased perinatal survival compared to not draining ($p=0.03$), but the finding was largely due to the marked improvement in the poor prognosis group ($p=0.03$). The poor prognosis group had a statistically significant increase in postnatal survival (elective termination and in utero death were excluded) with bladder drainage ($p=0.02$); the good prognosis group did not. Morbidity among survivors was similar, regardless of intervention or prognosis. The authors specifically note the lack of high quality evidence to reliably inform clinical practice [6].

Percutaneous fetal vesicoamniotic shunting, though less invasive than open surgery, still comes with risks. Complications are seen in up to 45 % of cases. There is a total perinatal loss rate of about 4 % per instance of shunt placement [42]. Shunt blockage is seen in 25 %, shunt migration in 20 %. The fetal limbs, with spontaneous movement, can sometimes entangle the external end of the shunt within the amniotic fluid and remove the shunt from the bladder. Shunt displacement can lead to urine ascites, with associated effects on intra-thoracoabdominal hemodynamics. Replacement of the vesicoamniotic shunt or even a fetal abdominal-amniotic shunt is sometimes necessary. The shunt can be deployed in inappropriate locations, such as limbs and other abdominal cavities. Iatrogenic gastroschisis through the shunt site has been reported. The Fetal Surgery Registry reported only 10 % of shunts were successfully placed in the 1980s, across multiple medical centers. Maternal life-threatening infections associated with fetal loss was reported in 3/159 cases. A more recent review in 2003 found that 206 of 210 shunts were successfully placed, with 9 major complications – 3 procedure related deaths, 4 chorioamnionitis, 1 fistulous tract, and 1 gastroschisis [6].

Different types of shunts and methods of shunting have been devised to prevent the shunt from malfunction or migration. Quintero et al. described a double-disk shunt, with the disks sitting on the inside of the fetal bladder and on the fetal abdominal skin, holding the shunt in place. The double-disk was an atrial septal occluder, used in combination with the standard vesicoamniotic shunt. They found the shunt could not be dislodged from its deployment site nor removed by the fetus. This new shunt does require a larger trocar, which may have an increase risk of premature rupture of membranes. Stone formation on the disk inside the fetal bladder is also a possible risk, though not seen in their study [42].

7.3.3 Fetal Cystoscopy

Fetal cystoscopy was first introduced by Quintero et al. in 1995 [44]. An advantage of fetoscopic intervention is its ability to allow for physiologic drainage of the obstructed bladder via endoscopic diagnosis and treatment of the obstruction, particularly in the case of posterior urethral valves [43]. Fetal cystoscopy allowed for correct diagnosis of the underlying pathology in 18/19 cases (94.7 %). To date, there are no studies comparing fetoscopy and vesicoamniotic shunting directly [22, 50, 53].

The procedure can be performed under general maternal and fetal anesthesia or local anesthesia. A trochar and curved sheath are introduced into the upper part of the fetal bladder, under ultrasonographic guidance. Once the fetoscope is inside the bladder, urine specimens can be collected for analysis. The fetoscope is then advanced towards to the bladder neck. The biggest challenge with fetal cystoscopy is entering into the posterior urethra. The vesicourethral angle becomes more acute with gestational age, making access increasingly difficult [2]. If posterior urethral valves are encountered, they can be treated at this time, either with hydroablation, disruption using a guide wire, or fulguration with a ND:YAG (neodymium-doped yttrium aluminum garnet) laser. Once the valves are ablated, the fetal bladder should empty, as the urine passes through the urethra. If a non-membrane-like structure is found, and it does not allow passage of fluid, urethral atresia is diagnosed and no attempts should be made to perforate the structure [49].

Risks of this procedure would be expected to be similar to other fetoscopic interventions. Preterm rupture of membranes and extreme prematurity was reported in 37 and 25 % [50]. There are few reports in the literature but thus far, there are no reports of fetal demise or peripheral bladder damage [49]. The biggest challenge with the fetoscopic approach is the instrumentation. The size of the patient, the size of the urethra, and the angle of access to the urethra necessitate specific surgical equipment, without which the procedure should not be performed.

7.4 Outcomes

The goals of fetal intervention for LUTO are to improve pulmonary function to allow for both, successful ventilation post nattily and improve renal outcomes and bladder function. Prevention of pulmonary hypoplasia is the primary goal of fetal intervention in the setting of LUTO. If oligohydramnios develops during the canalicular phase of lung development, around gestational week 20, the fetus will frequently have fatal pulmonary hypoplasia [21].

Relieving the obstruction is also performed with the goal of allowing normal nephrogenesis to proceed. In severe LUTO, histologically one finds early loss of the nephrogenic zone with formation of cortical cysts, a decrease in glomerular count and dysplastic structures [52]. One postulate is that relieving obstruction at 20–30 weeks gestation, when nephrogenesis is most active, may halt further renal damage and allow normal nephrogenesis to proceed [9]. The degree of renal damage is dependent upon the timing and severity of the obstruction. When oligohydramnios is found before 20 weeks gestation, the fetus would not be able to survive ex vivo and may warrant a vesicoamniotic shunt. Demonstrating fetal renal failure, there are cases where the vesicoamniotic shunt is in the correct position and yet, the urine output and amniotic fluid drops off. Review of outcomes in a case series of posterior urethral valve fetuses found 65 % of their patients who underwent fetal intervention developed postnatal renal failure. Their findings suggest prenatal intervention did not reverse the outcome of renal dysfunction; this may be because both the bladder and kidneys are primarily affected in bladder outlet obstruction; however, others have suggested that it is due to late drainage of the bladder, and attempts should be made to intervene earlier in pregnancy [22].

Similarly, bladder outcomes are relatively unchanged in studies comparing LUTO babies who underwent fetal shunting vs. postnatal management only. Urodynamic parameters in posterior urethral valve bladders are known to change as the patient ages. Holmes et al. found similar findings in their small series of PUV patients who underwent prenatal intervention [22]. Whether the patients have flaccid noncontractile bladders or thick fibrotic bladders, many ultimately require catheterization or reconstruction for appropriate urinary emptying and continence. The shunt will not prevent bladder wall fibrosis. An experiment was performed in sheep, with placement of vesicoamniotic shunts into fetal lambs with no evidence of obstructive uropathy [25]. On histologic examination of the bladders, the shunted bladder demonstrated increases fibrosis and distortion of muscle layers compared to control bladders. They found that the shunted bladder was worse from a histologic point of view than a nonshunted obstructed bladder. When a pressure regulated shunt was used [3], that maintained a continuous resistance between 15 and 54 mmHg, normal bladder development was preserved, reducing muscle hypertrophy and interstitial fibrosis. In support of Duckett's observations that putting a bladder on continuous drainage is more likely to lead to a small contractile bladder [11], Kitagawa et al.

concluded that some of the changes in the bladder wall after shunting are iatrogenic.

Crombleholme et al. demonstrated an improved survival rate for candidates of intervention in the good prognosis group (89 %) vs. the poor prognosis group (30 %), based on fetal urine electrolytes and renal cortical findings on ultrasound [8]. Coplen et al. reported that no evidence exists demonstrating the benefit of antenatal intervention in terms of renal function, and only a select number of cases will it benefit pulmonary function [7], and others reported a mortality rate of 79 % for interventions in fetuses with oligohydramnios [12]. A 2001 review of the University of San Francisco data suggest that fetal intervention helps in getting the pregnancy closer to term but may not prevent the sequelae of UTO, in terms of renal and bladder function [22].

A randomized controlled trial, Percutaneous Shunting in Lower Urinary Tract Obstruction (PLUTO), was designed to evaluate the efficacy and safety of vesicoamniotic shunting for LUTO [33]. This is a multinational, multicenter randomized controlled trial embedded within a comprehensive cohort study. Randomization was to vesicoamniotic shunt or conservative management without a shunt. Primary outcome measures are perinatal mortality and serum creatinine at 6 weeks of age. Secondary outcomes are to include renal and bladder function, termination and miscarriage rates, and resource usage. An update was presented in 2012. One hundred forty-five women were recruited; 31 were randomized. Sixteen pregnancies received vesicoamniotic shunt and 15 pregnancies were followed. 39 % of the randomized groups were alive at 28 days, 16 % opted for termination, 6 % miscarried at 24 weeks, and 36 % had neonatal death at less than 28 days. Analysis demonstrated an improved odds ratio of survival with shunting – OR 4.00 (95 % CI 1.11–14.35) [34]. Unfortunately, because of difficulty in recruiting patients, this study has been closed.

Conclusion

With the high morbidity and mortality associated with LUTO, fetal surgeons continue to strive to innovate in order to help these fetuses. Determining who, when, and where intervention is required remains a topic of debate and is currently difficult to assess in an evidence-based manner. Given the lack of well-controlled studies supporting intervention and the significant rate of fetal and the low but definite rate of maternal morbidity, fetal intervention should be restricted to centers of excellence, where ongoing research is being performed.

References

1. Adzick SN, Harrison MR, Glick PL, Flake AE (1985) Fetal urinary tract obstruction: experimental physiology. Semin Perinatol 9:79–90
2. Agarwal SK, Fisk NM (2001) In utero therapy for lower urinary tract obstruction. Prenat Diagn 21:970–976
3. Aoba T, Kitagawa H et al (2008) Can a pressure-limited vesico-amniotic shunt tube preserve normal bladder function? J Pediatr Surg 43:2250–2255
4. Bernardes LS, Aksnes G, Saada J et al (2009) Keyhole sign: how specific is it for the diagnosis of posterior urethral valves? Ultrasound Obstet Gynecol 34: 419–423
5. Biard JM, Johnson MP, Carr MC et al (2005) Long-term outcomes in children treated by prenatal vesicoamniotic shunting for lower urinary tract obstruction. Obstet Gynecol 106(3):503–508
6. Clark TJ, Martin WL et al (2003) Prenatal bladder drainage in the management of fetal LUTO: a systematic review and meta-analysis. Obstet Gynecol 102:367–382
7. Coplen DE, Hare JY, Zderic SA et al (1991) 10 year experience with prenatal intervention for hydronephrosis. J Urol 156:1142–1145
8. Crombleholme TM, Harrison MR, Golbus MS et al (1990) Fetal intervention in obstructive uropathy: prognostic indicators and efficacy of intervention. Am J Obstet Gynecol 162:1239–1244
9. Crombleholme TM, Harrison MR, Langer JC et al (1988) Early experience with open fetal surgery for congenital hydronephrosis. J Pediatr Surg 23:1114–1121
10. Deprest JA, Flake AW et al (2010) The making of fetal surgery. Prenat Diagn 30:653–667
11. Duckett JW (1997) Are valve bladders congenital or iatrogenic? Br J Urol 79:271–275
12. Elder JS, Duckett JW Jr, Snyder HM (1987) Intervention for fetal obstructive uropathy: has it been effective? Lancet 2:1007
13. Farrugia MK, Woolf AS (2010) Congenital urinary bladder outlet obstruction. Fetal Matern Med Rev 21:55–73
14. Freedman AL, Bokowski TP, Smith CA et al (1996) Fetal therapy for obstructive uropathy: specific outcome diagnoses. J Urol 156:720–723

15. Freedman AL, Johnson MP, Smith CA et al (1999) Long-term outcomes in children after antenatal intervention for obstructive uropathies. Lancet 354:374–377
16. Garne E, Loane M, Wellesley D et al (2009) Congenital hydronephrosis: prenatal diagnosis and epidemiology in Europe. J Pediatr Urol 5:47–52
17. Gilpin SA, Gosling JA (1983) Smooth muscle in the wall of the developing human urinary bladder and urethra. J Anat 137:503–512
18. Gloor JM (1995) Management of prenatally detected fetal hydronephrosis. Mayo Clin Proc 70:145–152
19. Golbus MS, Harrison MR, Filly RA et al (1982) In utero treatment of urinary tract obstruction. Am J Obstet Gynecol 142:383–388
20. Harrison M, Ross N, Hoall R, de Lorimer A (1983) Correction of congenital hydronephrosis in utero 1. The model: fetal urethral obstruction produces hydronephrosis and pulmonary hypoplasia in fetal lambs. J Pediatr Surg 18:247–256
21. Hislop A, Hey E, Reid L (1979) The lung in congenital bilateral renal agenesis and dysplasia. Arch Dis Child 54:32–39
22. Holmes N, Harrison MR, Baskin LS (2001) Fetal surgery for posterior urethral valves: long term postnatal outcomes. Pediatrics 108:36–42
23. Johnson MP, Bokowski TP, Reitleman C et al (1994) In utero surgical treatment of fetal obstructive uropathy: a new comprehensive approach to identify appropriate candidates for vesicoamniotic shunt therapy. Am J Obstet Gynecol 170:1770–1776
24. Johnson MP, Corsi P et al (1995) Sequential urinalysis improves evaluation of fetal renal function in obstructive uropathy. Am J Obstet Gynecol 173:59–65
25. Kitagawa H, Pringle KC et al (2007) Is a vesicoamniotic shunt intrinsically bad? Shunting a normal fetal bladder. J Pediatr Surg 42:2002–2006
26. Kumar S, Fisk NM (2003) Distal urinary obstruction. Clin Perinatol 30:507–519
27. Lissauer D, Morris RK, Kilby MD (2007) Fetal lower urinary tract obstruction. Semin Fetal Neonatal Med 12:464–470
28. Macdonald MS, Emery JL (1959) The late intrauterine and postnatal development of human renal glomeruli. J Anat 93:331–340
29. Mahony BS, Callen PW, Filly RA (1985) Fetal urethral obstruction: ultrasound evaluation. Radiology 157:221–224
30. Mann S, Johnson MP, Wilson RD (2010) Fetal thoracic and bladder shunts. Semin Fetal Neonatal Med 15:28–33
31. Manning FA, Harrison MR, Rodeck C (1986) Catheter shunts for fetal hydronephrosis and hydrocephalus. Report of the International Fetal Surgery Registry. N Engl J Med 315:336–340
32. Melo BF, Aguiar MB, Bouzada MCF et al (2012) Early risk factors for neonatal mortality in CAKUT: analysis of 524 affected newborns. Pediatr Nephrol 27:965–972
33. Morris RK, Kilby MD (2009) An overview of the literature on congenital LUTO and introduction to the PLUTO trial: percutaneous shunting in lower urinary tract obstruction. Aust NZ J Obstet Gynecol 49:6–10
34. Morris R, Kilby M (2012) The PLUTO trial: percutaneous shunting in lower urinary tract obstruction. Am J Obstet Gynecol 206:S14
35. Morris RK, Malin GL, Kjan KS et al (2009) Antenatal ultrasound to predict postnatal renal function in congenital lower urinary tract obstruction: systematic review of test accuracy. BJOG 116:1290–1299
36. Morris RK, Quinlan-Jones E et al (2007) Systematic review of accuracy of fetal urine analysis to predict poor postnatal renal function in cases of congenital urinary tract obstruction. Prenat Diagn 27:900–911
37. Nakayama DK, Harrison MR, deLorimier AA (1986) Prognosis of posterior urethral valves presenting at birth. J Pediatr Surg 21:43
38. Nicolini U, Spelzini F (2001) Invasive assessment of fetal renal abnormalities: urinalysis, fetal blood sampling and biopsy. Prenat Diagn 21:964–969
39. Paduamo L, Giglio L, Bambi B et al (1991) Clinical outcomes of prenatal echography positive for obstructive uropathy. J Urol 146:1094–1096
40. Park JM (2012) Chapter 111: Normal development of the Genitourinary tract. In: Wein AJ, Kavoussi LR et al (eds) Campbell-Walsh urology, 10th edn. Saunders, Philadelphia
41. Poutamo J, Vanninen R et al (2000) Diagnosing fetal urinary tract anomalies: benefits of MRI compared to ultrasonography. Acta Obstet Gynecol Scand 79: 65–71
42. Quintero RA, Castro LAG, Bermudez C et al (2010) In utero management of fetal LUTO with a novel shunt: a landmark development in fetal therapy. J Matern Fetal Neonatal Med 23:806–812
43. Quintero RA, Johnson MP, Munoz H et al (1998) In utero endoscopic treatment of posterior urethral valves: preliminary experience. Prenat Neonatal Med 3:208–216
44. Quintero RA, Johnson MP, Romero R et al (1995) In utero percutaneous cystoscopy in the management of fetal lower obstructive uropathy. Lancet 346(8974):537–540
45. Quintero RA, Shukla AR, Homsy YL, Bukkapatnam R (2000) Successful in utero endoscopic ablation of posterior urethral valves: a new dimension in fetal urology. Urology 55:774
46. Qureshi F, Jacques SM et al (1996) In utero fetal urine analysis and renal histology do correlate with the outcome in fetal obstructive uropathies. Fetal Diagn Ther 11:306–312
47. Reuss A, Wladirmiroff J et al (1987) Antenatal diagnosis of renal tract anomalies by ultrasound. Pediatr Nephrol 1:546–552
48. Robyr R, Benachi A, Daikha-Dahmane F et al (2005) Correlation between ultrasound and anatomical findings in fetuses with lower urinary tract obstruction in the first half of pregnancy. Ultrasound Obstet Gynecol 25:478–482
49. Ruano R (2011) Fetal surgery for severe LUTO. Prenat Diagn 31:667–674

50. Ruano R, Duarte S, Bunduki V et al (2010) Fetal cystoscopy for severe lower urinary tract obstruction – initial experience of a single center. Prenat Diagn 30:30–39
51. Sebire N, Kaisenbery CV, Rubio C, Snijders R, Nicolaides K (1996) Fetal megacystis at 10–14 weeks of gestation. Ultrasound Obstet Gynecol 8: 387–390
52. Shimada K, Hosokawa S (1996) Renal development in fetal hydronephrosis. Dialogues Pediatr Urol 2:2–3
53. Welsh A, Agarwal S, Kumar S et al (2003) Fetal cystoscopy in the management of fetal obstructive uropathy: experience in a single European centre. Prenat Diagn 23:1033–1041
54. Wiesel A, Queisser-Luft A et al (2005) Prenatal detection of congenital renal malformations by fetal ultrasonographic examination: an analysis of 709,030 births in 12 European countries. Eur J Med Genet 48:131–144
55. Wilkins IA, Chitkara U, Lynch L et al (1987) The non-predictive value of fetal urinary electrolytes: preliminary report of outcomes and correlations with pathologic diagnosis. Am J Obstet Gynecol 157:694–698
56. Yiee J, Wilcox DT (2008) Abnormalities of the fetal bladder. Semin Fetal Neonatal Med 13:164–170

Urological Imaging in the Newborn

8

Steven J. Kraus and Sara M. O'Hara

8.1 Introduction

In today's practice of pediatric urology, imaging of the abnormal urinary tract usually begins in utero, as a result of abnormal findings on a screening prenatal ultrasound (US) examination. Many abnormal fetuses are then imaged by fetal MRI, where available, for genetic counseling or in those centers where fetal surgeons can intervene prenatally. In the newborn period, imaging is performed with as little radiation exposure as is reasonably achievable (ALARA). Usually, this is easily achieved since the mainstay of imaging the newborn urinary tract is US. Voiding cystourethrography (VCUG) and radionuclide renography, with or without a diuretic, are relatively low-radiation-dose techniques when modified for pediatric patients and are utilized for specific indications. Sometimes neonatal magnetic resonance imaging (MRI) can be very helpful to further evaluate complex urinary tract anomalies but is not used unless other techniques are insufficient to define the abnormality or to evaluate extent of disease, such as in neonatal neoplasms.

S.J. Kraus, MD (✉) • S.M. O'Hara, MD
Department of Radiology,
Cincinnati Children's Medical Center,
MLC 5031, Cincinnati, OH 45229, USA
e-mail: steve.kraus@cchmc.org;
sara.ohara@cchmc.org

8.2 Imaging Techniques

8.2.1 Ultrasound

Because it is noninvasive, portable, and does not use ionizing radiation, ultrasound is the first choice for imaging the genitourinary tract in the newborn. Frequently prenatal images are also available for comparison. The urinary tract can be imaged from kidney to perineum sonographically, in supine, prone, or even upright position. Dynamic clips or sweeps through areas of pathology help document three-dimensional relationships, communications between dilated calyces in an obstructed collecting system versus cystic spaces in a multicystic dysplastic kidney—and help demonstrate peristalsis and movement within the urinary tract, ureteral jets or changing size of distal ureters in cases of vesicoureteral reflux. A range of ultrasound transducers are available to tailor the imaging exam to the patient size, depth of penetration needed, and skin surface window available. Smaller patients are best imaged with the highest frequency transducer that brings the area of interest into focus; this gives the best image detail or resolution. Small footprint transducers are ideal for imaging in between small ribs or adjacent to ostomies or unrepaired bladder exstrophy. Doppler techniques are valuable to differentiate between anechoic urine-filled spaces and blood-filled spaces. Assessment of renal perfusion, resistive indices, ureteral jets, and twinkle artifact are frequently used to answer clinical questions; these will be discussed in subsequent sections.

A.S. Chishti et al. (eds.), *Kidney and Urinary Tract Diseases in the Newborn*,
DOI 10.1007/978-3-642-39988-6_8, © Springer-Verlag Berlin Heidelberg 2014

8.2.2 Cystography

Cystography in neonates is usually performed to evaluate patients with prenatal hydronephrosis, hydroureter, or both, as well as for signs of bladder outlet obstruction, especially in boys, or to evaluate intravesical mass [5, 8]. Radionuclide cystography is insufficient to evaluate the complex anatomy that is often present in neonatal congenital anomalies of the bladder and ureterovesical junction such as duplication anomalies and diverticula. Cystosonography is becoming popular outside the United States, in Europe, and Canada; however, the contrast agents are not yet FDA approved for general use in the urinary tract in the United States; however, this technique is promising to replace the VCUG for many indications, further reducing the radiation burden to pediatric patients, especially neonates who are more susceptible to any deleterious effects of ionizing radiation. Typically the VCUG is performed after aseptic catheterization of the bladder and slow instillation of iodine-based water soluble contrast under intermittent fluoroscopic monitoring by a radiologist or other certified fluoroscopist. Images are obtained of the full bladder, the ureterovesical junction regions, especially if there is vesicoureteral reflux (VUR), evaluating the location of ureteral insertion relative to the bladder neck denoted by the urethral catheter and the grade of maximal reflux according to the international grading system. Any outpouching of contrast or any filling defect in the bladder contrast is also documented as well as contrast within the urethra during voiding. The female urethra can be imaged in the frontal projection with the catheter in; however, the male urethra should be imaged after removing the catheter, in a steep oblique projection to evaluate for posterior urethral valve (PUV) or other of the less common urethral anomalies. In patients with high-grade VUR, an image of the kidneys and ureters after voiding should document drainage of the refluxed contrast to evaluate for concomitant obstruction of the ureters at the ureterovesical junction which can be associated with high-grade vesicoureteral reflux (refluxing, obstructive megaureter). In addition, in patients with high-grade VUR, one should look for intrarenal reflux, a blush of contrast refluxing into the collecting ducts, a sign that is often seen in patients who may go on to develop renal scarring, especially in those who had pyelonephritis.

8.2.3 Radionuclide Renography

This nuclear medicine technique [14] is ideal to assess patients with hydronephrosis detected by US for suspected renal obstruction, especially after vesicoureteral reflux has been excluded by cystography. In addition, it can be used to assess differential renal function or the presence of the kidneys, if an ectopic kidney is suspected by US. The use of a diuretic after the initial phase of renography can be useful to differentiate urinary stasis from urinary obstruction. Since introduction of technetium-99m mercaptoacetyltriglycine (MAG3) in 1986, it has been the preferred radiopharmaceutical for assessing renal function because of its more efficient renal extraction compared to technetium-99m diethylenetriaminepentaacetic acid (DTPA). After injection of the MAG3, the patient is imaged for 20 min, acquiring serial images at standard intervals. If there are signs of potential obstruction after the first 20 min of baseline imaging, a diuretic is given IV and another 20–30 min of imaging is performed, similar to the baseline imaging. An automated T½ is calculated, that is, that time required to excrete ½ of the radiopharmaceutical that is present in the collecting system of the kidney due to the diuretic effect. Some centers have used MAG3 as a cortical agent as well, replacing technetium-99m dimercaptosuccinic acid (DMSA), since MAG3 has fairly good extraction, rivaling the sensitivity for detecting foci of pyelonephritis or scarring in some studies. DMSA is an excellent cortical agent, utilized to evaluate for pyelonephritis and renal scarring, to assess differential renal function, or to assess for the presence or absence of renal parenchyma in cases of suspected renal agenesis or renal ectopia [7].

8.2.4 MR Urography

This imaging technique is becoming a preferred technique because it does not expose the patient to potentially harmful radiation and can combine the advantages of cross-sectional imaging and functional imaging into a single exam. However, the technique is very sensitive to motion, which degrades the images. In newborns, one would try to avoid sedation by bundling the patient snuggly in warm blankets in the scanner and avoid motion by feeding the patient immediately prior to the exam hoping the patient will sleep through it. Contrast enhancement is required for obtaining functional information; however, administering IV MR contrast in patients with renal insufficiency is relatively contraindicated. Fast, fluid-sensitive MR sequences can nicely demonstrate anatomic details of complex urinary abnormalities, especially for preoperative planning, such as in patients with particularly complex duplication anomalies.

8.3 Normal Imaging Characteristics

8.3.1 Kidney

Neonatal kidneys have a distinctive appearance on US (Fig. 8.1). The cortex is much more echogenic in the neonatal period and retains this appearance for several weeks to months. The pyramids are quite hypoechoic and can be confused for hydronephrosis to the untrained eye. The kidneys should be of normal size, there are published standards available by gestational age. As a general benchmark, normal newborn kidneys range from 3.5 to 5 cm in length. Newborn kidneys often retain a lobulated contour called fetal lobation (Fig. 8.2), which corresponds to an individual calyx, pyramid, and surrounding cortex. Fetal lobation, like newborn echogenic cortex, may persist for months and some separation of lobes may persist indefinity. Kidneys on MRI (Fig. 8.3) are generally dark in signal intensity on T1 and bright on T2.

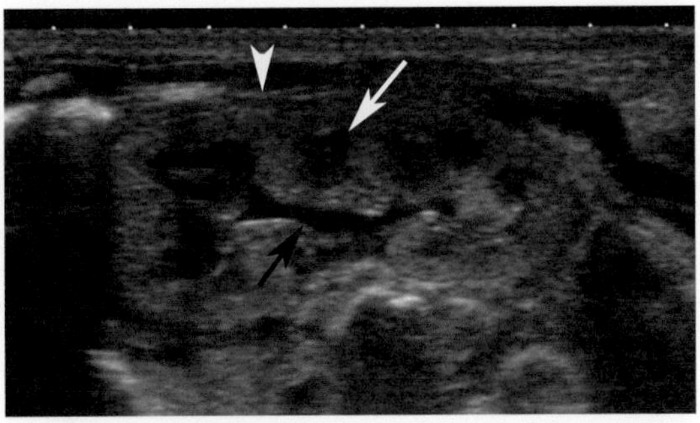

Fig. 8.1 Longitudinal sonographic image of the normal neonatal kidney in the prone position. The cortex is typically echogenic (*white arrowhead*) and the renal pyramids, hypoechoic (*white arrow*). A small amount of fluid in the renal pelvis is normal on prone views (*black arrow*)

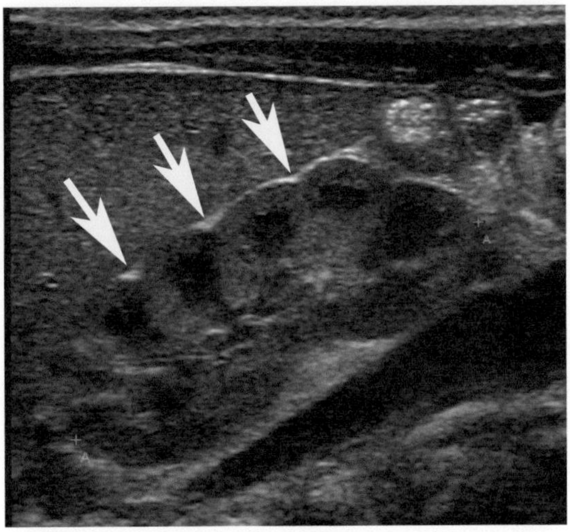

Fig. 8.2 Longitudinal sonographic image performed supine demonstrating fetal lobation. The *white arrows* represent the indentations in the renal cortex between the fetal lobes made up of the hypoechoic pyramid and its surrounding cortex. This configuration should not be mistaken for renal scarring

8.3.2 Bladder

The urinary bladder wall should be of uniform thickness, no greater than 5 mm thick in a decompressed state and no more than 3 mm at maximal capacity. The fluid within the bladder should be anechoic on US (Fig. 8.4) and of fluid intensity on MRI (Fig. 8.5). On a VCUG (Fig. 8.6), the

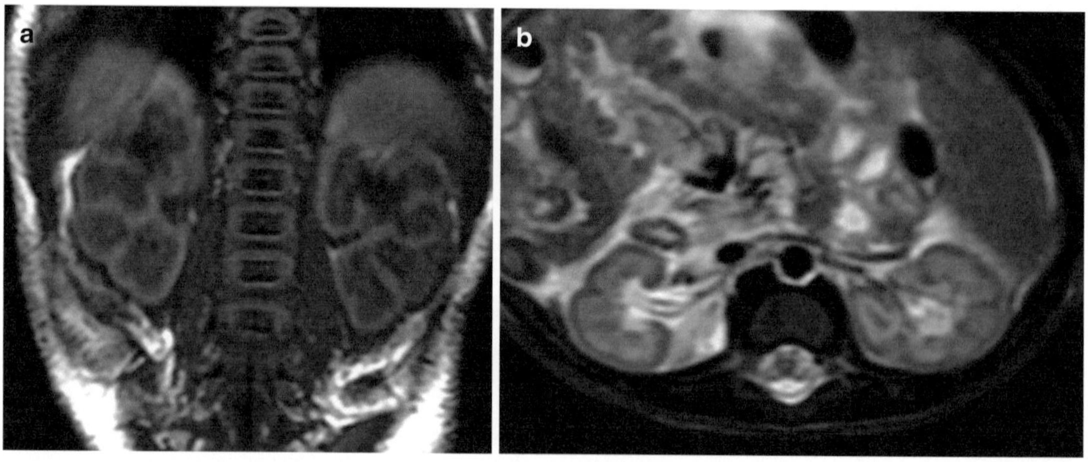

Fig. 8.3 MR images of the normal neonatal kidney; coronal T1 (**a**) shows kidneys which are of relatively dark signal intensity (with bright cortex and darker brighter medullary pyramids) compared to the axial T2 (**b**) images in which they are relatively brighter, with darker cortex and brighter medullary pyramids

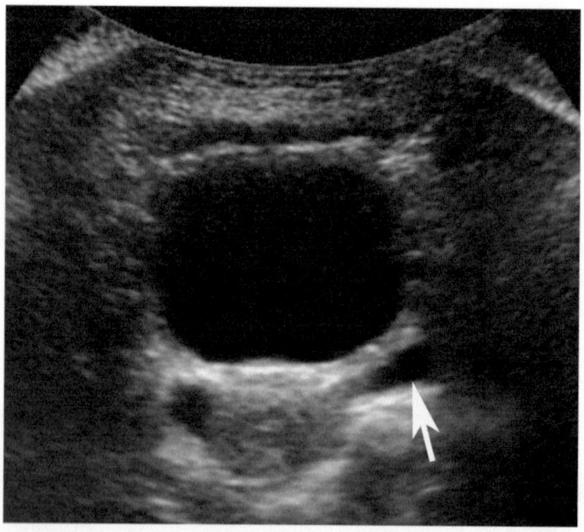

Fig. 8.4 Transverse sonographic image of the normal, distended urinary bladder showing anechoic fluid with no internal debris and no bladder wall thickening. Incidental mild dilation of the distal left ureter (*arrow*) can be seen in patients with VUR or UVJ narrowing

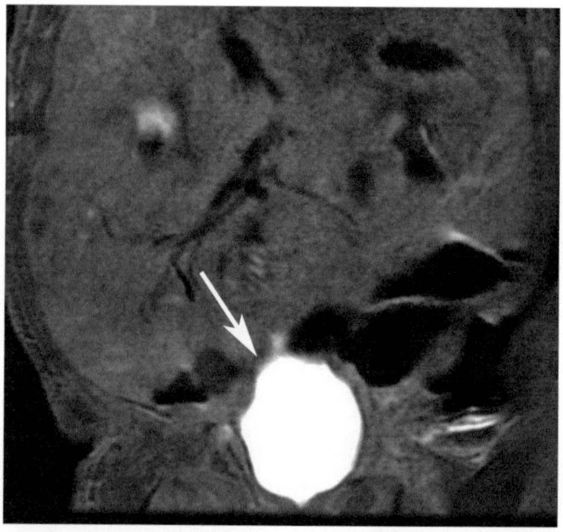

Fig. 8.5 Coronal T1-weighted MR image after IV contrast injection showing the urinary bladder full of high-intensity fluid (*arrow*). Without contrast, urine is dark intensity on T1 and bright intensity on T2

bladder should be smooth, and the base of the bladder should be almost touching the pubic symphysis. There should be no filling defects or outpouchings. Sometimes the lateral bases of the bladder bulge laterally and caudally into the inguinal canal; these are called "bladder ears," a normal variant appearance (Fig. 8.7). The normal bladder is usually wider than it is tall.

8.3.3 Urethra

The urethra is seen on US when imaged longitudinally on the perineum and is not distended unless imaged during urination. The lumen may [12] be hypoechoic with a thin echogenic mucosa (Fig. 8.8). On VCUG, one should visualize the entire urethra filled with contrast, preferably without a urethral catheter within it, especially in boys. In girls, one can image the urethra in the frontal projection (Fig. 8.9). However, the male urethra should be imaged in the oblique or lateral projection. Several normal landmarks are seen in the normal neonatal male urethra including the verumontanum, the valvulae colliculi, the subtle waist at the urethral sphincter, and contrast trapped within the prepuce in an uncircumcised male (Fig. 8.10).

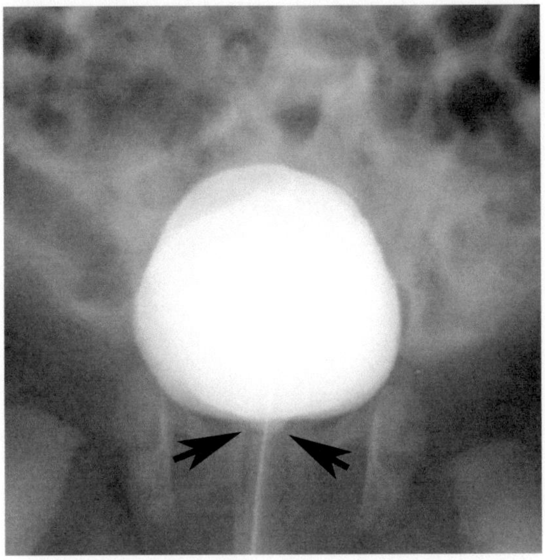

Fig. 8.6 Frontal, PA view of the normal, well-filled urinary bladder during a VCUG in a neonate. The patient is probably about to urinate as denoted by contrast distention of the bladder neck (*arrows*)

8.4 Fetal Imaging

Imaging of the fetal urinary tract is done routinely by US. It is not until about 11 weeks gestation that the fetal kidneys start making urine which then is the main source of normal amniotic fluid. Therefore, it is not until 11–12 weeks gestation that fetal obstructive uropathy can be detected (Fig. 8.11). Once obstructive uropathy is detected, fetal MRI is sometimes performed to better characterize the level of obstruction (Fig. 8.12) and to detect additional congenital anomalies. MRI of the fetus is performed in axial, coronal, and sagittal planes, predominantly utilizing fluid-weighted sequences, which can be performed rapidly since the fetus is frequently moving.

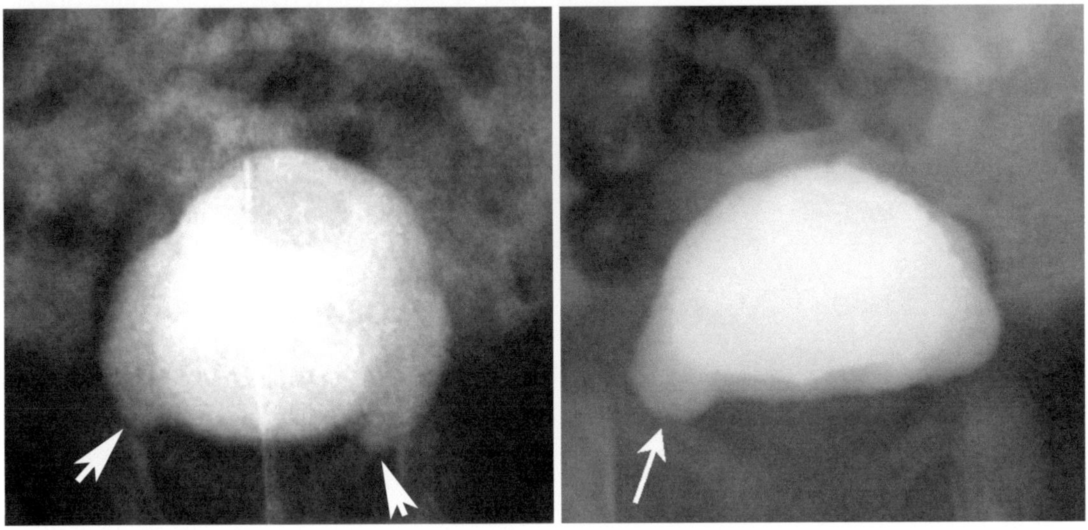

Fig. 8.7 Frontal view of the bladder during a VCUG shows bladder ears, (**a**) left more than right (*arrows*) and (**b**) unilateral right (*arrow*), a normal variant appearance which is transient, usually caused by Valsalva when the increased intra-abdominal pressure forces the lateral inferior aspects of the bladder toward the inguinal canal

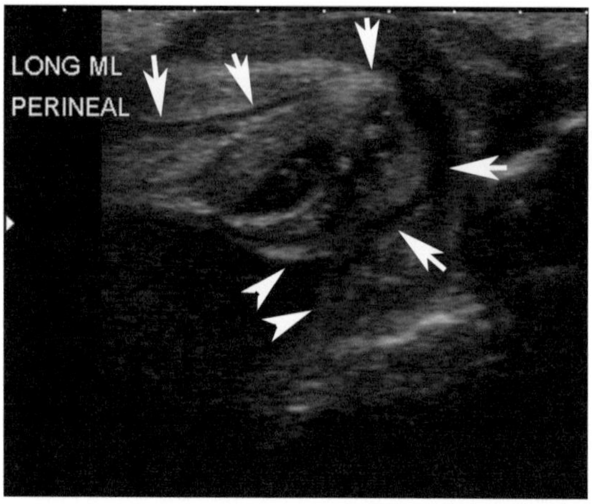

Fig. 8.8 Longitudinal perineal sonogram of an infant boy with showing the normal bladder outlet (*arrowheads*) and urethra (*arrows*), the transducers aligned ĉ base of bladder and penis

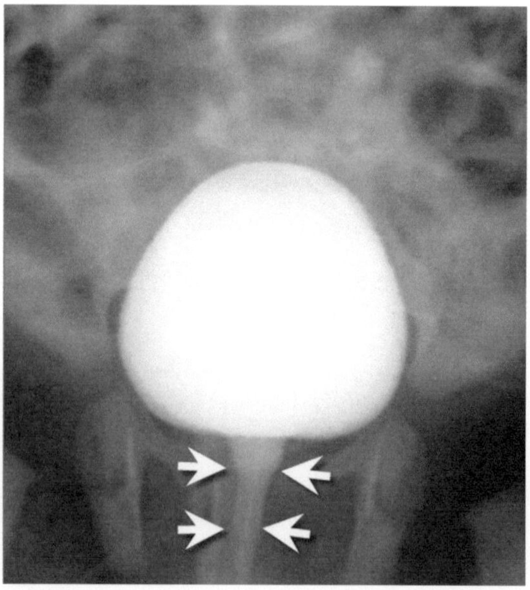

Fig. 8.9 Frontal view of bladder during voiding showing a normal appearance of the female urethra (*arrows*)

8.5 Congenital Anomalies

8.5.1 Renal Ectopia

During development of the fetus, the urinary tract and genital tract arise from the same primordial structures in the lower abdomen/pelvis. During the process, the kidneys undergo relative ascent and rotation to their final position in the retroperitoneum. Therefore, if one of the kidney's ascent is arrested, the location of the ectopic kidney can be anywhere from the pelvis to the expected location [16]. Occasionally, kidneys migrate excessively, above the renal fossa, resulting in an ectopic thoracic kidney. Possible associated renal abnormalities include hydronephrosis and vesicoureteral reflux. Ectopic kidneys are also more prone to traumatic injury or iatrogenic injury in this age of laparoscopic surgery.

8.5.1.1 Horseshoe Kidney

Estimated incidence is around 1 in 500 births, disregard changes SJK results from fusion of the lower poles of the kidneys during renal development as they are ascending from the pelvis. Because the lower poles are fused, the complete ascent of the kidneys to the normal expected position is arrested, the upper poles being somewhat more lateral than expected and the inferior portion of the kidneys forming a U or V shape. The long axis of each kidney is toward the ipsilateral shoulder rather than the opposite shoulder. This can be seen on US (Fig. 8.13), MRI (Fig. 8.14), or VCUG (Fig. 8.15). A third of individuals with this abnormality will have at least one other urinary anomaly or complication involving the cardiovascular system or central nervous system.

8.5.1.2 Crossed Fused Ectopia

Estimated incidence is 1 in 1,000 births. Crossed fused ectopia results from lack of ascent of the involved kidney. The two presiding theories for this abnormality include an abnormally situated umbilical artery preventing normal cephalic migration, or the ureteric bud extends to the opposite side and induces nephron formation in the contralateral metanephric blastema. The result is a single renal mass with two collecting systems located on one side of the abdomen (Fig. 8.16). Lack of a kidney in the renal fossa of the ectopic kidney results in failure of development of the extraperitoneal fascial layer of the side not occupied by renal tissue; this often results in bowel occupying the

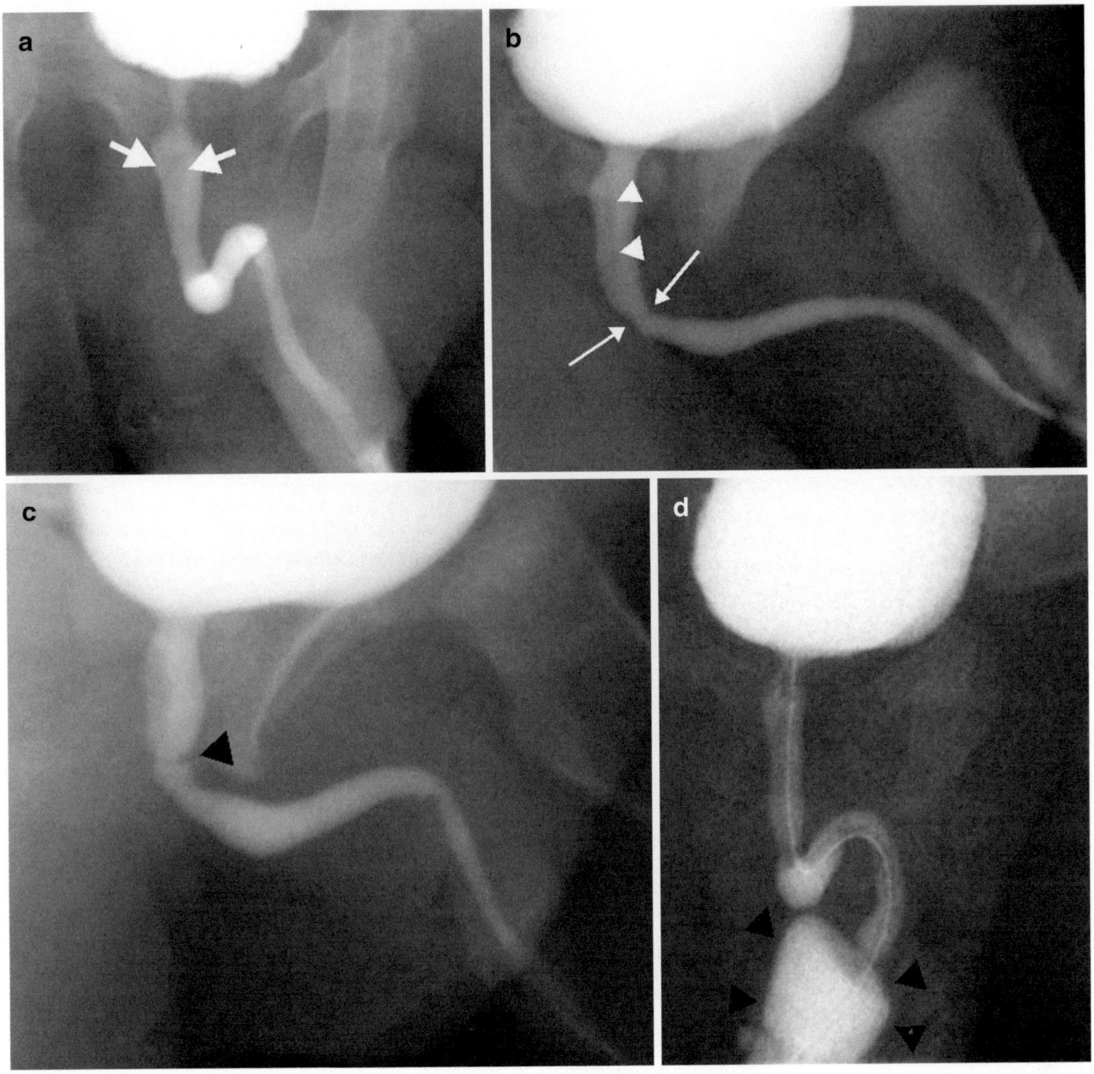

Fig. 8.10 Male urethra, normal anatomic variations of appearance. (**a**) Normal appearance of the urethra in near-AP projection showing the verumontanum en face (*black arrows*). (**b**) Standard oblique view of the urethra showing normal landmarks; the verumontanum (*white arrowheads*) and the slight narrowing of the urethra at the urethral sphincter (*white arrows*), also called the membranous urethra. (**c**) oblique view of the urethra showing a thin filling defect anteriorly (*arrowhead*) which represents the normal valuable colliculi. (**d**) AP view of the male urethra during voiding with the catheter still in showing contrast trapped within the prepuce (*black arrowheads*) in an uncircumcised patient

empty renal fossa due to relaxation of mesenteric supports, especially the splenic flexure when the left kidney is ectopically located on the right (Fig. 8.17).

8.5.1.3 Pelvic Kidney

Failure of ascent of one or both kidneys, which may be separate or fused (pancake kidney) in the pelvis (Fig. 8.18).

8.5.1.4 Pancake Kidney

Form of pelvic renal ectopia in which the kidneys are fused in the pelvis (Fig. 8.19). The kidney may have an atypical sonographic appearance due to abnormal lie in the pelvis or may appear similar in sonographic appearance in both longitudinal and transverse views, unlike the kidney in the usual position in the renal fossa which has a unique bean-shaped appearance on each view.

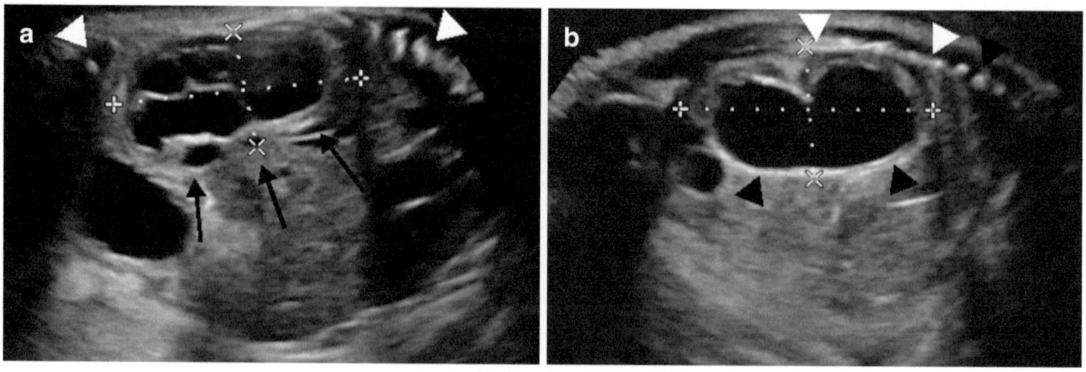

Fig. 8.11 Longitudinal prenatal US images of the fetal kidneys demonstrating severe hydronephrosis of the right (*black arrows*) (**a**) and left (*black arrowheads*) (**b**) kidney. *White arrowheads* denote fetal spine

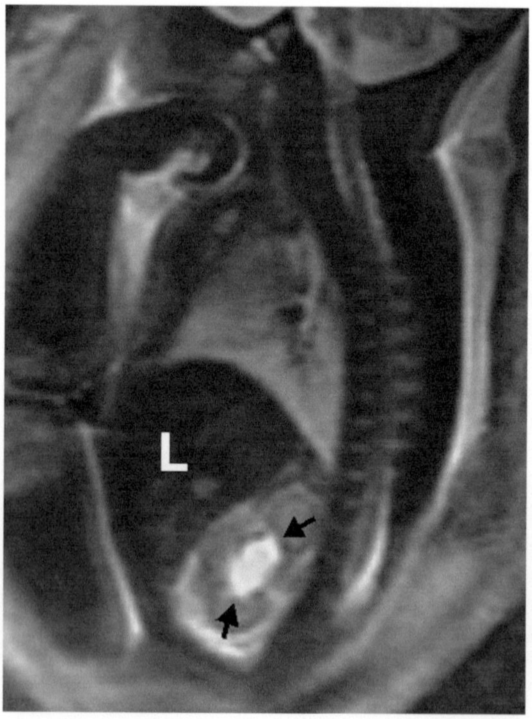

Fig. 8.12 Sagittal T2-weighted image from fetal MR shows high signal in the dilated right renal pelvis (*black arrows*) in this fetus with postnatal imaging which confirmed UPJ narrowing. *L* denotes the liver

8.5.2 Hydronephrosis +/− Hydroureter

Hydronephrosis and hydroureter are a common finding in the fetus and neonate. There are several etiologies to be considered in the differential diagnosis [11]. The most common causes include vesicoureteral reflux, ureteropelvic junction obstruction, ureterovesical junction obstruction, ureterocele/ureter duplication, posterior urethral valves in males, and some cases of a specific type of anorectal malformation in females, the cloaca.

8.5.2.1 Vesicoureteral Reflux

Vesicoureteral reflux is the most common cause of hydroureteronephrosis in the neonate. It may be quite severe, resulting in cortical thinning, and can be associated with renal dysplasia in a small percentage of patients. Early sonography (Fig. 8.20) and VCUG (Fig. 8.21) can allow differentiation of severe VUR from obstructive megaureter, and if obstruction is suspected, a nuclear medicine MAG3 diuretic renogram can be performed to assess for obstructive uropathy and assess differential renal function (Fig. 8.22). Often, one may see urothelial thickening of the intrarenal collecting system, renal pelvis and ureter on renal ultrasound.

8.5.2.2 Ureteropelvic Junction Obstruction

Ureteropelvic junction (UPJ) obstruction is one of the most common causes of moderate to severe hydronephrosis (pelvocaliectasis) without hydroureter in the neonate. Labile VUR can also cause moderate hydronephrosis. One may see urothelial thickening of the intrarenal collecting system, similar to patients with reflux (Fig. 8.23). Diuretic

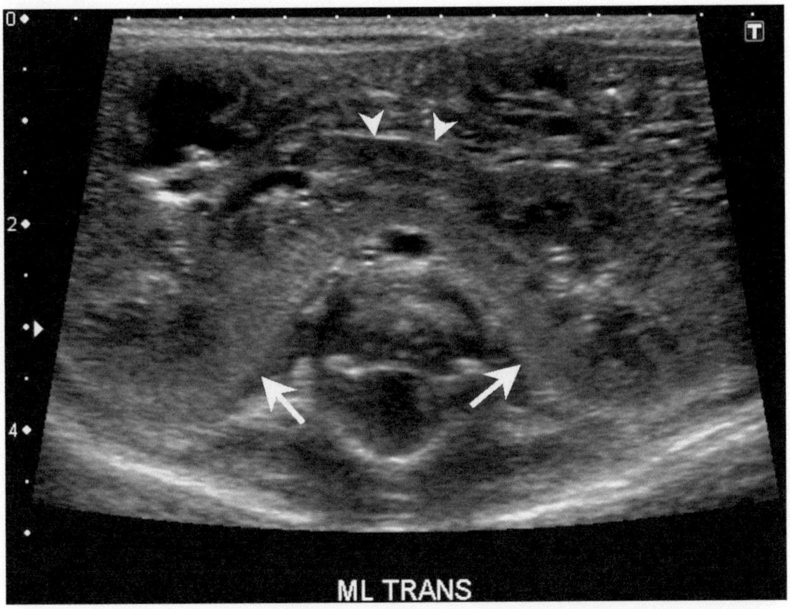

Fig. 8.13 Midline abdomen transverse US of a neonate demonstrating the isthmus (*arrowheads*) of renal parenchyma connecting the right and left renal moieties (*arrows*) in this patient with a horseshoe kidney

renography is often performed following US, showing delayed emptying of the intrarenal collecting system.

8.5.2.3 Ureterovesical Junction Obstruction

Ureterovesical junction (UVJ) obstruction is one of the less common causes of hydroureteronephrosis. It is most often due to primary megaureter, seen on imaging studies as short segment narrowing of the distal ureter (Fig. 8.24). It can be seen associated with VUR on a VCUG and is often bilateral, the degree of obstruction being of variable degree in the opposite renal moiety. There may be no associated reflux. A MAG3 diuretic renal scan may be performed to assess for urinary obstruction versus urinary stasis without obstruction (Figs. 8.22 and 8.25).

Obstruction of the distal ureters can also occur in females with anorectal malformation, specifically those born with a cloaca, a single perineal opening as described in Sect. (8.5.2.6).

8.5.2.4 Ureterocele/Ureteral Duplication

Multiple ureters/renal moieties result from the duplication or early division of the ureteral bud, each inducing corresponding nephrogenic blastema. Two, three, or more different renal units may form, dependent on the number of ureteric buds formed. According to the Weigert-Meyer rule, the lower pole ureter inserts orthotopically in the trigone and the upper pole ureters insert inferiorly and medially to the lower pole ureter. Most commonly, the ectopic ureters insert elsewhere in the bladder as a variation of normal and do not reflux or obstruct. However,

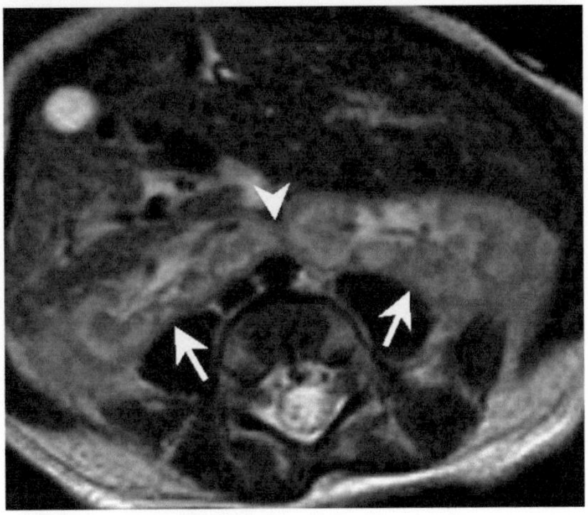

Fig. 8.14 Axial T2-weighted neonatal MR showing the isthmus (*arrowhead*) connecting the right and left renal moieties (*arrows*) in patient with horseshoe kidney

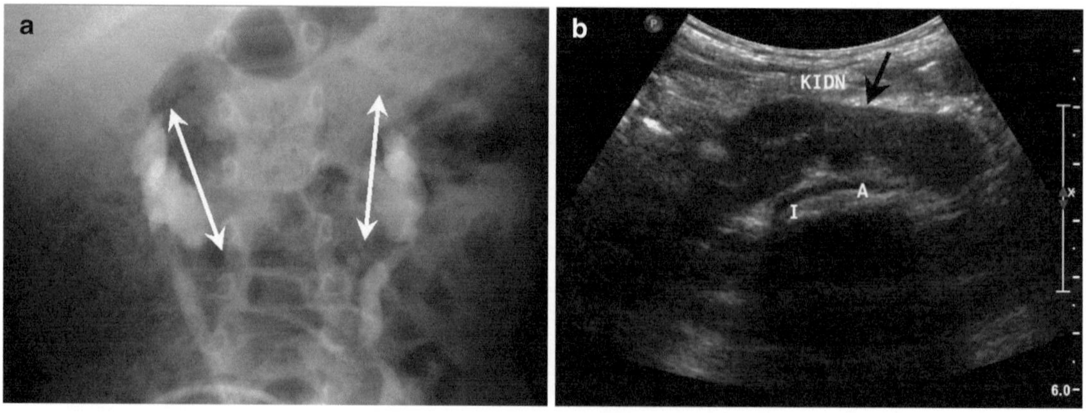

Fig. 8.15 (**a**) Frontal view of the contrast-filled ureters and single collecting systems from VCUG showing abnormal axis of both kidneys' (*double-headed white arrows*) upper poles pointing toward the ipsilateral shoulders and lower poles pointing toward each other. This is a characteristic appearance of VUR into both moieties of a horseshoe kidney. (**b**) Transverse abdomen US of the same patient showing an isthmus of parenchyma (*black arrow*) connecting the right and left lower poles of this horseshoe kidney. *I* inferior vena cava, *A* abdominal aorta

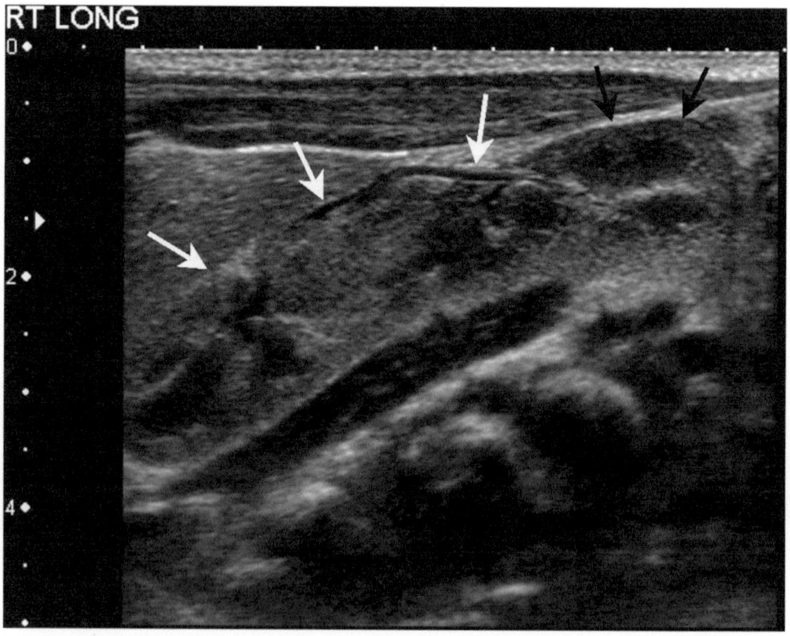

Fig. 8.16 Longitudinal US of the right renal fossa showing the upper pole of the left kidney (*black arrows*) fused to the right kidney (*white arrows*) in this patient with crossed fused ectopia. There was no renal tissue in the left renal fossa

sometimes the ectopic ureter is obstructed and the distal ureter dilates, prolapsing into the bladder as a ureterocele (Fig. 8.26). Sometimes the ureterocele can be so large that it prolapses toward the bladder base and can obstruct the urethra during voiding (Fig. 8.27). This is sometimes called a prolapsing cecoureterocele. Ureteroceles are easily detected by prenatal and postnatal renal ultrasound and sometimes are imaged by MRI, either prenatally or postnatally (Fig. 8.28).

The ectopic ureter can sometimes insert outside the bladder, into the urethra. In boys, the ureter usually inserts above the urethral sphincter so boys are continent; however, the ureter is therefore obstructed, causing upper pole hydronephrosis and hydroureter in almost all of these patients, except when the patient is urinating, at which time there may be reflux (Fig. 8.29). Ectopic ureters in boys may also insert into other structures such as the vas deferens, seminal vesicles, or prostate. In girls, the ectopic ureter can insert into the urethra below the urethral sphincter, causing constant wetting. Similar to boys, the ectopic ureter in girls can also insert outside the urinary tract, into the vagina, even onto the interlabial region or perineum, which can be detected clinically by physical exam. In both males and females, if there is upper pole hydronephrosis and no ureterocele, the upper pole ureter is ectopic, and either US or MRI of the urinary tract can usually define the anatomy, following the dilated ureter into the pelvis (Fig. 8.30).

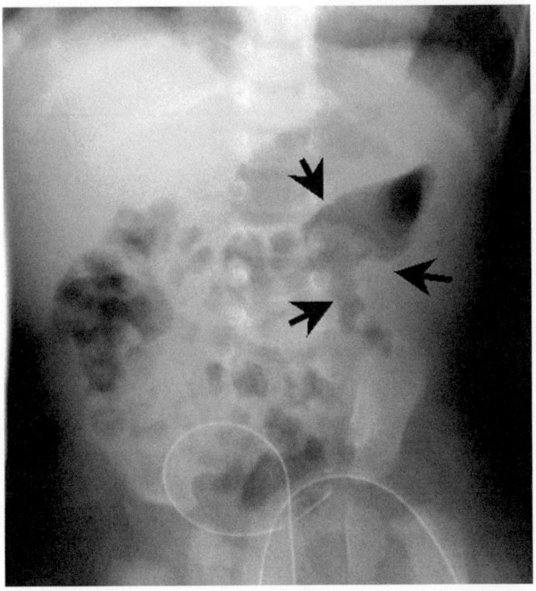

Fig. 8.17 AP radiograph of the abdomen showing splenic flexure of colon occupying the region of the left renal fossa (*arrows*), a sign that there is absence or ectopia of the left kidney

8.5.2.5 Posterior Urethral Valve (PUV)

Obstruction of the posterior urethra by posterior urethral valves, prominent plicae colliculi, is usually detectable prenatally, and with the advent of fetal surgery, prenatal imaging has become important not only for diagnosis but also for monitoring prenatal interventions. On US, the bladder wall is usually diffusely thickened, there may be bladder diverticula, and one may be able to document the dilated posterior urethra (Fig. 8.31) [12]. If there is VUR (Fig. 8.32), there

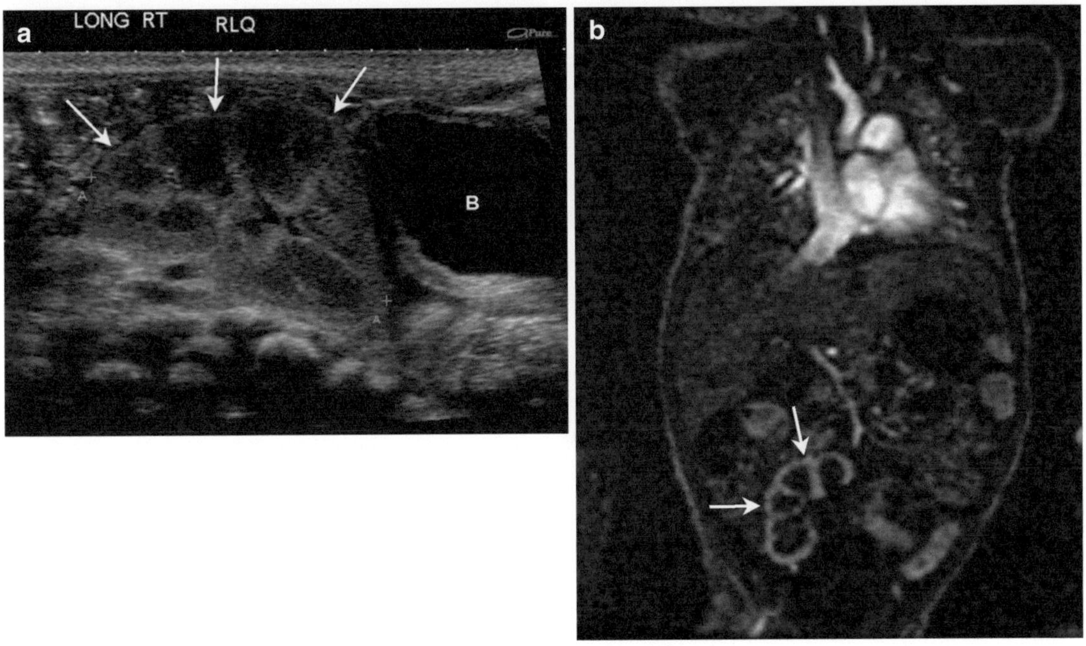

Fig. 8.18 Longitudinal US (**a**) and coronal MR image (**b**) of the pelvis of same patient as in Fig. 8.17 with congenital heart disease showing ectopic kidney within the pelvis (*arrows*); (*B*) bladder

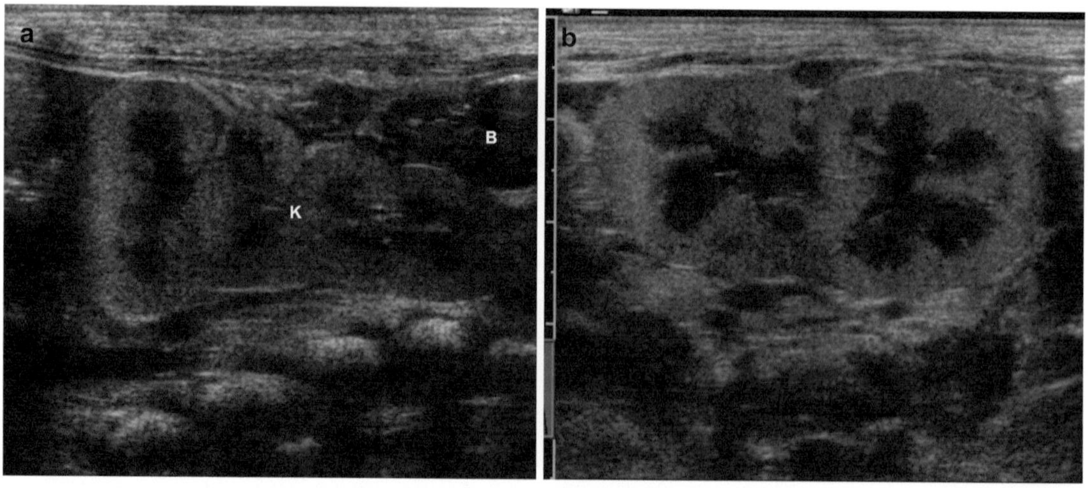

Fig. 8.19 (**a**) Longitudinal and (**b**) transverse US images of the pelvis in a neonate show similar appearance of the single pelvic kidney in both views, consistent with fused pancake kidney. The kidney (*K*) is low, abutting the urinary bladder (*B*), which is decompressed at the time of imaging

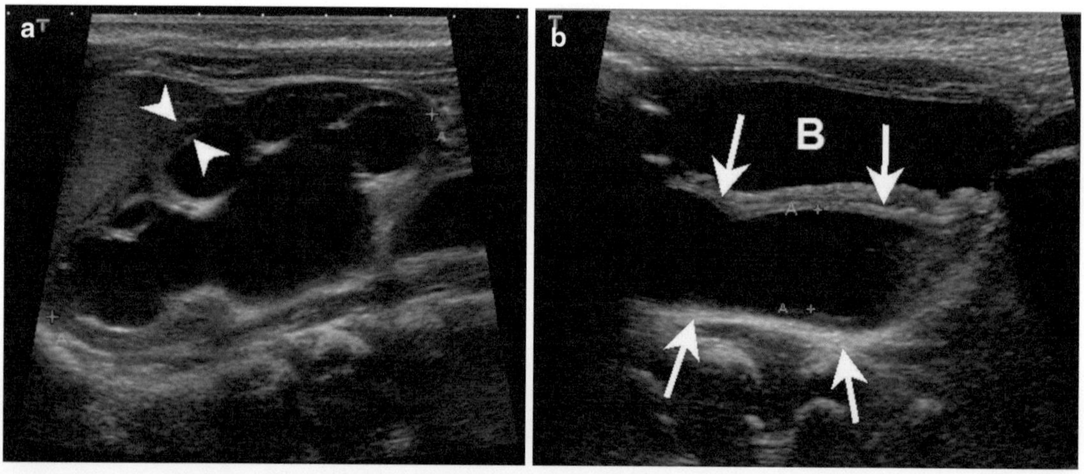

Fig. 8.20 Longitudinal US of the left kidney (**a**) and left UVJ (**b**) shows severe hydronephrosis associated with diffuse cortical thinning (*arrowheads*) and hydroureter with urothelial thickening (*arrows*). (*B*) bladder

is usually moderate to severe hydroureter and hydronephrosis (Fig. 8.33). Hydronephrosis may be so severe that the renal fornix may rupture, causing a perirenal urinoma or even urinary ascites detected as a fluid collection or ascites on US or MRI prenatally and/or postnatally (Fig. 8.34). In patients with little or no VUR, bladder outlet obstruction causes the most severe changes in the bladder, resulting in significant muscular hypertrophy and poor bladder function which may be permanent, tending to spare injury to the kidneys that usually results from severe VUR. In the setting of severe VUR, the bladder changes are often less severe, but the renal parenchyma often becomes thinned and/or dysplastic (Fig. 8.35). In the most severe cases, a forniceal rupture may be noted (Fig. 8.32c).

8.5.2.6 Anorectal Malformation (ARM)

Anorectal malformations include a spectrum of abnormalities involving formation of the rectal opening, resulting in misplacement of the rectal

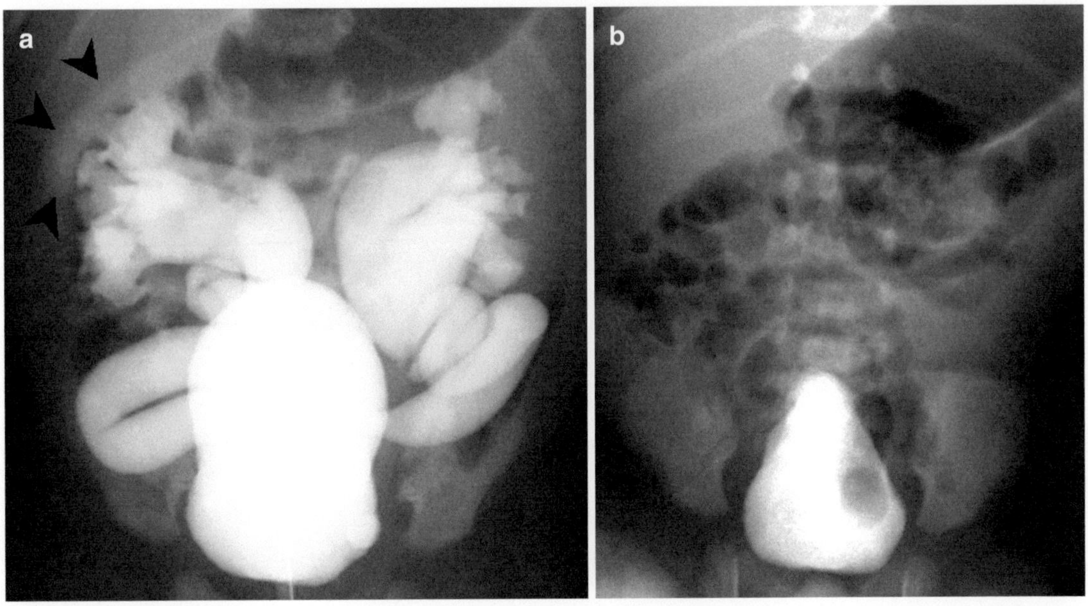

Fig. 8.21 Frontal spot images from VCUG in 2 patients with severe neonatal hydroureteronephrosis (HUN). (**a**) Grade 5 VUR with intrarenal reflux (*arrowheads*). (**b**) Lack of VUR on cyclic VCUG suggests non-refluxing primary megaureter as the etiology of patient's HUN. This can be confirmed with MAG3 diuretic renogram

opening. In some forms of imperforate anus, the rectal pouch is in the pelvis with or without a fistulous connection to the urinary tract in boys or formation of a single opening on the perineum in girls into which the rectum, vagina, and urethra open into, also called a cloaca. Patients with ARMs are at higher risk for genitourinary anomalies. The higher or more complex the malformation, the higher risk of associated urinary anomalies. Absent kidney, VUR, and hydronephrosis and hydroureter are some common abnormalities; crossed fused ectopia and horseshoe kidney are also fairly common. One of the most important abnormalities in girls with cloaca, in which the vagina becomes obstructed and enlarged, is called hydrocolpos [6]. The enlarged vagina often causes bilateral ureteral obstruction at the level of the bladder trigone (Fig. 8.36), causing obstructive uropathy that is best treated by vaginal drainage. If vaginal drainage is delayed, significant renal insufficiency can result, which is sometimes permanent. If hydrocolpos is not recognized as the cause of hydronephrosis and hydroureter, inappropriate and potentially damaging procedures such as surgical creation of a vesicostomy, ureterostomy, or percutaneous nephrostomy may be performed; unfortunately, these costly and unnecessary procedures would not treat the cause of obstructive uropathy. Simply draining the vagina is typically the only procedure necessary.

Therefore, in neonates with ARM, a renal and bladder US including detailed US of the pelvis to assess for genitourinary structures is necessary. Imaging to exclude a presacral mass, such as a teratoma (Fig. 8.37), which is sometimes associated with ARMs, is also paramount in making the correct and complete diagnosis during the neonatal period. In a patient with a scimitar, scooped out appearance of the distal sacrum, also called a hemi-sacrum, the presence of a sacral mass such as a teratoma or anterior meningocele should be suspected. The combination of a scimitar sacrum, presacral mass, and ARM is called Currarino's triad. If significant hydronephrosis and hydroureter is present in the absence of hydrocolpos, VUR may be suspected, and a VCUG may be helpful in the first weeks of life to exclude high-grade VUR and to assess for

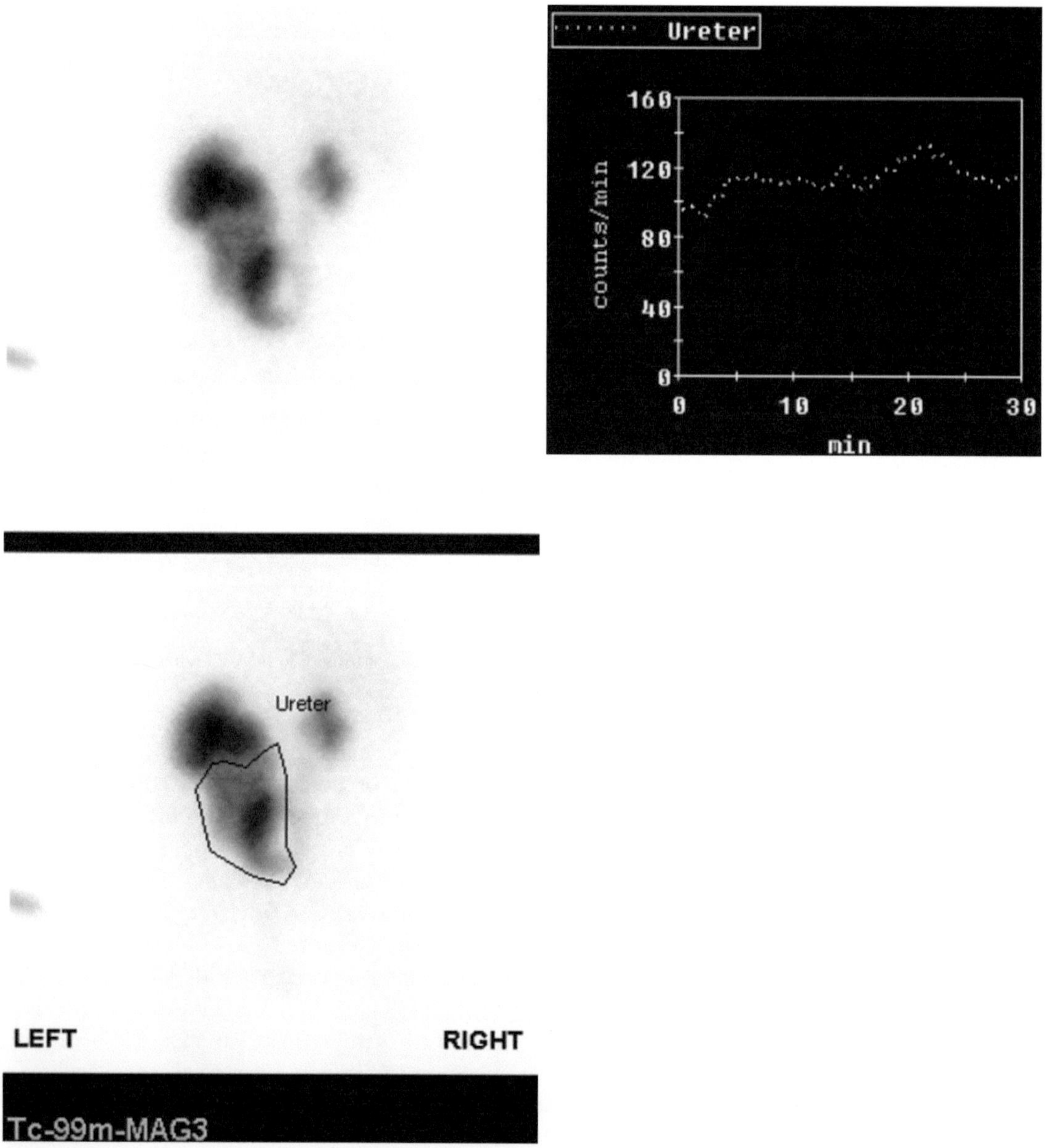

Fig. 8.22 Delayed posterior image of both kidneys and drainage curve of the left ureter from MAG3 diuretic renogram showing dilation and accumulation of radiotracer in the left intrarenal collecting system and left ureter (compared with the normal right moiety) and delayed flat drainage curve of the left ureter

possible neurogenic bladder in patients with more complex malformations since these patients have a higher association with significant sacral hypoplasia and intraspinal abnormalities such as tethered spinal cord.

8.5.3 Renal Cystic Disease (RCD)

The newest classification of RCD divides them into genetic and nongenetic etiologies [1]. With the advent of genetic characterization of disease

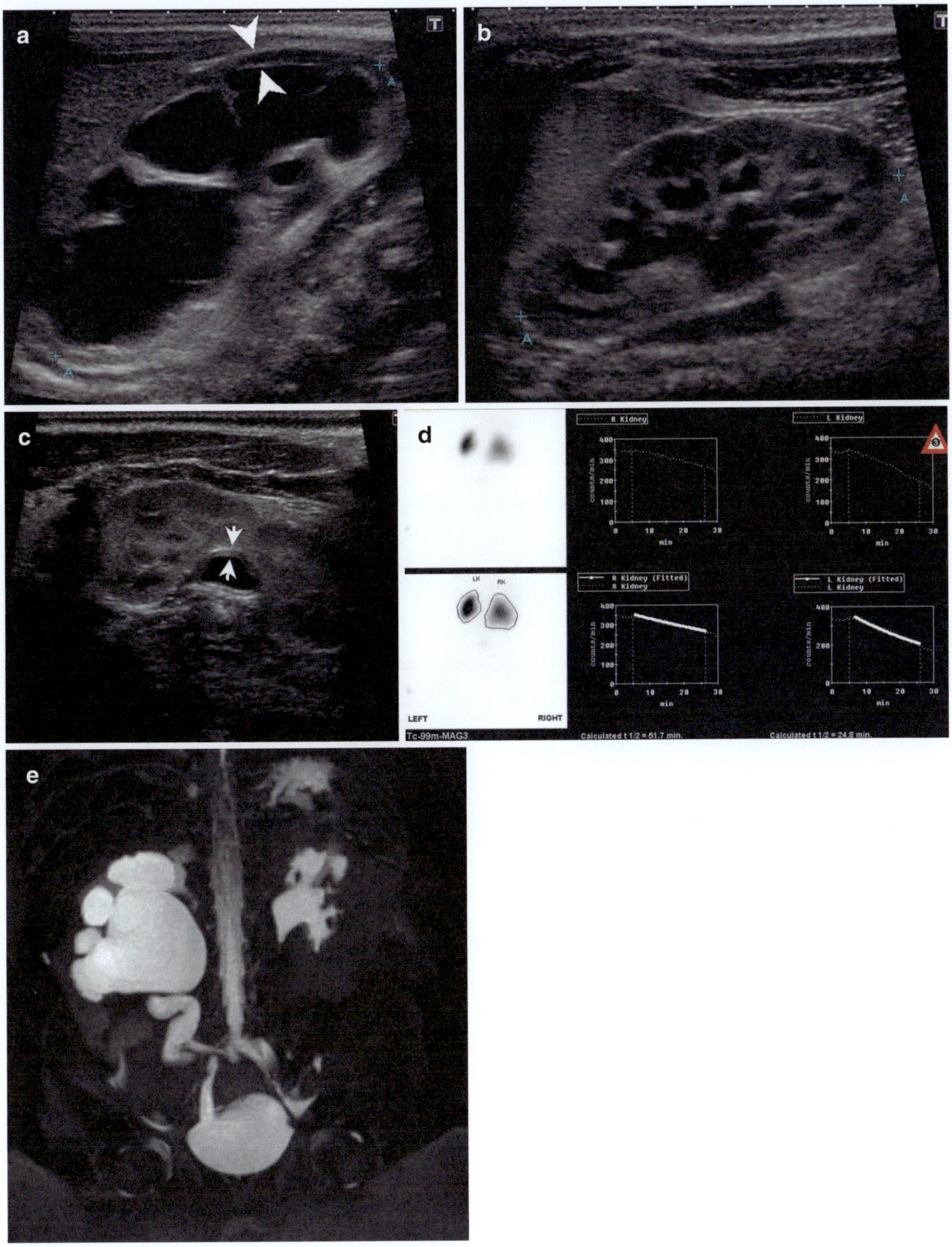

Fig. 8.23 UPJ obstruction. (**a**) Severe hydronephrosis of the right kidney with diffuse parenchymal thinning (*arrowheads*) and (**b**, **c**) mild to moderate hydronephrosis of the left kidney with moderate urothelial thickening (*short arrows*) of the renal pelvis. (**d**) Drainage curves from MAG3 renogram showing delayed drainage of both intrarenal collecting systems (T1/2>20 min) consistent with bilateral UPJ obstruction, right more severe than left. (**e**) Coronal T2-weighted MIP image from MR urogram in the sample nicely demonstrating the anatomy of the urinary tract in this patient with right UPJ obstruction

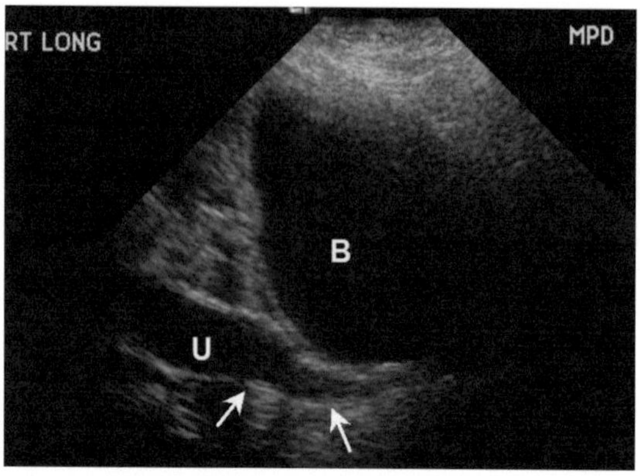

Fig. 8.24 Longitudinal US image of the right ureterovesical junction showing short segment tapered narrowing of the ureter (*U*) just above the ureteral insertion (*arrows*); (*B*) bladder

processes, many of these inherited renal cystic diseases such as autosomal recessive (infantile) polycystic kidney disease (ARPKD), autosomal dominant (adult) polycystic kidney disease (ADPKD), nephronophthisis-medullary cystic dysplasia complex (NMCDC), and medullary cystic dysplasia associated with syndromes (tuberous sclerosis and Von Hippel-Lindau syndrome) are now distinguishable by genes that code for a mutation of a protein in the cilia of the renal epithelium. This group of diseases is now sometimes referred to as ciliopathies. The nongenetic causes of RCD are most commonly the obstructive uropathies, which include

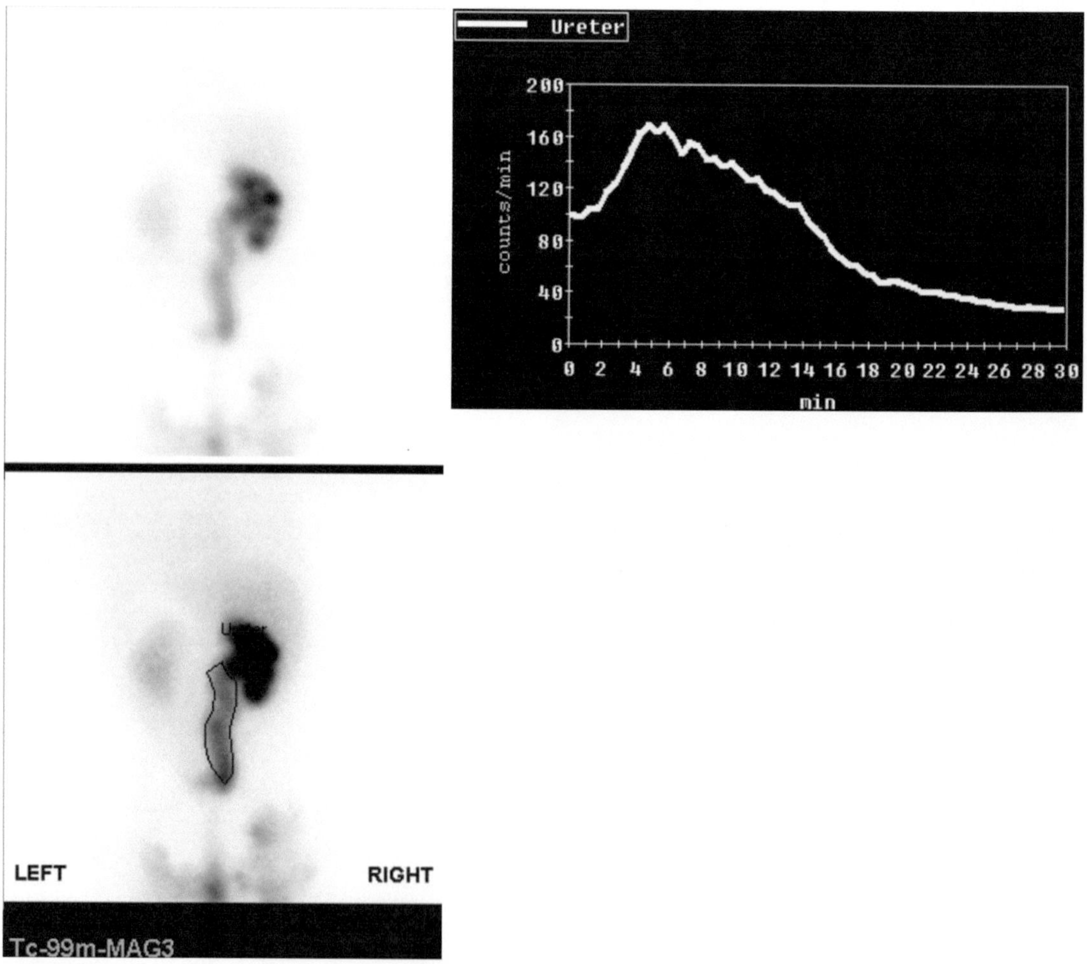

Fig. 8.25 Ureteral drainage curve of the right ureter from MAG3 diuretic renogram showing abnormal, borderline delayed drainage (T1/2 = 15.5 min)

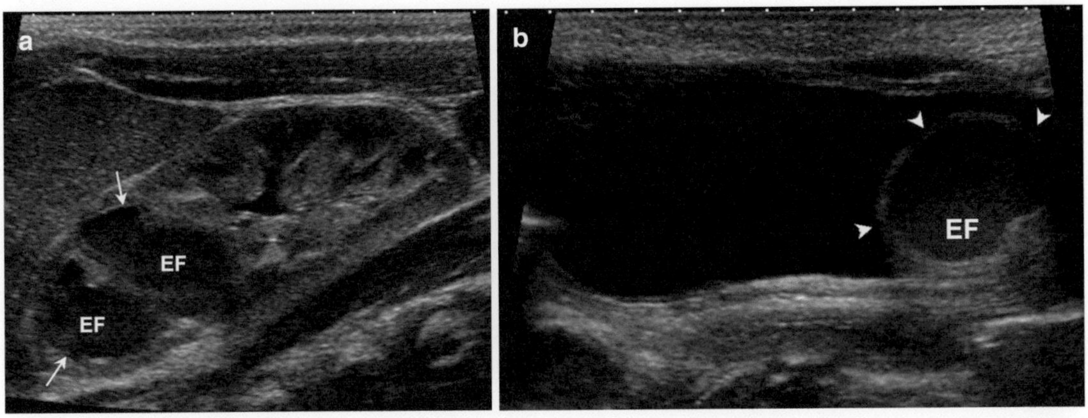

Fig. 8.26 (**a**) Longitudinal US image of the right kidney showing asymmetric upper pole pelvocaliectasis (*arrows*) with echogenic fluid (*EF*) within it. (**b**) Longitudinal US image of the right bladder showing a moderate-to-large-sized right ectopic ureterocele (*arrowheads*) also with echogenic fluid (*EF*) within it, which is the end of the obstructed right upper pole ureter, which enters the bladder ectopically, inferior and medial to the orthotopic lower pole ureteral insertion according to the Weigert-Meyer rule of urinary duplication anomalies. Echogenic fluid could be proteinaceous, hemorrhagic, or infectious

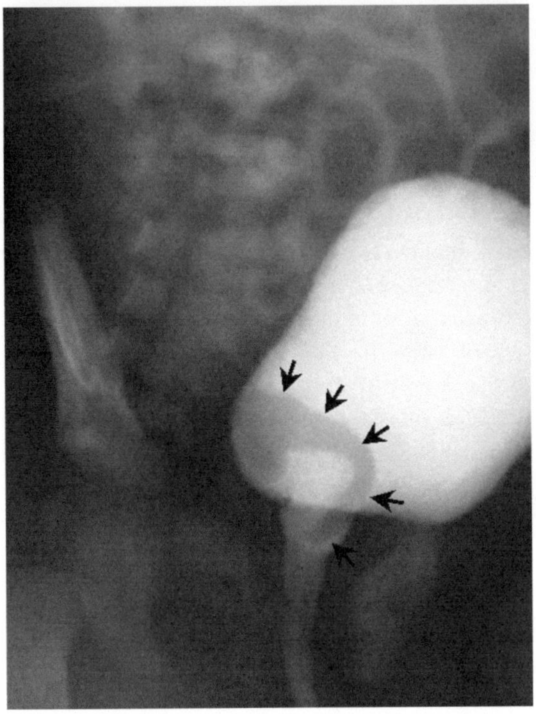

Fig. 8.27 Oblique spot image from the VCUG performed in the patient in Fig. 8.26 showing the urethra during voiding. There is prolapse of the ureterocele into the urethra (*arrows*), without overt signs of urethral obstruction such as bladder wall thickening or urethral dilation

posterior urethral valves, UVJ obstruction and UPJ obstruction, severe VUR, and multicystic dysplastic kidney (MCDK).

8.5.3.1 Genetic Renal Cystic Disease

ARPKD is the most common heritable RCD in infancy and childhood as compared to ADPKD which tends to occur in an older population. However, there is overlap and rarely ADPKD presents in the neonate with radiologic findings indistinguishable from ARPKD. The phenotypic expression of the disease is widely variable ranging from a severe form resulting in neonatal demise to a milder form which may not present for diagnosis until childhood or adolescence. The typical presentation in the neonate is that of bilateral flank masses due to symmetric, bilateral massive renal enlargement. On ultrasound, the massively enlarged kidneys of ARPKD are typically diffusely echogenic with poor corticomedullary differentiation, but without contour-deforming masses [1] (Fig. 8.38). In addition, about 45 % of these neonates also have liver abnormalities including an enlarged liver which may or may not be mildly echogenic, as well as intrahepatic and sometimes extrahepatic biliary dilation due to the same ciliary mutation within the biliary epithelial cells (Fig. 8.39). In severe cases, the urinary bladder may be empty due to poor renal function, and these neonates typically have oligohydramnios in the late prenatal period associated with pulmonary hypoplasia, abnormal facies, and high mortality (Potter's syndrome).

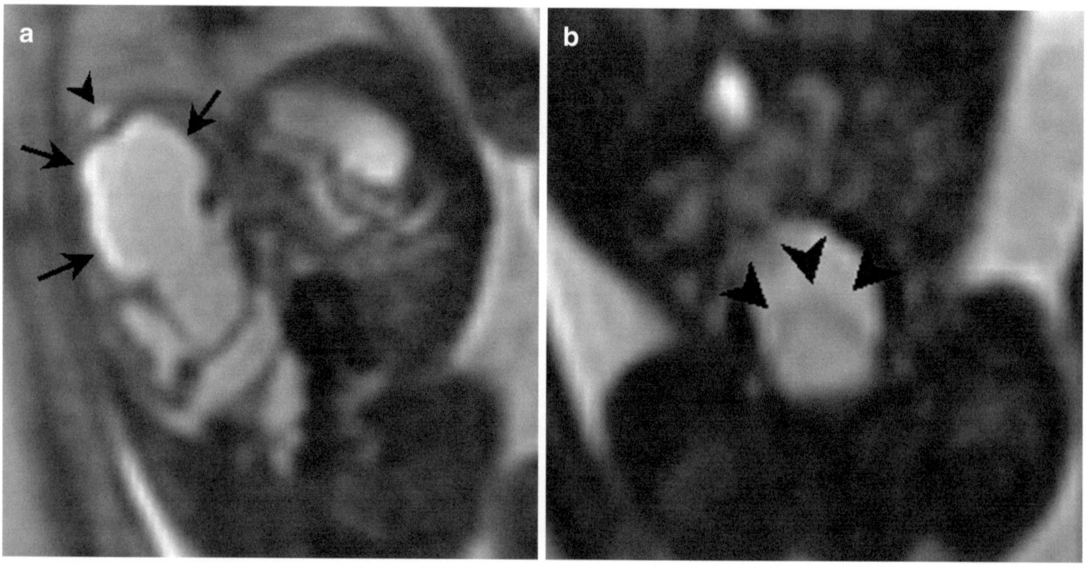

Fig. 8.28 Prenatal MR of patient with ectopic ureterocele. (**a**) Coronal T2-weighted images through the retroperitoneum show asymmetric dilation of the right collecting system (*black arrows*), the upper pole severely dilated compared to the lower pole, suggestive of urinary duplication anomaly. There may be cystic change of the upper pole parenchyma (*arrowhead*). (**b**) Coronal T2-weighted image of the pelvis shows a large ureterocele (*arrowheads*); on this image alone, without the images of the kidney, it would be difficult to determine if this was a right- or left-sided ureterocele

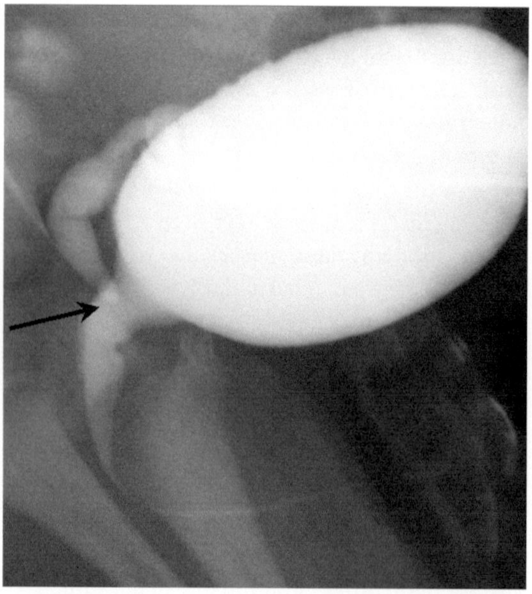

Fig. 8.29 VCUG in a male patient with a duplicated right urinary system and right upper pole hydroureteronephrosis. During voiding, there was reflux into the right upper pole ureter which is ectopically inserting into the junction of the bladder neck with the posterior urethra (*arrow*)

ADPKD more often presents later in childhood or adolescence, with numerous asymptomatic renal cysts incidentally discovered in one or both kidneys when performing an abdominal ultrasound for another indication.

8.5.3.2 Renal Dysplasia

Renal dysplasia, defined as abnormal metanephric differentiation, has a spectrum of presentation from aplasia to hypoplasia to multicystic dysplastic kidney (MCKD) and can be due to multiple etiologies including in utero drug exposure and genetic factors. Sometimes, abnormalities which affect other parts of the urinary tract can cause dysplasia, especially obstructive processes (Fig. 8.40). Specifically MCDK, a variant of renal dysplasia is one of the most frequently identified congenital anomalies of the urinary tract, characterized by the presence of multiple noncommunicating thin-walled cysts of various sizes, separated by abnormal looking renal parenchyma, the absence of a normal pelvicalyceal system, and lack of detectable renal function (Fig. 8.41). MCDK is presumably due to in utero

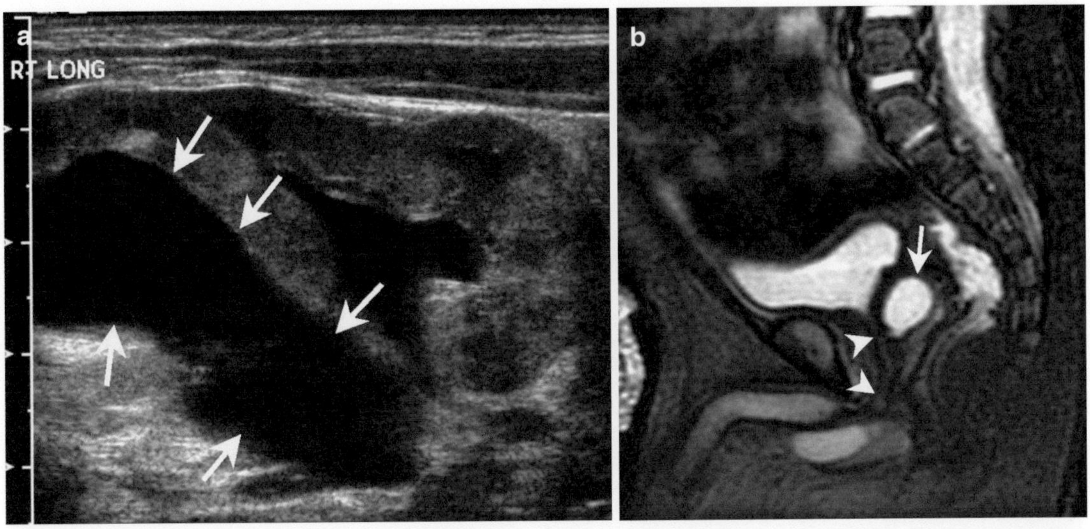

Fig. 8.30 (**a**) Longitudinal US of the right kidney showing asymmetric upper pole hydronephrosis and hydroureter (*arrows*) suggestive of a duplex kidney. No ureterocele was seen in the bladder (not shown). (**b**) Sagittal T2-weighted MR of the pelvis shows dilated fluid-filled distal ureter (*white arrow*) inserting into the posterior urethra (*arrowheads*)

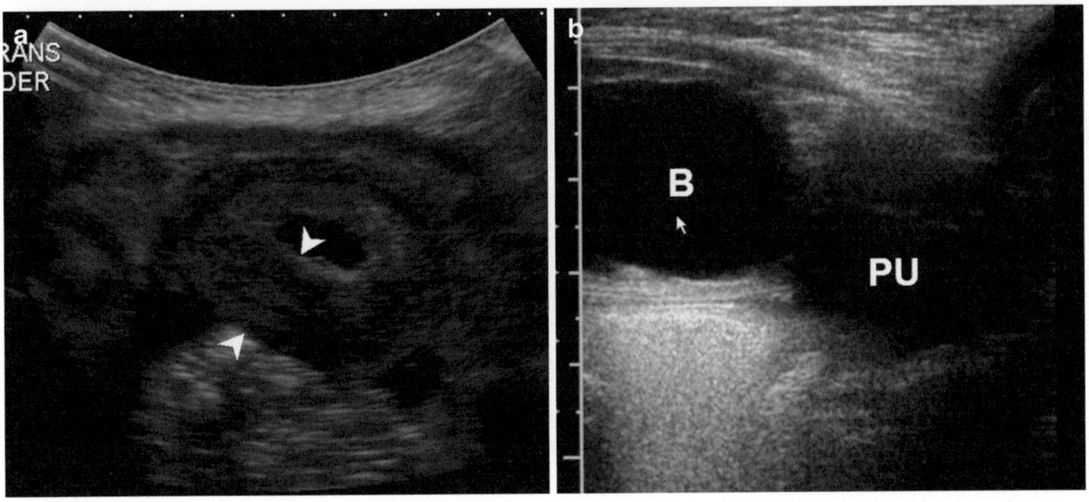

Fig. 8.31 (**a**) Transverse US image through the body of the urinary bladder in a patient with PUV showing marked bladder wall thickening (*arrowheads*). (**b**) Longitudinal perineal US of a different patient with PUV showing the partially filled and mildly thickened urinary bladder (*B*) and the dilated, fluid-filled posterior urethra (*PU*) inferior to the bladder base

high-grade obstruction of the ureter at or distal to the ureteropelvic junction. Other causes of urinary obstruction such as UVJ obstruction, UPJ obstruction, and PUVs can result in renal dysplasia though this type of dyplasia has a different natural history and treatment compared to MCDK. Even severe VUR can cause renal dysplasia (Fig. 8.42).

8.5.4 Renal Agenesis

Renal agenesis is a relatively common congenital anomaly, although its etiology is still unknown (4). It may be unilateral or bilateral. Bilateral renal agenesis is rare, occurring 1 in 10,000 births, and almost always results in fetal or neonatal

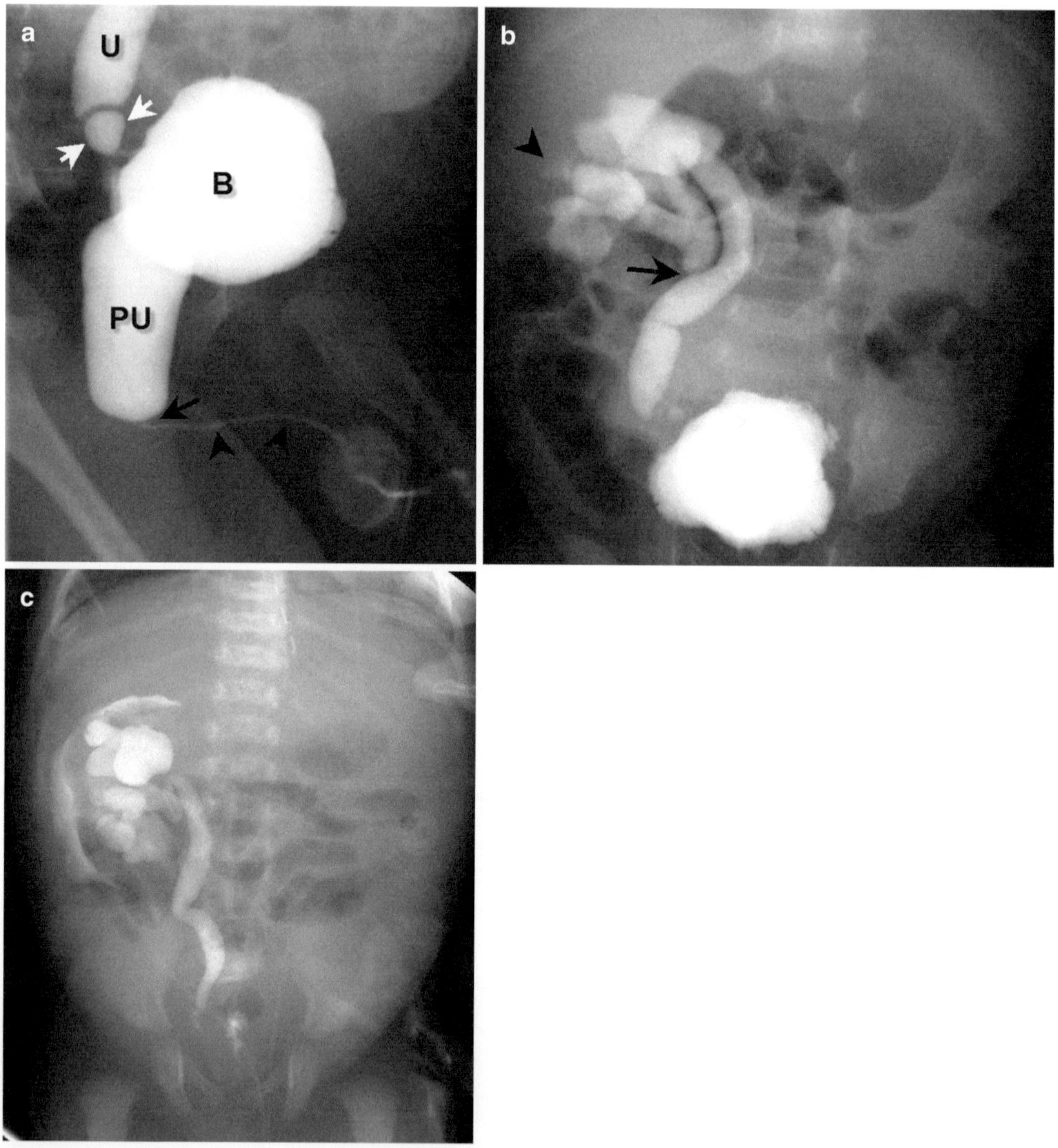

Fig. 8.32 (**a**) Oblique view of the urethra during voiding phase of VCUG showing the dilated posterior urethra (*PU*), linear lucency of prominent plicae or value (*black arrow*) between dilated posterior urethra and decompressed anterior urethra (*black arrowheads*), thickened, trabeculated urinary bladder (*B*) right periureteral or Hutch diverticulum (*arrows*), and dilated ureter (*U*) due to high-grade VUR. (**b**) Frontal view following voiding in same patient showing grade 5 VUR into bifid right ureter (*arrow*) with blush of intrarenal reflux (*arrowhead*). (**c**) A forniceal rupture seen on a VCUG of a different patient with urinary ascites, subsequents, dignosed with PUV, contrast seen in the perirenal space on the right

demise. Unilateral renal agenesis is usually discovered incidentally, associated with compensatory hypertrophy of the solitary kidney.

Renal agenesis is thought to result from the lack of induction of the metanephric blastema by the ureteric bud, possibly secondary to ureteric bud maldevelopment and/or a problem related to formation of the mesonephric duct. Infrequently, postnatal involution of an MCDK may result in a solitary kidney. Agenesis of a single kidney may be associated with ipsilateral genitourinary anomalies such as ipsilateral seminal vesicle

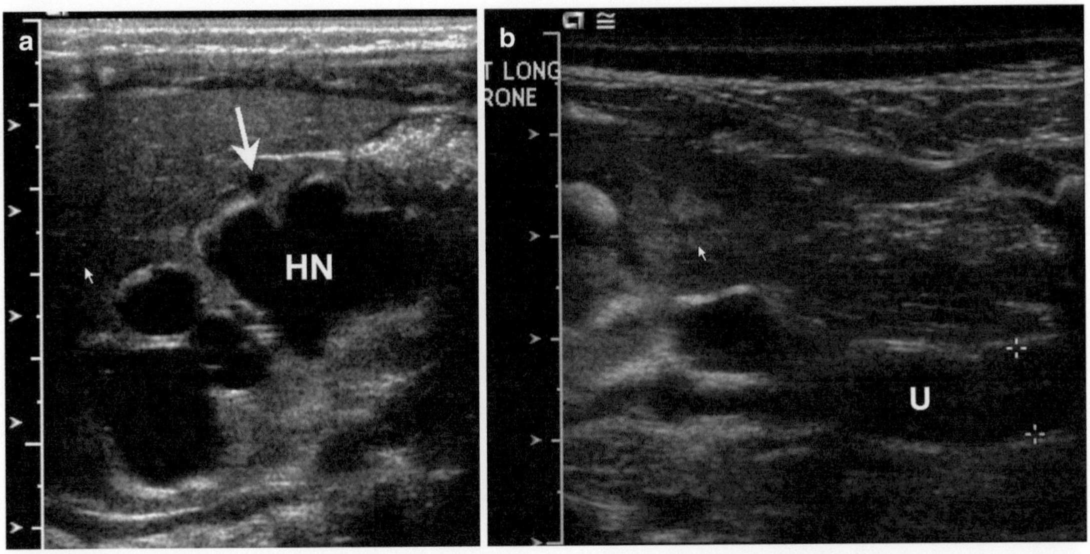

Fig. 8.33 Longitudinal images of the right kidney and right ureter in same patient as Fig. 8.32 showing severe hydronephrosis (*HN*) with (**a**) and moderate hydroureter (**b**). and a small cortical cyst (*white arrow*) are consistent with early renal dysplasia with in (*U*) this patient with PUV

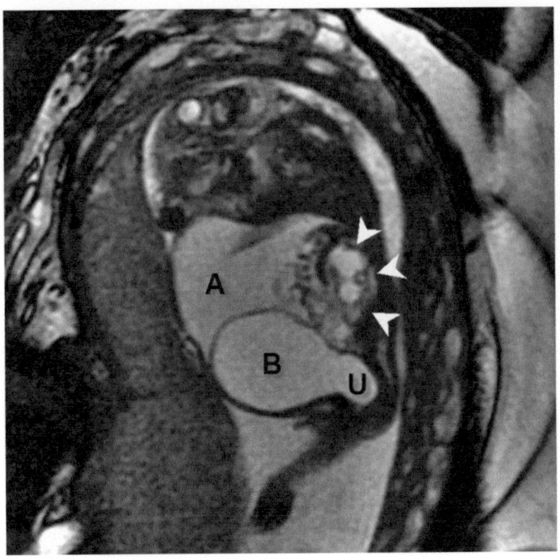

Fig. 8.34 Sagittal T2-weighted MR image of a fetus with findings of PUV including urinary ascites (*A*), a distended thick walled bladder (*B*); the dilated posterior urethra (*U*); and hydronephrotic, dysplastic kidney (*arrowheads*)

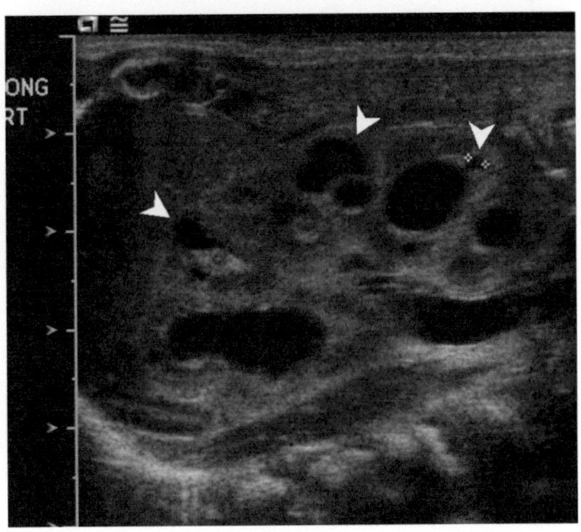

Fig. 8.35 Longitudinal US image of the right kidney in patient with PUV showing hydroureteronephrosis with abnormal increased echogenicity, loss of normal cortico-medullary differentiation of the renal parenchyma, and associated cortical cysts (*arrowheads*) consistent with renal dysplasia

hypoplasia and absence of the vas deferens or the VATER sequence of abnormalities. Associated ipsilateral adrenal agenesis is seen in 8–10 % of cases.

Imaging usually shows an empty renal fossa with compensatory hypertrophy of the contralateral kidney and no ectopic kidney elsewhere in the abdomen or pelvis on renal US; on radiography, one may see the colonic flexure occupying the expected location of the renal fossa on the side of the absent kidney, and at radionuclide imaging there will be no activity on the side of

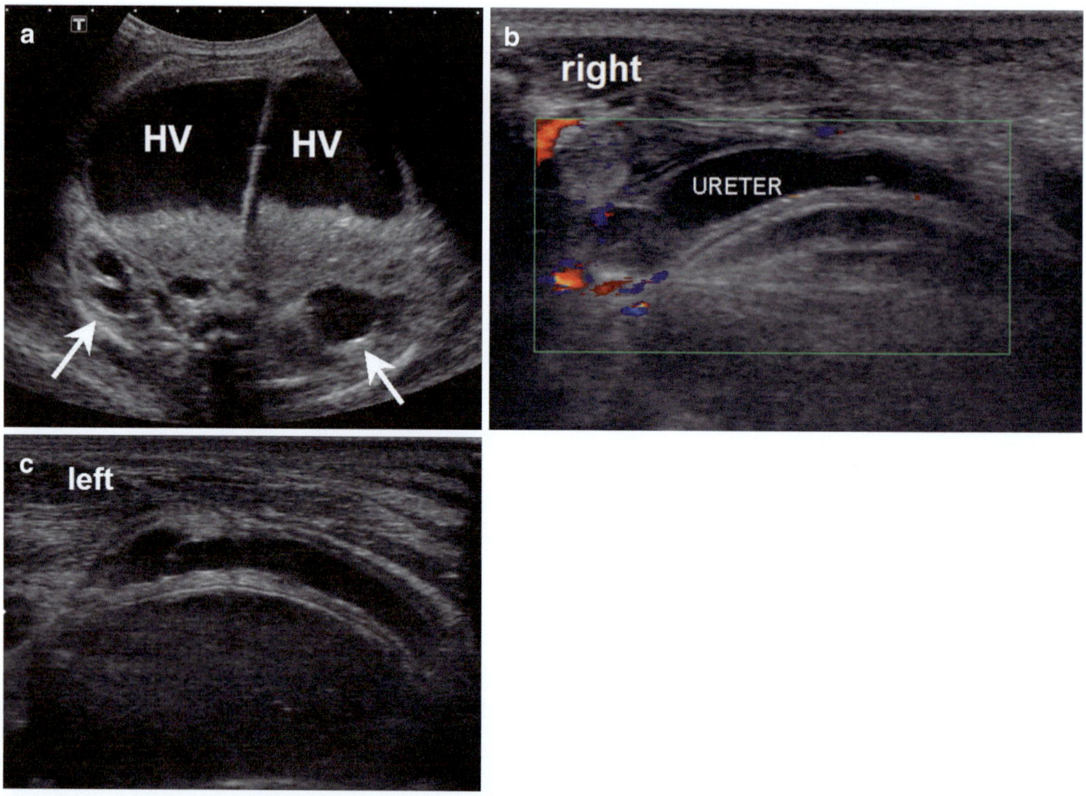

Fig. 8.36 (**a**) Transverse pelvic US of a newborn girl with a single perineal opening, and abdominal distention shows dilated fluid and debris filled hemivaginas (*HV*), also called hydrocolpos as well as associated bilateral moderate to severe pelvocaliectasis (*arrows*). (**b**, **c**) Longitudinal US images showing bilateral hydroureter which is caused by the dilated vagina compressing the ureters at the bladder trigone causing bilateral hydroureteronephrosis. This condition is treated simply by draining the dilated vagina(s)

agenesis (Fig. 8.43). As above, one may discover dilation of the ipsilateral ureter, hypoplasia of the ipsilateral seminal vesicle/uterine horn, or absence of the ipsilateral vas deferens. As in other renal abnormalities, there may be vesicoureteral reflux of the remaining solitary contralateral kidney; if there is hydronephrosis or hydroureter of the remaining renal unit, a cystogram should be considered to exclude vesicoureteral reflux.

8.6 Urinary Tract Infection (UTI)

Infection of the urinary tract can involve the lower urinary tract or the upper urinary tract [13]. Infection of the lower urinary tract usually involves the urethra or urinary bladder and is associated with dysuria, pyuria, and bacteriuria. Lower UTI is rarely associated with fever or other systemic symptoms. Conversely, infection of the upper urinary tract usually involves the renal pelvis or renal parenchyma and is associated with systemic symptoms such as fever, nausea, vomiting, an increase in WBC, and back pain. The goal of imaging in UTI is to detect anatomic abnormalities which predispose a child to UTI. Typically, the diagnosis of pyelonephritis is obvious clinically, and imaging the kidney to confirm the diagnosis is not necessary. In some instances, when pyelonephritis is suspected clinically but not confirmed clinically, an imaging test such as DMSA renal scan (Fig. 8.44) or MRI (Fig. 8.45) can be helpful to guide further work-up. Color Doppler US (Fig. 8.46) can sometimes make the diagnosis, but is not as sensitive as DMSA or MRI. Sometimes, computed tomography (CT) with intravenous (IV) contrast is performed for other reasons in older children and findings of pyelonephritis are seen. CT with IV contrast has similar sensitivity for detecting pyelonephritis as

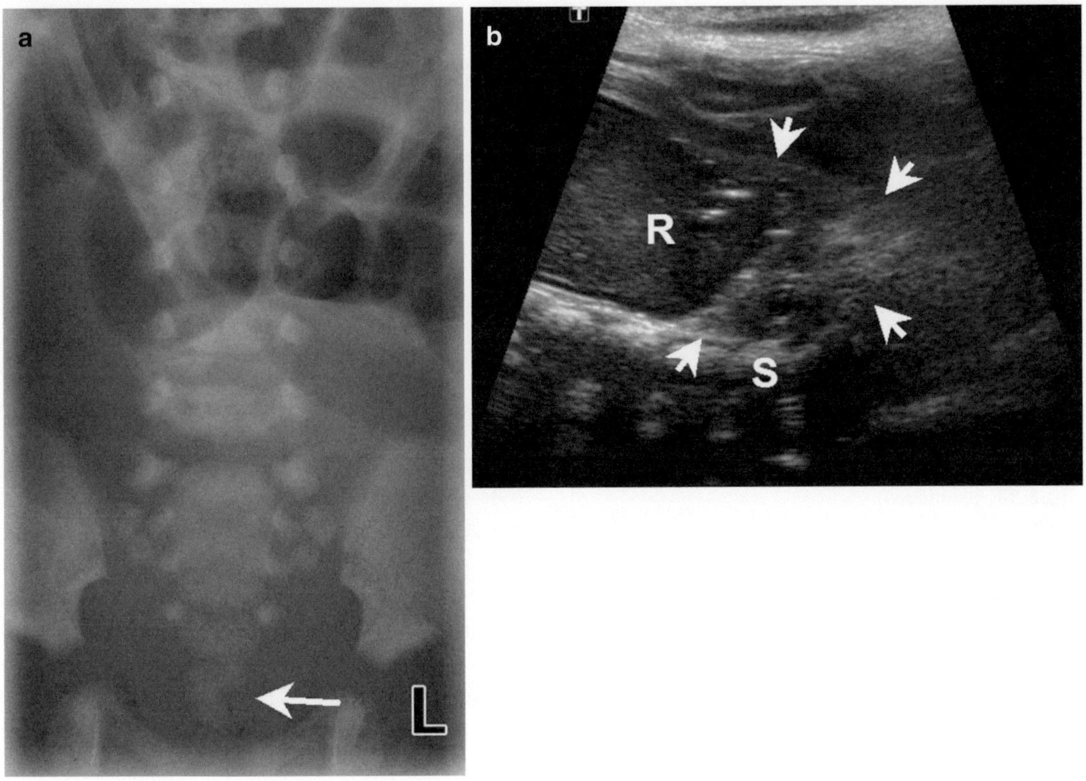

Fig. 8.37 (**a**) Frontal view of the lumbosacral spine in a neonate with distal bowel obstruction and imperforated anus shows a defect of the left fifth sacral segment (*arrow*) called a scimitar- or hemi-sacrum which, according to Currarino's triad, is highly associated with a presacral mass (*L*) indicates left side of paitent. (**b**) Longitudinal midline US of the pelvis in the same patient shows a solid and cystic mixed echogenicity mass (*arrows*) which is immediately anterior to the last sacral segment (*S*). At the time of anoplasty for imperforate anus, a benign sacral teratoma was resected. If undiscovered, this benign mass has the potential of becoming malignant later in life; (*R*) bladder dilated reatel pouch

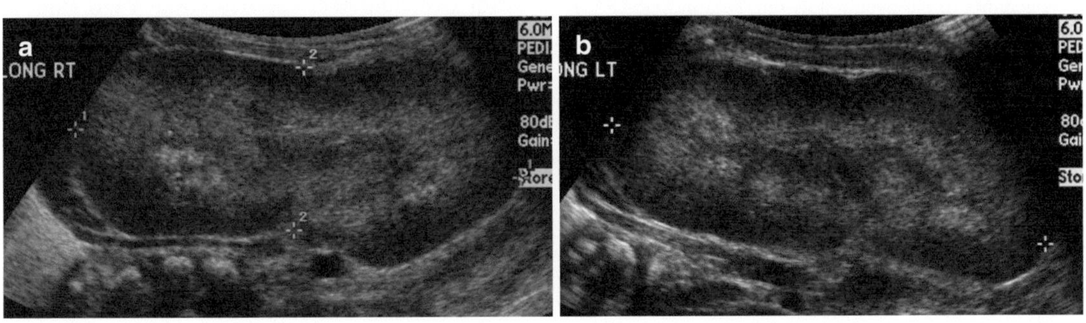

Fig. 8.38 (**a**, **b**) Longitudinal US images of the enlarged right and left kidney characterized by diffuse increased echogenicity, poor corticomedullary differentiation, and lack of contour-deforming abnormality. (**c**) Longitudinal US image of same kidney with higher-frequency linear transducer shows linear low echogenicity tubular structures radiating from the medulla to the cortex representing the dilated collecting ducts which are characteristic of ARPKD

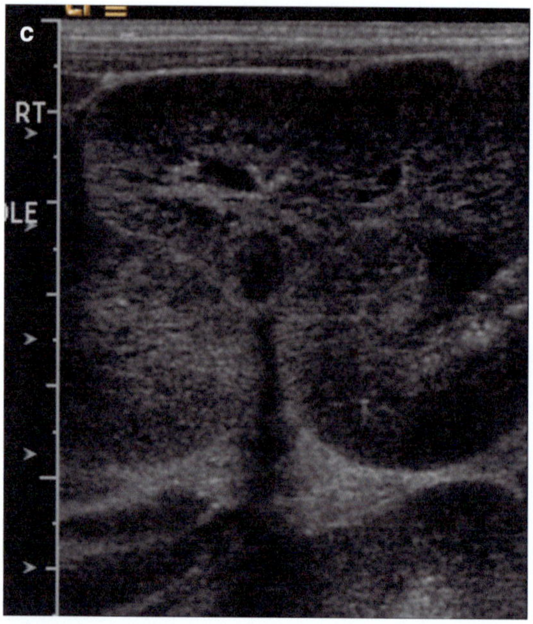

Fig. 8.38 (continued)

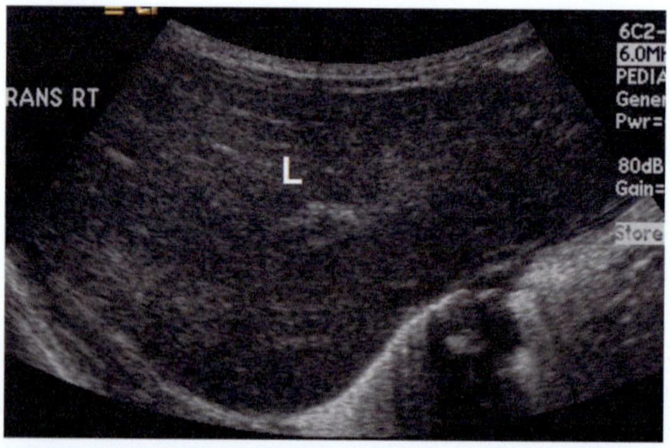

Fig. 8.39 Transverse US image of the liver (*L*) in this child with ARPKD showing diffusely heterogeneous echogenicity of the liver, not an uncommon finding since the abnormality of ciliary function of the renal tubule is also expressed in the biliary tubules but usually manifests later, in childhood rather than in the neonatal period

DMSA and MRI but at the cost of radiation exposure and is not utilized specifically for this indication in neonates.

A renal and bladder US can be performed at any time after the diagnosis of UTI is made and in most instances is normal. About 4 % of the time [3], an underlying anatomic renal anomaly is detected such as hydronephrosis (with or without hydroureter), a duplication anomaly with upper pole hydronephrosis with or without an ectopic ureterocele, bilateral hydronephrosis and bladder wall thickening in a male with posterior urethral valves, etc. In a female age 2 months to 2 years with a febrile UTI but no anatomic abnormalities and no findings to suggest pyelonephritis or renal scarring, no further work-up is suggested until a second febrile infection occurs, according to the current AAP guidelines for the management of UTI in children [15]. This is a change from the previous guidelines which recommended a cystogram after the first episode of UTI in the same age group [2]. A cystogram can diagnose vesicoureteral reflux (VUR). There are several types of cystogram. Voiding cystourethrography (VCUG) is an excellent test for detecting VUR and, if present, can characterize the ureterovesical junctions, the caliber of the ureters, the exact grade of reflux, the presence or absence of intrarenal reflux, the presence of duplication anomalies, and abnormalities of the urethra, anatomic details that are not usually detected by the direct or indirect radionuclide cystogram. Radionuclide cystography is performed similarly to the VCUG but characteristically shows the VUR with less anatomic detail but has been shown by several investigators to be more sensitive than VCUG in the diagnosis

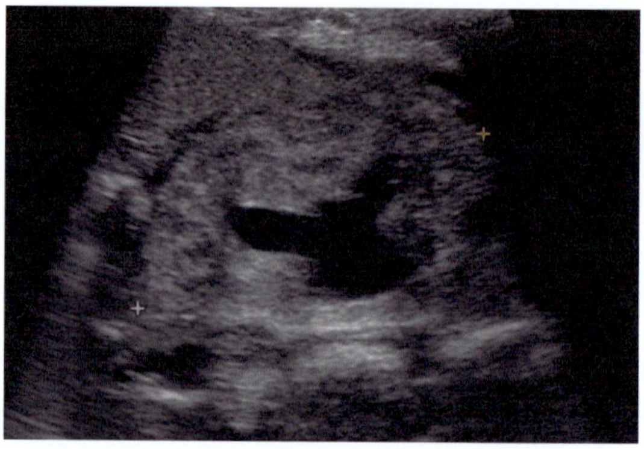

Fig. 8.40 Longitudinal US image of a small, echogenic left kidney in a newborn showing moderate hydronephrosis and poor corticomedullary differentiation of the renal parenchyma consistent with renal dysplasia, probably due to urinary obstruction in utero

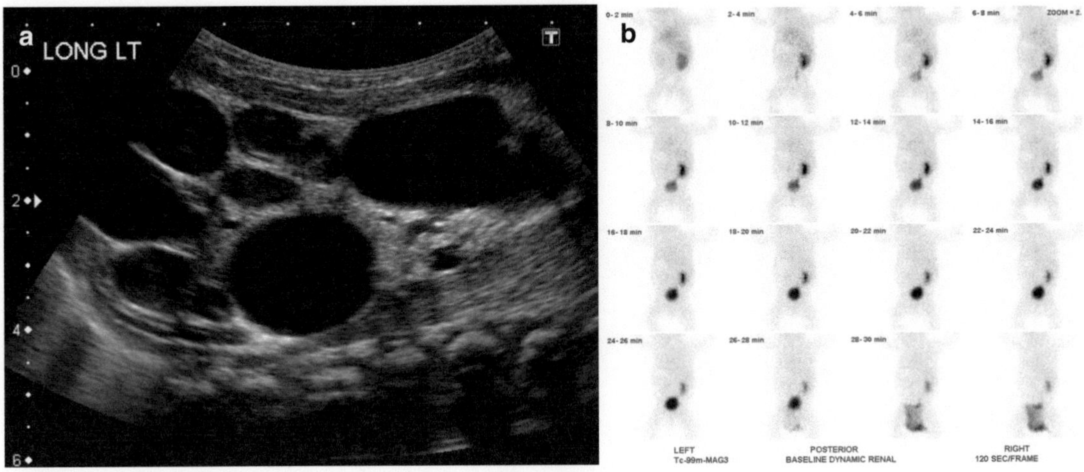

Fig. 8.41 (**a**) Longitudinal US image of the left kidney shows multiple thin-walled cysts of different size that do not communicate without normal intervening parenchyma consistent with MCDK. (**b**) An MAG3 nuclear medicine renogram in same patient shows no activity in the left renal fossa, supporting the diagnosis of MCDK

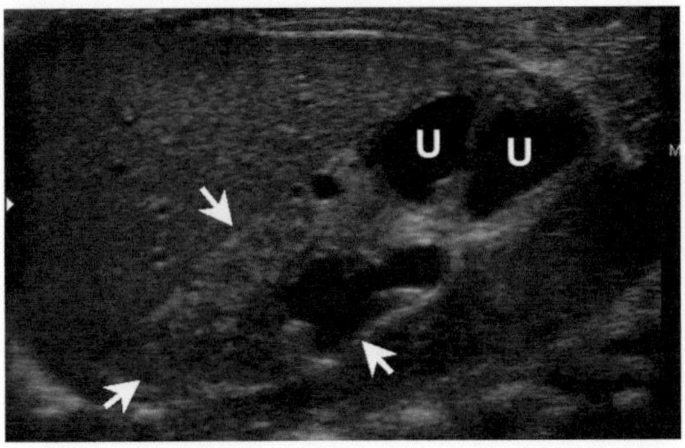

Fig. 8.42 Longitudinal US image showing a small dysplastic right kidney (*arrows*) demonstrating increased echogenicaly and cystic change with severe hydroureter (U) which was due to severe VUR discovered by VCUG in the neonatal period; (*U*) Ureter

of VUR. Cystosonography with intravesical contrast agents, performed outside the United States, especially in Europe, is a promising modality to detect VUR and characterize the anatomic details similar to VCUG but without the radiation dose risks. Note that ultrasound contrast agents are not yet FDA approved for pediatric use in the United States. This modality will most likely replace many VCUGs in the initial detection of VUR in girls, follow-up VUR in boys and girls, and in siblings of patients with VUR who are at higher than normal risk (50 vs 1–2 %) of having VUR.

8.7 Hypertension

Neonatal hypertension can be seen in various situations in the modern neonatal intensive care unit (NICU). It is especially common in neonates who have undergone umbilical artery catheterization, due to the increased risk of thromboembolism involving the aorta, the renal arteries, or both. However, most cases of neonatal hypertension are renal in origin, either renovascular such as renal vein thrombosis (RVT) or fibromuscular dysplasia; or due to mechanical compression of the renal arteries by tumors, hydronephrosis, or other masses; or due to parenchymal renal disease such as autosomal dominant or recessive polycystic renal disease, unilateral MCDK, UPJ obstruction, severe acute tubular necrosis, interstitial nephritis, cortical necrosis, or rarely by hemolytic uremic syndrome. Other causes include cardiac (aortic stenosis), endocrine (congenital adrenal hyperplasia, hyperaldosteronism, hyperthyroidism), and pulmonary disease. Neonatal hypertension is particularly common in premature infants with chronic lung disease of prematurity, patent ductus arteriosus, and intraventricular hemorrhage. In addition, there is a direct correlation between severity of illness in

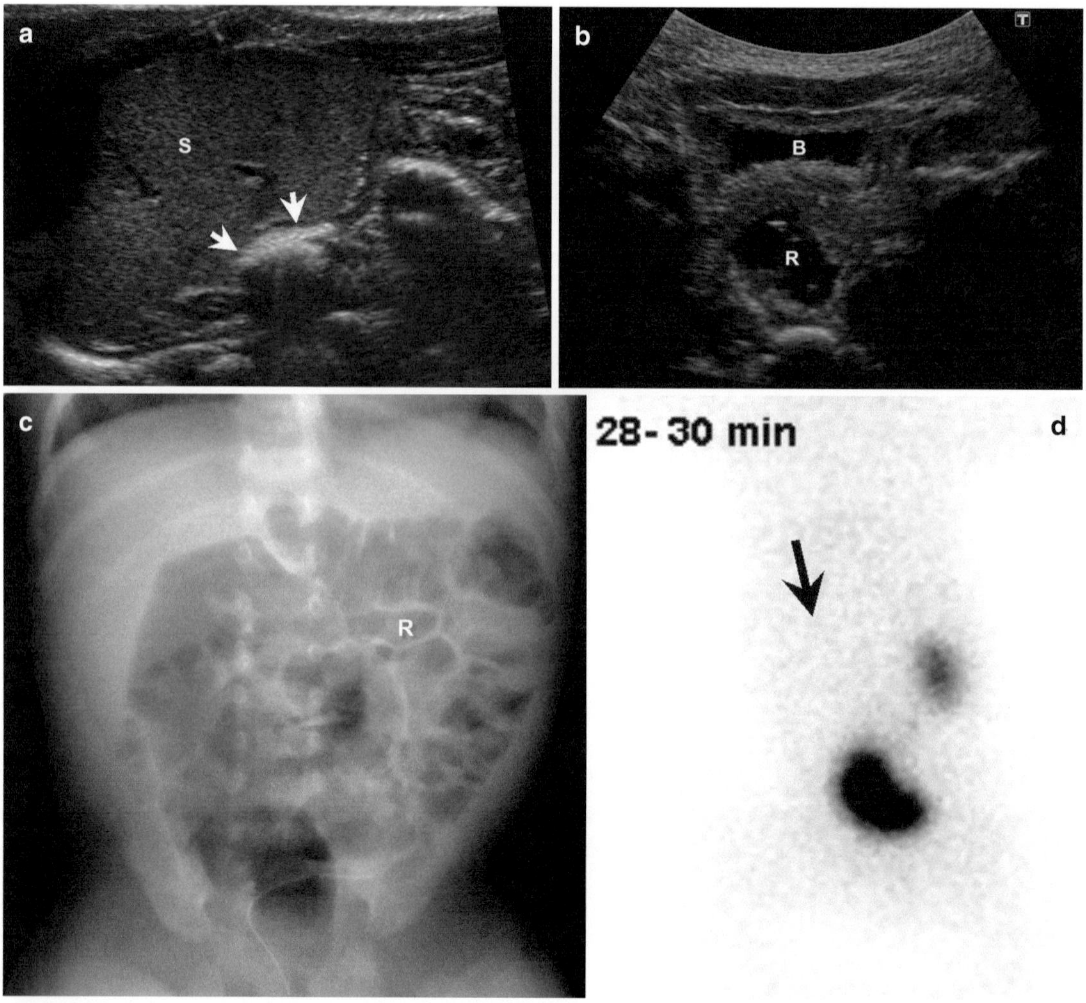

Fig. 8.43 Longitudinal US image of the left renal fossa (**a**) shows no renal tissue adjacent to the spleen (*S*), and instead, echogenic bowel gas (*arrows*) from the splenic flexus of the color is in its place, a known radiologic sign of renal agenesis. Transverse US image of the pelvis (**b**) shows the bladder (*B*) and rectum (*R*), but no evidence of renal ectopia. (**c**) AP scout image of the abdomen from a VCUG shows the splenic flexure occupying the renal fossa (*R*), and (**d**) NM MAG3 renal scan shows activity in a solitary right kidney, ruling out an ectopic position and confirming agenesis of the left kidney with no activity in the left renal fossa (*arrow*)

the NICU and development of neonatal hypertension; the more critically ill infants are at higher risk of developing hypertension.

Diagnosis of neonatal hypertension is made by blood pressure measurement. Etiologic work-up includes plasma renin activity and other laboratory evaluation. Imaging studies usually include a chest x-ray in patients who show signs of congestive heart failure or who have a heart murmur on physical exam. A renal ultrasound with Doppler is performed on all neonates with hypertension to help reveal possible correctable causes of hypertension such as RVT (Fig. 8.47), aortic or renal vein thrombi, congenital anatomic renal anomalies, neonatal abdominal masses (Fig. 8.48), or congenital parenchymal disease resulting from in utero insult, often resulting in a small dysplastic kidney (Fig. 8.49). Rarely, in neonates with severe blood pressure elevation, angiography via the umbilical artery catheter or by tradition femoral approach may be required to diagnose fibromuscular dysplasia that may be due to intrarenal renal artery branch abnormalities. CT and MR angiography do not offer sufficient resolution in

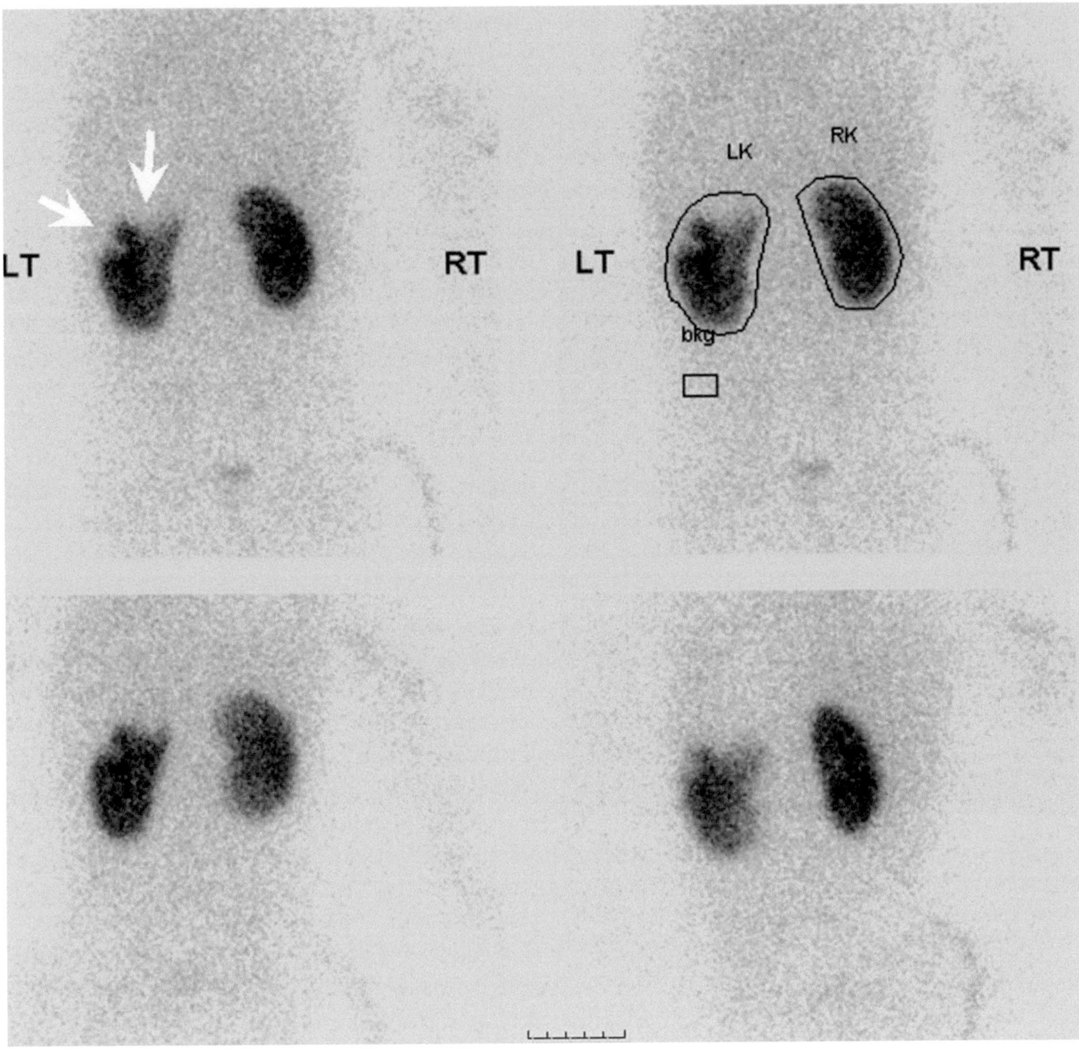

Fig. 8.44 Image from DMSA renal cortical scintigraphy shows a large defect of the upper pole and smaller wedge-shaped defect in the mid-pole (*arrows*) of the left kidney. In this patient with recent febrile UTI, this is consistent with focal pyelonephritis of the left kidney

the neonate, but can be helpful in the older, larger infants [10]. Nuclear scanning may demonstrate abnormalities of renal perfusion although obtaining diagnostic studies is sometimes difficult because of immature renal function.

8.8 Urinary Tract Neoplasms

The most common neonatal urinary tract neoplasm is mesoblastic nephroma, which has a variable behavior pattern and prognosis from fairly benign to malignant. The most aggressive form behaves like congenital fibrosarcoma. Chromosomal analysis can differentiate the benign from the aggressive forms. On imaging, these different varieties cannot be reliably distinguished, mandating surgical resection of these tumors. Other renal neoplasms that can present in the neonate include nephroblastomatosis (persistent renal blastema or nephrogenic rests), the very rare neonatal Wilms' tumor (especially in a patient with nephroblastomatosis), and, rarely, a malignant tumor such as a rhabdoid tumor, ossified renal tumor, or clear cell sarcoma of infancy [4].

Prenatal or postnatal US is the first line of imaging for renal masses. Once discovered, MRI is the best imaging modality to evaluate the extent of disease, involvement of surrounding structures, and for evaluation of spread to lymph nodes or solid organs of the abdomen. CT of the abdomen in the neonate offers less soft tissue differentiation and resolution and is not preferred over MRI. CT of the chest is utilized to evaluate for metastatic disease to the lungs.

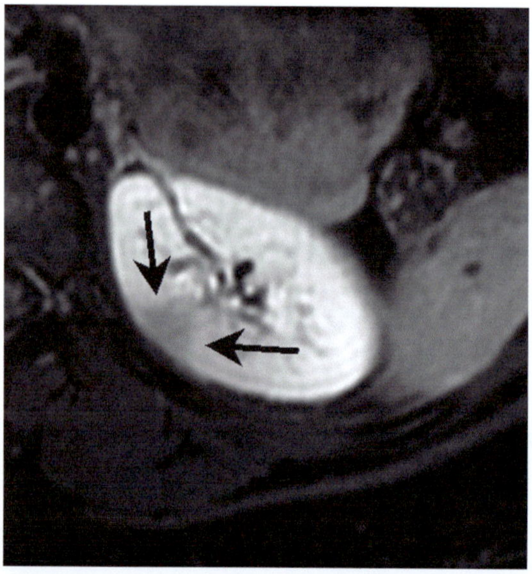

Fig. 8.45 Axial T1-weighted image of the left kidney after intravenous contrast administration with fat saturation shows a focal wedge-shaped region of poor perfusion of the posteromedial cortex (*arrows*) extending through the medulla in this patient with positive urine culture, consistent with a region of acute pyelonephritis

On US, mesoblastic nephroma typically appears as a large mass which often involves the renal sinus and usually is solid and vascular but may contain cystic regions and heterogeneous echogenicity due to areas of hemorrhage or necrosis (Fig. 8.50). The more aggressive forms may be larger with more cystic areas. On MRI, the mass appears similarly, low signal on T1, higher on T2, with variable enhancement (Fig. 8.51). There is often local infiltration of the perinephric tissues on imaging studies.

Nephroblastomatosis may have a variable appearance at imaging. On US, the first-line imaging modality, the kidney may be enlarged with a thick peripheral rind of low echogenicity or may be diffusely hypoechoic with poor corticomedullary differentiation (Fig. 8.52a). Alternatively, the kidney may have a number of homogeneously sized or variably sized hypoechoic nodules scattered in the cortex or medulla. On MRI, the preferred next imaging test, the abnormal renal blastema usually appears low intensity on T1- and T2-weighted images (Fig. 8.52b). If CT is performed, the

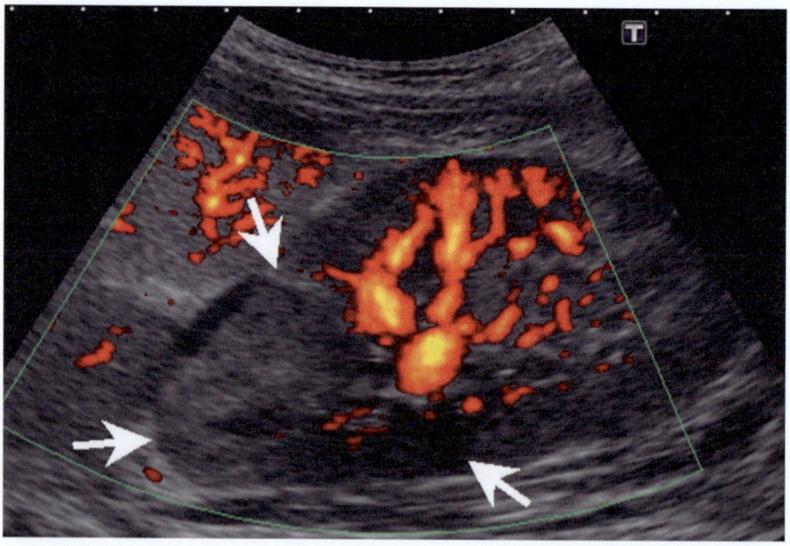

Fig. 8.46 Longitudinal color power Doppler US image of the left kidney showing a large region of absent perfusion involving most of the upper pole (*arrows*) in a patient being treated for febrile UTI, consistent with acute pyelonephritis

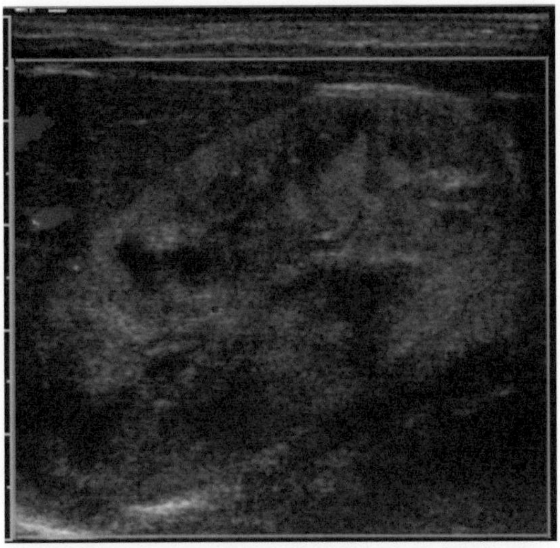

Fig. 8.47 Longitudinal color Doppler US image of the right kidney demonstrates heterogeneous echogenicity, loss of corticomedullary differentiation, and no significant blood flow and measured two times the volume of the normal left kidney, in this 1-day-old patient with documented inferior vena cava thrombus and right renal vein thrombosis

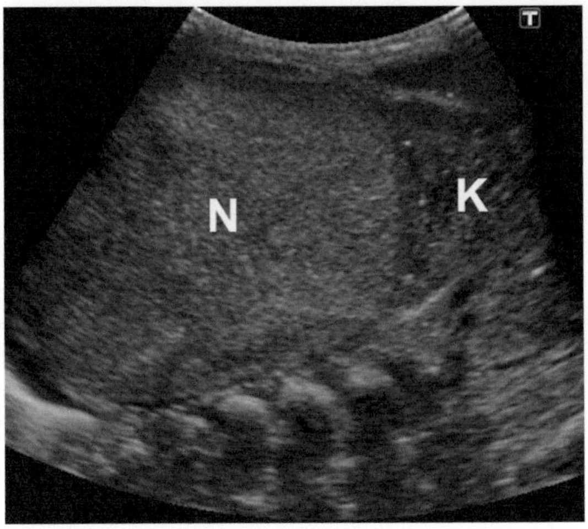

Fig. 8.48 Longitudinal US image of the large left neuroblastoma (*N*) in the left suprarenal region which is displacing the left kidney (*K*) inferiorly, and on other images, showed a stretched, compressed left renal vein, placing it at risk for thrombosis

nephrogenic rests appear as low-attenuation nodules or diffuse attenuation rind in contrast to the adjacent normally enhancing renal tissue. The key to diagnosing nephroblastomatosis is

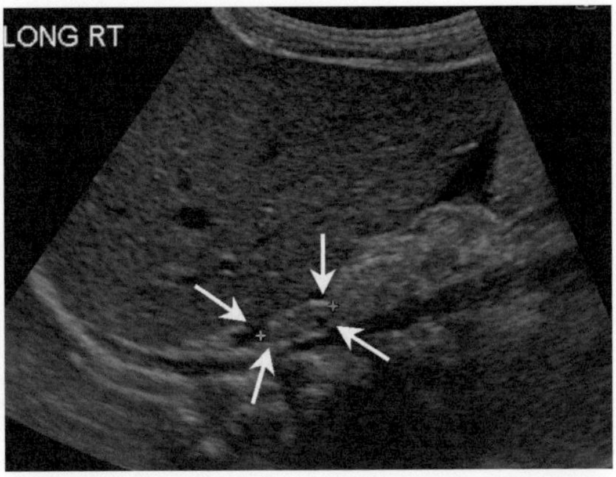

Fig. 8.49 Longitudinal US image of the small echogenic right kidney (*arrows*) in a patient with history of neonatal insult and refractory hypertension

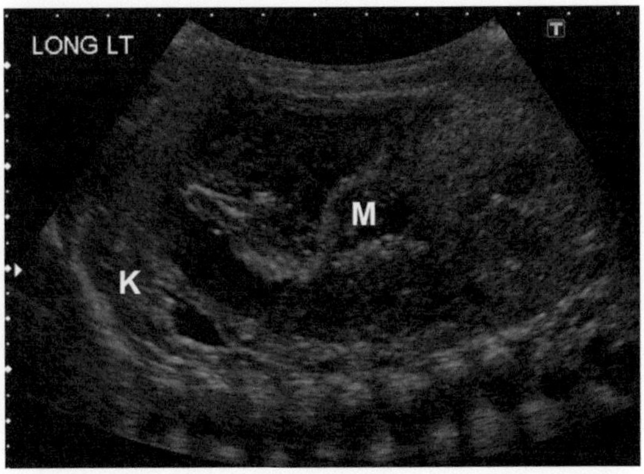

Fig. 8.50 Longitudinal US image of the left kidney showing a large mixed echogenicity mass (*M*) of the left kidney, sparing a narrow rind of normal appearing kidney (*K*) in the upper pole

the lack of enhancement on contrast-enhanced CT or MRI.

Wilms' tumor may arise in areas of nephrogenic rests, and therefore, it is these patients with nephroblastomatosis that are at higher risk of developing Wilms' tumor, which is a very rare occurrence in the neonate. Often, neonatal Wilms' tumor cannot be differentiated from mesoblastic nephroma. However, if there are areas of nephroblastomatosis in the ipsilateral or contralateral kidney, neonatal Wilms' tumor should be suspected. On US, the mass usually has heterogeneous echogenicity (Fig. 8.53a), and examination of the renal vein and inferior vena

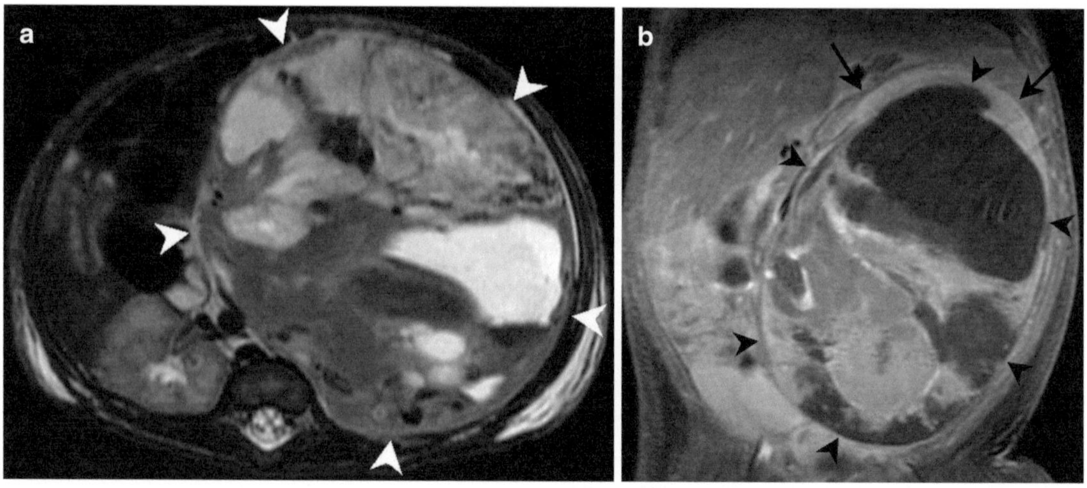

Fig. 8.51 Axial T2 (**a**) and coronal T1 with IV contrast (**b**) MR images of the same patient as Fig. 8.50 showing the mixed solid and cystic, heterogeneous signal intensity mass (*white arrowheads, a, black arrowheads, b*) centered in the left kidney. There is a small rind of normal renal signal in the upper pole (*arrows* in **b**). MR is more sensitive than US for detecting subtle abnormalities in the contralateral kidney, adenopathy, or distant metastases in other solid abdominal organs if they are present

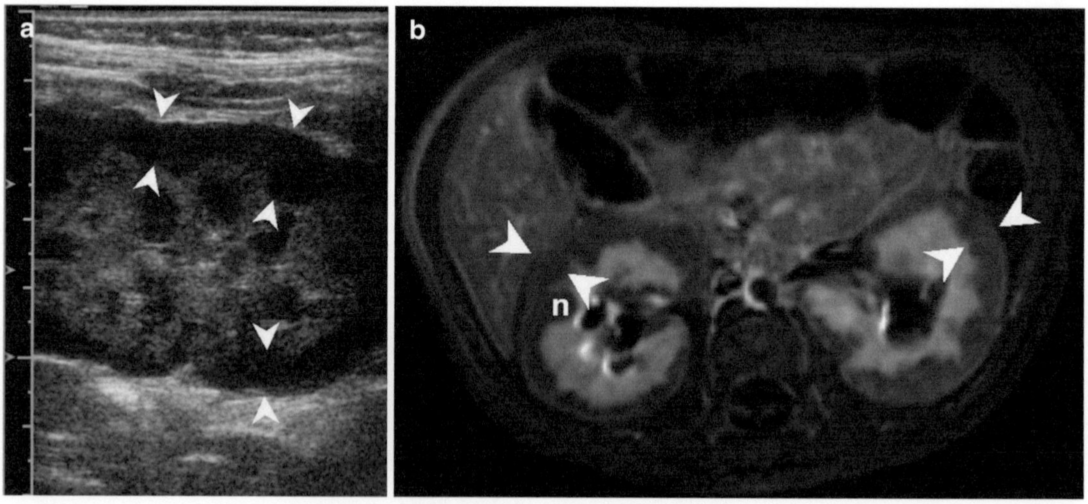

Fig. 8.52 (**a**) Longitudinal US image of the kidney shows a peripheral rind of low echogenicity surrounding the entire cortex (*arrowheads*) consistent with primitive renal blastema of nephroblastomatosis. (**b**) Axial T1-weighted MR image after IV contrast administration in the same patient showing similar findings as the US, non-enhancing, low signal intensity in the peripheral aspect of the cortex of both kidneys (*arrowheads*) representing nephroblastomatosis. Some areas may be quite nodular (*n*). Wilms' tumor has been found to develop in many patients with nephroblastomatosis and development of a larger mass-like lesion in these patients is highly suspicious for malignancy. Close interval follow-up imaging in these patients is recommended

cava (IVC) is critical to assess for tumor extension which could alter the surgical approach. Wilms' tumor has a propensity for intravascular extension and tumor thrombus. On MRI, not only can one visualize the predominantly low-intensity T1 and high-intensity T2 mass, but one

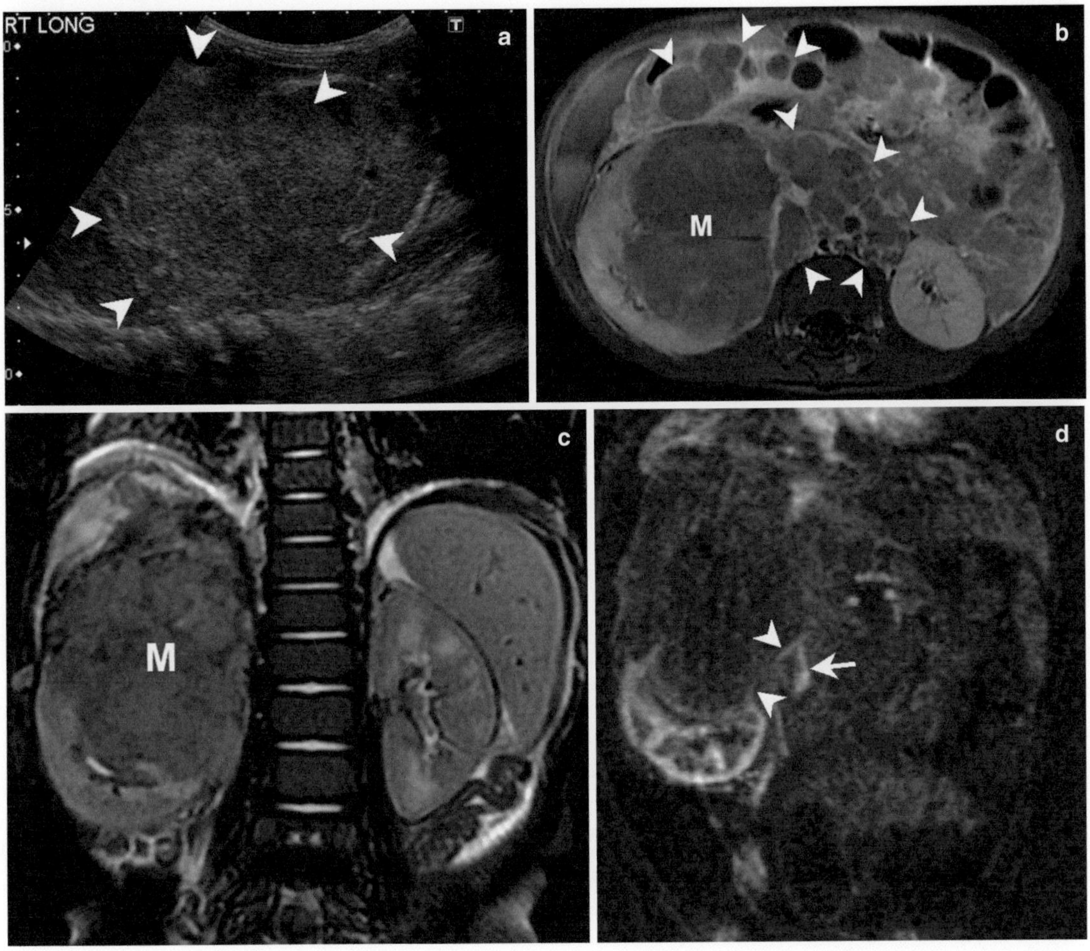

Fig. 8.53 (**a**) Longitudinal image from US of the right kidney showing a heterogeneous echogenicity, solid mass centered in the mid-pole of the right kidney (*arrowheads*), with some normal appearing renal parenchyma at the upper and lower aspects of the kidney. Axial (**b**) and coronal (**c**) T1-weighted MR images with IV contrast enhancement in same patient show large, heterogeneously low-signal-intensity solid mass (*M*) of the right kidney with extensive retroperitoneal and mesenteric adenopathy (*arrowheads*). (**d**) Coronal MR image showing patent but displaced IVC (*arrow*) and renal vein (*arrowheads*)

can assess local infiltration, nodal extent, renal vein and IVC involvement, and metastatic disease to other abdominal organs and visualized bones, especially with the use of IV contrast (Fig. 8.53b–d). CT is sometimes utilized to image a renal lesion due to the rapid acquisition of images, the ability to image the chest for metastatic disease at the same time, and this modality is usually more widely available; however, it exposes the neonate to ionizing radiation, and the resolution of soft tissues is less than an optimally performed MRI [9].

References

1. Avni F, Gare C, Cassart M et al (2012) Imaging and classification of congenital cystic renal disease. AJR Am J Roentgenol 198:1004–1013
2. Committee on Quality Improvement, Subcommittee on Urinary Tract Infection (1999) Practice parameter: the

diagnosis, treatment, and evaluation of the initial urinary tract infection in febrile infants and young children. Pediatrics 103:843–852
3. Gelfand M, Barr L, Abunku O (2000) The initial renal ultrasound examination in children with urinary tract infection: the prevalence of dilated uropathy has decreased. Pediatr Radiol 30(10):665–670
4. Isaacs H (2008) Fetal and neonatal renal tumors. J Pediatr Surg 43:1587–1595
5. Kraus S (2001) Genitourinary imaging in children. Pediatr Clin N Am 48:1381–1424
6. Levitt M, Pena A (2005) Pitfalls in the management of newborn cloacas. Pediatr Surg Int 21:264–269
7. Mishra A (2007) Renal agenesis: report of an interesting case. Br J Radiol 80:e167–e169
8. Riccabona M, Avni F, Blickman J et al (2009) Imaging recommendations in paediatric uroradiology. Pediatr Radiol 39:891–898
9. Riccabona M, Avni F, Dacher J et al (2010) ESPR Uroradiology task force and ESUR paediatric working group: imaging and procedural recommendations in paediatric uroradiology, Part III. Minutes of the ESPR uroradiology task force minisymposium on intravenous urography, uro-CT and MR-urography in childhood. Pediatr Radiol 40:1315–1320
10. Riccabona M, Lobo M, Papadopoulou F et al (2011) ESPR uroradiology task force and ESUR paediatric working group: imaging recommendations in paediatricUroradiology, Part IV. Minutes of the ESPR uroradiology task force mini-symposium on imaging in childhood renal hypertension and imaging of renal trauma in children. Pediatr Radiol 41: 030–944
11. Ringer S (2010) Hydronephrosis in the fetus and neonate: causes, management, and outcome. NeoReviews. http://neoreviews.aappublications.org/content/11/5/e236. Accessed 10 Feb 2012
12. Schoellnast H, Lindbichler F, Riccabona M (2004) Sonographic diagnosis of urethral anomalies in infants: value of perineal sonography. J Ultrasound Med 23:769–776
13. Shortliffe L (2011) Chapter 116: Infection and inflammation of the pediatric urinary tract. In: Wein J et al (eds) Campbell-Walsh urology, 10th edn. Saunders, Philadelphia
14. Shulkin B, Mandell G, Cooper J et al (2008) Procedure guideline for diuretic renography in children 3.0. J Nucl Med Technol 36(3):162–168
15. Subcommittee on Urinary Tract Infection and Steering Committee on Quality Improvement and Management (2011) Urinary tract infection: clinical practice guideline for the diagnosis and management of the initial UTI in febrile infants and children 2 to 24 months. Pediatrics. http://pediatrics.aappublications.org/content/early/2011/08/24/peds.2011-1330
16. Van Den Bosch C, Van Wijk J, Beckers G et al (2010) Urological and nephrological findings of renal ectopia. J Urol 183:1574–1578

Neonatal Urinary Tract Infection

9

Vimal Chadha and Uri S. Alon

Case Vignette

A 10-day-old male infant born to G1P1 mother at 35 weeks gestation (birth weight 1.93 kg) by cesarean section for non-reassuring heart tones is transferred from an outside hospital for the management of suspected sepsis. He had been inpatient at the outside facility for the management of hyperbilirubinemia and issues related with feeding. On the day of transfer, he had developed temperature instability and abdominal distension that was tender to touch. He had not been circumcised yet.

Initial laboratory evaluation revealed: hemoglobin 11.4 g/dL, WBC count 9,000, and platelet count 54,000/mm^3. Serum chemistries revealed normal electrolytes and creatinine of 0.4 mg/dL. Spinal tap resulted in clear CSF under normal pressure, 14 cells/mm^3 (22 % neutrophils), and normal protein and glucose levels; CSF culture remained sterile. Urinalysis revealed 2+ leukocyte esterase, negative nitrite, and 50–100 WBC and few bacterial rods per HPF. Blood culture and urine culture both grew *E. coli*. He was diagnosed with urosepsis and treated with IV cefepime for 21 days.

Imaging studies: Renal and bladder ultrasound revealed normal right kidney measuring 4.6 cm; left kidney measured 5.6 cm and showed moderate left hydroureteronephrosis (Fig. 9.1). Voiding cystourethrogram (VCUG) showed left grade IV VUR (Fig. 9.2). Initial ^{99m}Tc-DMSA scan revealed normal right kidney and multiple photopenic areas in the left kidney that were consistent with acute pyelonephritis (Fig. 9.3 Panel a). Four months later repeat ^{99m}Tc-DMSA scan showed persistence of photopenic areas on the left side suggesting scarring of the left kidney (Fig. 9.3 Panel b).

Following completion of his initial antibiotic therapy, he was prescribed continuous prophylactic antibiotic therapy, initially cephalexin (10 mg/kg/dose twice daily) that was later changed to nitrofurantoin (2 mg/kg once daily), when he was 4 months old. At age 11 months, he developed another episode of urosepsis and his urine and blood culture grew *Klebsiella pneumonia*. The bacterium was resistant to both nitrofurantoin and sulfamethoxazole/trimethoprim. He was hospitalized and treated with intravenous ceftriaxone.

V. Chadha, MD (✉) • U.S. Alon, MD
Department of Pediatric Nephrology, The Children's Mercy Hospitals and Clinics, University of Missouri at Kansas City School of Medicine, 2401 Gillham Road, Kansas City, MO 64108, USA
e-mail: vchadha@cmh.edu; ualon@cmh.edu

A.S. Chishti et al. (eds.), *Kidney and Urinary Tract Diseases in the Newborn*,
DOI 10.1007/978-3-642-39988-6_9, © Springer-Verlag Berlin Heidelberg 2014

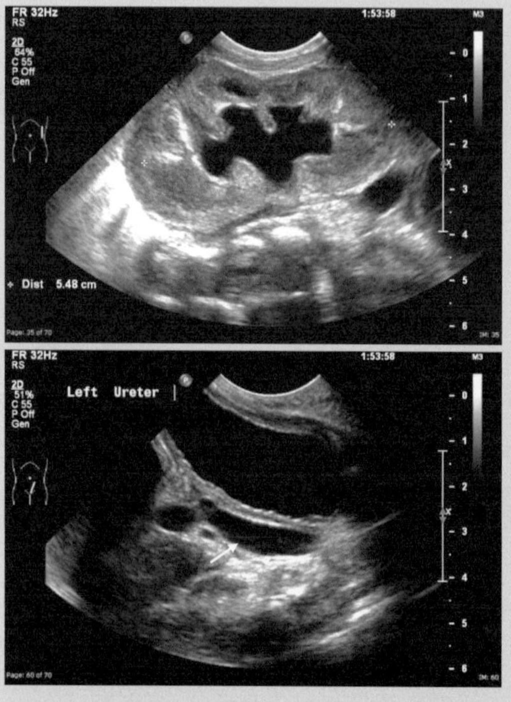

Fig. 9.1 Renal ultrasound of the patient described in the case vignette showing moderate hydronephrosis of left kidney (*upper panel*) and dilated left ureter (*arrow*) in the lower panel

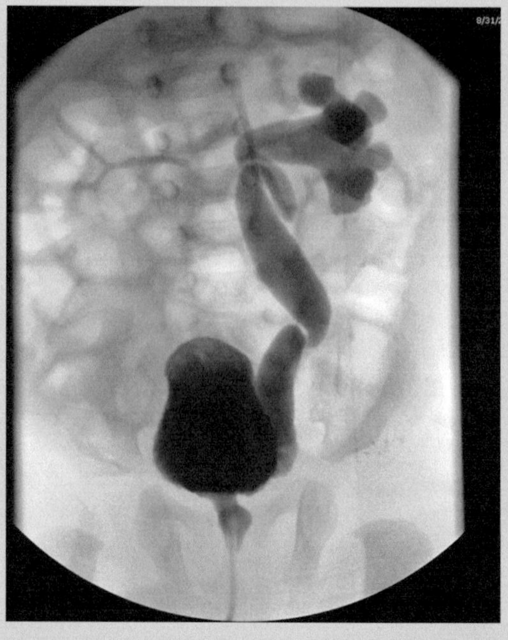

Fig. 9.2 VCUG of the patient described in the case vignette showing grade IV VUR on the left side

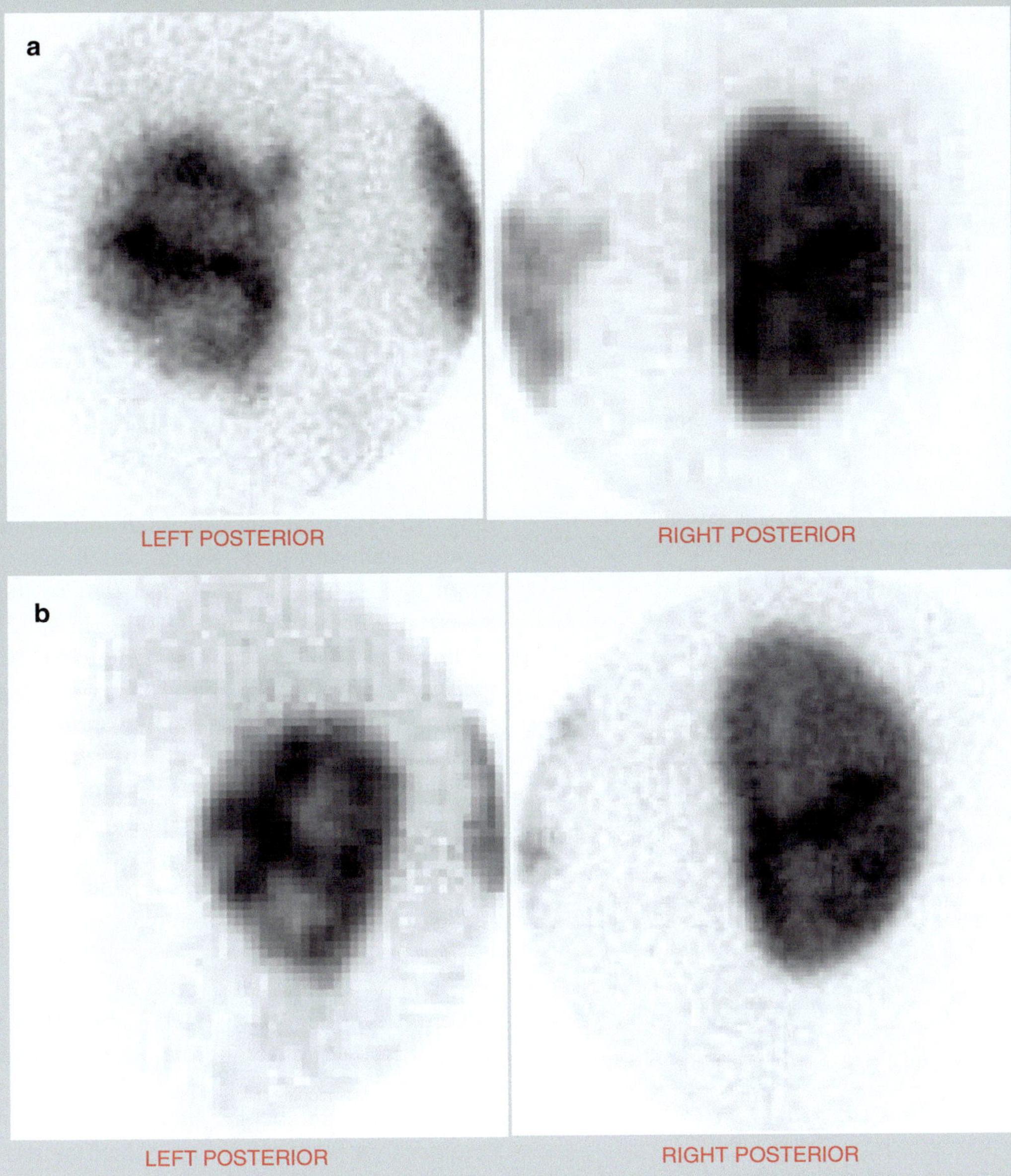

Fig. 9.3 ^{99m}Tc-DMSA scan of the patient described in the case vignette: (Panel **a**) at the time of admission showing multiple photopenic areas in left kidney consistent with acute pyelonephritis, and (Panel **b**) 4 months later there were no changes seen in the radiotracer uptake on the left side suggesting chronic renal damage (scarring). Split renal function was 72 % on right and 28 % on left side. It should however be noted that the possibility of left renal dysplasia associated with high-grade reflux on that side cannot be ruled out

Core Messages

- Initial episodes of urinary tract infection occur more commonly in infancy than at any other age, male newborns are at higher risk, and even more so those who are uncircumcised.
- In young infants, fever is the only consistent symptom/sign of UTI and most of the UTIs are diagnosed during sepsis evaluation.
- Even infants with another source of fever may still have UTI.
- Urine specimen for culture should be obtained by either bladder catheterization or suprapubic aspiration.
- Associated bacteremia is common but likely does not alter the outcome.
- Total duration of therapy is 10–14 days and can be completed in part with oral antibiotics as outpatient.
- Widespread application of prenatal ultrasonography has reduced the prevalence of previously unsuspected obstructive uropathy in infants.
- The need to obtain VCUG and the role of prophylactic antimicrobial therapy after initial febrile UTI is being increasingly questioned, thus influencing the way we manage UTI, especially in infants older than 2 months of age.

9.1 Introduction

Urinary tract infection (UTI) is one of the most common bacterial illnesses in febrile infants younger than 60 days of age. It usually involves the upper urinary tract (pyelonephritis) and delay in therapy can lead to permanent renal damage. During early infancy, UTI is more common in boys, and uncircumcised males have the highest rates of UTI. The male-to-female ratio starts reversing by 4–6 months of age, and by 1 year of age, UTI is three times more common in girls than in boys. In febrile young infants, the diagnosis of UTI is made during sepsis evaluation as there are no specific symptoms or signs of UTI at this age. All febrile newborns <29 days of age and ill appearing 29–60 days old, undergoing sepsis evaluation (that must include urinalysis and culture), are hospitalized and treated with intravenous antibiotics until completion of sepsis work-up. Those with uncomplicated UTI are treated for 10–14 days and part of therapy can be completed with oral antibiotics as outpatient.

Over the last decade the management of children with a febrile UTI has become quite controversial. Conventionally, all children following an episode of UTI were investigated using renal ultrasound and voiding cystourethrogram (VCUG), aiming to identify renal anomalies, obstructive uropathy, and vesicoureteral reflux (VUR). Children with VUR of any grade were treated with prophylactic antibiotics, and surgical intervention was considered in those cases with breakthrough infections in spite of prophylactic treatment. This paradigm has been questioned in recent years by many investigators. Firstly, the widespread application of prenatal ultrasonography has clearly reduced the prevalence of previously unsuspected obstructive uropathy in infants; accordingly the yield of actionable findings revealed by renal-bladder ultrasound (RBUS) is relatively low (1–2 %) [2, 23, 25, 69]. Secondly, the most recent studies do not support the use of antimicrobial prophylaxis to prevent febrile recurrent UTI in infants without VUR or with grades I to IV VUR, thereby questioning the need for obtaining routine VCUG after the first UTI [10, 17, 37, 42, 48]. Accordingly, the American Academy of Pediatrics (AAP) recently published the newly revised guidelines on diagnosis and management of initial UTI in febrile infants and children 2–24 months of age [9]. It should be noted that the guidelines excluded infants <2 months of age, because of special considerations in this age group that may limit application of evidence derived from the studies focused on 2- to 24-month-old children. While the information in this chapter is mainly focused on infants <2 months, the material form of new AAP guidelines and other studies in older infants has been incorporated where appropriate.

9.2 Epidemiology

Initial episodes of urinary tract infection occur more commonly in infancy than at any other age [26, 66]. Infants with UTI typically present in the second week after birth, as UTI is an unusual occurrence during the first 3 days after birth [63]. In febrile infants, the reported prevalence of UTI has ranged from 4.1 to 9 % [5, 11, 47, 71]. In a recent meta-analysis of 14 articles that reported prevalence of UTI in febrile infants <24 months of age, the pooled prevalence of UTI was 7.0 % (CI: 5.5–8.4 %) [54]. The variability in prevalence is likely attributable to differences among studies in age, sex, and race of subjects; methods of urine collection; and criteria for the diagnosis of UTI. When analyzed for effects of gender and age, the meta-analysis found that prevalence rates were highest among uncircumcised male infants <3 months of age and females <12 months of age [54]. Four studies that reported UTI prevalence by race found that UTI rates were higher among white infants at 8.0 % (CI: 5.1–11.0) than among black infants 4.7 % (CI: 2.1–7.3) [54]. Among infants aged ≤2 months undergoing sepsis evaluation, the 4.6 % prevalence of UTI was fairly similar to 5.9 % in infants aged >2 months in whom UTI was suspected because there was no other source of fever. However, febrile infants with no apparent source of fever were twice (7.5 %) as likely to have UTI compared to those (3.5 %) with a possible source of fever such as otitis media [22]. Nevertheless the important lesson here is that even in infants suspected or found to have another source of fever, UTI may still coexist.

As mentioned before, in the first 6 months of life, more boys than girls present with UTIs and the incidence is greater in uncircumcised boys [68, 71]. Zorc et al. [71] reported on the clinical and demographic factors associated with UTI in febrile (≥38.0 °C) infants ≤60 days of age using a prospective multicenter cohort from eight pediatric emergency departments during consecutive bronchiolitis seasons. Overall, 9 % of the 1,025 infants were diagnosed with UTI and uncircumcised male infants had the highest rate (21 %), compared with females (5 %) and circumcised males (2.3 %). The odds ratio of UTI being associated with uncircumcised state was 10.4 (95 % CI 4.7–31.4).

9.3 Pathophysiology

UTI has multifactorial etiologies and represents an altered balance between the host and the pathogen (*vide infra*). As in many other diseases, biological susceptibility plays an important role in the cause of neonatal UTIs as, for instance, Lewis blood group negative children have higher incidence of UTI. Abnormal genitourinary anatomy can contribute to and complicate the clinical course of UTI. While hematogenous spread of bacteria to the urinary tract can occur, it is rare, and most UTIs start in the urinary bladder and then ascend to produce pyelonephritis. The ascent of infection to the upper tract can take place via two major mechanisms: (1) bacterial adherence properties that help them migrate upstream and (2) the presence of VUR that showers the renal pelvis with infected urine, thus allowing seeding of the renal parenchyma. If inflammation of renal parenchyma is not treated promptly, it can lead to tissue damage resulting in renal scarring.

9.3.1 Predisposing Host Factors

9.3.1.1 Vesicoureteral Reflux

The previously accepted concept that VUR is almost always the key factor in acquired renal injury secondary to a urinary tract infection is no longer accepted. This is based on the fact that less than half of the children who incur renal damage secondary to pyelonephritis have VUR; conversely, reflux itself does not cause UTI as many children with VUR diagnosed as part of evaluation of prenatally detected hydronephrosis never develop UTI. However, infants with VUR who get UTI are more likely to get pyelonephritis, and in the presence of VUR, less virulent bacteria can gain access to the upper urinary tract [34]. Furthermore, the risk of renal damage in children with high-grade VUR (grades III to V) is 4–6 times greater than the risk in those with grade

I or II VUR and 8–10 times greater than the risk in those without VUR [29]. The relationship of VUR with UTI and renal damage has become more complex with the realization that some kidneys with high-grade reflux have elements of dysplasia and scarring even before any infection has been documented. In many of these cases, the parenchymal damage took place already in utero.

9.3.1.2 Innate Immunity

Despite its proximity to fecal flora, the urinary tract, with the exception of urethral meatus, is usually sterile. The precise mechanism by which the urinary tract maintains sterility is not well understood. A recent study has shown that ribonuclease 7 (RNase 7) is a novel antimicrobial peptide that is expressed in the human urinary tract and plays an important role in the innate immunity of the human uroepithelium [59]. Further studies are needed to see if alteration of this innate immunity plays a part in recurrence and severity of UTIs in certain individuals.

9.3.2 Agent Virulence

The most common bacteria infecting the urinary tract are usually *Escherichia coli*. The bacterial fimbriae mediate adherence to epithelial cells of the urinary tract and also cause agglutination of P-type red blood cells. Both these properties are important for bacterial virulence. The red blood cell agglutination can be blocked by sugars like mannose; therefore, mannose-resistant *E. coli* are more virulent than those that are mannose sensitive and predominate as pyelonephritogenic strains. Mannose resistance is mediated by P-fimbriae that recognizes specific carbohydrate receptors (Gal1–4 Gal) on the uroepithelium and can cause ascending infection in the absence of VUR [34]. K antigen is a capsular polysaccharide covering bacteria that shields them from phagocytosis and exists in greater quantities in pyelonephritogenic strains. Plos et al. [44] documented that children with UTI carry P-fimbriated *E. coli* in their fecal flora more often than healthy controls both at diagnosis (86 % vs. 29 %) and during infection-free intervals. The fecal carriage of P-fimbriated *E. coli* was also higher in children who were P-1 blood group positive (88 %) than those with P-2 blood group (40 %).

9.4 Microbiology

As in older children, the most common bacteria causing UTI in infants are Gram-negative bacteria belonging to the family Enterobacteriaceae, with *E. coli* being the most common pathogen. Other Gram-negative bacteria that are responsible for UTI include *Klebsiella*, *Enterobacter*, *Citrobacter*, *Proteus*, *Pseudomonas*, and *Serratia* species. Infection with Gram-positive organisms is less common and *Enterococcus* is the most common Gram-positive organisms isolated. Organisms such as *Lactobacillus* spp, micrococcus, diphtheroids, coagulase-negative staphylococci, and *Corynebacterium* spp are usually not considered clinically relevant isolates for otherwise healthy, 2- to 24-month-old children. The spectrum of the causative bacteria is usually similar regardless of whether or not the child has VUR [40].

9.5 Clinical Presentation

Symptoms of a febrile UTI are very nonspecific, particularly in young infants. Apart from fever, which is consistently present in infants with UTI, other nonspecific symptoms and signs such as vomiting, diarrhea, irritability, poor feeding, and jaundice, singly or in combination, may be present but cannot accurately predict the presence of UTI. Some authors recommend that UTI should always be included in the differential diagnosis of fever during the first year of life, even when a source of fever is unequivocal.

9.5.1 Focal Bacterial Nephritis

Focal bacterial nephritis also known as acute lobar nephronia affects one or more of the renal lobules and is an uncommon presentation of UTI [30, 62].

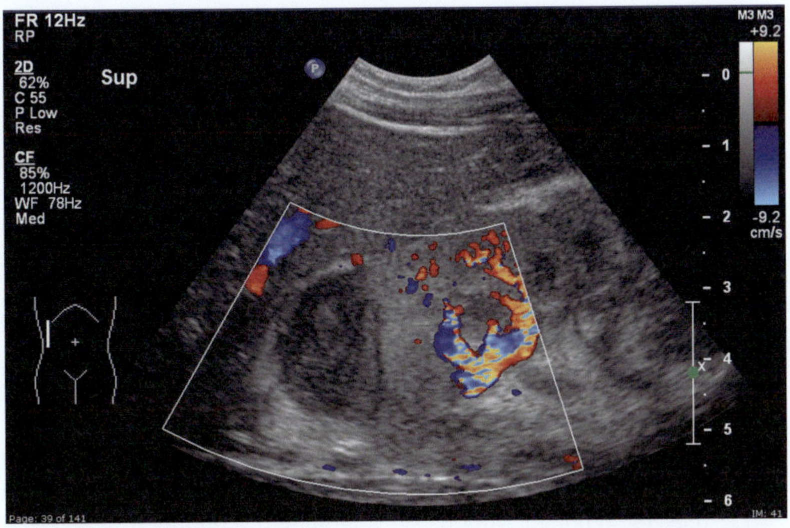

Fig. 9.4 Renal abscess: this 3-month-old infant presented with high-grade fever of 1 day duration. Urinalysis was positive for leukocyte esterase and nitrites. Urine culture grew *Citrobacter freundii* (>10,000 CFU per mL); blood culture no growth. Renal ultrasound performed 2 days later revealed abscess in the superior pole of right kidney

These patients may not have any pyuria. The diagnosis is suspected on imaging studies such as renal ultrasound (Fig. 9.4) and can be confirmed by computerized tomography in doubtful cases.

9.6 Diagnosis

Urine culture from an appropriately collected urine specimen is the most important diagnostic test to establish the diagnosis of UTI. The results of urinalysis (dipstick and microscopic examination) are helpful but cannot substitute urine culture to document the presence of UTI. The physician managing young febrile infants must ensure that a urine specimen is obtained for both culture and urinalysis before treatment with an antimicrobial agent is initiated. The importance of this cannot be overemphasized, as a study conducted almost 20 years ago found that over half of the 1,600 pediatricians, family practitioners, and emergency medicine physicians surveyed reported that they would treat a highly febrile 4-month-old infant with an antibiotic without first obtaining a urine culture specimen [27]. It is the authors' impression though that nowadays many more physicians, taking care of febrile infants, do obtain a urine culture before antimicrobial treatment is started.

9.6.1 Urine Collection Methods

The most common method of urine collection in older children and adults "midstream clean catch" is not practical in young infants, and bagged specimens are frequently contaminated with very high false-positive culture rates. Namely, a urine specimen obtained by urine bag is an acceptable method to rule out an infection but often an inadequate one to positively diagnose one. Therefore, and in order not to delay the start of antimicrobial treatment, bladder catheterization is the procedure of choice to collect urine for culture in febrile young infants. Less commonly, and especially in the newborn with urethral and other anatomic abnormalities of the external genitalia, suprapubic aspiration is indicated (*vide infra*).

9.6.1.1 Suprapubic Aspiration

Suprapubic aspiration of the bladder is the most reliable technique to identify bacteriuria that is uncontaminated by perineal flora. The technique is relatively simple and safe in young infants as urinary bladder is an abdominal organ at this age and not covered by peritoneum. The procedure should be performed in infants who have not voided in at least the hour prior to procedure and have a full bladder as assessed by palpation or percussion. One has to be very gentle during this examination as stimulation can initiate voiding. The suprapubic area is cleaned with an antiseptic solution, and a 1.5-inch, 22-gauge needle attached to a syringe is inserted perpendicular to the abdominal wall, approximately one centimeter above the pubic symphysis, and advanced under negative pressure until urine sample is obtained. The procedure can stimulate urination in many infants resulting in high failure rate. Reported success rates for obtaining urine by suprapubic aspiration have ranged from 23 to 90 % [12, 32, 45], with better results when the procedure is performed under ultrasonographic guidance [6, 19].

Despite its reported simplicity, suprapubic aspiration is associated with more pain than bladder catheterization and complications can happen [14, 31]. Minor complications such as microscopic hematuria are common, while major complications such as gross hematuria, intestinal perforation, and abdominal wall abscess are rare. As a result, suprapubic aspiration is rarely practiced outside the neonatal intensive care unit and is becoming a lost art. However, there may be no acceptable alternative to suprapubic aspiration in certain situations such as abnormalities of the external genitalia and urethra.

9.6.1.2 Bladder Catheterization

Transurethral bladder catheterization is a safe and effective method for obtaining urine samples for culture in most infants. The procedure is performed by observing all aseptic precautions. The infant is held with thighs in abducted (frog-leg) position. In uncircumcised boys the foreskin of the glans is retracted gently to permit complete visualization of the urethral meatus; the foreskin must be repositioned at the end of the procedure to prevent paraphimosis. The anterior urethra is cleansed thoroughly with povidone-iodine solution, and the penis is held perpendicular to the abdomen with the nondominant hand (which is henceforth considered contaminated) and gentle traction is applied to straighten the urethra. A 4- or 5-French catheter lubricated with sterile jelly is inserted through the urethral meatus with the dominant hand until urine returns. It is not uncommon to feel slight resistance as the catheter passes through the external bladder sphincter. This can be overcome by maintaining gentle pressure as the spasm will relax; the catheter should never be forced at this point. In female infants, the urethra may be difficult to visualize and an assistant is often needed to separate the labia majora. If the catheter is inadvertently placed in the vagina, it should be left in place to serve as a landmark for subsequent attempts.

The first few drops should be allowed to fall outside the sterile container, because they may be contaminated by bacteria in the distal urethra. Specimen contamination can occur in uncircumcised male infants and in female infants in whom the urethra is not well visualized and several attempts are required to pass the catheter.

9.6.1.3 Clean Voided Bag Specimens

While the noninvasiveness of this method of urine collection appeals to many physicians, nurses, and parents, this method should never be used for obtaining urine specimen for culture because of very high false-positive rates (*vide infra*). It should be noted that even if contamination from the perineal skin is minimized by cleansing, rinsing, and drying before application of the collection bag, there may be significant contamination from the vagina in girls or the prepuce in uncircumcised boys, the two groups at highest risk of UTI. Therefore, a "positive" culture result from a specimen collected in a bag cannot be used to document a UTI, and confirmation requires culture of a specimen collected through catheterization or suprapubic aspiration. Because there may be substantial delay in obtaining a second specimen, many clinicians prefer to obtain a definitive urine specimen through catheterization initially. However, if the clinician determines that the infant does not require immediate antimicrobial therapy, then often a urine collection bag affixed to the perineum can be used to collect urine specimen to rule out diagnosis of UTI by checking for leukocyte esterase and nitrites. To minimize the possibility of contamination, it is recommended that the mother checks on the bag every 10 min and that the bag is replaced by a new one every 30 min. As aforementioned, in essence a negative culture rules out a UTI whereas a positive one requires further confirmation.

9.6.2 Urinalysis

Because urine culture results are not available for at least 24 h, there is considerable interest in other urine tests that may be helpful in diagnosing those children who might have UTI thus enabling initiation of presumptive therapy. In contrast to urine specimen collected for culture, urinalysis can be performed on any specimen, including one collected from a bag applied to the perineum. However, the specimen must be fresh (<1 h after voiding with maintenance at room temperature or <4 h after voiding with refrigeration), to ensure sensitivity and specificity of the urinalysis. The tests that have received the most attention are biochemical analyses of leukocyte esterase and nitrite through a dipstick method and urine microscopic examination for white blood cells (WBCs) and bacteria.

9.6.2.1 Leukocyte Esterase

The test detects "esterase" (an enzyme released by white blood cells) and indicates presence of white blood cells in the urine (pyuria). Hoberman et al. [24] reported a sensitivity of 52.9 % in detecting the presence of ≥10 leukocytes/mm^3. The specificity of this test in general is low; therefore, positive leukocyte esterase by no means confirms the diagnosis of UTI.

9.6.2.2 Nitrites

Dietary nitrates are converted to nitrites by bacteria, and positive urinary nitrite test has very high specificity (98 %) in diagnosing UTI. However, a nitrite test is not a sensitive marker of UTI in children, particularly infants, who empty their bladders frequently as conversion from nitrates to nitrites usually requires ~4 h of reaction time. Furthermore, only Gram-negative bacteria convert nitrates to nitrites; therefore, negative nitrite test results have little value in ruling out UTI [21].

9.6.2.3 Microscopic Examination

The diagnostic accuracy and the interpretation of microscopic urinalysis are influenced by the preparation of the specimen (centrifuged vs. uncentrifuged) and the method of quantifying and reporting. Stamm [61], defined pyuria as the presence of ≥10 leukocytes/mm^3 in uncentrifuged urine. In young febrile children in whom urine specimen was obtained by catheterization, Hoberman et al. [24] showed that a count of <10 leukocytes/mm^3 was almost invariably associated with a sterile culture, whereas a count of ≥10 leukocytes/mm^3 had a sensitivity of 91 % and a low false-positive rate of 3.4 % in identifying urine culture results of ≥50,000 colony-forming units (CFUs) per ml. In urinary sediment from a centrifuged (10 mL at 2,000 rpm for 5 min) specimen, the usual threshold for significant pyuria is ≥5 WBCs per high-power field (~25 WBCs per μL). The absence of pyuria can help differentiate true UTI from asymptomatic bacteriuria in infants with concurrent febrile infection from another source.

9.6.3 Urine Culture

"Significant" bacteriuria in urine culture has been the sole gold standard for the diagnosis of UTI. However, limitations of urine culture include uncertainty concerning the magnitude of a "significant" bacterial colony count, and inability to differentiate asymptomatic bacteriuria from infection. Urine culture results are considered positive or negative on the basis of the number of CFUs that grow on the culture medium. Definition of significant colony counts with regard to the method of collection considers that the distal urethra and periurethral area are commonly colonized by the same bacteria that may cause UTI; therefore, a low colony count may be present in a specimen obtained through voiding or catheterization even when bacteria are not present in the bladder urine. On the other hand, asymptomatic bacteriuria (≥10^6 bacteria/L in urine specimens obtained by suprapubic aspiration) has been reported in 0.9 and 2.5 % of female and male infants, respectively [65]. In majority of these infants, the bacteriuria is spontaneously cleared in a few months [64]. The concept that >100,000 CFUs per mL indicates a UTI was based on morning collections of urine from adult women, with comparison of specimens from women without symptoms and women considered clinically to have pyelonephritis; while the former had bacterial counts <10,000 CFUs per mL, women with pyelonephritis had ≥100,000 CFUs per mL with only 1 % of the women having bacterial counts between 10,000 and 100,000 CFUs per mL [28]. It is important to realize that definitions of positive and negative culture results are operational and not absolute. The time the urine resides in the bladder (bladder incubation time) is an important determinant of the magnitude of the colony count. Accordingly, in most instances, an appropriate threshold to consider bacteriuria "significant" in infants and children is the presence of at least 50,000 CFUs per mL of a single urinary pathogen in specimen obtained by catheterization [24]. For specimens collected by suprapubic aspiration, usually >1,000 CFU per mL of bacterial count is considered significant. As mentioned before, cultures of urine specimens collected in a bag applied to the perineum have an unacceptably high false-positive rate and are valid only when they yield negative results.

For urine culture results to be reliable, urine specimens should be processed as expeditiously as possible. If the specimen is not processed promptly, then it should be refrigerated to prevent the growth of organisms that can occur in urine at room temperature; for the same reason, specimens that require transportation to another site for processing should be transported on ice.

9.6.4 Blood Culture and Spinal Tap

In comparison to older children, UTI in infants is more commonly associated with bacteremia, occurring in 4–22.7 % of cases. Presence of bacteremia is inversely related to age and is usually limited to those <6 months old, and these patients are more likely to have abnormal RBUS and VCUG [4, 13, 43]. While blood culture is routinely obtained in all infants <29 days old as a part of sepsis evaluation, it should also be obtained in older infants who appear ill at initial examination. Presence of bacteremia might require prolonged intravenous antibiotic therapy but usually there are no adverse consequences in terms of outcome. In infants <3 months of age, the risk of coexisting bacterial meningitis with UTI is very low (<1 %) but sterile pleocytosis can be seen in up to 3 % of patients [52].

9.6.5 Miscellaneous Tests

The commonly obtained laboratory tests such as WBC count, C-reactive protein, and erythrocyte sedimentation rate (ESR) have not shown high degree of accuracy in confirming the diagnosis of acute pyelonephritis in young (<2 years old) febrile children with UTI [16]. Therefore, other special tests such as urine interleukin-1β and serum procalcitonin have been investigated and have shown promising results for early detection of acute pyelonephritis but currently remain a research tool [41, 55].

9.7 Management

9.7.1 Antibiotic Therapy

The goals of treatment of acute UTI are to eradicate the acute infection, to prevent complications, and to reduce the likelihood of renal damage. All febrile infants <29 days of age who usually undergo full sepsis evaluation (complete blood count with differential, blood culture, cerebrospinal fluid analysis with culture, and urinalysis with culture) are hospitalized, and treatment is initiated with broad-spectrum intravenous antibiotics such as ampicillin along with cefotaxime. It should be noted that bacterial susceptibility to antimicrobial agents is highly variable across geographic areas; therefore, initial therapy should be guided by local sensitivity patterns [18, 70]. Once the diagnosis of UTI is confirmed, the antibiotic is changed according to the culture results and treatment is continued for 10–14 days. While in the past, all newborns used to receive intravenous antibiotics for complete duration of therapy, currently, many of them are discharged home with PO antibiotic (usually cefixime) after variable length of inpatient intravenous therapy (Personal communication with Section of Infectious Diseases, Children's Mercy Hospital, Kansas City, MO; 2012). The majority of infants without any underlying genitourinary abnormality will become afebrile within 48–72 h of therapy [3]. The length of intravenous therapy and hospital stay is determined by the severity of illness, non-*E. coli* UTI (e.g., *Pseudomonas*), presence of bacteremia, obstructive genitourinary anomaly, abnormal kidney function, response to therapy, and questionable parental compliance.

Most experimental and clinical data support the concept that delays in the institution of appropriate treatment of pyelonephritis increase the risk of renal damage [58, 67]. For these reasons, all infants who have sustained a febrile UTI should have a urine specimen obtained at the onset of subsequent febrile illnesses, so that a UTI can be diagnosed and treated promptly.

Older infants (1–3 months old) with UTI who are well appearing at initial examination, have no history of genitourinary abnormalities or previous UTI, are not dehydrated, have no respiratory distress or concomitant acute disease, were born at term, and do not have congenital heart, lung, or metabolic disease are at very low risk of adverse events and can be treated with brief hospitalization or ambulatory intravenous antibiotics followed by oral therapy [49].

Whether given to neonates or older infants, when aminoglycosides are used, it is important to monitor their blood level and concomitant kidney function, thus avoiding or detecting in its early stage acute kidney injury that is not uncommon in this patient population.

9.7.2 Prophylactic Antibiotic Therapy

Over the last decade, the practice of using prophylactic antibiotics in patients with VUR to prevent recurrence of febrile UTIs has been challenged. A number of studies in recent years have failed to show their usefulness in children older than 24 months with VUR grades I to IV [10, 17, 37, 42, 48]. The AAP subcommittee that worked on the 2011 Clinical Practice Guidelines requested the raw data on 2- to 24-month-old infants from six researchers and their analysis on this group of 1,091 infants failed to detect any significant benefit of prophylactic antibiotics in infants with grades I–IV VUR [9]. Accordingly, both National Institute for Health and Care Excellence (NICE) [39] and current American Academy of Pediatrics (AAP) guidelines recommend that prophylactic antibiotic treatment should not be routinely used. However, these recommendations are not applicable for infants <2 months of age and those with grade V reflux. The results of the currently ongoing RIVUR (Randomized Intervention for Children with Vesicoureteral Reflux) study may put an end to this debate.

Currently, due to the high risk of UTI recurrence at a young age (*vide infra*), it is our practice to keep all newborns and young infants, who had a UTI, with or without the presence of VUR, on prophylaxis for 6 months. Until age 2 months, the infants receive cephalexin to be replaced then by sulfamethoxazole/trimethoprim. Due to the high rate of resistance of community *E. coli* to ampicillin, which in some places reaches 50 %, it is important to avoid using this drug as first-line prophylaxis [1].

9.7.3 Circumcision

Uncircumcised male infants <2 months old have one of the highest incidence of UTIs; the impact of uncircumcised state on risk of UTI decreases by 1 year of age. A meta-analysis conducted by Singh-Grewal et al. [56] that included 402,908 boys showed that circumcision was associated with a significantly reduced risk of UTI (OR = 0.13, 95 % CI 0.08–0.20, $p<0.001$). Because circumcision is not a benign procedure, these authors determined that the net clinical benefit of circumcision is likely only in boys at high risk of UTI such as those with posterior urethral valves or high-grade reflux. However, this assessment was critiqued by Schoen [50], who had earlier reported that newborn circumcision not only results in a 9.1-fold decrease in incidence of UTI during the first year of life but also markedly lowers the UTI-related costs and rate of hospital admissions, thus supporting newborn circumcision as a valuable preventive health measure, particularly in the first 3 months of life [51].

9.8 Imaging Studies

9.8.1 Ultrasound

The purpose of renal-bladder ultrasound (RBUS) is to detect anatomic abnormalities that might help in the management of current UTI and/or help plan further evaluation and long-term follow-up. In addition, RBUS also provides an evaluation of the renal parenchyma and an assessment of renal size that can be used to monitor renal growth. The widespread application of prenatal ultrasonography has clearly reduced the prevalence of previously unsuspected obstructive uropathy in infants and the yield of actionable findings is relatively low (1–2 %), thereby questioning the utility of RBUS in evaluation of the infant or child with a first febrile UTI [2, 23, 25, 69]. Furthermore, in the vast majority of those found to have an abnormal finding, no intervention was required. However the above studies did not pinpoint on the neonate population, and due to the possible association of UTI at this age with a missed congenital anomaly, the practice is still to obtain an ultrasound in neonates with UTI. Images of urinary bladder should always be included so as not to miss findings such as ureterocele or diverticulum (Fig. 9.5).

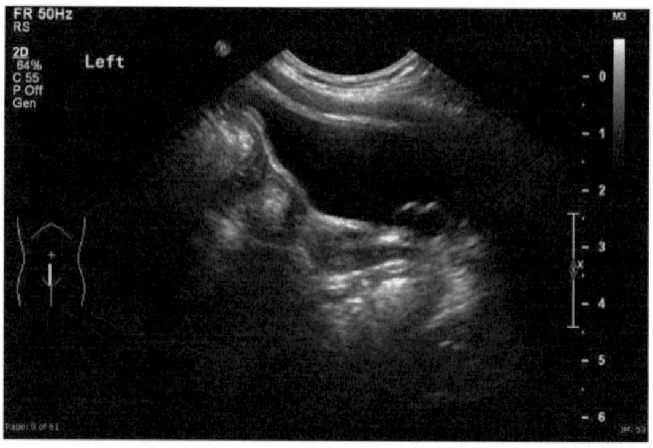

Fig. 9.5 Ureterocele: This 2-month-old female infant presented with fever. Urine culture grew *E. coli* (>10^5 CFU per mL). Renal and bladder ultrasound revealed left ureterocele (*arrow*) and hypoplastic left kidney (not shown). VCUG (not shown) revealed grade III VUR on right side

9.8.2 Voiding Cystourethrogram

The whole premise behind detecting VUR by VCUG is to prevent UTI recurrence (and renal damage) by prophylactic antibiotics or an antireflux procedure. Recent evidence has shown that VUR is neither necessary nor sufficient for the development of renal scarring, and many cases of scarring do occur in children without VUR. Furthermore, as the role of prophylactic antimicrobial therapy in preventing febrile UTI (and renal damage) in infants with grades I to IV VUR has become controversial, current AAP Clinical Practice Guidelines do not recommend obtaining VCUG routinely after the first UTI. The committee also concluded that the proportion of infants with grade V VUR among all infants with first febrile UTI is small (1 %) and these infants will likely show the abnormality on RBUS, prompting obtaining VCUG. Most nephrologists will usually obtain VCUG if renal and bladder ultrasound reveals significant hydronephrosis, solitary kidney, renal dysplasia or scarring, abnormal ureteral or bladder anatomy, suggestion of obstructive uropathy, and in other atypical or complex clinical circumstances. At the same time it is important to note that a normal ultrasound does not rule out the presence of VUR [57]. Because of the high prevalence of VUR in siblings (27.4 %) and offsprings (35.7 %) [57], VCUG may be indicated for infants with a family history of VUR. Although high-grade (IV–V) V VUR is less common [9, 38] than low-grade (I–III) VUR, identification of the former is important as it places these infants in high-risk category who are at greater risk of UTI recurrence and renal damage (Fig. 9.2). These infants should be closely monitored and investigated for UTI when they present with febrile illness.

9.8.3 Radionuclide Scintigraphy

Technetium-labeled dimercaptosuccinic acid (^{99m}Tc-DMSA) is taken up by the cells of the straight and convoluted parts of the proximal tubules and provides functional image of proximal renal tubular mass. Areas of inflammation, or those damaged by scarring, or areas with dysplasia are seen as focal defects associated with volume loss or contraction of the renal cortex (Fig. 9.3) [35]. A ^{99m}Tc-DMSA renal scan is highly sensitive in detecting the focal hypoperfusion and edema of acute inflammation (pyelonephritis) as well as subsequent scarring of inflamed parenchymal areas and is considered a "gold standard" for diagnosing pyelonephritis. This test is helpful in neonates and infants in whom the diagnosis is unclear based on the clinical findings. The findings on nuclear scans rarely affect acute clinical management and do not predict risk of future scarring; therefore, nuclear scanning is not recommended as part of routine evaluation of infants with their first febrile UTI. However, the ^{99m}Tc-DMSA scanning is useful in research, because it ensures that all subjects in a study have confirmed pyelonephritis to start with and it permits assessment of later renal scarring as an outcome measure.

9.8.4 Magnetic Resonance Urography

Magnetic resonance urography (MRU) is a relatively new technology that offers major advantages in evaluation of genitourinary abnormalities. It integrates exquisite anatomical information with a variety of functional data and avoids ionizing radiation and iodinated contrast agents [7]. Using DMSA scan as the reference standard, a gadolinium-enhanced T1 sequence MRU was found to have 100 % sensitivity and 78 % specificity for the detection of renal scarring [8]. In addition, MRU can distinguish among acute pyelonephritis (area of compromised perfusion with interstitial edema), renal scarring (parenchymal defect), and renal dysplasia [20]. However, at this point, its cost, limited availability, and need for patient sedation limit its widespread application.

9.9 Prognosis

9.9.1 Risk of Recurrence

A retrospective study from Finland revealed that roughly one-third of boys and girls who had their first episode of UTI under 1 year of age and were not receiving prophylactic antibiotics had recurrence of UTI over a follow-up period of 3 years; in 86 % of the cases the first recurrence occurred within 6 months of the primary UTI. The study excluded children with genitourinary abnormalities and none of the boys in this study were circumcised. It also found that the recurrence-free interval was shorter and recurrent UTIs occurred more often in children with grades III–V VUR than in those with grades I–II VUR (log rank test $p=0.0005$) [40].

9.9.2 Risk of Scarring and CKD

In a study conducted 25 years ago it was estimated that each episode of febrile UTI can lead to a 5 % risk of new renal scar formation and risk of scarring increases with number of recurrences [26]. It is generally believed that the risk of renal parenchymal damage from UTI as manifested by subsequent renal scarring is strongly related to age at the time of UTI, being highest in infancy and declining markedly with age [46]. Several studies have reported an increased risk of scarring with delayed and inadequate treatment [15, 36, 67]. Hoberman et al. [23] reported on renal scan findings in 309 children (1–24 months old); 61 % of the children had findings compatible with acute pyelonephritis and renal scarring was noted in 9.5 % of the 89 % children who had repeat scans. The degree of VUR was significantly associated with a higher incidence of renal scarring ($p=0.007$). Similarly, Montini et al. [38], reported changes of pyelonephritis on initial DMSA scans in 54 % of 300 children ≤2 years of age with scarring developing in 15 % of cases on repeat DMSA scans. A recently published meta-analysis of 33 articles that included 4,891 children (0–18 years old) revealed that 57 % (CI: 50–64) of children with first UTI had changes consistent with acute pyelonephritis on the acute-phase DMSA renal scan and 15 % (CI: 11–18) had evidence of renal scarring on the follow-up DMSA scan, 5–24 months after an initial episode of UTI. Children with VUR were significantly more likely to develop pyelonephritis (RR, 1.5; CI, 1.1–1.9) and renal scarring (RR, 2.6; CI 1.7–3.9) compared with children with no VUR. Furthermore, children with VUR grades III or higher were more likely to develop scarring than children with lower grades of VUR (RR, 2.1; CI, 1.4–3.2) [53]. On the other hand, it has been shown that children who have a normal ultrasound at presentation continue to demonstrate intact anatomy on follow-up studies irrespective of recurrence of UTIs [33]. It is also evident that the vast majority, if not all those who in the past where diagnosed with reflux nephropathy due to infection, sustained the renal parenchymal damage already in utero. Several studies indeed showed that UTI per se is not a frequent cause of chronic renal failure in childhood [60].

Conclusion

Many studies regarding UTI have been conducted on infants older than 30 or 60 days but there is only a paucity of such studies in the neonate. In general it seems agreeable by all that once appropriate urine sample is obtained, prompt antibiotic treatment should be provided, at least for several days by the intravenous route, and ultrasound of the urinary tract performed. Common sense should guide the need for a VCUG especially when taking into consideration the fact that only a minority of patients may benefit from long-term prophylaxis. On the other hand, a 6-month prophylaxis in all neonates recovering from acute UTI might be less invasive and more cost effective.

References

1. Alon U, Davidai G, Berant M et al (1987) Five-year survey of changing patterns of susceptibility of bacterial uropathogens to trimethoprim-sulfamethoxazole and other antimicrobial agents. Antimicrob Agents Chemother 31:126–128
2. Alon US, Ganapathy S (1999) Should renal ultrasonography be done routinely in children with first urinary tract infection? Clin Pediatr 38:21–25
3. Bachur R (2000) Nonresponders: prolonged fever among infants with urinary tract infections. Pediatrics 105:e59–e62
4. Bachur R, Caputo GL (1995) Bacteremia and meningitis among infants with urinary tract infections. Pediatr Emerg Care 11:280–284
5. Bauchner H, Phillip B, Dashefsky B et al (1987) Prevalence of bacteriuria in febrile children. Pediatr Infect Dis J 6:239–242
6. Buys H, Pead L, Hallett R et al (1994) Suprapubic aspiration under ultrasound guidance in children with fever of undiagnosed cause. Br Med J 308:690–692
7. Cerwinka WH, Kirsch AJ (2010) Magnetic resonance urography in pediatric urology. Curr Opin Urol 20:323–329
8. Chan YL, Chan KW, Yeung CK et al (1999) Potential utility of MRI in the evaluation of children at risk of renal scarring. Pediatr Radiol 29:856–862
9. Clinical Practice Guideline (2011) Urinary tract infection: clinical practice guideline for the diagnosis and management of the initial UTI in febrile infants and children 2 to 24 months. Pediatrics 128:595–610
10. Craig J, Simpson J, Williams G (2009) Antibiotic prophylaxis and recurrent urinary tract infection in children. N Engl J Med 361(18):1748–1759
11. Crain EF, Gershel JC (1990) Prevalence of urinary tract infection in febrile infants younger than 8 weeks of age. Pediatrics 86:363–367
12. Djojohadipringgo S, Abdul Hamid RH, Thahir S et al (1976) Bladder puncture in newborns: a bacteriological study. Paediatr Indones 16:527–534
13. Doré-Bergeron MJ, Gauthier M, Chevalier I et al (2009) Urinary tract infections in 1- to 3- month old infants: ambulatory treatment with intravenous antibiotics. Pediatrics 124:16–22
14. El-Naggar W, Yiu A, Mohamed A et al (2010) Comparison of pain during two methods of urine collection in preterm infants. Pediatrics 125:1224–1229
15. Fernandez-Menendez JM, Malaga S, Matesanz JL et al (2003) Risk factors in the development of early technetium-99m dimercaptosuccinic acid renal scintigraphy lesions during first urinary tract infection in children. Acta Paediatr 92:21–26
16. Garin EH, Olavarria F, Araya C et al (2007) Diagnostic significance of clinical and laboratory findings to localize site of urinary infection. Pediatr Nephrol 22:1002–1006
17. Garin EH, Olavarria F, Garcia N et al (2006) Clinical significance of primary vesicoureteral reflux and

urinary antibiotic prophylaxis after acute pyelonephritis: a multicenter, randomized, controlled study. Pediatrics 117(3):626–632
18. Gaspari RJ, Dickson E, Karlowsky J et al (2005) Antibiotic resistance trends in pediatric uropathogens. Int J Antimicrob Agents 26:267–271
19. Gochman RF, Karasic RB, Heller MB (1991) Use of portable ultrasound to assist urine collection by suprapubic aspiration. Ann Emerg Med 20:631–635
20. Grattan-Smith JD, Little SB, Jones RA (2008) Evaluation of reflux nephropathy, pyelonephritis and renal dysplasia. Pediatr Radiol 38:s83–s105
21. Hellerstein S, Alon U, Warady BA (1992) Letter. Urinary screening tests. J Pediatr Infect Dis 11:56–57
22. Hoberman A, Chao HP, Keller DM et al (1993) Prevalence of urinary tract infection in febrile infants. J Pediatr 123:17–23
23. Hoberman A, Charron M, Hickey RW et al (2003) Imaging studies after a first febrile urinary tract infection in young children. N Engl J Med 348:195–202
24. Hoberman A, Winberg J, Roberts KB et al (1994) Pyuria and bacteriuria in urine specimens obtained by catheter from young children with fever. J Pediatr 124:513–519
25. Jahnukainen T, Honkinen O, Ruuskanen O et al (2006) Ultrasonography after the first febrile urinary tract infection in children. Eur J Pediatr 165:556–559
26. Jodal U (1987) The natural history of bacteriuria in childhood. Infect Dis Clin N Am 1:713–729
27. Jones RG, Bass JW (1993) Febrile children with no focus of infection: a survey of their management by primary care physicians. Pediatr Infect Dis J 12:179–183
28. Kass E (1956) Asymptomatic infections of the urinary tract. Trans Assoc Am Phys 69:56–64
29. Keren R (2007) Imaging and treatment strategies for children after first urinary tract infection. Curr Opin Pediatr 19:705–710
30. Klar A, Hurvitz H, Berkun Y et al (1996) Focal bacterial nephritis (lobar nephronia) in children. J Pediatr 128:850–853
31. Kozer E, Rosenbloom E, Goldman D et al (2006) Pain in infants who are younger than 2 months during suprapubic aspiration and transurethral bladder catheterization: a randomized controlled study. Pediatrics 118:e51–e56
32. Leong YY, Tan KW (1976) Bladder aspiration for diagnosis of urinary tract infection in infants and young children. J Singapore Paediatr Soc 18:43–47
33. Lowe LH, Patel MN, Gatti JM et al (2004) Utility of follow-up renal sonography in children with vesicoureteral reflux and normal initial sonogram. Pediatrics 113:548–550
34. Majd M, Rushton HG, Jantausch B et al (1991) Relationship among vesicoureteral reflux, P-fimbriated *Escherichia coli*, and acute pyelonephritis in children with febrile urinary tract infection. J Pediatr 119: 578–585
35. Merrick MV, Uttley WS, Wild SR (1980) The detection of pyelonephritic scarring in children by radioisotope imaging. Br J Radiol 53:544–556
36. Miller T, Phillips S (1981) Pyelonephritis: the relationship between infection, renal scarring, and antimicrobial therapy. Kidney Int 19:654–662
37. Montini G, Rigon L, Zucchetta P et al (2008) Prophylaxis after first febrile urinary tract infection in children? A multicenter, randomized, controlled, non-inferiority trial. Pediatrics 122(5):1064–1071
38. Montini G, Zucchetta P, Tomasi L et al (2009) Value of imaging studies after a first febrile urinary tract infection in young children: data from Italian renal infection study I. Pediatrics 123:e239–e245
39. Mori R, Lakhanpaul M, Verrier-Jones K (2007) Diagnosis and management of urinary tract infection in children: summary of NICE guidance. Br Med J 335:395–397
40. Nuutinen M, Uhari M (2001) Recurrence and follow-up after urinary tract infection under the age of 1 year. Pediatr Nephrol 16:69–72
41. Pecile P, Miorin E, Romanello C et al (2004) Procalcitonin: a marker of severity of acute pyelonephritis among children. Pediatrics 114:e249–e254
42. Pennesi M, Travan L, Peratoner L et al (2008) Is antibiotic prophylaxis in children with vesicoureteral reflux effective in preventing pyelonephritis and renal scars? A randomized, controlled trial. Pediatrics 121(6):e1489–e1494
43. Pitetti RD, Choi S (2002) Utility of blood cultures in febrile children with UTI. Am J Emerg Med 20:271–274. doi:10.1053/ajem.2002.33786
44. Plos K, Connell H, Jodal U et al (1995) Intestinal carriage of P fimbriated Escherichia coli and the susceptibility to urinary tract infection in young children. J Infect Dis 171:625–631
45. Pryles CV, Atkin MD, Morese TS et al (1959) Comparative bacteriologic study of urine obtained from children by percutaneous suprapubic aspiration of the bladder and by catheter. Pediatrics 24:983–991
46. Pylkkänen J, Vilska J, Koskimies O (1981) The value of level diagnosis of childhood urinary tract infection in predicting renal injury. Acta Paediatr Scand 70:879–883
47. Roberts KB, Charney E, Sweren RJ et al (1983) Urinary tract infection in infants with unexplained fever: a collaborative study. J Pediatr 103:864–867
48. Roussey-Kesler G, Gadjos V, Idres N et al (2008) Antibiotic prophylaxis for the prevention of recurrent urinary tract infection in children with low grade vesicoureteral reflux: results from a prospective randomized study. J Urol 179(2):674–679
49. Schnadower D, Kuppermann N, Macias CG et al (2010) Febrile infants with urinary tract infections at very low risk for adverse events and bacteremia. Pediatrics 126:1074–1083
50. Schoen EJ (2005) Circumcision for preventing urinary tract infections in boys: North American view. Arch Dis Child 90:772–773
51. Schoen EJ, Colby CJ, Ray GT (2000) Newborn circumcision decreases incidence and costs of urinary tract infections during the first year of life. Pediatrics 105:789–793

52. Shah SS, Zorc JJ, Levine DA et al (2008) Sterile cerebrospinal fluid pleocytosis in young infants with urinary tract infections. J Pediatr 153:290–292
53. Shaikh N, Ewing AL, Bhatnagar S et al (2010) Risk of renal scarring in children with a first urinary tract infection: a systematic review. Pediatrics 126:1084–1091
54. Shaikh N, Morone NE, Bost JE et al (2008) Prevalence of urinary tract infection in childhood. Pediatr Infect Dis J 27:302–308
55. Sheu JN, Meng-Chi C, Sun-Long C et al (2007) Urine interleukin-1β in children with acute pyelonephritis and renal scarring. Nephrology 12:487–493
56. Singh-Grewal D, Macdessi J, Craig J (2005) Circumcision for the prevention of urinary tract infection in boys: a systematic review of randomized trials and observational studies. Arch Dis Child 90:853–858
57. Skoog SJ, Peters CA, Arant BS et al (2010) Pediatric vesicoureteral reflux guidelines panel summary report: Clinical Practice Guidelines for screening siblings of children with vesicoureteral reflux and neonates/infants with prenatal hydronephrosis. J Urol 184:1145–1151
58. Smellie JM, Poulton A, Prescod NP (1994) Retrospective study of children with renal scarring associated with reflux and urinary infection. Br Med J 308:1193–1196
59. Spencer JD, Schwaderer AL, DiRosario JD et al (2011) Ribonuclease 7 is a potent antimicrobial peptide within the human urinary tract. Kidney Int 80:174–180
60. Sreenarasimhaiah S, Hellerstein S (1998) Urinary tract infections per se do not cause end-stage kidney disease. Pediatr Nephrol 12:210–213
61. Stamm WE (1983) Measurement of pyuria and its relation to bacteriuria. Am J Med 75:53–58
62. Steele BT, Petrou C, DeMaria J (1990) Renal abscess in children. Urology 36:325–328
63. Visser VE, Hall RT (1979) Urine culture in the evaluation of suspected neonatal sepsis. J Pediatr 94:635–638
64. Wettergren B, Jodal U (1990) Spontaneous clearance of asymptomatic bacteriuria in infants. Acta Paediatr Scand 79:300–304
65. Wettergren B, Jodal U, Jonasson G (1985) Epidemiology of bacteriuria during the first year of life. Acta Paediatr Scand 74:925–933
66. Winberg J, Andersen HJ, Bergstrom T (1974) Epidemiology of symptomatic urinary tract infection in childhood. Acta Paediatr Scand 252(Suppl):1–20
67. Winter AL, Hardy BE, Alton DJ et al (1983) Acquired renal scars in children. J Urol 129:1190–1194
68. Wisewell TE, Hachey WE (1993) Urinary tract infections and the uncircumcised state: an update. Clin Pediatr 32:130–134
69. Zamir G, Sakran W, Horowitz Y et al (2004) Urinary tract infection: is there a need for routine renal ultrasonography? Arch Dis Child 89:466–468
70. Zhanel GG, Hisanaga TL, Laing NM et al (2005) Antibiotic resistance in outpatient urinary isolates: final results from the North American Urinary Tract Infection Collaborative Alliance (NAUTICA). Int J Antimicrob Agents 26:380–388
71. Zorc JJ, Levin DA, Platt SL et al (2005) Clinical and demographic factors associated with urinary tract infection in young febrile infants. Pediatrics 116:644–648

Posterior Urethral Valves

10

Shumyle Alam

Case Study

A 24-year-old G2P0A1 patient presents to our fetal care center for multidisciplinary evaluation due to ultrasound findings of oligohydramnios, bilateral hydronephrosis, and cystic changes of the kidneys due to suspected bladder outlet obstruction. At 20 weeks of gestation a fetal MRI demonstrated a normal central nervous system, normal heart, normal GI tract, and no limb abnormalities. She is here with her mother and her husband to discuss options. Her first pregnancy was complicated with anhydramnios and loss of the fetus at 14 weeks.

She meets with representatives from nephrology, fetal care, transplant surgery, urology, high-risk obstetrics, and social work. Mom states that she wants every measure taken to bring the fetus to term. Successful amniotic shunt placement and amnioinfusion were performed at 21 weeks. An amnioinfusion port was placed and the baby was electively delivered via C-section at 36 weeks.

The 2,100 g baby was transferred to the NICU after delivery and was on room air after delivery with Apgar's of 8 and 9. The birth serum creatinine (SCr) is 3.2 mg/dL. A non-balloon catheter was placed in the urethra and put to drainage. An ultrasound performed 24 h after birth demonstrated markedly hydronephrotic dysplastic kidneys. A voiding cystourethrogram confirmed valves and high-grade bilateral reflux with a small trabeculated bladder. The renal profile at 24 h revealed a SCr of 4.1 mg/dL. The hydronephrosis gradually improved with drainage, but the cystic changes persisted. At 3 weeks the baby was taken to the OR and valves were ablated. Clean intermittent catheterization (CIC) was initiated and the SCr stabilized to 2.5 g/dL. Urine output remained brisk at 4–5 mL/kg/h.

Over the course of the next few weeks, two episodes of UTI and sepsis occurred and the baby was unable to maintain adequate oral intake. He was taken to the OR at 3 months of age for placement of a G-tube and a peritoneal dialysis catheter. He was finally discharged home at 4 months on peritoneal dialysis and gastrostomy-tube feeds and CIC. His discharge weight is 3,200 g. The workup for a living-related kidney donor transplant was initiated.

S. Alam, MD
Urogenital Center, Division of Pediatric Urology, Cincinnati Children's Medical Center, 3333 Burnet Ave, Cincinnati, OH 45229-3039, USA
e-mail: shumyle@yahoo.com

A.S. Chishti et al. (eds.), *Kidney and Urinary Tract Diseases in the Newborn*,
DOI 10.1007/978-3-642-39988-6_10, © Springer-Verlag Berlin Heidelberg 2014

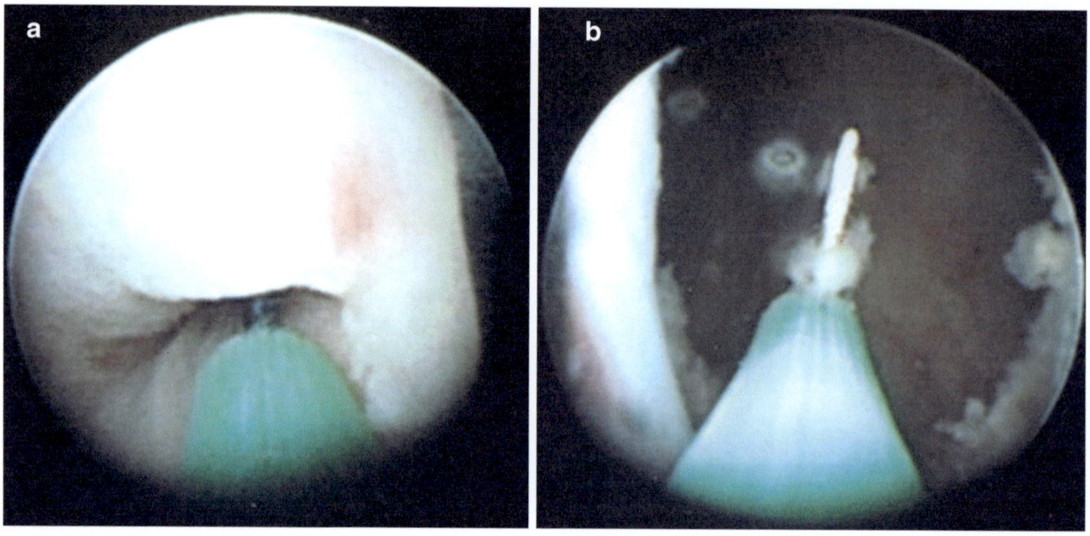

Fig. 10.1 (**a**) Appearance of PUV seen with a cystoscopy. (**b**) Appearance after ablation of the PUV

10.1 Introduction

The above scenario seems a bit futuristic, but is beginning to occur more frequently in institutions with fetal care centers. Posterior urethral valves (PUVs) are the most common cause of obstructive uropathy in males and previously had a progression rate to end-stage renal disease (ESRD) of 50 % [3]. That paradigm may be changing. Improvements in neonatal intensive care, dialysis, and transplantation have allowed some quaternary centers to become comfortable with neonatal ESRD management in these infants. These resource-intense patients require a multidisciplinary approach to management and pose many new ethical and medical dilemmas. The following chapter will serve as an overview of posterior urethral valves with a focus on the concerns of this growing new population of neonates.

The incidence of PUV is reported between 1/4,000 and 1/8,000 live births, but the actual incidence may be higher as some afflicted fetuses suffer in utero demise [21]. PUV can cause renal dysplasia with resulting renal insufficiency that can be progressive. Often PUV is diagnosed prenatally due to the widespread use of prenatal ultrasound.

Prenatal ultrasound is the screening modality of choice for identification of abnormalities of the genitourinary tract [4]. Bilateral hydronephrosis in a male fetus with any evidence of oligohydramnios should alert the physician for a possible bladder outlet obstruction [3]. Unfortunately the ultrasound alone is not able to accurately predict postnatal renal function [2]. Often the fetus with poor renal function either did not survive in utero or die shortly after birth. Typically these were cases of severe oligohydramnios or anhydramnios. This chapter will focus on fetal management on PUV with special consideration given to the neonate with ESRD.

10.1.1 Anatomy

Posterior urethral valves are defined as obstructing or partially obstructing tissue arising from the floor of the urethra. They are continuous with the verumontanum and the divide in the bulbomembranous urethra just proximal to the urethral sphincter [7]. Typically they appear as "sails" at the 5 o'clock and 7 o'clock positions. The leaflets can appear as an obstructing membrane. The definitive treatment is valve ablation achieved with transurethral resection (Fig. 10.1).

The valves are not normal tissue and cause obstruction of anterograde flow of urine from the bladder. The degree of obstruction tends to correlate with the severity of bladder and renal involvement, although PUV remains a spectrum of disease without a good predictive model regarding disease severity. Diligence of the workup and management of the neonate are the most effective way to prevent future complications.

The most severely affected infants with PUV may benefit from evaluation in a fetal care center where more sophisticated imaging modalities such as fetal MRI and assessment of the amniotic fluid can be performed [22]. A multidisciplinary team approach can be utilized for pre- and postnatal management as well as the formulation of a comprehensive birth plan. Survival in the early postnatal period for these infants depends on the prenatal management, resources of the NICU, and the birth hospital.

In a fetus diagnosed with PUV, evidence of in utero renal insufficiency can be detected by decreased amniotic fluid and abnormal fetal urine electrolytes. The resulting oligohydramnios is a cause of pulmonary hypoplasia [22]. In the past, the pulmonary issues have led to poorer outcomes in these infants. Advances in in utero fetal treatment and neonatal critical care have improved the outcome in afflicted infants by optimizing pulmonary function. This has resulted in improved perinatal survival. Unfortunately, the interventions have not improved renal function, so although infants survive, they quickly progress to ESRD.

There is a defined rate of progression to ESRD observed in some children with PUV. There is no clear timeline for progression, and the variables leading to eventual renal failure are poorly defined [18, 22]. ESRD develops in 13–42 % of patients diagnosed with PUVs [15, 18]. The management of these infants has improved over time most likely due to early diagnosis. The recent improvement in perinatal outcomes in severely afflicted neonates has created a new cohort of infants who have ESRD from the onset of life, and as a result, new challenges have arisen.

Prenatal screening ultrasound identifies hydronephrosis readily, and a prenatal consultation can be performed with just the pediatric urologist in the case where amniotic fluid is preserved. The benefit of this meeting would be to create a birth plan such that the infant is quickly transported to a children's hospital for management. This also allows for a postnatal testing plan to be created expediting care after delivery.

10.1.2 Goals of Management

Early valve ablation with bladder cycling and the stabilization of the upper tracts is the mainstay of therapy in uncomplicated PUV. Infants are treated in the first few days of life and the bladder allowed to cycle normally once the obstructing leaflets are ablated. The infants are watched carefully and the upper tracts followed for the development of hydronephrosis and vesicoureteral reflux (VUR). The goal of management is to prevent progression of renal injury and preserve bladder function.

Renal transplantation is the treatment of choice for pediatric patients with ESRD and PUV as it promotes growth and development. Transplantation in these neonates presents some challenges. These patients have a unique set of anatomic and functional concerns, and the provider must create novel solutions to problems that we traditionally had months or even years to solve. Now we have an unforgiving timeline to adhere to in order to allow these infants to survive. Much of the ability to address these concerns is dependent on the neonatal management of these infants.

10.2 Neonatal Management

Though a birth plan is critical for both the survival and long-term care of PUV with ESRD, the infant with preserved renal function and PUV is easier to manage. Though there exist a subset of patients with "missed valves" which is simply delayed presentation, this chapter will focus on neonatal PUV management with a special focus on infants with ESRD and PUV.

10.2.1 PUV Management in Infants with Normal Renal Function

The treatment of PUV in the neonatal period is relatively straightforward. Often the diagnosis is suspected prenatally and the child is transferred to a children's hospital shortly after birth. A renal ultrasound should be performed 24 h after birth to avoid the pitfall of under

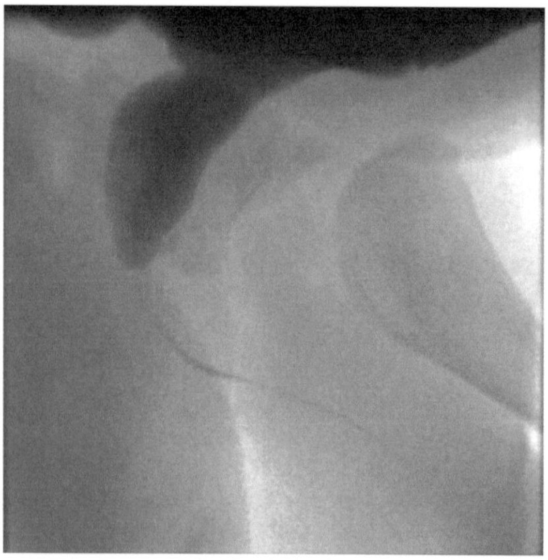

Fig. 10.2 The appearance of the posterior urethral valve on a voiding image from a VCUG

recognizing hydronephrosis as the infant is physiologically dehydrated. A measurement of SCr should also be delayed as an early sample is more reflective of maternal values. A non-balloon urinary catheter is inserted to allow unobstructed drainage of urine. The balloon may irritate the bladder and trigger unwanted spasms which can worsen hydronephrosis [13]. The diagnosis of valves is confirmed with a radiographic voiding cystourethrogram (VCUG). Care must be taken to observe the voiding phase to capture the valve (Fig. 10.2).

Endoscopic valve ablation can be performed safely even in cases where the infant is less than 2,500 g. The relative safety is due to the availability of small endoscopes. Coexisting anesthesia concerns must be taken into consideration before ablation despite the technical ability to operate on the smallest of infants. If the bladder is not draining appropriately with the catheter, the infant is too small, or due to unavailability of appropriate endoscopes, a temporary urinary diversion with a vesicostomy may be performed. This is becoming a less frequent scenario in most centers, and there is controversy regarding the long-term bladder outcomes following diversion. There is literature to both support and condemn a diversion in PUV [11].

Once the valves are ablated, practices vary regarding timing of removal of catheter with some practitioners advocating immediate voiding afterwards. Long-term outcome data regarding standard practices for catheter removal do not exist.

The appropriate imaging and lab studies for the follow-up of treated infants are poorly documented. Significant variation exists with regard to timing of studies and the interpretation of the clinical significance of upper tract dilation. Recently Coleman et al. described a novel way to predict renal outcome measuring SCr velocity [5]. This exciting new study is perhaps a way to begin to standardize testing and follow-up of infants with PUV. The addition of a predictive variable may have another impact on the ability to standardize the interpretation of upper tract changes seen on imaging.

As mentioned previously, the progression to ESRD can be seen in up to 50 % of PUV patients. The reason is that the entire urinary tract proximal to the valves is affected. Hydronephrosis, vesicoureteral reflux (VUR), or cystic changes to the kidneys are obvious on imaging. Subtle changes such as loss of bladder compliance and the development of high pressures in the bladder may portend long-term deterioration of renal function [24]. Long-term follow-up is critical for success from both a nephron-urologic standpoint.

10.2.2 PUV Management in Infants with ESRD

The management of the PUV infant with ESRD is not well documented and will be the primary focus of this chapter as they represent a new group of patients presenting to the NICU. This is due to the impact of fetal care centers with their interventions increasing the number of pulmonary survivors with ESRD from obstructive uropathy [23].

Care of patients with PUV and ESRD is focused on supportive measures that will allow the patient to progress to renal transplantation. When the affected individual is a neonate, the timeline for definitive management becomes somewhat unforgiving. The infant with ESRD is subject to delays in growth and development, nutritional concerns, need for stable dialysis access, increased risks of infection and hospitalization, and the technical limitations to transplant regarding vascular anatomy and abdominal domain.

The infant with PUV and ESRD has the added burden of structural and functional abnormalities of the genitourinary tract. This is a relatively new phenomenon as severely affected infants with ESRD and bladder outlet obstruction often did not survive the perinatal period. Affected infants often were born with enough renal function to allow early childhood transplant and correction of any structural or functional issues prior to transplant. Now, early identification of at risk infants and prenatal interventions including a delivery plan has resulted in the observation of increased survival and the creation of a new cohort of patients.

After stabilization of the infant, a multidisciplinary approach to care with the combined input of the neonatology, nephrology, transplant surgery, and urology is helpful for the management of this resource-intense group of patients. Dialysis is often necessary in the early prenatal term, and this decision needs to be carefully planned and coordinated with the team.

10.3 Renal Replacement Therapy in PUV with ESRD

In infants, hemodialysis is technically challenging and is associated with high morbidity. A review of infant hemodialysis patients in the UK suggested line complications (thrombosis and infection), anemia with transfusion requirements, and inadequate dialysis as common morbidities [32]. Peritoneal dialysis can be achieved with relative ease and is convenient for parents as the treatment can be administered at home. Associated issues impacting peritoneal dialysis include inguinal hernia, abdominal wall defects, and leaking catheters.

Dialysis access concerns are multiple. The infant obviously must not have any intra-abdominal process such as necrotizing enterocolitis (NEC). Patent processus if large should be corrected; otherwise, PD cycling may prove difficult. If a G-tube is necessary, timing should coincide with the placement of the dialysis catheter. If done later, a period where dialysis is held may be necessary. Despite marginal clearance, if the infant makes urine, it may allow for a short time frame where PD can be held.

10.3.1 Nutritional Concerns

Nutrition is another difficult issue to address. Growth in the neonatal time period is rapid (1.5 cm/month) and requires significant calories [6]. Infants with renal failure very often are unable to consume the required nutrition with traditional oral feeding. An additional complication in this cohort of patients is the fixed urine output seen in obstructive uropathy [8]. In some cases urine output is so high that the majority of intake must be water to prevent dehydration, which greatly impacts feeding.

Many infants will benefit from a G-tube placement. Often nutritional and calorie goals are not met, and a feeding tube is placed for management. It is most common that the G-tube is placed after a trial of nasogastric feeding. Recombinant growth hormone is also considered for infants that have not achieved adequate growth after nutritional supplementation [28].

Consideration should be given to placement of G-tube utilizing direct visualization technique. When needed, this can be done with laparoscopic placement of the peritoneal dialysis catheter. Visualization of the placement of the G-tube ensures that the arcade along the greater curvature is preserved. This would allow for the consideration of future gastrocystoplasty.

The stomach serves as a valuable segment to preserve for bladder reconstruction in this population for several reasons. First is the setting of diminished GFR, acidosis is generally not a concern with the stomach [29, 31]. Avoiding acidosis is important for growth and development. Secondly, the anatomic features of the stomach with its outer muscular layer allow for reimplantation of the Mitrofanoff and the ureter in both continent and anti-refluxing manners [29]. This is most pertinent when the bladder is so hypertrophied and thickened that it is resistant to medical management to

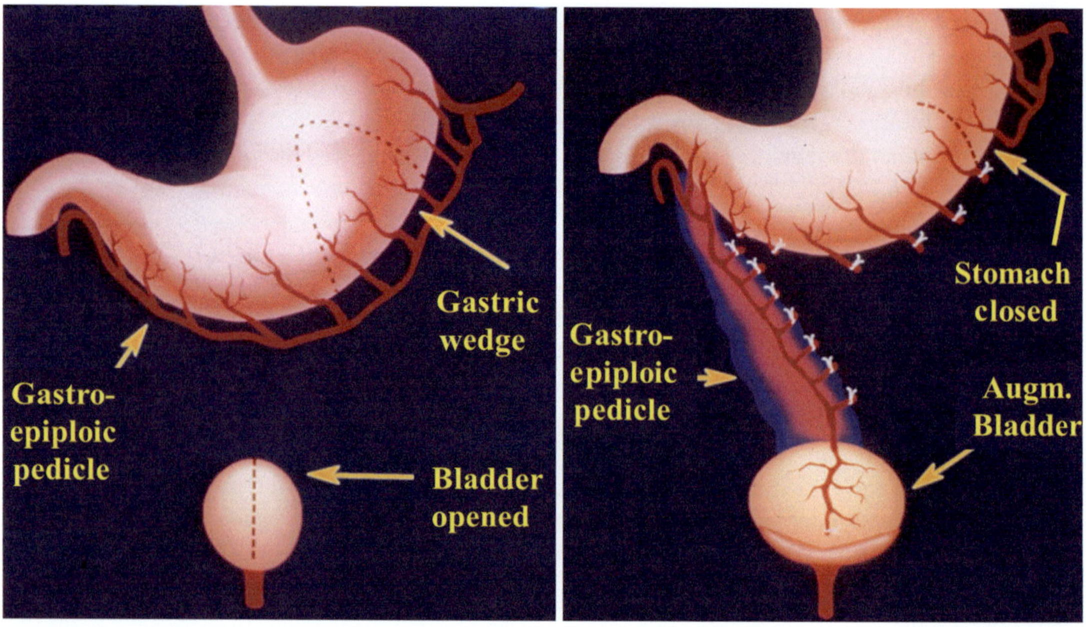

Fig. 10.3 Technique for gastrocystoplasty utilizing vessels along the greater curvature

improve compliance. This is not to suggest that all patients with ESRD and PUV undergo a gastric augment but rather that all reconstructive options be preserved in these complex patients. Placement of a G-tube such that the arcade on the greater curvature is interrupted limits this option as a gastric segment will only reach the pelvis based on the right gastroepiploic vessel (Fig. 10.3).

The important point to understand regarding the management of the PUV infant is the long-term implications of each individual intervention. An incorrectly placed dialysis catheter can irreversibly harm the vessels impacting future access and/or transplant. A transperitoneal approach for urologic reconstruction can limit PD access and success. Catheter placement in PUV is not a benign procedure and can lead to lifelong morbidity (Fig. 10.4). A multidisciplinary team can assist in understanding these long-term concerns.

10.4 Anatomic Concerns

Structural and functional abnormalities of the GU tract are a significant concern in the infant with PUV irrespective of the degree of renal injury. Functional abnormalities can lead to long-term renal deterioration and progression of disease.

Hydronephrosis, VUR, and bladder diverticula remain the primary anatomic concerns in these infants. In the past reconstructive surgery was performed prior to transplant or in an effort to slow or stop progression of renal injury. Progression to ESRD though defined occurred over the course of months to years. This allowed for reconstruction including reimplantation, nephrectomy, urinary diversion, Mitrofanoff creation, and occasionally augmentation.

The bladder can be a significant source of ongoing morbidity in the patient with PUV. The primary problem has to do with bladder compliance. Bladder compliance is defined as the relationship between the changes of the bladder pressure as volume increases. Poorly compliant bladders demonstrate increased pressure with filling. Histopathology confirms both detrusor hypertrophy and fibrosis of the bladder in infants with valves [9, 16]. This leads to lack of compliance of the bladder which may be permanent without aggressive management or a way for the bladder to relieve the pressure [14].

Large bladder diverticuli can also prohibit effective emptying of urine and cause stasis. This

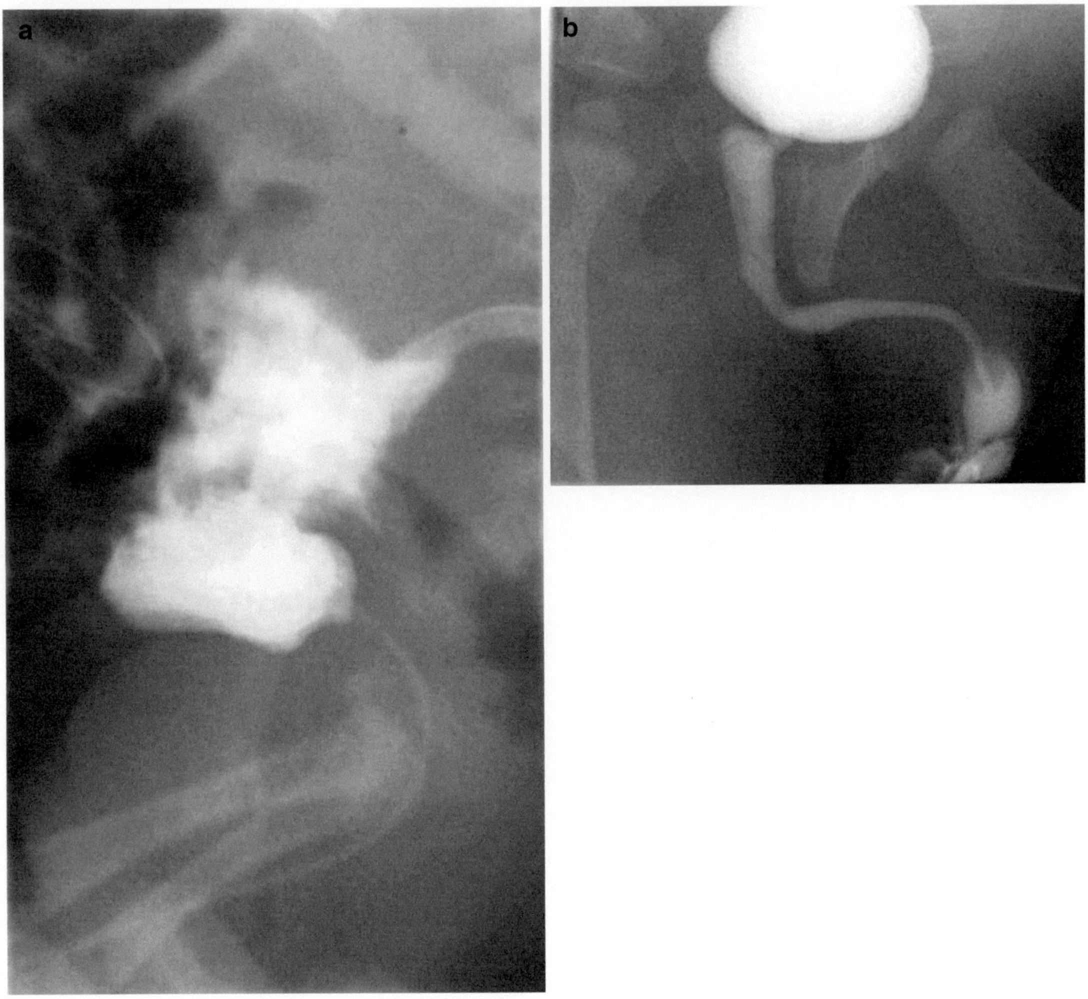

Fig. 10.4 (**a**) A catheter placed in an infant with ESRD and PUV had perforated the posterior urethra. (**b**) A follow-up VCUG after 2 years, unfortunately urethral catheterization is not possible without general anesthesia cystoscopy and guide wire placement of a catheter

in turn increases the risks of infection, debris, stones, and worsening bladder disease (Fig. 10.5). All of these functional concerns can be detected on radiographic imaging. As the child gets older, a functional assessment of the urinary tract may be performed with urodynamic studies. These are rarely helpful in the neonate.

10.4.1 Medical Management

PUV infants with ESRD present some unique challenges. Transperitoneal surgery is not feasible in the PD-dependent child, which severely limits reconstructive options. Early reimplantation of the massively refluxing ureter is not only technically difficult in the infant, but the individual renal moieties may have such poor function that the results would not be satisfactory. Often the bladder has poor compliance which is a concern for graft survival after transplant [30].

Interventions are limited to diversion in the form of a vesicostomy or clean intermittent catheterization (CIC) with anticholinergic use in these patients. The Cincinnati Children's Urology algorithm is to perform CIC and titrate to the maximally tolerated dose of oxybutynin (0.2 mg/kg/dose). Even in the setting of high-grade VUR, medical management may result in positive bladder outcomes (Fig. 10.6).

Caution must be exercised regarding this management strategy, if urine output is low. Bladder compliance in the setting of oliguria has not been observed to greatly improve suggesting a need for urine production to allow bladder cycling. In the anuric child with ESRD and neurogenic bladder, some have suggested bladder cycling with the instillation of sterile saline or water and anticholinergics. This strategy may not be successful in the presence of high-grade VUR.

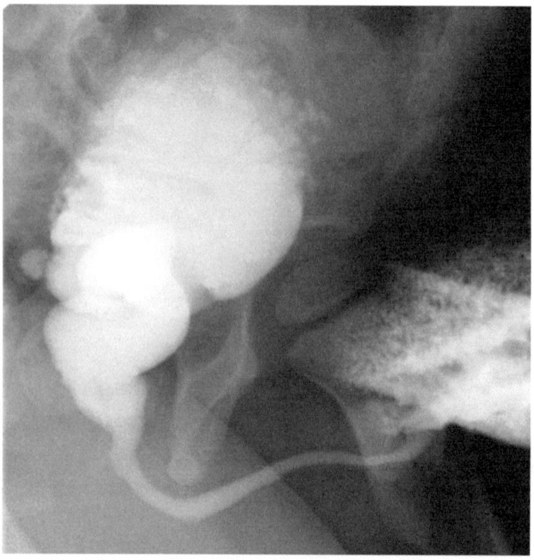

Fig. 10.5 The typical appearance of diverticula and trabeculations in a noncompliant bladder in PUV

In the PUV infant without renal failure but with CKD, care must be taken to protect the kidneys from further damage. These infants are typically voiding after valve ablation, and imaging must be performed to ensure adequate drainage. A repeat ultrasound and labs are often necessary to determine adequate bladder emptying.

10.4.2 Surgical Management

Surgical management of the infant is limited to valve ablation or diversion in the infant with preserved renal function and PUV. Reimplantation of the ureters for treatment of VUR is not advised as a primary management strategy in PUV. In some cases the medical management of the bladder results in resolution of the VUR, this can include valve ablation alone [12].

Dilating VUR is of significant concern in these patients, and native nephrectomies at the time of transplant can performed for this reason. Grade III VUR to the native kidneys or greater is associated

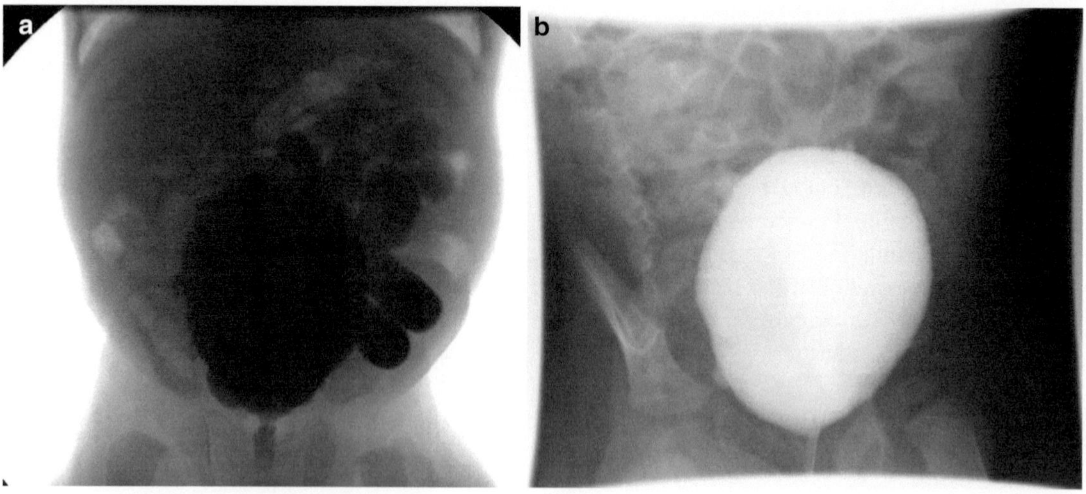

Fig. 10.6 (**a**) The "valve bladder" with high-grade reflux and severe renal damage. (**b**) After a trial of intermittent catheterization and oxybutynin

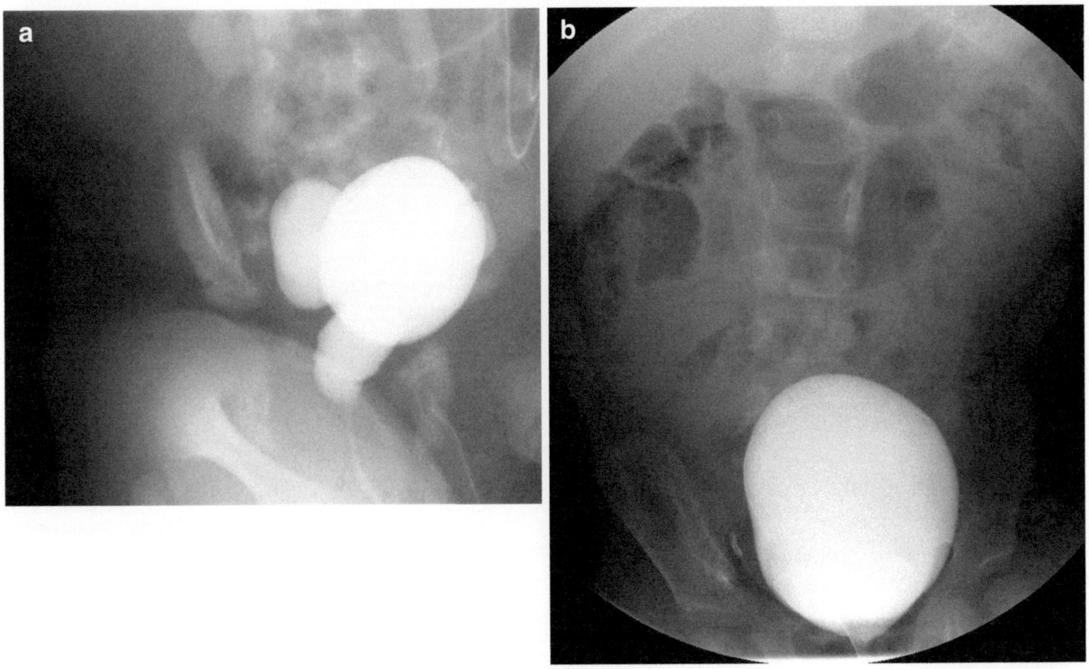

Fig. 10.7 (**a**) The appearance of the bladder on VCUG before transplant. (**b**) Ipsilateral native nephrectomy and ureterectomy performed at time of transplant. Image taken 6 months post-op with patient on CIC and no left sided surgery

with risk to the graft [1, 26]. Planned nephrectomy before transplant is not advised unless hypertension, proteinuria, or infectious concerns. Very often ipsilateral native nephrectomy can be performed at the time of transplant. The contralateral side can be addressed after the child has recovered from transplant (Fig. 10.7).

High-grade VUR in the child with preserved renal function must be carefully assessed. A functional study of the upper tracts is suggested with either nuclear study to assess function. Tc-99m diethylenetriamine pentaacetic acid (DTPA) is a cortical binding agent helpful for calculation of GFR and differential function. A 99mTc mercaptoacetyltriglycine (Mag-3) study will allow for differential function as well and may be helpful if concomitant obstruction is suspected [27]. It is critical that this test is performed with the bladder decompressed as high-grade reflux can cause the appearance of ureteropelvic junction obstruction (UPJO). In general if the bladder is treated the degree of VUR will likely diminish with time.

Another commonly encountered phenomenon is the so-called "pop-off" mechanism where the high-grade VUR will subtend a nonfunctional kidney. This generally allows for the contralateral kidney to be relatively preserved. Other "pop-off" mechanisms can be a large bladder diverticulum, a forniceal rupture, or a bladder rupture. This can be a renal protective phenomenon but requires immediate intervention except in the case associated with isolated VUR [14].

The bladders of PUV infants with valves are initially noncompliant and thickened. These are typically the worst bladders to work with from a reimplantation standpoint. In order to improve compliance, infants can be placed on clean intermittent catheterization (CIC) and anticholinergics (oxybutynin and a dose of 0.2 mg/kg/dose given every 8 h) [17]. Improving bladder compliance also facilitates the ability to perform non-refluxing ureteral anastomosis for the graft which may have long-term benefit for graft survival [25].

Among infants where urine output and upper tract function are preserved, compliance will improve with time [19]. This natural progression of the bladder should not be allowed to the detriment of the upper tracts. If SCr remains normal and the follow-up ultrasounds are stable, it is a reasonable strategy to follow in select cases.

Conclusion

The long-term prognosis of PUV suggests a spectrum of disease. There is a suggestion that early detection will improve long-term outcome for children without renal failure [20]. Unfortunately, there is no data suggesting an improvement in renal outcome with prenatal treatment.

The literature regarding long-term outcomes in ESRD with PUV is lacking. An excellent review by Fine et al. suggests that the long-term graft survival in patients with valves is no worse than other patients with ESRD [10]. Limitations of their study were poor urologic follow-up, no urodynamic data, limited radiographic data, and documentation of only voiding dysfunction. Curiously enough, they note improved graft survival in patients with a vesicostomy, a suggestion that bladder compliance and pathologic voiding may have a role in graft demise.

Further study will lead to improved renal survival in severely affected neonates with PUV. Aggressive multidisciplinary management in the neonatal period may improve outcomes in the future. With time and the development of disease registries, we may come closer to improved outcomes in these fragile resource-intense patients.

References

1. Basiri A, Otookesh H et al (2006) Does pre-transplantation antireflux surgery eliminate post-renal transplantation pyelonephritis in children? J Urol 175(4):1490–1492
2. Bernardes LS, Salomon R et al (2011) Ultrasound evaluation of prognosis in fetuses with posterior urethral valves. J Pediatr Surg 46(7):1412–1418
3. Casella DP, Tomaszewski JJ et al (2012) Posterior urethral valves: renal failure and prenatal treatment. Int J Nephrol 2012:351067
4. Clayton DB, Brock JW III (2012) Prenatal ultrasound and urological anomalies. Pediatr Clin North Am 59(4):739–756
5. Coleman R, King T et al (2013) Posterior urethral valves: creatinine velocity, a new early predictor of renal insufficiency. J Pediatr Surg 48(2):384–387
6. Csaicsich D, Russo-Schlaff N et al (2008) Renal failure, comorbidity and mortality in preterm infants. Wien Klin Wochenschr 120(5–6):153–157
7. Dewan PA (1997) Congenital posterior urethral obstruction: the historical perspective. Pediatr Surg Int 12(2–3):86–94
8. Dinneen MD, Duffy PG et al (1995) Persistent polyuria after posterior urethral valves. Br J Urol 75(2): 236–240
9. Ewalt DH, Howard PS et al (1992) Is lamina propria matrix responsible for normal bladder compliance? J Urol 148(2 Pt 2):544–549
10. Fine MS, Smith KM et al (2011) Posterior urethral valve treatments and outcomes in children receiving kidney transplants. J Urol 185(6 Suppl):2507–2511
11. Godbole P, Wade A et al (2007) Vesicostomy vs. primary ablation for posterior urethral valves: always a difference in outcome? J Pediatr Urol 3(4):273–275
12. Hassan JM, Pope JCt et al (2003) Vesicoureteral reflux in patients with posterior urethral valves. J Urol 170(4 Pt 2):1677–1680, discussion 1680
13. Jordan GH, Hoover DL (1985) Inadequate decompression of the upper tracts using a Foley catheter in the valve bladder. J Urol 134(1):137–138
14. Kaefer M, Keating MA et al (1995) Posterior urethral valves, pressure pop-offs and bladder function. J Urol 154(2 Pt 2):708–711
15. Kibar Y, Ashley RA et al (2011) Timing of posterior urethral valve diagnosis and its impact on clinical outcome. J Pediatr Urol 7(5):538–542
16. Kim KM, Kogan BA et al (1991) Collagen and elastin in the obstructed fetal bladder. J Urol 146(2 (Pt 2)): 528–531
17. Kim YH, Horowitz M et al (1997) Management of posterior urethral valves on the basis of urodynamic findings. J Urol 158(3 Pt 2):1011–1016
18. Klaassen I, Neuhaus TJ et al (2007) Antenatal oligohydramnios of renal origin: long-term outcome. Nephrol Dial Transplant 22(2):432–439
19. Koff SA, Mutabagani KH et al (2002) The valve bladder syndrome: pathophysiology and treatment with nocturnal bladder emptying. J Urol 167(1):291–297
20. Kousidis G, Thomas DF et al (2008) The long-term outcome of prenatally detected posterior urethral valves: a 10 to 23-year follow-up study. BJU Int 102(8):1020–1024
21. Krishnan A, de Souza A et al (2006) The anatomy and embryology of posterior urethral valves. J Urol 175(4):1214–1220
22. Lissauer D, Morris RK et al (2007) Fetal lower urinary tract obstruction. Semin Fetal Neonatal Med 12(6):464–470

23. Mann S, Johnson MP et al (2010) Fetal thoracic and bladder shunts. Semin Fetal Neonatal Med 15(1): 28–33
24. McGuire EJ (1994) Bladder compliance. J Urol 151(4):965–966
25. Neuhaus TJ, Schwobel M et al (1997) Pyelonephritis and vesicoureteral reflux after renal transplantation in young children. J Urol 157(4):1400–1403
26. Ohba K, Matsuo M et al (2004) Clinicopathological study of vesicoureteral reflux (VUR)-associated pyelonephritis in renal transplantation. Clin Transplant 18(Suppl 11):34–38
27. Othman S, Al-Hawas A et al (2012) Renal cortical imaging in children: 99mTc MAG3 versus 99mTc DMSA. Clin Nucl Med 37(4):351–355
28. Rees L (2002) Management of the infant with end-stage renal failure. Nephrol Dial Transplant 17(9): 1564–1567
29. Sumfest JM, Mitchell ME (1994) Gastrocystoplasty in children. Eur Urol 25(2):89–93
30. Taghizadeh AK, Desai D et al (2007) Renal transplantation or bladder augmentation first? A comparison of complications and outcomes in children. BJU Int 100(6):1365–1370
31. Traxel E, DeFoor W et al (2011) Low incidence of urinary tract infections following renal transplantation in children with bladder augmentation. J Urol 186(2):667–671
32. Wedekin M, Ehrich JH et al (2010) Renal replacement therapy in infants with chronic renal failure in the first year of life. Clin J Am Soc Nephrol 5(1):18–23

11 Neonatal Obstructive Uropathy

Brian A. VanderBrink

Core Messages

- Obstructive uropathy describes a condition where renal function has been adversely affected by impairment of flow of urine within the collecting system. This condition can be congenital, acquired, reversible, and irreversible.
- The majority of neonatal obstructive uropathy is diagnosed based upon findings on prenatal ultrasounds; however, the majority of fetuses with evidence of prenatal renal/ureteral dilation will not require any type of surgical intervention.
- Percutaneous nephrostomy tube is an effective means of decompressing the obstructed urinary tract in the clinically unstable neonate while awaiting definitive surgical reconstruction at a later time.

Case Vignette

A 25-day-old male presents to the emergency room with history of fever and repetitive emesis for the past 2 days. The mother states he has not been feeding well and his emesis occurs shortly after feedings. He was born full term via Cesarean section for breech presentation. His neonatal course has been uncomplicated. There is no family history of urologic problems.

The patient had a history of unilateral left sided prenatal hydronephrosis. This was detected at 20 weeks and was observed on every ultrasound obtained throughout the pregnancy. The hydronephrosis increased in its severity with an anterior posterior renal pelvic diameter of 22 mm at 34 weeks. There was no evidence of ureteral dilation or bladder distension. He was lost to follow-up postnatally until presenting to the emergency room with the above complaints.

His physical examination reveals a child that is responsive but not overly active. His temperature is 102 °F with a pulse of 170 bpm and blood pressure of 100/50. His abdomen reveals no any palpable mass in the right upper quadrant, but there is tenderness to palpation and fullness to the left upper quadrant. He is circumcised with an orthotopic urethral meatus and normal penis. Both testicles are descended. The lumbosacral region is normal to inspection and palpation.

B.A. VanderBrink, MD
Division of Urology, Nationwide Children's Hospital URO, 555 South 18th Street Suite 6D, Columbus, OH 43205, USA
e-mail: brian.vanderbrink@nationwidechildrens.org

A.S. Chishti et al. (eds.), *Kidney and Urinary Tract Diseases in the Newborn*,
DOI 10.1007/978-3-642-39988-6_11, © Springer-Verlag Berlin Heidelberg 2014

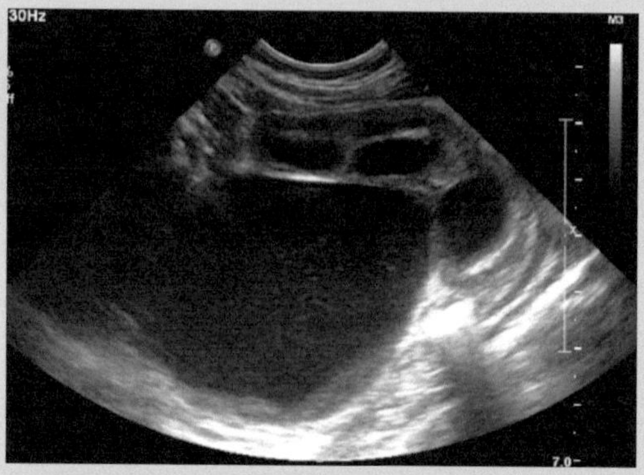

Fig. 11.1 Ultrasound appearance of severe left hydronephrosis and layering echogenic debris within the renal pelvis in a febrile neonate

An abdominal radiograph shows normal air gas pattern and no signs of intestinal obstruction. There is medial deviation of the left upper quadrant abdominal contents. An abdominal ultrasound was performed given concern over possible pyloric stenosis and there was no evidence of pyloric hypertrophy. There was severe left hydronephrosis and layering echogenic debris within the renal pelvis (Fig. 11.1). There was no left ureteral dilation. The right kidney and ureter were normal. The bladder was not distended. A catheterized urine specimen is sent for urinalysis and is without abnormality. A CBC shows a leukocyte count of 20,000. Serum creatinine is 0.3 mg/ dL.

The diagnosis of left ureteropelvic junction (UPJ) obstruction with obstructive pyelonephritis is made. IV fluid resuscitation is begun

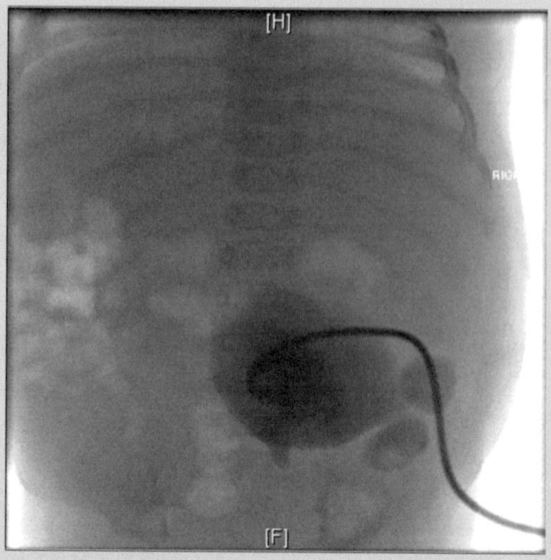

Fig. 11.2 Percutaneous nephrostogram performed at the time of urgent nephrostomy tube placement to treat obstructive pyelonephritis. This revealed high-grade UPJ obstruction that was treated with open pyeloplasty after successful treatment of infection

and broad-spectrum antibiotics administered. A percutaneous nephrostomy is placed which reveals high-grade UPJ obstruction and turbid fluid is drained (Fig. 11.2). The patient defervesces within 24 h of the procedure and is discharged home with nephrostomy tube to complete a 2-week course of antibiotics. A diagnostic nephrostogram confirms the initial findings of stenosis at the UPJ. He underwent a dismembered pyeloplasty 4 weeks after initial presentation. His surgery was uncomplicated; he made a full recovery and has done well without any recurrent clinical problems.

11.1 Introduction

Obstructive uropathy describes a condition where renal function has been adversely affected by impairment of flow of urine within the collecting system. This condition can be congenital, acquired, reversible, and irreversible. Peters proposed a similar definition for congenital urinary obstruction in children of "a condition of impaired urinary drainage which, if uncorrected, will limit the ultimate functional potential of a developing kidney" [33]. Obstructive uropathy is an important cause of end-stage renal disease in newborns and children [39]. Identification of obstruction and relief of it can minimize its deleterious effect on renal function. This seems obvious, however current clinical criteria, in the form of laboratory or radiographic investigations, to recognize this category of patients is challenging.

Table 11.1 Society of fetal urology hydronephrosis grading system

SFU grade	Central renal complex	Renal parenchymal thickness
Grade 1	Slight splitting	Normal
Grade 2	Evident splitting, complex confined within renal border	Normal
Grade 3	Wide splitting pelvis dilated outside renal border, calices dilated	Normal
Grade 4	Further dilatation of pelvis and calices	Thin

Contemporary congenital cases of obstructive uropathy are diagnosed based upon the widespread use of prenatal ultrasonography. Ultrasound abnormalities of the urinary tract have reportedly been detected in up to 4.5 % of prenatal ultrasounds performed [11, 16]. The majority of these radiographic anomalies are hydronephrosis [29]. The severity of the hydronephrosis can vary, and the Society of Fetal Urology (SFU) has developed a grading system (Table 11.1) [27]. Additional obstructive uropathies diagnosed based upon prenatal ultrasounds, besides hydronephrosis secondary to ureteropelvic junction (UPJ) obstruction, can be megaureters as a result of ureterovesical junction (UVJ) obstruction, ectopic ureter, or ureterocele.

The majority of prenatally detected urinary tract abnormalities will not require any surgical intervention [28]. However, there can be cases of prenatally detected unilateral or bilateral severe urinary tract dilation that can cause concern in the neonatal period where any intervention aside from observation may be appropriate.

11.2 Diagnosis

11.2.1 History

The initial step in the evaluation of the neonate with potential obstructive uropathy will be obtaining a prenatal history. If obstructive uropathy is suspected as a result of prenatal ultrasonography, there are important data variables from the ultrasound to guide in diagnosis and subsequent management of the neonate. Specifically answers to the following questions can be critical to arriving at the correct diagnosis and subsequent appropriate treatment:

- What is degree of dilation?
  Prenatal transverse anteroposterior (AP) renal pelvic diameter has predictive value in determining the likelihood of postnatal surgery. Fetuses with an AP renal pelvic diameter of greater than 20 mm have a greater than 90 % of intervention, whereas fetuses with a diameter less than 10 mm have low probability [9].
- Are one or both kidneys hydronephrotic?
  Bilateral hydronephrosis can obviously be more challenging because there is no contralateral "normal" kidney to perform compensatory renal function when a unilateral obstruction is present. However, bilateral hydronephrosis is not an absolute indication for operative intervention. Close monitoring urine output and serum creatinine is essential in the scenario of severe bilateral hydronephrosis as prompt intervention may be necessary.
- Is there associated ureteral dilation?
  Ureteral dilation may signify a transient physiologic process as a result of diuresis, vesicoureteral reflux, or obstruction. Neonatal ureteral obstruction is most commonly the result of the presence of a ureterovesical junction obstruction or ureterocele. A ureteral duplication can be seen and if seen usually associated with hydroureteronephrosis of the upper pole moiety as a result of a distal ureteral obstructive process such as ectopic ureter or ureterocele. However, a ureterocele can be observed in single or duplex collecting systems.

Knowledge of the sonographic appearance of the bladder is critical in interpreting the pathophysiology of the dilated ureter. For example, a distended bladder with accompanying ureteral dilation can be due to vesicoureteral reflux; however, obstruction can also be the cause. Conversely, an empty bladder does not rule out reflux to be the cause of the hydroureter unless the fetus voided shortly before image acquisition and the dilated ureter a result of refluxed urine from the bladder.

- What is the status of the bladder? Is it empty, thickened, and distended? Is an ureterocele identified?
  As stated in the previous section, knowledge of the bladder is crucial to correctly interpret the collecting system dilation. Bilateral hydroureteronephrosis with a distended and thickened bladder in a male fetus is highly compatible with a diagnosis of posterior urethral valves.
- What is the amniotic fluid volume? Is there oligohydramnios?
  Children with a history of oligohydramnios may have pulmonary difficulties as a result of poor lung development. Respiratory assistance is given as clinically indicated. A frequent etiology of oligohydramnios is renal dysplasia, and thus oligohydramnios can be a predictor of poor postnatal renal function in addition to poor lung function.

  A postnatal history of feeding intolerance may be related to severe hydronephrosis that can result in recurrent emesis from either direct compression of gastrointestinal tract or further distention of collecting system. In this uncommon neonatal scenario, a palpable mass is nearly universal. The neonate with an obstructed upper urinary tract can present with urinary tract infection manifested by fever, lethargy, and at times turbid fluid exiting the introitus of female representing infected urine.

11.2.2 Physical Examination

Inspection of the neonate will be the first portion of the physical examination. The infant with significant renal dysfunction as a result of an obstructive uropathy and accompanying oligohydramnios can result in labored breathing. Hydronephrosis can be appreciated as a palpable abdominal mass in severe cases as described in the previous section. An interlabial mass in the female may be a result of a prolapsed ureterocele (Fig. 11.3). Bladder outlet obstruction as a result of an ureterocele can result in bladder distension and a palpable suprapubic mass.

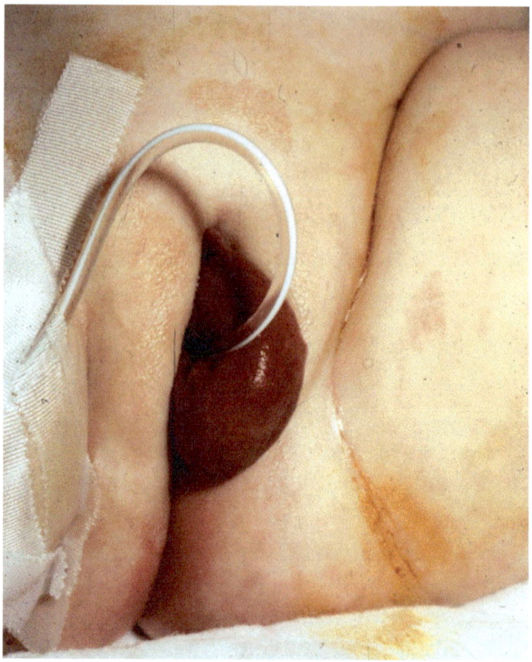

Fig. 11.3 Photograph of female neonate that presented with vomiting and interlabial mass secondary to vascular congested prolapsed ureterocele. The catheter is draining the bladder placed adjacent to the prolapsed ureterocele and reduction of the ureterocele with transurethral incision performed after adequate resuscitation

11.3 Imaging

A renal ultrasound is the preferred initial radiographic imaging test of choice to assess the urinary tract because of its widespread availability and lack of radiation. There is a physiologic degree of intravascular volume depletion in the immediate newborn period. Therefore, in certain cases of prenatally detected unilateral hydronephrosis, it is recommended to delay the initial postnatal ultrasound until at least 48 h to minimize false-negative findings or understaging which has been reported to occur in up to 44 % [44]. The severity of neonatal hydronephrosis and the appearance of the renal parenchyma are easily assessed using ultrasound and graded using the SFU grading system [27]. Differentiation of severe hydronephrosis from cystic dysplasia can be challenging at times, and additional imaging such as nuclear scan can clarify this. As outlined

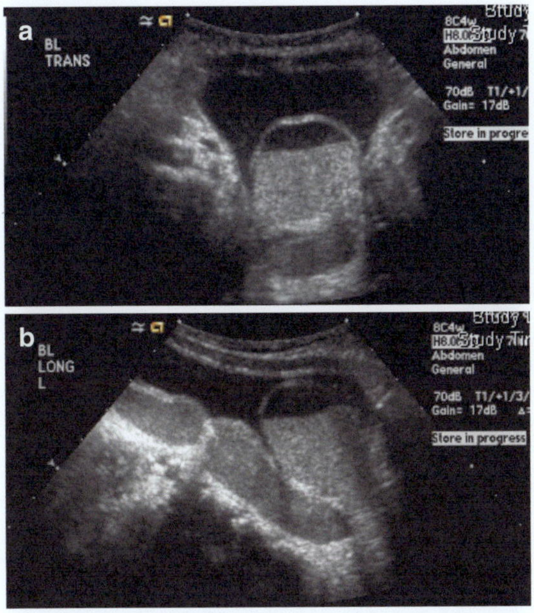

Fig. 11.4 (**a**) Transverse and (**b**) longitudinal ultrasound appearances of echogenic debris within an infected obstructed ureterocele

above it is essential to obtain images of the bladder as well as kidneys to determine if the bladder is distended, if a ureterocele is present, or if a dilated ureter is present. The neonate with an infected obstructed ureterocele can demonstrate hyperechoic debris on sonographic images of the bladder (Fig. 11.4). The ureterocele found with a duplex system is associated with the upper pole, and the renal parenchyma can have a cystic dysplastic appearance on ultrasound which may help determine if extirpative or reconstructive surgical approach is selected.

A voiding cystourethrogram (VCUG) is mandatory in cases of megaureter to exclude the presence of vesicoureteral reflux (VUR). However, there is the scenario of an obstructed, refluxing megaureter where both processes can be present and beneficial to know prior to treatment. Identification of coexistent VUR and excluding urethral anomalies is another reason to perform VCUG.

Nuclear imaging renogram provides valuable information with respect to differential function of the kidneys. A decision to intervene may be based upon decreased differential function of the hydronephrotic renal unit and concern that the hydronephrosis may be a result of significant obstruction. Diuretic renography is an extremely useful imaging investigation to discern whether a dilated collecting system is a result of an obstructed or nonobstructed process. Hydrational status of the patient, urethral catheterization, the timing of diuretic, dosage of diuretic, and data analysis can all affect the results or interpretation of the renogram. Therefore, the SFU has proposed the "well-tempered" renogram to standardize the procedure in an attempt to minimize these technical variables and create a uniform [8].

Due to their dependence on glomerular filtration, radionucleotide tracers have been deemed to be unreliable in the neonatal period due to immature renal function, a reduced glomerular filtration rate, and reduced responsiveness to a diuretic stimulus. Several investigators have assessed the reliability of a diuretic renogram in the neonatal period. Chung et al. found that in 17 neonates that underwent diuretic renal scans and followed clinically [7], there was no statistically significant difference between neonatal and follow-up differential function and response to diuretic stimulation revealed no statistically significant difference as the patients aged. Similarly the mean drainage times for normal non-hydronephrotic kidneys were similar when comparing those performed as neonates and at follow-up. The authors concluded to refute each of the criticisms against the use of diuretic renography to evaluate neonatal hydronephrosis and demonstrate its reliability in neonates. While maturation of the glomerular filtration takes several weeks, delaying the diuretic renogram, when clinically appropriate, may eliminate any confounding variables. However, the renogram should not be delayed when its results will impact the clinician's decision to intervene based on possibly diminished differential function that could be ameliorated with relief of obstruction.

Percutaneous antegrade pyeloureterography is helpful to define the anatomy, however mandates the use of sedation or general anesthetic to be safely performed. The length of stenotic segment can be accurately delineated prior to embarking upon operative intervention with either retrograde ureteropyelography or antegrade nephrostogram.

11.4 Treatment

The hydronephrotic kidney or dilated ureter is a radiographic finding that must be interpreted to determine whether a surgical procedure is appropriate. These imaging results are not absolute indications for intervention. A simple classification scheme of collecting system dilation would be obstructing or nonobstructing. Unfortunately in the clinical setting, this classification scheme is not this dichotomous or simplistic. The "holy grail" of urology is identifying the neonate with asymptomatic urinary tract dilation who will benefit from intervention with respect to limiting, or improving, renal function as a result of correcting the obstruction from those patients that will not benefit.

Unilateral ureteral obstruction during early development in the experimental setting has been shown to result in impaired growth and development of the kidney [6, 35]. Experimentally, relief of the obstruction has been shown to attenuate, but unfortunately not reverse the observed decrease in number of nephrons in the affected renal unit [5]. Clinically a similar lack of significant improvement in differential renal function following pyeloplasty has also been shown to be true [26, 30].

11.4.1 Nonoperative Management of Hydronephrosis

The observation of similar preoperative and postoperative differential renal function has led many to advocate for an observational approach to the management of neonatal hydronephrosis as there appears to be limited "recoverable" function. Proponents of this surveillance strategy publish their experience in nonoperative treatment and have shown that approximately 75 % of neonates with history of prenatal hydronephrosis will not require immediate or any surgery [18, 42]. There is an essential requirement for regular follow-up when embarking upon an observational protocol. During this observational period, renal ultrasound and diuretic renograms are used to identify as early as possible of renal deterioration reflected as either progression of hydronephrosis or decreasing differential function, respectively. Prompt surgical intervention is necessary for these signs of deterioration to prevent progressive deterioration and potentially restore function.

11.4.2 Nonoperative Management of Hydroureteronephrosis

Similar principles apply to the management of antenatally detected dilated ureter as are applied to the management of hydronephrosis. Initial attempts at observation can be entertained when clinically appropriate. Several reports have shown that resolution of the hydroureteronephrosis and/or avoidance of surgery can be expected in up to 80 % of patients whose megaureters were identified prenatally [4, 31]. According to Lee et al. the risk of urinary tract infection during the first year of life is higher in cases of obstructive hydroureteronephrosis (47 %) compared to obstructive hydronephrosis (13 %) [25]. Periodic renal ultrasound and diuretic renograms are once again used to identify signs of renal deterioration reflected as either progression of hydronephrosis or decreasing differential function, with surgical intervention enacted swiftly.

The patient who has a megaureter associated with an ureterocele is also a candidate for a nonoperative approach [10, 13]. Ureteroceles with nonobstructed duplex systems have better preservation of renal function and a high rate of natural resolution of hydronephrosis and reflux. Ureteroceles associated with MCD or completely nonfunctioning upper pole moieties may never require surgical management.

11.4.3 Operative Management of Hydronephrosis Without Hydroureter

In the neonate with severe hydronephrosis secondary to UPJ obstruction and decreased differential renal function is a clinical situation that warrants serious consideration of surgical correction. Pyeloplasty can be safely performed in the neonatal period; however, deferring the procedure may decrease the risk of general anesthesia as the child continues to mature from a cardiovascular and pulmonary perspective. Success rates and the incidence of complications have not been reported to be higher when the pyeloplasty has been performed in the neonatal period compared to when the child is older [19, 21]. Hanna commented that frequently encountered wide caliber of the neonatal ureter below the UPJ may contribute to a technically easier pyeloplasty to perform relative to the older child where the ureteral diameter is not as wide [14]. Surgical complications of urine leak, persistent/recurrent obstruction have been reported to be less than 5 % of patients undergoing open pyeloplasty in modern series [2, 38].

At times the differential function of the hydronephrotic obstructed kidney may reveal extremely poor function, 10 % or less. Management of the kidney with UPJ obstruction and associated poor function in the neonate is controversial and options include reconstruction or removal of the affected kidney. Reconstruction becomes a viable alternative because of reports of significant increase in differential renal function with relief of the obstruction [1, 12, 43]. Percutaneous nephrostomy tube placement is an easy and effective means to decompress the kidney and assessing the kidney's function devoid of obstruction while avoiding the risks of a potentially ineffective pyeloplasty. Gupta et al. described their experience of placing percutaneous nephrostomy in 20 patients who presented with UPJ obstruction and a split differential renal function of less than 10 % [12]. The nephrostomy tube remained in situ for at least 4 weeks and renography repeated 4 weeks after decompression. If no improvement in the split renal function had occurred, nephrectomy was performed; otherwise, pyeloplasty was performed. Twelve of 17 kidneys with unilateral UPJO improved after PCN drainage and underwent pyeloplasty with the split differential renal function increasing to 29 % from baseline where all kidneys were ≤10 %.

The scenario of infection and urinary tract obstruction is a potentially lethal one and merits emergent treatment. Decompression of the obstructed renal pelvis in the form of percutaneous nephrostomy tube is the most expeditious technique to achieve relief of the obstruction [23, 41]. Broad-spectrum intravenous antibiotics and aggressive intravenous resuscitation are essential components to proper treatment to minimize the systemic effects of this serious infection.

11.4.4 Operative Management of Hydroureteronephrosis

11.4.4.1 Operative Management of Primary Obstructed Megaureter in the Neonate

Once again similar principles apply to the clinical decision-making process on whether surgery is necessary for cases of obstructed megaureter. Accepted indications for immediate intervention include the presence of symptoms or infection, whereas poor drainage and decreased renal function can reasonably be initially observed. Operative treatment options are more numerous with an isolated distal obstructive process compared to obstruction at the level of the UPJ.

Definitive surgical treatment of primary obstructed megaureters typically involves ureteral reimplantation, which is technically challenging in the neonate because of the significant size discrepancy between the dilated distal ureter, small bladder template, and need for ureteral tailoring [34]. Cutaneous ureterostomy is an effective method of alleviating the distal obstruction and allowing the neonate to grow to adequate size while awaiting definitive reconstruction at a later time. End cutaneous ureterostomy has been used and can minimize the need for ureteral tailoring in subsequent ureteral reimplantation in approximately 75 % of cases [20, 36]. Loop cutaneous ureterostomy is another surgical technique performed through a Gibson incision that does not disturb the distal ureteral anatomy near the ureterovesical junction [32].

Surgical complications of ureterostomy include stomal stenosis and inadequate drainage. The incidence of stomal stenosis following end cutaneous ureterostomy has been reported to occur more frequently than loop cutaneous ureterostomy because of the division of the ureter from the bladder with end ureterostomy. Kaefer and colleagues have proposed an alternative surgical treatment strategy that simultaneously avoids the problem of stomal stenosis while addressing the distal ureteral obstruction with the creation of an intentional refluxing ureteral reimplant as an internal diversion of the primary obstructed megaureter [17, 24]. The definitive non-refluxing ureteral reimplantation is deferred until after the child is older than 1 year and is maintained on daily antibiotic prophylaxis for high-grade reflux. Kaefer described this technique in 10 children who underwent surgery at 2 months of age with all patients demonstrating improved drainage postoperatively. Five patients have subsequently undergone uncomplicated ureteral reimplantation with the remainder awaiting reconstruction.

11.4.4.2 Operative Management of Primary Obstructed Ureterocele in the Neonate

Ureteroceles can be associated with either single or duplicated ureteral collecting system. The ureterocele that is obstructed and non-refluxing can adversely affect the renal function of the moiety it is associated with. Presenting symptoms of an infected ureterocele can be fever, lethargy, and even sepsis. Emergent decompression in the form of transurethral incision is preferable as this avoids the challenges of maintaining a percutaneous nephrostomy tube in the neonate. A low transverse incision achieves decompression while minimizing the risk of de novo vesicoureteral reflux [37, 40]. However, there may be technical challenges of transurethral instrumentation in the patient population with the smallest commercially available resectoscope being too large for the male neonatal urethra. In this circumstance percutaneous drainage of the obstructed renal moiety is always an alternative method of drainage in the septic patient to eliminate causing iatrogenic injury to the urethra.

The obstructed ureterocele associated with ureteral duplication can be unobstructed by performing ipsilateral ureteroureterostomy [3, 22]. The ureteroureterostomy can be performed either proximally or distally. The advantage of performing an ipsilateral ureteroureterostomy is avoiding operating on the small bladder of the neonate or infant while eliminating the need for ureteral tailoring and its attendant operative risks. The ability to treat bladder pathology in the older through the same incision is one advantage of a distal, or low, ureteroureterostomy compared to a proximal ureteroureterostomy. Surgical complications include urine leak, persistent obstruction of the hydronephrotic upper pole moiety, or de novo obstruction of the lower pole ureter. The success rate of this type of "upper tract" approach as a single procedure for the successful treatment of obstructed ureterocele has been reported to range from 100 to 4 % in one study [15]. The presence of high-grade reflux into one moiety or vesicoureteral reflux into more than one moiety, regardless of the grade of reflux, was strongly associated with the need for further surgery.

Conclusion

Neonatal hydronephrosis and hydroureter is diverse spectrum that poses significant diagnostic dilemma for the clinician. The overwhelming majority of these patients are asymptomatic with a partial obstruction. Differentiating between the children who benefit from aggressive surgical intervention from those patients that may experience spontaneous resolution and observation appropriate is inadequate based upon current diagnostic imaging modalities.

However, when the patient has been diagnosed with obstructive uropathy, there should be no delay in seeking relief of the obstructive process and minimize its deleterious effects on kidney function regardless of the patient's age. A variety of methods to decompress the hydronephrotic collecting system exist each with their advantages and disadvantages. Temporary urinary diversion may be indicated prior to pursuing more definitive surgical reconstruction based upon the clinical scenario.

References

1. Audry G, Boyer C, Grapin C et al (1996) The value of split renal function in severe neonatal and infant pelviureteric obstruction managed by percutaneous nephrostomy. Eur J Pediatr Surg 6:274–276
2. Chacko JK, Koyle MA, Mingin GC et al (2006) The minimally invasive open pyeloplasty. J Pediatr Urol 2:368–372
3. Chacko JK, Koyle MA, Mingin GC et al (2007) Ipsilateral ureteroureterostomy in the surgical management of the severely dilated ureter in ureteral duplication. J Urol 178:1689–1692
4. Chertin B, Pollack A, Koulikov D et al (2008) Long-term follow up of antenatally diagnosed megaureters. J Pediatr Urol 4:188–191
5. Chevalier RL, Kim A, Thornhill BA et al (1999) Recovery following relief of unilateral ureteral obstruction in the neonatal rat. Kidney Int. 55: 793–807
6. Chung KH, Chevalier RL (1996) Arrested development of the neonatal kidney following chronic ureteral obstruction. J Urol 155:1139–1144
7. Chung S, Majd M, Rushton HG et al (1993) Diuretic renography in the evaluation of neonatal hydronephrosis: is it reliable? J Urol 150:765–768
8. Conway JJ, Maizels M (1992) The "well tempered" diuretic renogram: a standard method to examine the asymptomatic neonate with hydronephrosis or hydroureteronephrosis. A report from combined meetings of The Society for Fetal Urology and members of The Pediatric Nuclear Medicine Council – The Society of Nuclear Medicin. J Nucl Med 33:2047–2051
9. Dhillon HK (1998) Prenatally diagnosed hydronephrosis: the Great Ormond Street experience. Br J Urol 81:39–44
10. Direnna T, Leonard MP (2006) Watchful waiting for prenatally detected ureteroceles. J Urol 175: 1493–1495
11. Dremsek PA, Gindi K, Voitl P et al (1997) Renal pyelectasis in fetuses and neonates: diagnostic value of renal pelvis diameter in pre- and postnatal sonographic screening. AJR Am J Roentgenol 168:1017–1019
12. Gupta DK, Chandrasekharam VV, Srinivas M et al (2001) Percutaneous nephrostomy in children with ureteropelvic junction obstruction and poor renal function. Urology 57:547–550
13. Han MY, Gibbons MD, Belman AB et al (2005) Indications for nonoperative management of ureteroceles. J Urol 174:1652–1655
14. Hanna MK (2000) Antenatal hydronephrosis and ureteropelvic junction obstruction: the case for early intervention. Urology 55:612–615
15. Husmann DA, Ewalt DH, Glenski WJ et al (1995) Ureterocele associated with ureteral duplication and a nonfunctioning upper pole segment: management by partial nephroureterectomy alone. J Urol 154: 723–726
16. Ismaili K, Hall M, Donner C et al (2003) Results of systematic screening for minor degrees of fetal renal pelvis dilatation in an unselected population. Am J Obstet Gynecol 188:242–246
17. Kaefer M (2008) The refluxing ureteral reimplant: an ideal method for avoiding cutaneous ureterostomy in cases of obstructed megaureter. Presented at the American Academy of Pediatrics, Boston, Massachusetts (Abstract)
18. Karnak I, Woo LL, Shah SN et al (2009) Results of a practical protocol for management of prenatally detected hydronephrosis due to ureteropelvic junction obstruction. Pediatr Surg Int 25:61–67
19. King LR, Coughlin PW, Bloch EC et al (1984) The case for immediate pyeloplasty in the neonate with ureteropelvic junction obstruction. J Urol 132: 725–728
20. Kitchens DM, DeFoor W, Minevich E et al (2007) End cutaneous ureterostomy for the management of severe hydronephrosis. J Urol 177:1501–1504
21. Koyle MA, Ehrlich RM (1988) Management of ureteropelvic junction obstruction in neonate. Urology 31:496–498
22. Lashley DB, McAleer IM, Kaplan GW (2001) Ipsilateral ureteroureterostomy for the treatment of vesicoureteral reflux or obstruction associated with complete ureteral duplication. J Urol 165:552–554
23. Laurin S, Sandström S, Ivarsson H (2000) Percutaneous nephrostomy in infants and children. Acad Radiol 7:526–529
24. Lee SD, Akbal C, Kaefer M (2005) Refluxing ureteral reimplant as temporary treatment of obstructive megaureter in neonate and infant. J Urol 173: 1357–1360
25. Lee JH, Choi HS, Kim JK et al (2008) Nonrefluxing neonatal hydronephrosis and the risk of urinary tract infection. J Urol 179:1524–1528
26. MacNeily AE, Maizels M, Kaplan WE et al (1993) Does early pyeloplasty really avert loss of renal function? A retrospective review. J Urol 150:769–773
27. Maizels M, Reisman ME, Flom LS et al (1992) Grading nephroureteral dilatation detected in the first year of life: correlation with obstruction. J Urol 148: 609–614
28. Maizels M, Mitchell B, Kass E et al (1994) Outcome of nonspecific hydronephrosis in the infant: a report from the Registry of the Society for Fetal Urology. J Urol 152:2324–2327
29. Mandell J, Blyth BR, Peters CA et al (1991) Structural genitourinary defects detected in utero. Radiology 178:193–196
30. McAleer IM, Kaplan GW (1999) Renal function before and after pyeloplasty: does it improve? J Urol 1999(162):1041–1044
31. McLellan DL, Retik AB, Bauer SB et al (2002) Rate and predictors of spontaneous resolution of prenatally diagnosed primary nonrefluxing megaureter. J Urol 168:2177–2180

32. Mor Y, Ramon J, Raviv G et al (1992) Low loop cutaneous ureterostomy and subsequent reconstruction: 20 years of experience. J Urol 147(6):1595–1597
33. Peters CA (1995) Urinary tract obstruction in children. J Urol 154:1874–1883
34. Peters CA, Mandell J, Lebowitz RL et al (1989) Congenital obstructed megaureters in early infancy: diagnosis and treatment. J Urol 142:641
35. Peters CA, Carr MC, Lais A et al (1992) The response of the fetal kidney to obstruction. J Urol 148:503–509
36. Rabinowitz R, Barkin M, Schillinger JF et al (1977) Surgical treatment of the massively dilated ureter in children. Part I. Management by cutaneous ureterostomy. J Urol 117:658
37. Rich MA, Keating MA, Snyder HM III et al (1990) Low transurethral incision of single system intravesical ureteroceles in children. J Urol 144:120–121
38. Salem YH, Majd M, Rushton HG et al (1995) Outcome analysis of pediatric pyeloplasty as a function of patient age, presentation and differential renal function. J Urol 154:1889–1893
39. Seikaly MG, Ho PL, Emmett L et al (2003) Chronic renal insufficiency in children: the 2001 Annual Report of the NAPRTCS. Pediatr Nephrol 18: 796–804
40. Tank ES (1986) Experience with endoscopic incision and open unroofing of ureteroceles. J Urol 136: 241–242
41. vanSonnenberg E, Wittich GR, Edwards DK et al (1987) Percutaneous diagnostic and therapeutic interventional radiologic procedures in children: experience in 100 patients. Radiology 162:601–605
42. Ulman I, Jayanthi VR, Koff SA (2000) The long-term follow-up of newborns with severe unilateral hydronephrosis initially treated nonoperatively. J Urol 164: 1101–1105
43. Wagner M, Mayr J, Häcker FM (2008) Improvement of renal split function in hydronephrosis with less than 10 % function. Eur J Pediatr Surg 18:156–159
44. Wiener JS, O'Hara SM (2002) Optimal timing of initial postnatal ultrasonography in newborns with prenatal hydronephrosis. J Urol 168:1826

Structural Anomalies of the Bladder and External Genitalia

12

Lauren N. Hendrix and Ali M. Ziada

12.1 Introduction

Genitourinary tract anomalies are some of the most common forms of congenital anomalies. A thorough appreciation of embryology as well as sexual differentiation is imperative to understanding these disease processes and their related assessment and management techniques. The scope of these anomalies and the manner in which they present is vast; therefore, we have attempted to present these disease processes in a concise yet comprehensive manner. The underlying common theme is the goal of the practitioner to provide refunctionalization of the urinary tract and/or genitalia in these patients.

12.2 Bladder Anomalies

Genitourinary anomalies are commonly diagnosed in the perinatal period, but congenital bladder anomalies are relatively rare. Usually these anomalies are caused by outlet obstruction or are part of a more serious syndrome. When detected prenatally, these anomalies are usually separated into dilated or nondilated anomalies.

L.N. Hendrix, MD
Division of Urology, University of KY,
Lexington, KY 40536, USA

A.M. Ziada, MD (✉)
Pediatric Urology, University of Kentucky
Medical Center, 740 South Limestone Street,
Suite B 219, Lexington, KY 40536, USA
e-mail: ali.ziada@uky.edu

12.2.1 Dilated Bladder Anomalies

The presence of a large or dilated bladder usually suggests either a functional or mechanical outlet obstruction. Examples of obstructive causes of dilation include posterior urethral valves, urethral atresia, or other causes of extrinsic obstruction. Nonobstructive causes of a dilated bladder might be neurologic disorders in which the patient is unable to empty the bladder and congenital megacystis in which vesicoureteral reflux and continuous cycling of urine between the upper and lower tracts causes bladder dilation [1].

12.2.2 Nondilated Bladder Anomalies

Cloacal and bladder exstrophy result in the nonvisualization of the bladder in a fetus due to incomplete closure of the bladder template [2]. This can be distinguished from bladder hypoplasia by the presence of normal levels of amniotic fluid. Bladder hypoplasia can be due to a number of causes including bypass of urine due to ureteral ectopia, abnormalities of kidney development with decreased urine production, or decreased bladder outlet resistance such as in severe epispadias. Complete bladder agenesis is extremely rare; there have been only 60 reported cases in English literature [3]. This is incompatible with life unless the ureters are drained ectopically [4].

A.S. Chishti et al. (eds.), *Kidney and Urinary Tract Diseases in the Newborn*,
DOI 10.1007/978-3-642-39988-6_12, © Springer-Verlag Berlin Heidelberg 2014

12.2.3 Other Bladder Anomalies

Other bladder anomalies that are detected postnatally are usually compatible with life and only detected incidentally. Congenital bladder diverticula are herniations of the bladder mucosa between defects in the smooth muscle fibers [5]. They may be caused by bladder outlet obstruction or congenital defects. Most diverticula are asymptomatic, so the true incidence is difficult to determine [6]. However, patients with symptomatic diverticula and associated genitourinary dysfunction such as vesicoureteral reflux should undergo surgical intervention.

Bladder and urethral duplication can occur as complete or incomplete and may be associated with duplications of the external genitalia and gastrointestinal tract [7].

12.2.4 Urachal Anomalies

The urachus serves as a form of bladder drainage through the umbilical cord that obliterates prior to birth in normal development. The urachus is a tubular structure that extends from the dome of the bladder to the anterior abdominal wall and is flanked by the umbilical arteries on either side. When this structure fails to obliterate, one of four anomalies occurs based on the extent of failed obliteration to include the following: patent urachus, umbilical-urachal sinus, urachal cyst, or vesicourachal diverticulum [8]. Males tend to outnumber females, from 1.2:1 to 2:1 [9, 10].

A completely patent urachus presents with drainage from the umbilicus, delayed cord stump healing, or an erythematous cord stump [11]. Ultrasound can support this diagnosis by identifying a fluid-filled structure from the dome of the bladder to the level of the cord stump. A patent urachus may also present with infection or abscess – the most common organisms being *Staphylococcus aureus, Escherichia coli, Enterococcus, Citrobacter,* and *Proteus* [9]. A patent urachus should be treated with surgical excision with the addition of antibiotic coverage if it is associated with infection.

An umbilical-urachal sinus occurs when the urachus obliterates at the level of the bladder but remains patent at the umbilicus resulting in a continuously draining sinus. This must be differentiated from a fully patent urachus, usually done with ultrasonography. The treatment is surgical excision [8].

A urachal cyst is comprised of a portion of urachus that remains tubularized without connection to either the bladder or the umbilicus. This cyst can intermittently drain into the bladder or the umbilicus and may present as an umbilical abscess or a UTI. If left unrecognized, an infected urachal cyst can perforate into the peritoneal cavity, causing peritonitis [12]. Again, ultrasonography is used for diagnosis, but may require other imaging such as CT or MRI in older patients to better evaluate the extent of the disease. Traditional treatment entails initial surgical drainage and antibiotics with subsequent surgical excision of the entire urachal remnant [13].

A vesicourachal diverticulum occurs when the urachus obliterates almost completely with the exception of a portion near the bladder dome. Typically, these lesions are asymptomatic as they tend to have a wide neck that prevents stone formation or infection from occurring within the diverticulum. They are usually diagnosed incidentally on radiographic imaging for other purposes. There is no need for intervention for this particular finding unless the patient is symptomatic, such as with development of infection or stones within a small-necked diverticulum [14].

12.3 Neuropathic Bladder

12.3.1 Myelomeningocele

Myelomeningocele is the most common of all myelodysplasias or spinal dysraphisms in children and is the most common cause of neuropathic bladder dysfunction in children [14]. Development of the spinal canal begins on the 18th day of gestation and closes in a caudad to cephalad fashion, complete by day 35. Mesoderm in-growth over the developing spinal cord is necessary for closure of the canal; otherwise, an open lesion is noted, most often in the lumbosacral area with decreasing incidence in the thoracic and cervical regions [15].

Neural injury and associated lower urinary tract dysfunction are related to an exposed spinal cord and tension on the spinal cord as the spinal cord comes to its final location in the canal during fetal development [16]. The conus medullaris is almost always involved due to the high relative incidence of lumbar and lumbosacral defects [15]; therefore, nerve roots originating from this area that would normally innervate the bladder are almost always involved and cause varying degrees of dysfunction. Other related features that may affect urologic management include the following: hydrocephalus, paralysis/mobility, and spinal deformities [15].

Hydrocephalus is a typical finding in these patients, with severity directly correlated to the extent of spinal cord involvement. More pronounced intellectual disabilities tend to go hand-in-hand with more pronounced physical disabilities. Patients with severe disabilities often lack the physical capabilities and cognitive skills necessary to perform clean intermittent catheterization (CIC) or deploy an artificial urinary sphincter, thereby precluding these common interventions and introducing challenges for caregivers. Spinal deformity such as kyphoscoliosis and mobility limitations must also be taken into consideration for planning of long-term management strategies. Fortunately, the trend toward early closure of the spinal defect has recently been demonstrated to decrease the incidence of hydrocephalus and may improve neurologic function in patients with myelomeningoceles [16].

12.3.1.1 Assessment

The bony spinal lesion is not predictive of the extent of the spinal cord lesion and resultant neurologic and lower extremity dysfunction [17], so thorough neonatal assessment is imperative. Renal ultrasonography and measurement of post-void residual urine are assessed as early as possible. If the patient demonstrates inability to empty satisfactorily or has evidence of upper tract deterioration such as loss of kidney parenchyma, CIC should be initiated [18]. A serum creatinine, urinalysis, and culture should also be obtained [15].

Urodynamic studies (UDS) and voiding cystourethrogram (VCUG) are delayed until the spinal defect has been closed, and it is prudent to transport the patient and position him or her appropriately for the study [19]. These studies provide vast amounts of information including radiologic appearance of the upper and lower urinary tracts, identification of patients at risk for renal impairment due to bladder dysfunction, or outflow obstruction. They also provide anatomic and functional baselines to which future studies can be compared. As high as 15–20 % of patients have abnormal GU tract radiologic findings, usually due to spinal shock or bladder outlet obstruction [14]. UDS provide information about bladder and urethral sphincter function that may categorize patients as having either high or low risk for upper tract deterioration.

12.3.1.2 Management

As previously mentioned, CIC is an essential component of GU tract management in a significant number of patients with neuropathic bladders. Indications include detrusor muscle-external urethral sphincter dyssynergia, elevated bladder pressures, and/or grade III or higher vesicoureteral reflux [14]. This intervention has been shown to prevent upper tract deterioration, provides continence in a majority of patients, and reduces the need for bladder augmentation [20].

In patients with vesicoureteral reflux (VUR) secondary to high bladder pressures from neuropathic dysfunction, CIC lowers intravesical voiding pressures. When coupled with anticholinergic pharmacotherapy, this can serve to lower detrusor filling pressures and increases bladder compliance which may result in resolution of reflux [20].

The goal of therapy is to maintain bladder stability as well as stable renal function via adequate bladder capacity, a compliant detrusor muscle, periodic emptying at a low pressure, and continence. When this cannot be achieved by CIC and anticholinergic medications, a variety of surgical procedures are available to meet specific needs as follows:

- Failure to perform CIC due to body habitus, mobility issues, discomfort, or anatomic concerns – surgical creation of a catheterizable channel or vesicostomy on the lower abdomen.
- Detrusor noncompliance or impaired/high-pressure bladder capacity – bladder augmentation (reserved for refractory cases in older patients).
- Conduit urinary diversions are no longer the first-line surgical in managing these patients and are reserved for severely debilitated patients or those who have failed other modalities.

12.3.2 Spina Bifida Occulta

Occult spinal dysraphism, or spina bifida occulta, is a group of congenital defects of spinal column formation that do not result in an open defect. These make up about 10 % of all congenital spinal dysraphisms and include tethered cord, lipomeningocele, diastematomyelia, and intraspinal cysts [21]. A majority of these patients have a normal neurologic exam in the neonatal period, but may later develop signs of neurologic impairment such as gait abnormalities, decreased perineal sensation, voiding dysfunction, or back pain during periods of rapid growth. An underlying spinal cord defect is often signaled by a cutaneous lesion such as a dimple, tuft of hair, or abnormal gluteal cleft in 90 % of these patients [22].

Forty to ninety percent of spina bifida occulta patients have some variety of voiding dysfunction on urodynamic testing [14, 23]. The defect may be of upper or lower motor neuron origin or a combination of the two. Early detection with MRI and early intervention allow reversal or at least stabilization of the lesion.

12.3.3 Sacral Agenesis

Sacral agenesis is defined as the absence of two or more vertebral bodies and is often associated with a variety of anorectal anomalies. Evaluation of the bony spine, and spinal cord if indicated, should therefore be performed in any patient with anorectal malformations or if clinical suspicion exists, e.g., patients with buttock wasting, especially in infants of diabetic mothers or mothers with gestational diabetes. The extent of vertebral deformity is not predictive of the spinal cord lesion or associated voiding dysfunction, and a reported 25 % of these children have no signs of neurologic dysfunction on urodynamic testing [24]. However, 35 and 40 % show an upper or lower motor neuron deficit, respectively [24]. In these patients, upper tract imaging and cystography are indicated, especially in the setting of a history of urinary tract infections. Management depends on the neurologic deficit with goals of protecting renal function and achieving appropriate quality of life endpoints such as continence.

12.4 Exstrophy-Epispadias Complex

The exstrophy-epispadias complex is a spectrum of abnormalities thought to arise from maldevelopment of the lower abdominal wall during the early part of gestation that includes the following:

- Bladder exstrophy – open bladder plate (always associated with a bifid clitoris in females and an epispadic urethra in both sexes)
- Cloacal exstrophy – both the bladder and bowel are open plates on the low abdominal wall
- Primary penile epispadias – partial or complete open plate of the urethra on the dorsal surface of the penis, comprised of three subtypes based on location of the opening of the urethra without associated exstrophy:
  - Glandular epispadias – opening is located distally on the glans penis.
  - Penile epispadias – opening is located at any location on the shaft of the penis.
  - Pubic or penopubic epispadias – opening is located at the junction of the base of the penis and the abdominal wall.

These are relatively rare defects, with incidence of each as follows: 1 in 10,000 to 1 in 50,000 for bladder exstrophy; 1 in 120,000 for primary epispadias; and 1 in 300,000 for cloacal exstrophy [25, 26]. It occurs predominantly in males, with a reported male to female ratio from 2:1 to 6:1 [25, 27]. This condition represents a challenge to pediatric urologists given its low incidence and complex surgery needed to correct bladder and genital deformities.

There are many hypotheses regarding the etiology and embryologic defects that occurs to cause exstrophy. Current theories include failure of migration of mesoderm to the cloacal membrane [28], persistence of the cloacal membrane [29], and failure of the lateral body wall folds to meet in the midline [30]. There appears to be a familial component as the risk of bladder exstrophy in the offspring of a parent with exstrophy is about 1 in 100 [31]. Other theories regarding the etiology of exstrophy such as genetic defects and perinatal exposure are currently being explored [32, 33].

Prenatal diagnosis is possible as early as 18 weeks' gestation with fetal ultrasound. Sonographic features include inability to visualize urine in the fetal bladder, a bulging bladder plate or an apparent lower abdominal mass, a foreshortened penis, widening of the pubic ramus, and a low-set umbilicus [2]. These defects can easily be confused with other abdominal wall defects such as omphalocele or gastroschisis, but the use of 3D ultrasonography and MRI has improved diagnostic accuracy. The importance of prenatal diagnosis is for parental counseling and possible preparation for delivery at a specialized exstrophy center to allow for timely surgical intervention.

12.4.1 Bladder Exstrophy

Classic bladder exstrophy is exposure of the bladder plate and urethra beneath a low-set umbilicus. Associated maldeveloped structures include split rectus abdominis muscles, an open pelvic ring or pubic diastasis, and a foreshortened penis or bifid clitoris as the corporal bodies must traverse the pubic diastasis to meet in the midline (Fig. 12.1a, b). In males, testes are usually in a normal scrotal position, but the anus may be located

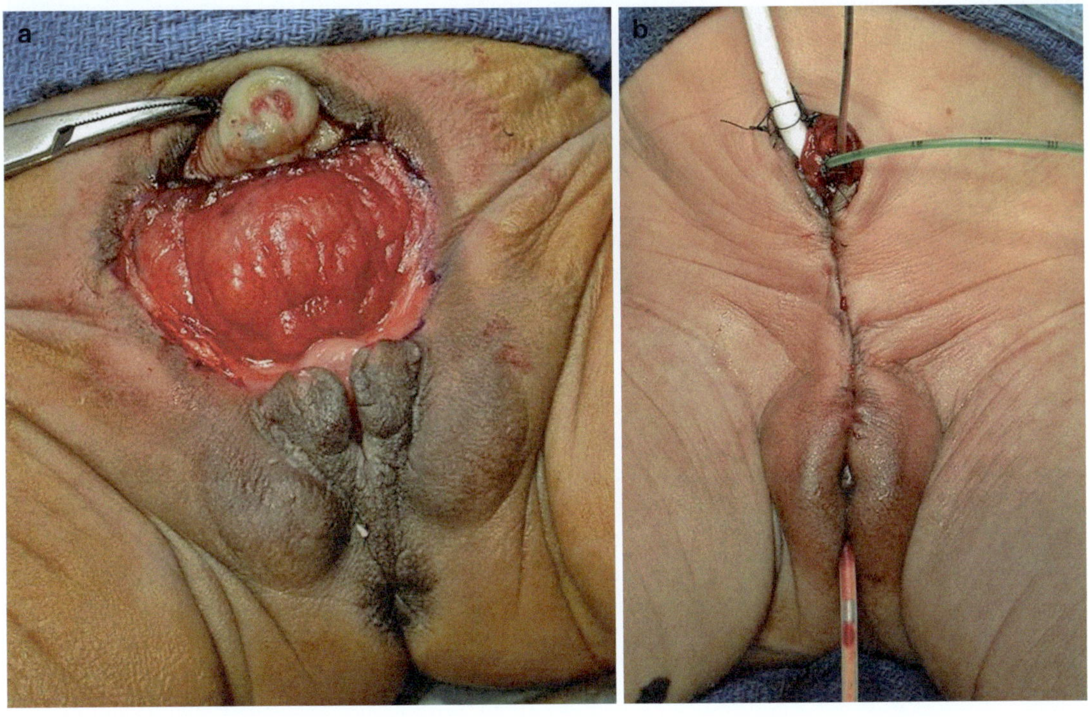

Fig. 12.1 (**a**) Bladder exstrophy and epispadias in a female. Note the exposed bladder plate and bifid clitoris. (**b**) The same patient after exstrophy closure

more anteriorly due to failure of development of both the lower abdominal wall and pelvic ring.

There are typically few associated anomalies with the exception of inguinal hernia, which occurs in up to 80 % of boys and 15 % of girls [34]. These babies are usually born full term without many significant medical comorbidities, so emergent surgical intervention is usually not warranted. However, timing of bladder closure is controversial, with some advocating immediate closure and others advocating delayed closure based on findings that later closure does not negatively affect overall bladder growth rates [35].

12.4.2 Cloacal Exstrophy

Unlike classic bladder exstrophy and epispadias, children born with cloacal exstrophy are often born prematurely and may be affected by the following associated anomalies: sacral agenesis or spinal dysraphism with related neurologic findings, cyanotic heart disease, renal agenesis or ectopia, orthopedic deformities of the lower extremities and pelvis, and small bowel defects such as malrotation or duodenal atresia [35]. Children born with cloacal exstrophy should have thorough evaluation to identify these possible comorbidities. Repair of life-threatening deformities such as cardiovascular or bowel defects may necessitate delay of exstrophy repair. In this case, the bladder and/or bowel plates are protected from desiccation or injury by cling wrap, and the umbilical stump is tied off to avoid trauma from clamps.

Severe genital deformities in males with cloacal exstrophy have historically presented a difficult challenge to both parents and pediatric urologists. If the genitalia could not be reconstructed to a functional and cosmetically acceptable male form, patients were assigned to female gender. In this case, they would also undergo simultaneous bilateral orchidectomy with vaginoplasty at a later date. Newer surgical techniques allow for better approximation of the corporal bodies in penile reconstruction, reducing the need for gender reassignment [36].

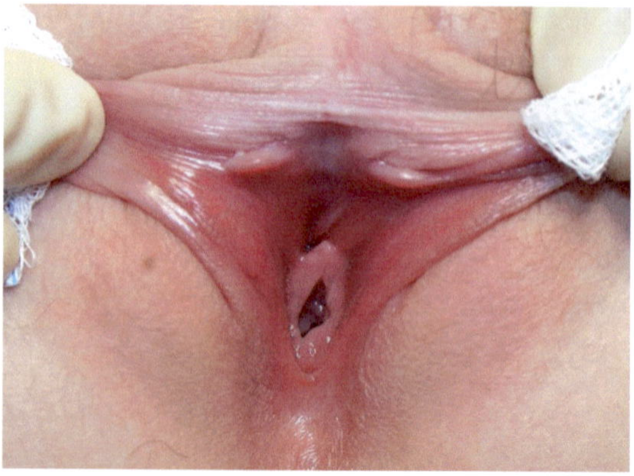

Fig. 12.2 Female epispadias. Note the bifid clitoris

12.4.3 Epispadias

Primary epispadias is rarely detected prenatally, but is usually detected at birth in males. Seventy percent of male epispadic patients have complete epispadias and associated incontinence due to incompetent sphincter mechanisms [37]. However, the meatus may be located at any point along the penile shaft; the more distal the meatus, the less likely the patient to have associated bladder neck and sphincter defects with incontinence. Associated anomalies include dorsal chordee in males, pubic diastasis, inguinal hernia, and vesicoureteral reflux.

Females may have delayed diagnosis as this is a rare entity and may be missed during routine examinations. These patients usually present later in life with stress incontinence or failure to complete toilet training (Fig. 12.2). Surgical repair is aimed at restoring normal voiding and continence as well as providing acceptable cosmesis.

12.4.4 Treatment and Outcomes

Though bladder exstrophy-epispadias is not a lethal anomaly, it has many obvious hygiene and social implications for pursuing repair. On the other hand, some cases of untreated cloacal exstrophy can result in death due to dehydration, malnutrition, and electrolyte abnormalities [38]. The goals of reconstruction are closure of the abdominal wall defect with or without closure of the pelvic ring, urinary continence, preservation of the upper tracts, functional and aesthetically acceptable genitalia, and low-pressure urine storage. Staged reconstruction is usually required to obtain these outcomes in more severe cases [39].

Rates of urinary continence vary by both defect and use of differing definitions of the term. Most authors reporting continence rates do not specify whether this means complete continence, continence with catheterization and/or meds, or applies to daytime versus nighttime continence [40].

Sexual function and libido is usually preserved in cases of bladder exstrophy and epispadias, though fertility in males with exstrophy can be significantly reduced due to disruption of the ejaculatory ducts during lower tract reconstruction or retrograde ejaculation. Female fertility is preserved but may require surgical augmentation of the introitus to allow vaginal intercourse [41]. Fertility and sexual function in cloacal exstrophy repair is dependent on whether gender reassignment has occurred and whether phallic reconstruction in boys is successful. Girls tend to have normal fertility rates; delivery by Caesarian section is recommended [41].

Kidney damage can be detected in up to 25 % of patients as a result of reflux, recurrent infections, and vesicoureteral reflux [42]. However, the rate of renal insufficiency is estimated to be only about 10 % [37].

12.5 Hypospadias

Hypospadias is an association of features that results from abnormal development of the ventral portion of the penis. This typically presents with an abnormal ventral opening of the urethral meatus with or without hypoplasia of the corpus spongiosum and urethra, ventral chordee or curvature of the penis, and an incomplete, hooded prepuce. This incomplete penile development is thought to occur as a result of altered androgen influence via decreased production by the fetal testis, decreased androgen sensitivity in the developing tissues, or early cessation of androgen stimulation prior to completion of genital development [43].

12.5.1 Incidence and Etiology

Hypospadias is a relatively common anomaly with a reported incidence of 0.3–0.8 %, though there is some variation in data reported from different countries [44]. The incidence appears to be increasing in the USA, England, Hungary, and Norwegian countries [45]. Proposed theories for the increasing incidence are related to the known effects of androgens on development of hypospadias. Environmental contamination with estrogens from insecticides, pharmaceuticals, and plant estrogens might explain the rising incidence and increasing numbers of more severe forms of hypospadias [46]. The familial rate of hypospadias is about 4–10 %, which suggests that hereditary factors may be responsible for the defect [47].

There is an association between undescended testicles and hypospadias, with an overall incidence of approximately 7 % [48]. In a large number of these patients, there is an underlying genetic or phenotypic sexual abnormality, so disorders of sexual development should be investigated. This is especially true in cases of severe proximal hypospadias and/or bilateral cryptorchidism [49].

12.5.2 Classification

Standard classification of hypospadias is based on anatomic location of the urethral meatus. As hypospadias is the result of arrested development of the ventral portion of the penis, the meatus can be located anywhere along this surface, from the perineum to the glans (Fig. 12.3). This may also be associated with absence of the frenulum, incomplete fusion of the urethral plate and corpus spongiosum, as well as lack of development of the ventral portion of foreskin. Planning surgical intervention should take into account both the location of the urethral meatus as well as need for reconstruction or correction of these associated abnormal features.

12.5.3 Assessment

Patients tend to present with ventral chordee (curvature) of the penis, hooded foreskin, and

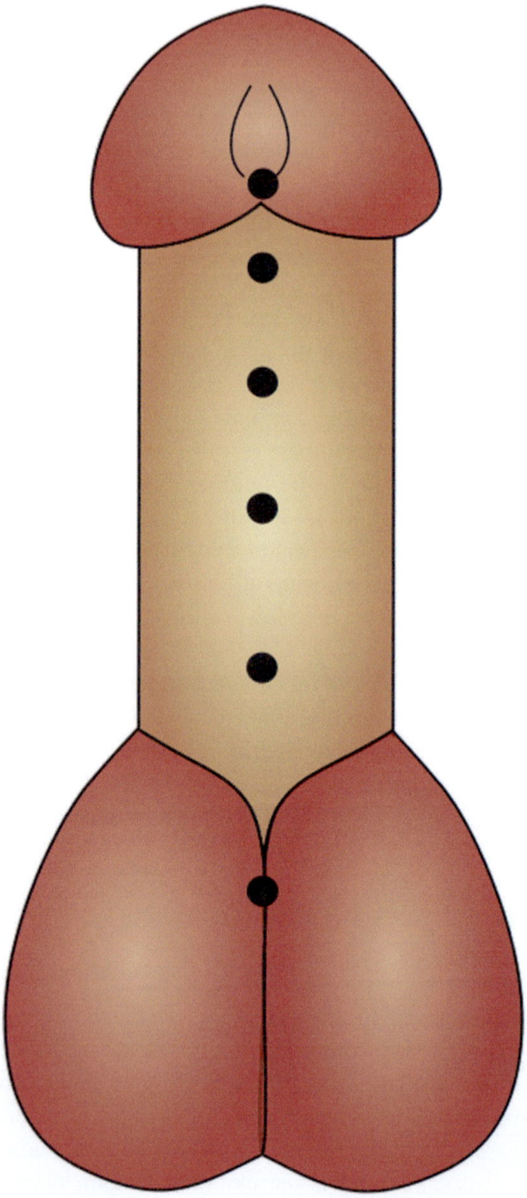

Fig. 12.3 Classification of hypospadias from most distal to proximal: glanular, coronal, distal, mid shaft, proximal, and perineal (Illustration courtesy of David A. Hamilton, Jr., M.D)

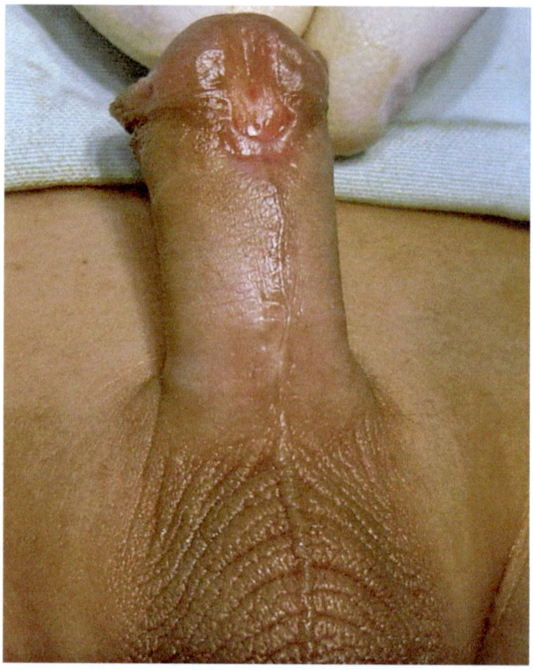

Fig. 12.4 Distal, or coronal, hypospadias

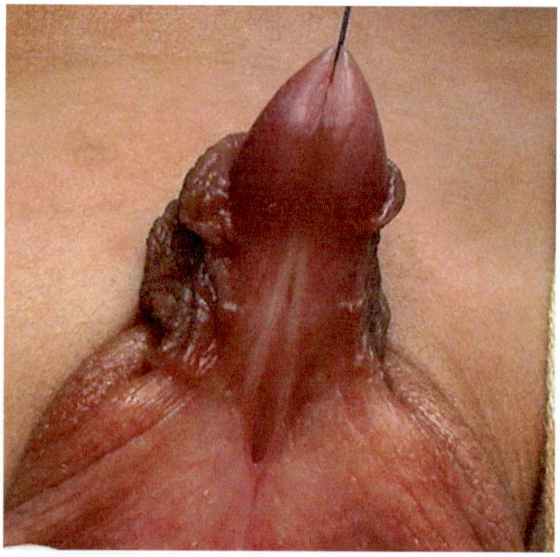

Fig. 12.5 Proximal, or penoscrotal, hypospadias

a stenotic ventral meatus. However, it is not uncommon for a patient to have incidental diagnosis of hypospadias at the time of circumcision when development of the prepuce has not been altered. The urethral meatus may be located in a variety of positions as previously mentioned, but 70–80 % of boys with hypospadias have a meatus located on the glans or distal shaft of the penis (Fig. 12.4), 20–30 % will have a mid-shaft location, and the remainder will have more severe defects with proximal location such as scrotal or perineal [50] (Fig. 12.5). If a patient presents with severe proximal hypospadias or hypospadias and cryptorchidism, a karyotype should be obtained and evaluation for disorders of sexual development (DSD) should be undertaken as there is an association between endocrine dysfunction in hypospadias and DSD [50].

12.5.4 Management

The optimal timing of surgical intervention is controversial. The American Academy of Pediatrics Section on Urology recommends that the repair be complete by age 6–12 months as this allows correction of the defect before awareness of it causes long-term emotional or psychosexual impairment [51].

There are a variety of methods for hypospadias repair, and the techniques have been evolving over the last several decades. Despite numerous options for approaching the repair, the goals of repair are urethroplasty, correction of chordee or ventral curvature, and management of the foreskin either by circumcision or reconstruction.

12.6 Abnormalities of the Testis and Scrotum

12.6.1 Cryptorchidism

Cryptorchidism, or undescended testes (UDT), is the most common male endocrine gland disorder in children with reported rates from 2 to 8 % in full-term boys and up to 30 % in preterm males [52]. Testicular descent occurs in the seventh month of fetal life and depends on a multitude of factors including activation of gene SRY, appropriate gonadal differentiation, development of the gubernaculum, and a variety of hormones including testosterone and insulin-like hormone 3 (INSL3). Descent occurs in two phases, transabdominal and inguinoscrotal, and is usually complete by the time of birth [53]. Given the multitude of factors involved in testis development and descent, it is not surprising that the pathogenesis is also considered to be multifactorial with both genetic and environmental influences.

12.6.1.1 Definitions

True cryptorchidism can be confused with other entities of abnormal testis position. For clarification purposes, normal scrotal position is the positioning of the midpoint of the testis at or below the midscrotum. The following are descriptions of abnormal scrotal positioning:

- Undescended testis – the absence of one or both testes in a normal scrotal position; may be a palpable or nonpalpable testis
- Vanishing testis – a testis that was lost due to vascular compromise, i.e., torsion, may occur in utero
- Agenesis – the complete absence of testis development
- Secondary/acquired cryptorchidism – testes that are suprascrotal after previous documentation of normal position, such as after inguinal hernia repair
- Retractile testes – testes that are easily manipulated into a normal scrotal position but are usually located in retracted position, such as is seen with an increased cremaster muscle reflex [52]

12.6.1.2 Assessment and Management

Accurate evaluation of the scrotum and testes requires examination in the supine, seated, and upright positions. A warm environment, warm hands, and abduction of the thighs help to decrease elicitation of the cremaster reflex, or testicular elevation due to contraction of the cremaster muscle. Repeated examinations also help to decrease this reflex. Seventy-five to eighty percent of cryptorchid testes are palpable and a majority of cases, reported from 60 to 70 %, are unilateral [52]. Palpable testes are usually present along the line of descent, but may be located in ectopic positions such as perineal, peripenile, lower abdominal wall, or femoral.

In the case of nonpalpable testes, surgical exploration is the gold standard of diagnosis and also allows for definitive management. Ultrasonography, CT, and MRI have been used for diagnosis, but the reported accuracy rates for identification of cryptorchid testes is highest in the inguinal region, which is the most easily palpable undescended testis. Accuracy drops to less than 50 % when the UDT is in an abdominal location. Therefore, exam under anesthesia and laparoscopic or open exploration provides opportunity for both diagnosis and orchidopexy if a viable testis is found [54].

12.6.2 Hydroceles and Hernias

Development of the processus vaginalis and inguinal canal begins in the third trimester in both sexes, though more prominent development of the processus vaginalis is noted in males to allow transinguinal passage of the testis into the scrotum [55]. The processus becomes obliterated within and just distal to the inguinal canal, then known as the funicular process, but remains patent around the testis to become the tunica vaginalis. Incomplete closure of the processus vaginalis may result in a symptomatic hernia in 1–5 % of newborns or hydrocele in 2–5 % of newborn males [56]. The incidence of hernias and hydroceles is nine times greater in males than in females [57].

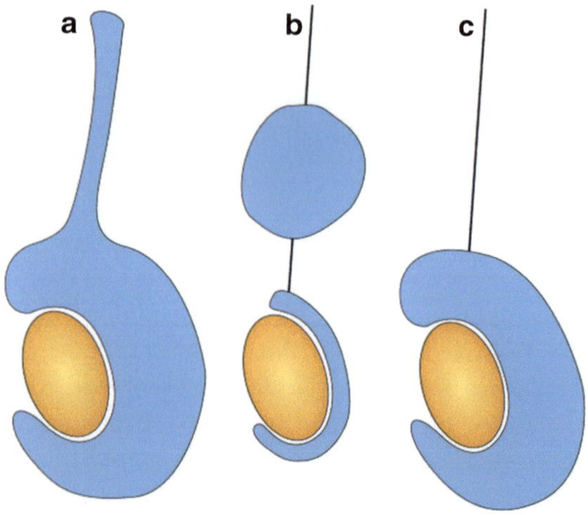

Fig. 12.6 Classification of hydroceles: (**a**) Communicating hydrocele (**b**) Encysted hydrocele or spermatic cord hydrocele (**c**) Noncommunicating hydrocele (Illustration courtesy of David A. Hamilton, Jr., M.D)

12.6.2.1 Hydroceles

Hydroceles present as a spectrum of anatomic varieties depending on the presence and location of processus vaginalis obliteration. The spectrum includes (1) communicating hydrocele with complete patency of the processus vaginalis with passage of intraperitoneal fluid; (2) encysted hydrocele with obliteration proximal to the testis, i.e., spermatic cord hydrocele; and (3) noncommunicating hydroceles that usually occur later in life and are due to accumulation of fluid around the testis with or without a patent processus vaginalis (Fig. 12.6).

Assessment

Most hydroceles present as a painless scrotal or inguinal swelling. Communicating hydroceles are usually fluctuant and may appear larger at the end of the day or with increased activity. Encysted hydroceles of the cord may be confused with an incarcerated inguinal hernia as they appear to be "nonreducible." Rarely is a hydrocele accompanied by pain, so other causes of an acute scrotum must be ruled out. However, in some cases, incarceration of the hydrocele sac can occur with associated symptoms of nausea, vomiting, and fever just as is seen with an incarcerated hernia [58].

Transillumination of the hydrocele classically differentiates it from a hernia, but this is not reliable in infants as a hernia may also transilluminate in bright light. However, if a groin swelling fluctuates with changes in position or stretching of the cord, or if there is a blue coloration to the swelling, this is suggestive of a hydrocele. Hernias are more likely to extend up toward the inguinal canal, are typically reducible, may have palpable crepitus of bowel contents, and may be exacerbated with Valsalva maneuvers.

Management

As most congenital hydroceles resolve spontaneously within the first year of life, conservative management is recommended. Surgical intervention is recommended when the hydrocele persists greater than 12 months or if the hydrocele presents later in childhood.

12.6.2.2 Hernias

The major difference between a hydrocele and a hernia is the size of the opening of the processus vaginalis. If the opening is large enough to allow passage of abdominal viscera in addition to peritoneal fluid, this is an indirect inguinal hernia. The incidence of inguinal hernias is 1–5 % across both sexes with a male to female ratio as high as 9:1 [55]. There is an increased occurrence of right-sided hernias and unilaterality, and these may occur in up to 30 % of premature infants [55]. Indirect inguinal hernias are the vast majority of pediatric hernias, though direct and femoral hernias can also occur. Indirect and direct inguinal hernias both present as a groin bulge and so must be delineated at the time of surgery. However, a femoral hernia usually presents as an upper or medial thigh bulge. It has been reported that up to 20 % of indirect inguinal hernias are associated with hydroceles [53].

The risk factors for congenital inguinal hernias include having a first-degree relative with history of congenital inguinal hernias, especially if this relative is female. There is overlap of risk factors with cryptorchidism that include low birth weight, bladder exstrophy, cystic fibrosis, connective tissue disorders, epididymal anomalies, and posterior urethral valves [59]. Inguinal hernia is also a component of over 200 syndromes and is more common in patients with ventriculoperitoneal shunts and other disorders causing increased intra-abdominal fluid such as peritoneal dialysis [52].

Assessment

As previously mentioned, inguinal hernias and hydroceles can be clinically difficult to distinguish. An inguinal hernia is typically unique from a hydrocele in that it may extend into and above the inguinal canal and can be elicited by maneuvers that increase intra-abdominal pressure such as crying or laughing. A hernia may also be reducible versus ballotable or fluctuant like a hydrocele. The "silk glove" sign is indicative of a hernia and is elicited by palpating the cord over the pubis that results in a sensation of the layers of the hernia sac slipping over one another [60]. Though not routinely used, ultrasonography of the scrotum and inguinal canal can be used to differentiate inguinal hernia from hydrocele and allows visualization of the testis. Ultrasonography is also useful in determining if an associated condition such as cryptorchidism or testis tumor with secondary hydrocele is present.

An incarcerated hernia is evident by inability to reduce the contents of a known hernia, whereas a strangulated hernia is incarcerated with compromised blood flow resulting in ischemia and necrosis of the hernia contents with associated systemic signs such as nausea, vomiting, fever, and even shock. Incarceration and strangulation are indications for urgent and emergent surgical intervention, respectively. Risks of delayed intervention include bowel necrosis, sepsis, and even death.

Management

Unlike neonatal hydroceles, the rate of spontaneous resolution of indirect inguinal hernias is low. Therefore, elective repair of the defect is recommended with either an open or laparoscopic approach. Cases of incarceration and strangulation are, as previously mentioned, repaired in an urgent or emergent fashion. If associated ipsilateral cryptorchidism is present, delay for observation of spontaneous testicular descent is not recommended; both entities can be surgically corrected in the same procedure.

The traditional inguinal approach for hernia/hydrocele repair is preferred due to its high success rate and low morbidity. There is a 0.7–1 % recurrence rate related to increased hernia size, poor surgical technique, or comorbid conditions that affect wound healing [61]. There is a potential need for later operation in the instance that a persistent or secondary hydrocele occurs without spontaneous resolution. There has been an increase in laparoscopic hernia/hydrocele repairs over the last several years with reported rates of recurrence similar to open approaches with improved pain control [62].

Selective exploration or repair of the contralateral side in cases of unilateral inguinal hernia is a matter of debate as there is no consensus recommendation and current practice varies widely among surgeons [63]. However, with use of laparoscopic technique, it is commonplace to visually inspect the contralateral inguinal ring while repairing a hernia and does not add morbidity to the case as an open contralateral inguinal dissection could.

12.6.3 Varicoceles

12.6.3.1 Etiology

A scrotal varicocele is an abnormal tortuosity and dilatation of the veins of the pampiniform plexus of the spermatic cord. It is a common finding in otherwise normal males but has been linked to subfertility. The exact effect on fertility is unclear as a reported 85 % of men with varicoceles have fathered children [64], yet the incidence in male partners of infertile couples is as high as 30 % [55].

Although varicocele is considered a congenital lesion, it is rarely diagnosed before school age as progression of size and severity is related to increased Tanner stage. The reported incidence in this age group is similar to that reported in adults, ranging from 8 to 16 % [61]. Factors predisposing children to varicoceles include varicocele in a first-degree relative, an ectomorph body habitus, and intrinsic venous abnormalities [65]. Almost 90 % of varicoceles occur on the left side, reflecting the differences in venous anatomy with the left gonadal vein draining into the left renal vein and the right gonadal vein draining directly into the inferior vena cava. Several patterns of intrinsic and anatomic venous abnormalities have been described:

- Incompetency or absence of valves
- Anomalous venous drainage, i.e., between gonadal and retroperitoneal veins
- Abnormal point of entry of gonadal vein into the left renal vein with resultant turbulent/decreased flow

12.6.3.2 Assessment and Classification

Varicoceles are typically detected during routine examination or the patient may present with scrotal swelling or discomfort. The typical description of the exam finding is that of a "bag of worms" in the scrotum. The standard grading system is as follows:

- Subclinical – neither palpable nor visible but detectable by Doppler ultrasonography
- Grade I – palpable only with Valsalva maneuver
- Grade II – palpable at rest but not visible
- Grade III – palpable and visible at rest

12.6.3.3 Associated Pathology

The presence of a varicocele is associated with an increase in scrotal temperature that may be related to altered testicular growth, spermatogenesis, and semen quality [66]. These relationships are unclear, however, as definite links between these parameters and fertility have not been clearly established. Some specifically reported abnormalities include testicular hypotrophy, abnormal tubular maturation or tubular degeneration, altered Leydig cell number, exaggerated LH and FSH response to GnRH, and poor semen quality [63]. Interestingly, higher varicocele grade has not been definitively linked to inferior semen parameters [65].

12.6.3.4 Management

Despite the unclear link between the pathologic findings associated with varicocele in adolescence and potential for later reproductive ability, the current indications for surgical intervention are pain and significant hypotrophy of one or both testes in infants, with the additional indication of improving fertility in teenagers and adults [65].

There are various approaches to surgical intervention including microsurgical varicocelectomy, laparoscopic or open varicocelectomy, and sclerotherapy or embolization with the common goal of ligation of venous outflow. Laparoscopic and microsurgical approaches are associated with the lowest incidence of both recurrence and hydrocele, especially when employing lymphatic-sparing techniques [64].

12.6.4 Testicular Torsion

The sudden onset of swelling, pain, and/or tenderness of the scrotum or scrotal contents is referred to as an "acute scrotum." Testicular torsion accounts for 80–90 % of male patients' age 13–21 presenting with an acute scrotum. There is a bimodal distribution of torsion with peaks within the first year of life and in early adolescence with an overall incidence of 3.8 per 100,000 [67]. An extensive differential diagnosis of causes of the acute scrotum exists, but testicular or spermatic cord torsion is a surgical emergency and requires intervention within 6 h of onset to avoid long-term sequelae related to reduction or cessation of blood flow to the testis.

Spermatic cord or testicular torsion occurs in one of two ways: intravaginal or extravaginal. Intravaginal spermatic cord torsion occurs when the testis twists within the tunica vaginalis. This is more common in teenage boys and is predisposed by the bell-clapper deformity in which the tunica completely or partially fails to fuse to the epididymis, allowing incomplete attachment of testis/epididymis to the scrotum. Bell-clapper deformity was identified in 12 % of males in an autopsy series, but torsion occurs at a much lower incidence of 0.009 % [68]. The inciting event is unknown in most patients but may include cold temperature, sudden movement, trauma, or rapid growth of the testis at puberty.

Extravaginal torsion occurs most commonly in the perinatal period. This is due to rotation of the entire cord, testis, and tunica vaginalis before the fixation has been established between the dartos and the tunica vaginalis. This is more common while the patient remains in utero, but has also been described at several months of age. We will focus the further attention of this section on perinatal, or extravaginal, torsion.

12.6.4.1 Etiology and Assessment

Postulated risk factors include large birth weight, difficult delivery, or a family history of torsion [69]. Typical exam findings include induration of the scrotal skin or testis and scrotal edema, erythema, and/or discoloration. Patients may present with pain, but are usually asymptomatic making timely diagnosis difficult. Hydroceles may coexist, further complicating accurate diagnosis.

Ultrasound is the imaging modality of choice to diagnose torsion, especially with the use of Doppler to detect vascular flow. Sensitivity and specificity for accurately diagnosing torsion are reported as high as 100 and 95 %, respectively, in some series [70]. If, however, imaging is nondiagnostic, surgical exploration is advocated in lieu of delaying or avoiding treatment.

12.6.4.2 Management

Most cases of extravaginal torsion are not salvageable as they occur during the prenatal period while the fetus remains in utero. However, partial or complete salvage is possible in some cases if emergent surgery is performed; this is the most prudent approach to minimize loss of testicular tissue. Contralateral exploration and orchidopexy should be performed at the same time as emergent detorsion/orchidopexy.

12.7 Disorders of Sex Development

Disorders of sex development (DSD), previously known as intersex disorders, are due to one of the following mechanisms: chromosomal defects, abnormal gonadal development, or defects in sex hormone production or sex hormone receptors. These infants present at birth with ambiguous genitalia. Associated medical conditions such as congenital adrenal hyperplasia and adrenal insufficiency may also be present and require urgent intervention. In the cases when an urgent underlying medical condition is not present, disorders of sex development warrant a thorough investigation from a multidisciplinary team including a pediatric endocrinologist, a pediatric urologist, a radiologist, and a geneticist. Support and counseling for the parents should also be available, and assignment or registration of gender should be delayed until a formal diagnosis has been made [71].

12.7.1 Normal Sexual Differentiation

Precursors of gonads and external genitalia are present in an identical state in both 46XX and 46XY embryos until gestational week 6. Development down a phenotypic female pathway occurs passively unless the presence of certain genes and hormones activates male differentiation. In this case, the presence of *SRY* (sex-determining region Y) on the Y chromosome in addition to secretion of Mullerian inhibitory substance (MIS) and testosterone is responsible

Table 12.1 Revised nomenclature for disorders of sex development (DSD)

Previous nomenclature	Current nomenclature	Presentation
Intersex	Disorders of sex Development (DSD)	(See below)
Female pseudohermaphrodite	46 XX DSD	Virilization of 46XX fetus
Male pseudohermaphrodite	46XY DSD	Incomplete virilization of 46XY fetus
True Hermaphrodite	Ovotesticular DSD	Both ovary and testis present; variable genotype and phenotype
Gonadal dysgenesis	Gonadal dysgenesis (unchanged)	Loss of one pair of sex chromosomes, e.g., 45X or 45X/46XY; variable genotype and phenotype

for the early development of male internal and external genitalia with regression of female characteristics [72].

12.7.2 Classification

As previously mentioned, the origin of DSD can be chromosomal defects, abnormal gonadal development, or endocrine dysfunction. The most commonly seen forms of DSD are as follows (see Table 12.1):

- 46XX DSD – virilization of a 46XX fetus due to exposure to virilizing agents such as testosterone
- 46XY DSD – incomplete virilization of a 46XY fetus
- Ovotesticular DSD – both ovarian and testicular tissue are present; phenotype and genotype are highly variable
- Gonadal dysgenesis – a spectrum of gonadal and genital abnormalities that occurs due to the loss of one of a pair of sex chromosomes, e.g., 45X or 45X/46XY mosaicism

12.7.2.1 46XX DSD

46XX DSD is composed almost entirely of 46XX females with normal gonads and internal genitalia but ambiguous external genitalia. Congenital adrenal hyperplasia is by far the most common cause of 46XX DSD and accounts for a vast majority of cases of ambiguous genitalia in the West. This disorder can result from one of three enzymatic defects in the pathway for adrenal production of cortisol and aldosterone that in turn causes increased adrenocorticotropic hormone (ACTH) production with resultant overproduction of androgens (see Fig. 12.7). The most common defect is 21-hydroxylase deficiency that results in elevated 17α-hydroxyprogesterone and can be associated with life-threatening hyponatremia. 11ß-hydroxylase deficiency is associated with hypernatremia, hypokalemia, and severe virilization. 3ß-hydroxysteroid dehydrogenase deficiency is the least common of the three defects and is similar to 21-hydroxylase deficiency but with less severe virilization [72, 73, 76].

Prenatal diagnosis is possible, and suppression of ACTH with dexamethasone has been successfully reported in cases. However, if diagnosis is made at birth, management includes replacement of necessary substrates, management of electrolyte imbalances, and female assignment with feminizing genitoplasty if indicated [73–75].

Less common causes of 46XX DSD include deficiency of estrogen synthetase that normally synthesizes estrogens from androgen precursors and exposure of the fetus to maternal androgens from androgen secreting tumors of the adrenals or ovaries.

12.7.2.2 46XY DSD

Male infants with 46XY DSD exhibit varying degrees of incomplete virilization due to defects in androgen production and metabolism or defective androgen receptors. Defective testosterone production is rare, but may be due to testicular dysgenesis or an enzymatic defect in the biosynthetic pathway. Testosterone conversion to its more potent form dihydrotestosterone (DHT) is regulated by the enzyme 5α-reductase. A deficiency in this enzyme is most common in consanguine communities in the Dominican Republic and may appear to be normal phenotypic

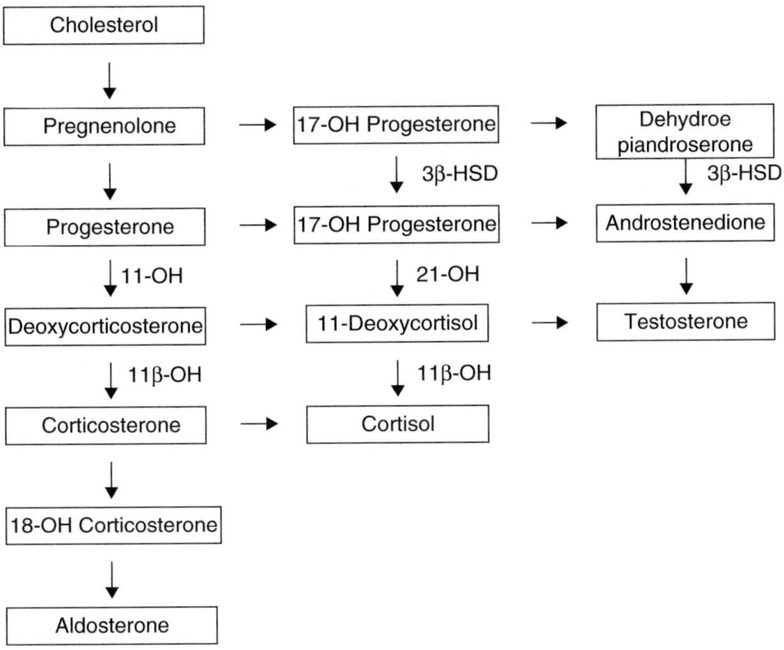

Fig. 12.7 Sites of enzyme deficiency in congenital adrenal hyperplasia

females until virilization occurs at puberty with increased levels of testosterone that overcome the DHT deficiency [74, 76].

Androgen insensitivity syndrome is characterized by tissue resistance to testosterone with resultant female phenotypic external genitalia. However, the presence of MIS still drives internal genitalia and gonadal differentiation down a normal male pathway. This condition is usually discovered when investigating causes of primary amenorrhea or if a testis is found during herniorrhaphy in a female patient. On the other hand, MIS deficiency or MIS receptor insensitivity results in normal male external genitalia with persistent Mullerian structures [74].

12.7.2.3 Gonadal Dysgenesis

Dysgenesis or abnormality of the development of the gonads can lead to a variety of genotypic and phenotypic presentations depending on the presence of any normal functioning gonadal tissue. For example, a 45XO (Turner syndrome) female will have normal female internal and external genitalia since no tissue with a Y chromosome is present. However, mixed gonadal dysgenesis with 45X/46XY mosaicism results in a broad spectrum of gonadal and external phenotypes due to the presence of both X and Y chromosomes with incomplete function of the dysgenetic gonads with an associated increase in malignancy risk in these gonads [74].

12.7.2.4 Ovotesticular DSD

Previously known as true hermaphroditism, ovotesticular DSD is a variation of gonadal dysgenesis in which both testicular and ovarian tissue are present in an individual, and in some cases, within the same gonad. The external genitalia are invariably ambiguous. This is virtually a diagnosis of exclusion and sometimes relies on macroscopic or microscopic examination of the gonads. Gender assignment proves difficult in this population and usually requires hormone supplementation and surgical reconstruction [75].

12.7.3 Assessment

Evaluation of neonates with ambiguous genitalia should include a physical exam that focuses on the degree of virilization, the presence of palpable gonads, and identification of other congenital abnormalities. History should include details of the pregnancy as well as a thorough family history with attention to any defects present in siblings [75].

Initial laboratory evaluations should include karyotype, serum electrolytes, and 17-hydorxyprogesterone levels. A more detailed evaluation might include a steroid assay, serum testosterone levels, MIS levels, and even DNA analysis to identify specific gene mutations [77].

Diagnostic imaging is useful for identifying gonads or internal genitalia via ultrasonography. Ultrasound is the primary modality for imaging internal organs. Genitograms, or contrast studies performed through a catheter placed into the urethra, vagina, or opening of the urogenital sinus, are helpful to determine the presence of internal genitalia such as the uterus, fallopian tubes, or even the vasa deferentia [78].

Direct visualization via surgical methods is sometimes indicated. Endoscopy of the lower genitourinary tract, such as vaginoscopy or cystourethroscopy, and laparoscopy are useful minimally invasive procedures. However, there is still an indication for laparotomy in some instances when identification of the gonads and/or biopsy of gonads is not possible through less invasive means [75, 77].

12.7.4 Management

After medical stabilization of the patient when indicated, the next most important step in management of a child with DSD is gender assignment. This should be delayed until a formal diagnosis has been established. Each case must be tailored to the patient's particular features including genital appearance, fertility potential, familial or cultural preferences, and surgical and/or medical requirements.

Female assignment is almost invariably advised in cases of 46XX DSD as most patients have normal female internal genitalia and gonads. Female gender assignment is also often advised in cases of 46XY DSD with the exception of those patients that have a positive response to androgen stimulation. In mixed gonadal dysgenesis and ovotesticular DSD, gender assignment is variable but usually depends on the presence of functional gonadal tissue. Female assignment is more common for this group unless sufficient androgen response and external male genitalia is present, though practice varies widely among practitioners. Orchidopexy in patients assigned male gender is necessary to enable examination of the testes, and orchiectomy in patients assigned female gender is advised given the increased risk of malignancy in these gonads [79, 80].

Once gender assignment has been completed, hormonal and surgical therapy can then be pursued. As previously mentioned, a multidisciplinary team including pediatric endocrinology, pediatric urology, radiology, genetics, and psychiatry/counseling for the parents is often necessary to address all aspects of management of these children.

References

1. Burbige KA, Lebowitz RL, Colodny AH et al (1984) The megacystis-megaureter syndrome. J Urol 1131:1133
2. Gearhart JP, Ben-Chaim J, Jeffs RD et al (1995) Criteria for the prenatal diagnosis of classic bladder exstrophy. Obstet Gynecol 85:961
3. Weight CJ, Chand D, Ross JH (2006) Single system ectopic ureter to rectum subtending solitary kidney and bladder agenesis in newborn male. Urology 68:1344
4. Graham SD (1972) Agenesis of bladder. J Urol 107:660–661
5. Garat JM (1987) Malformaciones vesicales. In: Garat R, Gosálbez R (eds) Urología Pediátrica. Salvat, Barcelona, pp 287–313
6. Barrett D, Malek R, Kelalis P (1976) Observations on vesical diverticulum in childhood. J Urol 116(2): 234–236
7. Gyftopoulos K, Wolffenbuttel KP, Nijman RJ (2002) Clinical and embryologic aspects of penile duplication and associated anomalies. Urology 60:675–679
8. Frimberger DC, Kropp BP (2012) Sect. XVII, Chapter 125: Bladder anomalies in children. In: Wein AJ, Kavoussi LR et al (eds) Campbell Walsh urology, vol 4, 10th edn. WB Saunders Elsevier, Philadelphia, pp 3379–3388
9. Mesrobian HGO, Zacharias A, Balcom AH, Cohen RD (1997) Ten years of experience with isolated urachal anomalies in children. J Urol 158:1316–1318
10. Ashley R, Inman B et al (2001) Urachal anomalies: a longitudinal study of urachal remnants in children and adults. J Urol 178(4):1615–1618
11. Schiesser M, Lapaire O, Holzgraeve W, Tercanli S (2003) Umbilical cord edema associated with patent urachus. Ultrasound Obstet Gyenecol 22:646–647

12. Campanale RP, Krumbach RW (1955) Intraperitoneal perforation of infected urachal cyst. Am J Surg 90:143–145
13. Iuchtman M, Rahav S, Zer M, Mogilner J, Siplovich L (1993) Management of urachal anomalies in children and adults. Urology 42:426–430
14. Bauer SB (2008) Neurogenic bladder: etiology and assessment. Pediatr Nephrol 23:541–551
15. Steinbrecher HA, Malone PS et al (2008) Chapter 13: Neuropathic bladder. In: Thomas DFM, Duffy PG, Rickwood AMK (eds) Essentials of paediatric urology. Informa Healthcare UK Ltd., London, pp 171–187
16. Danzer E, Johnson MP, Adzick NS (2012) Fetal surgery for myelomeningocele: progress and perspectives. Dev Med Child Neurol 54(1):8–14
17. Szulc A (2011) Classification of patients with myelodysplasia according to the level of neurosegmental lesion as a basis of motor function assessment. Ortop Traumatol Rehabil 13(2):113–123
18. Frimberger D, Cheng E, Kropp BP (2012) The current management of the neurogenic bladder in children with spina bifida. Pediatr Clin North Am 59(4):757–767
19. Yeung CK, Sihoe JDY, Bauer SB (2007) Chapter 123, Sect. XVII: Voiding dysfunction in children: non-neurogenic and neurogenic. In: Wein AJ, Kavoussi LR et al (eds) Campbell Walsh urology, vol 4, 9th edn. WB Saunders Elsevier, Philadelphia, pp 3625–3628
20. Edelstein RA, Bauer SB, Kelly MD et al (1996) The long-term urologic response of neonates with myelodysplasia treated proactively with intermittent catheterization and anticholinergic therapy. J Urol 154(4):1500–1504
21. James CM, Lassman LP (1972) Spinal dysraphism: spina bifida occulta. Appleton, New York
22. Pierre-Kahn A, Zeral M, Renier D et al (1997) Congenital lumbosacral lipomas. Childs Nerv Syst 13:298–334
23. Sarica K, Erbagci A, Yagci F, Yurtseven C (2003) Multidisciplinary evaluation of occult spinal dysraphism in 47 children. Scand J Urol Nephrol 37:329–334
24. Wilmshurst JM, Kelly R, Borzyskowski M (1999) Presentation and outcome of sacral agenesis: 20 years' experience. Dev Med Child Neurol 41:806–812
25. Lancaster PAL (1987) Epidemiology of bladder exstrophy: a communication from the International Clearinghouse for Birth Defects monitoring systems. Teratology 36:221
26. Cuckow P (2008) Chapter 15: Bladder exstrophy and epispadias. In: Thomas DFM, Duffy PG, Rickwood AMK (eds) Essentials of paediatric urology. Informa Healthcare UK Ltd., London, pp 199–211
27. Shapiro E, Jeffs RD, Gearhart JP, Lepor H (1985) Muscarinic cholinergic receptors in bladder exstrophy: insights into surgical management. J Urol 134:309
28. Marshall VF, Muecke E (1968) Congenital abnormalities of the bladder. In: Handbuch der Urologie. Springer, New York, p 165
29. Johnston JH, Kogan SJ (1974) The exstrophic anomalies and their surgical reconstruction. Curr Probl Surg 46:1–39
30. Sadler TW, Feldkamp ML (2008) The embryology of the body wall closure: relevance to gastroschisis and other ventral body wall defects. J Med Genet 148:181–185
31. Ives E, Coffey R, Carter CO (1980) A family study of bladder exstrophy. J Med Genet 17:139
32. Gambhir L, Höller T, Müller M et al (2008) Epidemiological survey of 214 families with bladder exstrophy-epispadias complex. J Urol 179:1539–1543
33. Wood HP, Trock BP, Gearhart JP (2003) In vitro fertilization and the cloacal-bladder exstrophy-epispadias complex: is there an association? J Urol 169:1512–1515
34. Connolly JA, Peppas DS, Jeffs RD, Gearhart JP (1995) Prevalence in repair of inguinal hernia in children with bladder exstrophy. J Urol 154:1900
35. Baradaran N, Cervellione RM, Stec AA et al (2012) Delayed primary repair of bladder exstrophy: ultimate effect on growth. J Urol 188:2336–2342
36. Nerli RB, Shirol SS, Guntaka A et al (2012) Genital reconstruction in exstrophy patients. Indian J Urol 28(3):280–285
37. Gearhart JP, Jeffs RD (1998) The bladder exstrophy-epispadias complex. In: Walsh PC et al (eds) Campbell's urology, 7th edn. WB Saunders, Philadelphia, p 1939
38. Bischoff A, Calvo-Garcia MA, Baregamian N et al (2012) Prenatal counseling for cloaca and cloacal exstrophy – challenges faced by pediatric surgeons. Pediatr Surg Int 28(8):781–788
39. Stec AA, Baradaran N, Schaeffer A et al (2012) The modern staged repair of classic bladder exstrophy: a detailed postoperative management for primary bladder closure. J Pediatr Urol 8(5):549–555
40. Lloyd JC, Spano SM, Ross SS et al (2012) How dry is dry? A review of definitions of continence in the contemporary exstrophy/epispadias literature. J Urol 188(8):1900–1904
41. Ansari MS, Cervellione RM, Gearhart JP (2010) Sexual function and fertility issues in cases of exstrophy epispadias complex. Indian J Urol 26(4):595–597
42. Ben-Chaim J, Docimo SG, Jeffs RD et al (1996) Bladder exstrophy from childhood into adult life. J R Soc Med 89(1):39–46
43. Borer JG, Retik AB (2007) Chapter 125, Sect. XVII: Hypospadias. In: Wein AJ, Kavoussi LR et al (eds) Campbell Walsh urology, vol 4, 9th edn. WB Saunders Elsevier, Philadelphia, pp 3703–3743
44. Palmert MR, Dahms WT (2006) Abnormalities of sexual differentiation. In: Fanaroff A, Martin RJ, Walsh MC (eds) Neonatal–perinatal medicine diseases of the fetus and infant, 8th edn. Mosby, Philadelphia, pp 1565–1566
45. Paulozzi LJ, Erickson JD, Jackson RJ (1997) Hypospadias trends in two US surveillance systems. Pediatrics 100:831–834
46. Gray LE Jr, Ostby J, Furr J et al (2004) Toxicant-induced hypospadias in the male rat. Adv Exp Med Biol 545:217–241

47. Abdullah NA, Pearce MS, Parker L et al (2007) Birth prevalence of cryptorchidism and hypospadias in northern England, 1993–2000. Arch Dis Child 92(7):576–579
48. Weidner IS, Moller H, Jensen TK, Skakkebaek NE (1999) Risk factors for cryptorchidism and hypospadias. J Urol 161:1606–1609
49. Cox MJ, Coplen DE, Austin PF (2008) The incidence of disorders of sexual differentiation and chromosomal abnormalities of cryptorchidism and hypospadias stratified by meatal location. J Urol 180:2649–2652
50. Snodgrass WT, Shukla AR, Canning DA (2007) Chapter 71, Sect. VI: Hypospadias. In: Docimo SG, Canning DA, Khoury AE (eds) Kelalis-King-Belman textbook of pediatric urology, 5th edn. Informa Healthcare UK Ltd., London, pp 1205–1238
51. Schultz JR, Klykylo WM, Wacksman J (1983) Timing of elective hypospadias repair in children. Pediatrics 71:342
52. Kolon TF (2007) Chapter 74, Sect. VI: Cryptorchidism. In: Docimo SG, Canning DA, Khoury AE (eds) Kelalis-King-Belman textbook of pediatric urology, 5th edn. Informa Healthcare UK Ltd., London, pp 1295–1301
53. Virtanen HE, Cortes D et al (2007) Development and descent of the testis in relation to cryptorchidism. Acta Paediatr 96:622–627
54. Tasian GE et al (2011) Diagnostic imaging in cryptorchidism: utility, indications and effectiveness. J Pediatr Surg 46(12):2406–2413
55. Barthold JS (2012) Chapter 132, Sect. XVII: Abnormalities of the testis and scrotum and their management. In: Wein AJ, Kavoussi LR et al (eds) Campbell Walsh urology, vol 4, 10th edn. WB Saunders Elsevier, Philadelphia, pp 3557–3596
56. Clarke S (2010) Pediatric inguinal hernia and hydrocele: an evidence-based review in the era of minimal access surgery. J Laparoendosc Adv Surg Tech A 20(3):305–309
57. Lau ST, Lee YH, Caty MG (2007) Current management of hernias and hydroceles. Semin Pediatr Surg 16(1):50–57
58. Ringert RH (1998) The acute scrotum. Z Arztl Fortbild Qualitatssich 92(5):343–348
59. Heikkla J, Taskinen S et al (2008) Posterior urethral valves are often associated with cryptorchidism and inguinal hernias. J Urol 180(2):715–717
60. Luo CC, Chao HC (2007) Prevention of unnecessary contralateral exploration using the silk glove sing (SGS) in pediatric patients with unilateral inguinal hernia. Eur J Pediatr 166(7):667–669
61. Vogels HD, Bruijnen CJ, Beasley SW (2009) Predictors of recurrence after inguinal herniotomy in boys. Pediatr Surg Int 25(3):235–238
62. Dutta S, Albanese C (2009) Transcutaneous laparoscopic hernia repair in children: a prospective review of 275 hernia repairs with minimum 2-year follow-up. Surg Endosc 23(1):103–107
63. Wang KS (2012) Assessment and management of inguinal hernia in infants. Pediatrics 130(4):768–773
64. Safarinejad MR (2008) Infertility among couples in a population-based study in Iran: prevalence and associated risk factors. Int J Androl 31(3):303–314
65. Diegidio P, Jhaveri JK, Ghannam S et al (2011) Review of current varicocelectomy techniques and their outcomes. BJU Int 108(7):1157–1172
66. Ficarra V, Crestani A, Novara G et al (2012) Varicocele repair for infertility: what is the evidence? Curr Opin Urol 22(6):489–494
67. Zhao LC, Lautz TB, Meeks JJ et al (2011) Pediatric testicular torsion epidemiology using a national database: Incidence, risk of orchiectomy and possible measures toward improving the quality of care. J Urol 186(5):2009–2013
68. Caesar RE, Kaplan GW (1994) Incidence of the Bell-clapper deformity in an autopsy series. J Urol 44(1):114–116
69. Schenck FX, Bellinger MF (2007) Chapter 127, Sect. XVII: Abnormalities of the testes and scrotum and their surgical management. In: Wein AJ, Kavoussi LR, Novick AC, Partin AW, Peters CA (eds) Campbell Walsh urology, vol 4, 9th edn. WB Saunders Elsevier, Philadelphia, pp 3776–3781
70. Sandor L, Gajda T, Aranyi V et al (2011) Role of ultrasonography in the urgent differential diagnosis of acute scrotum. Orv Hetil 152(23):909–1012
71. Wu H, Snyder HM (2007) Sect. VI, Chapter 68: Intersex. In: Docimo SG, Canning DA, Khoury AE (eds) Kelalis-King-Belman textbook of pediatric urology, 5th edn. Informa Healthcare UK Ltd., London, pp 1147–1160
72. Lottman H, Thomas DFM (2008) Chapter 20: Disorders of sex development. In: Thomas DFM, Duffy PG, Rickwood AMK (eds) Essentials of paediatric urology. Informa Healthcare UK Ltd., London, pp 275–293
73. Lee P, Schober J, Nordenstrom A et al (2012) Review of recent outcome data of disorders of sex development (DSD): emphasis on surgical and sexual outcomes. J Pediatr Urol 8(6):611–615
74. Guerra-Junior G, Latronico AC, Hiort O et al (2012) Disorders of sex development and hypogonadism: genetics, mechanism, and therapies. Int J Endocrinol 2012: 820373
75. Romao RL, Pippi Salle JL, Wherrett DK (2012) Update on the management of disorders of sex development. Pediatr Clin North Am 59(4):853–869
76. Massanyi EZ, Dicarlo HN, Miqeon CJ et al (2013) Review and management of 46 XY disorders of sex development. J Pediatr Urol 9:368–379
77. Hughes IA (2008) Disorders of sex development: a new definition and classification. Best Pract Res Clin Endocrinol Metab 22:119–134
78. Chavhan GB, Parra DA, Oudjhane K et al (2008) Imaging of ambiguous genitalia: classification and diagnostic approach. Radiographics 28(7):1891–1904
79. Josso N, Audi L, Shaw G (2011) Regional variations in the management of testicular or ovotesticular disorders of sex development. Sex Dev 5(5):225–234
80. Barthold JS (2011) Disorders of sex differentiation: a pediatric urologist's perspective of new terminology and recommendations. J Urol 185(2):393–400

Urinary Tract Malignancies of Infancy and Young Childhood

13

John D'Orazio, Samantha Michaels, John Romond, and Joseph Pulliam

Core Messages

- Urinary tract masses occur very rarely in neonates and young infants. When they do, they are more likely to be mesoblastic nephromas rather than more aggressive and more malignant disorders. Therefore, urinary tract masses, in general, are associated with a more favorable outcome when diagnosed in very young children.
- Very young presentation of malignancy can be an indication of an inherited cancer predisposition syndrome.
- Urinary tract malignancies of infancy may be diagnosed prenatally (e.g., ultrasonography) or may present clinically (usually in the setting of gross hematuria or abdominal mass).
- Malignancies that involve the urinary tract of infants and very young children are embryologically distinct from the typical carcinomas that affect adults. Malignant urinary tract tumors of infancy and young usually respond better to therapy than those in adults.
- Due to their small size, sensitive developmental stage, and metabolic characteristics, there are unique challenges that arise when treating very young infants for cancer.

Case Vignette

A 3-month-old infant was taken to his pediatrician for evaluation of a firm abdominal mass first noticed by his mother during his bath. His pre- and postnatal histories were unremarkable, including normal gestational screening ultrasounds. He had a history of gastroesophageal reflux since birth which had been treated with proton pump inhibitors and dietary interventions. The baby's pediatrician confirmed the presence of a large left-sided non-tender abdominal mass. Imaging studies revealed a 4.7 × 5.5 × 6 cm well-defined mass arising from the anterior aspect of the left kidney and displacing adjacent structures without obvious direct invasion (Fig. 13.1). The contralateral kidney was uninvolved, and there was no evidence of metastatic spread to the lung. The child underwent

J. D'Orazio, MD, PhD (✉)
Pediatric Hematology-Oncology, The Markey Cancer Center, University of Kentucky College of Medicine, Combs Research Bldg. Rm. 204 800 Rose Street, Lexington, KY 40536-0096, USA
e-mail: jdorazio@uky.edu

S. Michaels, MD • J. Romond, MD • J. Pulliam
Department of Pediatrics, University of Kentucky, 800 Rose Street MN118, Lexington, KY 40536, USA
e-mail: samantha.michaels@uky.edu; john.romond@uky.edu

A.S. Chishti et al. (eds.), *Kidney and Urinary Tract Diseases in the Newborn*, DOI 10.1007/978-3-642-39988-6_13, © Springer-Verlag Berlin Heidelberg 2014

left radical nephrectomy with regional lymph node dissection. Pathologic examination of the mass revealed a Wilms tumor with favorable histology, confined to the kidney. Surgical margins and regional lymph nodes were uninvolved. Because the tumor was small, localized, and completely resected without peritoneal spillage, the patient's disease was classified as "Very Low Risk" according to the National Wilms Tumor Study Group (NWTSG), and he did not require further treatments such as radiation therapy or chemotherapy. The child has been followed by close observation with interval imaging studies monitoring for local or metastatic relapse. He is thriving and without evidence of disease, now roughly 30 months after presentation.

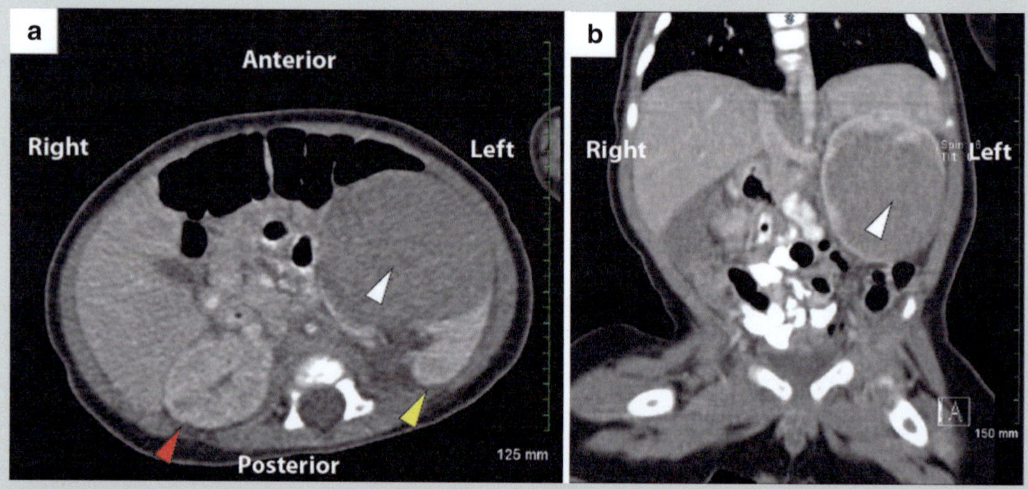

Fig. 13.1 Wilms tumor in the 3-month-old male described in our introductory vignette. Shown are transverse (**a**) and coronal (**b**) magnetic resonance (*MR*) images of the patient's abdomen. Note the large, fairly homogeneous mass (*white triangles*) arising from the anterior aspect of the left kidney and compressing normal renal architecture (*yellow triangle*). There was no evidence of either contralateral renal abnormality (*red triangle*) or pulmonary metastasis (not shown)

13.1 Introduction

The function of the urinary tract is to filter the blood of impurities, produce and eliminate urine from the body, and maintain electrolyte homeostasis. The urinary tract consists of two kidneys that lie retroperitoneally in the abdomen, each drained by a ureter that empties into the bladder that collects and stores urine before expelling urine through the urethra. Disorders of the development of the urinary tract, such as anatomic renal anomalies or posterior urethral valves or faulty implantation of the ureters to the bladder, are relatively much more common than malignancies of the urinary tract; however, cancers of the urinary system do sometimes present in infancy and may arise from any urinary tract structure. In this review, we will describe various malignancies that involve the urinary tract of infants, consider them in the greater context of childhood malignancies, discuss various genetic syndromes that predispose to such cancers, and outline some of the challenges of treating infants and very young children with anticancer therapy.

13.2 Cancer of the Urinary Tract: A Comparison Between Adults and Children

In general, tumors of the urinary system correlate with age, with the great majority of renal and bladder tumors presenting in adults (Fig. 13.2). Nonetheless, urinary system malignancies do affect infants and young children and unlike those malignancies of the urinary tract diagnosed in adults are often highly treatable and associated with a good clinical outcome. One reason for the great discrepancy in prognosis between urinary tract tumors of children and adults is that those of adults are pathologically distinct from those affecting infants and young children. Epithelial cancers such as bladder cancer predominate in adults, and their development is heavily influenced by environmental risk factors, particularly cigarette smoke and/or chronic exposure to certain chemicals such as aromatic amines, diesel fumes, and reagents used in the manufacture of leather, rubber, and textiles. Urinary tract tumors of childhood, in contrast, tend not to be linked with environmental exposures but rather with dysregulated genetic processes that control embryonic development of normal tissues [122]. Childhood urinary tract malignancies tend to be embryonal cancers rather than carcinomas and as such may be inherently less aggressive and more treatment responsive than those diagnosed in adults.

13.3 Cancer Among Infants

Although it may seem unlikely that babies would be at risk of cancer, malignancies of infants (typically thought of as patients under a year of age) account for about 10 % of the total number of cancers diagnosed in children under the age of 15 years [59]. In fact, the age of peak overall cancer incidence is actually in the first year of life (Fig. 13.3), with the cancer incidence rate of infants (roughly 235 per million) being over 10 % higher than that of the next highest age group [59]. Most cancers of infancy present beyond 1 month of life; neonatal tumors (from birth through 1 month of life) are exceptionally unusual. In a 40-year retrospective analysis at a major cancer center, for example, only about 15 % of children diagnosed with malignant solid tumors under the age of 1 year presented with their disease in the first 30 days of life [150].

Most tumors of very young children arise either from the hematopoietic system or from embryonic/developing tissues. The pattern of cancers diagnosed in infancy is different than that of the general pediatric population. Neuroblastoma, an embryonal malignancy of the adrenal cortex and sympathetic nervous system, is overrepresented among infants and accounts for almost a third of malignancies in this age group [59]. In contrast, neuroblastomas make up only about a tenth of cancers in the general pediatric population. Retinoblastoma, fibrosarcoma, and hepatoblastoma are other solid tumors overrepresented in the very young. Acute leukemias, on the other hand, are underrepresented in infants. As a group, acute leukemias are the most commonly diagnosed cancers of childhood; however, they account for less than 20 % of malignancies in infants (Fig. 13.4). Similarly, lymphomas and bone tumors – among the most common solid tumors of school-age children and adolescents – occur very rarely in infants. Altogether, urinary tract malignancies (particularly renal tumors) make up about 10–15 % of tumors diagnosed in infancy [59].

Outcome for infants with cancer is variable and depends on the particular type of cancer, stage of disease at diagnosis, clinical factors, and therapeutic response. Prognosis for infants with cancer tends to be worse than for older children, even for the same diagnosis. The most obvious example is that of pediatric acute lymphoblastic leukemia (ALL). Infant ALL is much more difficult to cure than standard childhood ALL, in part because many cases are associated with the MLL (11q23) gene rearrangement that renders leukemias treatment refractory and prone to relapse. Similarly, many solid tumors, including rhabdomyosarcoma, CNS ependymomas, and PNETs, are associated with a poorer prognosis if diagnosed in infants. It is not clear whether these differences related to different molecular mechanisms of disease in tumors of

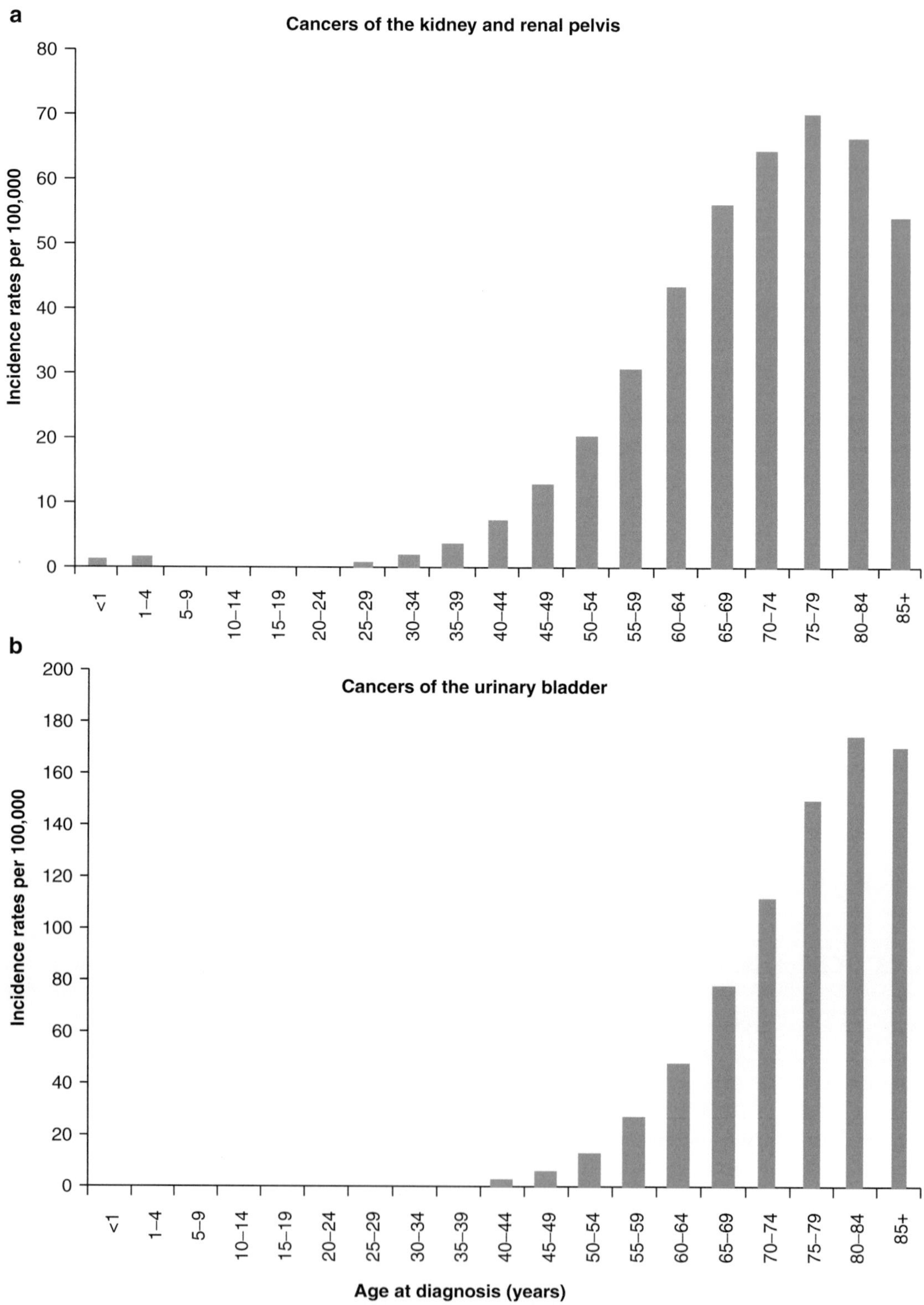

Fig. 13.2 Age-specific incidence rates for cancers of (**a**) the kidney and renal pelvis and (**b**) the urinary bladder, 2004–2008, NCI SEER data [59, 99]. Note the marked increase in urinary tract malignancies with age

Fig. 13.3 Age-specific cancer incidence rates for all pediatric cancers (**a**) and for pediatric renal tumors (**b**), 2004–2008, NCI SEER data [59, 99]. Note the relatively high incidence of cancer in infants (**a**) and the relatively high incidence of kidney tumors (mostly Wilms tumor) in the very young (**b**)

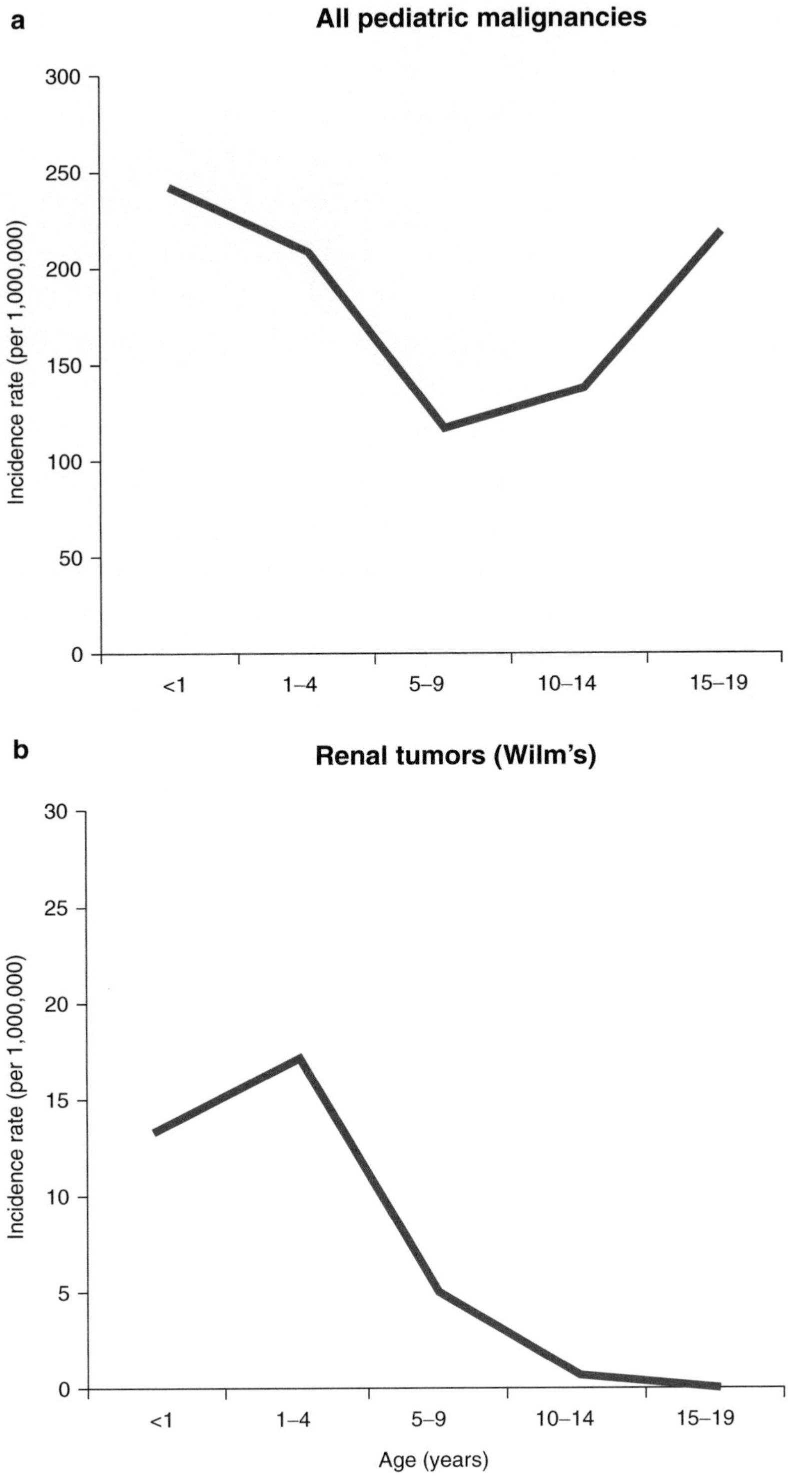

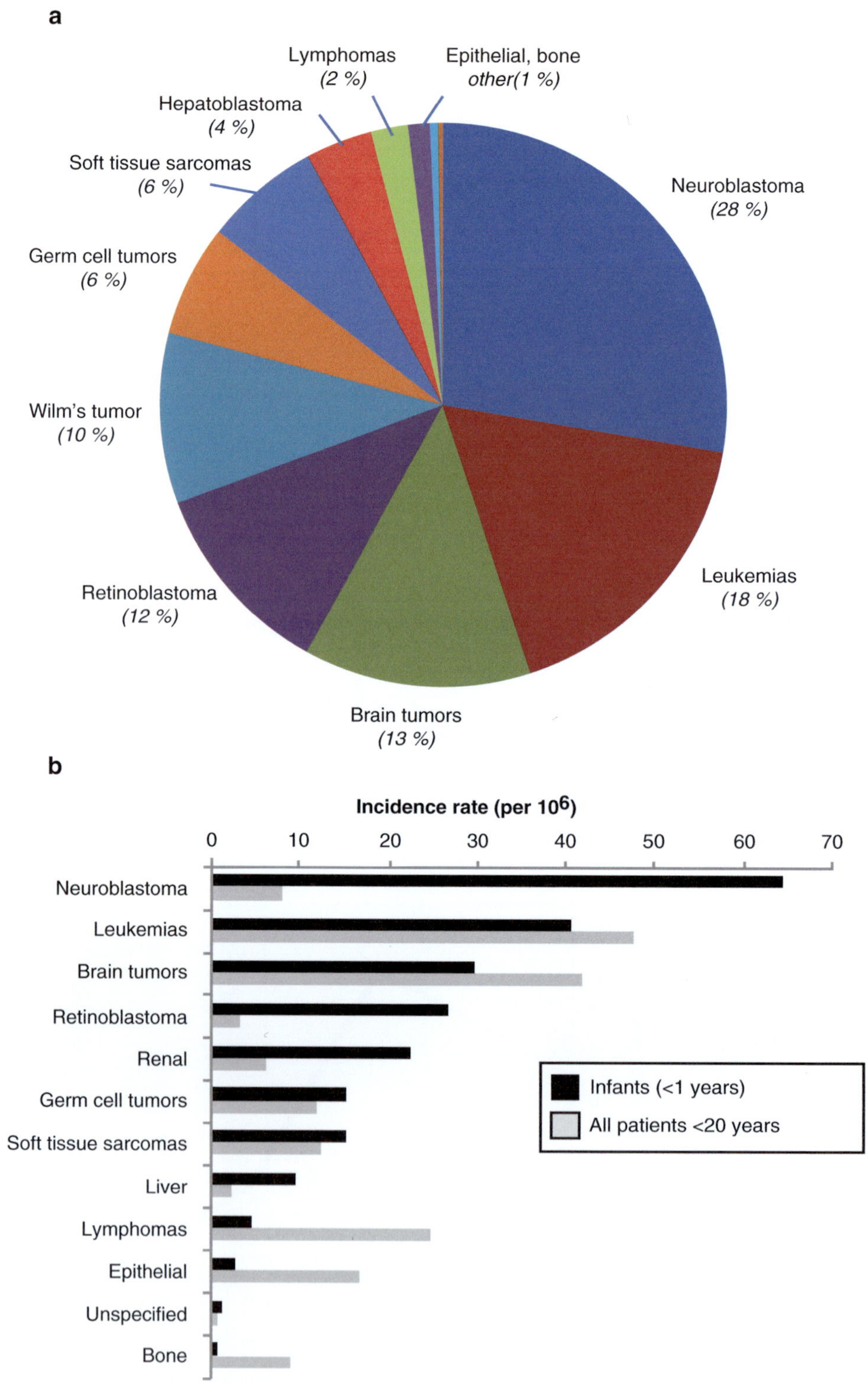

Fig. 13.4 Malignancies of infancy. (**a**) Frequency of cancer types diagnosed among patients less than 1 year of age at diagnosis. (**b**) Incidence rates (per million) of tumors in infants (*black bars*) compared with those for the total pediatric population (patients <20 years old, *gray bars*). Values represent combined NCI SEER data from 1976 to 1984 and 1986 to 1994, all races, both sexes [59]. Note the overrepresentation of neuroblastomas, retinoblastomas, and renal tumors in infants

the very young making cure more difficult or to the increased toxicity of therapy in the young. Neuroblastoma, however, is the major exception to this trend. Very young age (less than 12–18 months) at diagnosis is actually a favorable prognostic risk factor, correlating with more benign biological features and particularly a normal copy number of the N-myc oncogene. When the N-myc oncogene is amplified, neuroblastomas behave much more aggressively and are much more treatment refractory. Expansion of the N-myc gene tends to correlate with age at presentation, thus neuroblastomas in neonates and infants have a much better clinical outlook and usually require less intensive therapy for effective management. The 5-year survival rate for infants with neuroblastoma is over 80 % but is only 40–50 % in children more than 12–18 months at diagnosis [96].

Tumors have been described for both the upper (kidney, ureters) and lower (bladder, urethra) urinary system in infants [45, 79, 82, 109, 137, 141]. Renal tumors are the most common; however, like tumors in other anatomic regions, they can be either benign or malignant. In fact, the most common renal tumor in neonates is congenital mesoblastic nephroma which behaves in a benign manner and is treated successfully with surgical resection alone [71, 73]. Among neonates, congenital mesoblastic nephromas outnumber malignant kidney tumors by roughly a 4-to-1 margin [66, 123]. Considering malignant tumors of the infant kidney, Wilms tumor is the most frequent, accounting for about 10 % of all malignancies diagnosed in infants under a year of age (Fig. 13.4). Nonetheless, Wilms tumors are relatively unusual in neonates [7, 13, 16], peaking in incidence between the ages of 1 and 4 years (Fig. 13.3). In one analysis of over 3,000 children enrolled on National Wilms Tumor Studies, there were only four cases of Wilms tumor diagnosed in infants 30 days old or younger [66, 123]. Radiologic and pathologic diagnostic interpretations are critically important to differentiate benign versus malignant disease since therapy is usually markedly different.

13.4 Clinical Presentation of Urinary Tract Malignancies in Infants

With the widespread use of antenatal sonography and other imaging modalities, imaging of the fetal urinary system is feasible [29], and many tumors of the urinary tract are diagnosed even before birth (Fig. 13.5) [27, 47, 68, 90]. Some tumors can be easily distinguished as abnormal masses on ultrasound, distinct from their normal tissues of origin. Others appear as unilateral enlargement of a kidney caused either by impairment of urine outflow by a tumor or by growth of a mass in the kidney itself. Nonetheless, there are many nonmalignant causes of unilateral renal enlargement, including hydronephrosis from urinary outflow obstruction and cystic renal disease. Further modalities such as magnetic resonance imaging may be useful to distinguish between malignant and nonmalignant processes and to evaluate the contralateral kidney for premalignant abnormalities such as nephroblastomatosis [72, 81]. As with solid tumors of adulthood, detecting tumors as rapidly as possible facilitates early diagnosis of tumors at lower, more treatable stages of disease [64]. When not identified prenatally, most urinary tract tumors of infants and young children come to medical attention because of symptoms caused by the presence of the mass itself and its physical interference with normal structures and organ function. Many abdominal tumors (like the one in our clinical vignette) are first appreciated as asymptomatic masses palpated either by a caretaker or the pediatrician. Others may come to attention because of associated signs or symptoms such as hematuria, vomiting, polyuria, or hypertension [122]. Proteinuria, azotemia, or electrolyte disturbances can also be a feature of urinary tract malignancies.

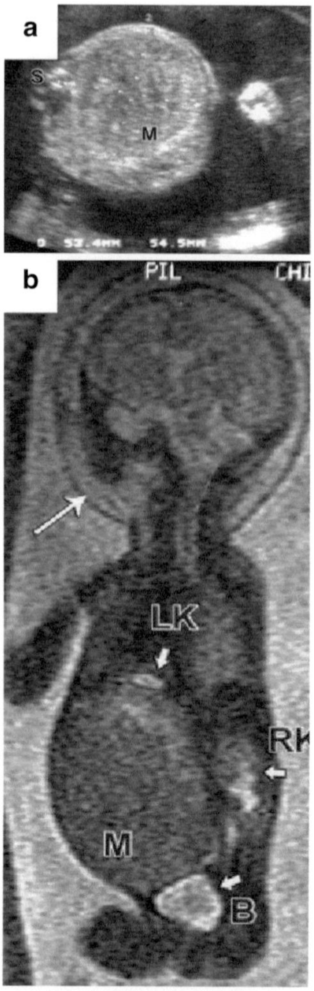

Fig. 13.5 Prenatal detection of a renal mass in a 22-week fetus by sonography (**a**) and confirmatory MRI (**b**). (**a**) Large mass (*M*) in the fetal abdomen (*S* spine). (**b**) Renal mass (*M*) with displacement of the left kidney (*LK*); *RK* right kidney, *B* bladder, *arrow* scalp edema. The mass proved to be a benign congenital mesoblastic nephroma (Images used with permission from Chen et al. [27])

The approach to the infant suspected of having a tumor of the urinary tract typically includes renal/abdominal imaging, a urinalysis, and basic bloodwork including a complete blood count (CBC), serum electrolytes, BUN and creatinine, and a hepatic function panel [47, 67, 77, 115, 150]. If a mass is documented, then further studies including either resection or biopsy and evaluation for metastatic disease are indicated to complete tumor identification and staging. Because workup and staging can have significant implications for therapy and prognosis, it is recommended that evaluation and management of urinary tract masses be performed by experienced pediatric oncology medical, radiologic, and surgical teams.

Table 13.1 Clinical characteristics of inherited cancer syndromes

Cancers at a young age (including infancy)
Multiple primary tumors of the same type over time
Multiple family members affected by cancer
Family history of similar tumor type
Bilateral or multiple foci of disease
Rare cancers in unusual anatomic locations
Constellation of tumors or clinical findings consistent with a specific cancer syndrome

13.5 Cancer Syndromes Involving the Urinary Tract

Familial cancer syndromes are characterized by heritable predisposition to one or more types of malignancy. These conditions are caused by the inheritance of a genetic mutation that causes a person to be at increased risk of cancer. There are numerous examples of familial cancer syndromes, each caused by a defective cancer-relevant gene and each associated with a specific pattern of cancer risk. Individuals with inherited loss of function mutation of one allele of the p53 tumor suppressor gene, for example, have the "Li-Fraumeni syndrome" and are at risk for sarcomas, leukemias, brain tumors, breast cancer, and adrenocortical carcinoma [54, 80]. In contrast, persons with neurofibromatosis type I have a defective NF1 gene and are at risk for optic pathway gliomas, myelogenous leukemia, and malignant peripheral nerve sheath tumors [88]. Each cancer syndrome is associated with unique cancer risk, and cancers of the urinary tract, especially Wilms tumor, feature prominently among familial cancer syndromes of infancy and childhood. Clinical "clues" to familial cancer syndromes (Table 13.1) include presentation of malignancy at a very young age; therefore inherited cancer predisposition should be considered as a possibility in any affected neonate or young infant [35].

Table 13.2 Cancer syndromes that predispose to Wilms tumor

WAGR	Wilms tumor, Aniridia, Genitourinary malformations, and mental Retardation
Denys-Drash syndrome	Intersex disorders (ambiguous genitalia), progressive nephropathy, Wilms tumor
Frasier syndrome	Streak gonads, ambiguous genitalia, renal failure, gonadoblastoma, Wilms tumor
Beckwith-Wiedemann syndrome	Omphalocele; macroglossia; gigantism; organomegaly; hemihypertrophy; genitourinary, cardiac, and/or musculoskeletal abnormalities; hearing loss; mild developmental delay; and cancer (Wilms tumor, hepatoblastoma, rhabdomyosarcoma, adrenocortical carcinoma)
Perlman syndrome	Polyhydramnios, macrosomia, macrocephaly, dysmorphic facies, visceromegaly, nephroblastomatosis, and Wilms tumor

There are at least five distinct clinical entities which predispose infants and children to Wilms tumor (Table 13.2) including Beckwith-Wiedemann syndrome, WAGR (Wilms tumor, Aniridia, Genitourinary anomalies, and mental Retardation) syndrome, Denys-Drash syndrome, Perlman syndrome, and Frasier syndrome [4, 44, 50, 60, 93, 120, 142]. Many Wilms tumor cancer syndromes involve mutation or epigenetic silencing of pertinent tumor suppressor genes on chromosome 11 [58, 119]. The first gene associated with Wilms tumor was mapped to chromosome 11p13 and named WT1 [61]. WT1 is a zinc finger transcription factor involved in the regulation of renal cell growth, differentiation, and apoptosis [40]. Genetic defects in WT1 underlie WAGR syndrome, Frasier syndrome, and Denys-Drash syndrome [30, 48, 89]. WT1 function can be lost either by mutation, alternative splicing, or genomic imprinting, depending on the syndrome. WT2 is another Wilms tumor-associated gene located on chromosome 11 (at 11p15) that, when defective through aberrant genetic imprinting, causes Beckwith-Wiedemann syndrome (BWS). BWS is a clinical overgrowth syndrome characterized by omphalocele, gigantism, macroglossia, visceromegaly, and an increased risk of embryonal tumors including Wilms tumor and hepatoblastoma [46, 113, 129, 144]. Wilms tumors associated with cancer syndromes tend to occur earlier and more often than Wilms tumors in the general pediatric population. One study found that the average age of presentation of Wilms tumor was 22 months in children with a predisposition syndrome compared to 39 months for sporadic cases [22]. Actual risk of Wilms tumor varies according to the cancer syndrome. Children with Beckwith-Wiedemann syndrome, for example, have up to a 7.5 % chance of developing Wilms tumor, whereas essentially 100 % of patients with WAGR will develop Wilms tumor by 7 years of age [120].

Once a patient has been identified with a cancer syndrome that predisposes him/her to development of Wilms tumor, then she/he should be regularly screened for malignancy with regular physical examination, urinalysis, and imaging. Wilms tumors can double in size each week [12]; thus early detection of tumors facilitates diagnosis of malignancy at earlier stage of disease, improving prognosis and reducing intensity of therapy [35, 107]. In general, children with identified cancer syndromes should undergo serial screening with abdominal/renal ultrasound every 3 months through 7–10 years of age [41]. Importantly, diagnosis of a child with an inherited cancer syndrome carries a variety of implications for that child, his/her parents, and other members of the family. Confirmatory genetic testing, formal cancer genetic counseling, and development of a rational cancer surveillance plan are all critical aspects of management [28, 63, 112].

13.6 Tumors Involving the Infant Urinary System

13.6.1 Mesoblastic Nephroma

Originally thought to be a Wilms tumor variant, mesoblastic nephroma was later described to be distinct from Wilms [15]. It is now appreciated to be an incompletely malignant tumor, with a low propensity for metastatic spread [97]. Rather, mesoblastic nephromas exhibit features of benign hamartomas, but they can grow to massive sizes and invade local

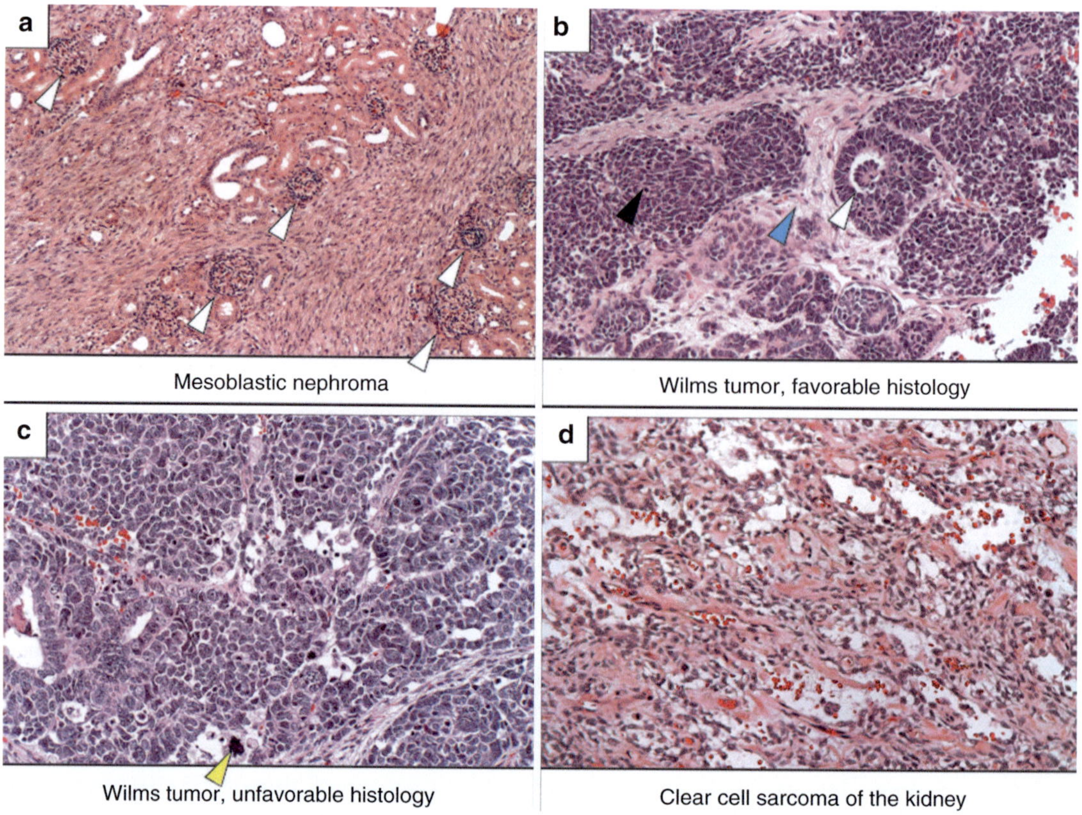

Fig. 13.6 Histologic characteristics of various renal tumors of infancy in order of increasing clinical aggressiveness. (**a**) Mesoblastic nephromas retain many features of the kidney. These proliferative tumors which behave in a benign manner are composed of sheets of fibrous or mesenchymal stroma with scattered renal tubules and glomeruli (*white triangles*). (**b**) "Favorable histology" Wilms tumors retain differentiated characteristics of the kidney and typically contain blastemal (*black triangle*), stromal (*blue triangle*), and glomerular (*white triangle*) elements. (**c**) "Unfavorable histology" or "anaplastic" Wilms tumors are less differentiated and more aggressive, exhibiting features of hyperdiploid mitotic figures (*yellow triangle*), nuclear enlargement, and/or hyperchromasia. (**d**) Clear cell sarcoma of the kidney (*CCSK*) contains sarcomatous features including the presence of spindle-shaped tumor cells and mucopolysaccharide-rich cytoplasm, imparting a "clear cell" appearance to the cells. Note the progressive loss of renal differentiation with increased aggressiveness of malignancy

structures. In addition, there are reports of distant spread and local recurrences after resection particularly among the "cellular" histologic subtypes [11, 55]. Mesoblastic nephroma is characteristically a disease of the very young infant. In fact, it is the most common renal tumor identified in neonates and young infants with one study finding over 85 % being diagnosed in infants younger than 4 months of age [122]. Cases can be identified either prenatally on routine sonography [147] or because of clinical signs/symptoms such as the presence of a flank mass, hematuria, hypertension, hyperbilirubinemia, or emesis [73]. Mesoblastic nephroma tumors have a homogeneous rubbery fibroid-like character and are composed of sheets of fibrous or mesenchymal stroma with scattered renal tubules and glomeruli [122] (Fig. 13.6). Most cases can be cured by surgery alone provided that tumors can be completely excised [51]. In general there is no role for chemotherapy or radiotherapy.

13.6.2 Wilms Tumor

Wilms tumor is the most common malignant kidney tumor in children [138]. Affecting roughly 1 in every 100,000 children, Wilms tumor is somewhat more common in children of African

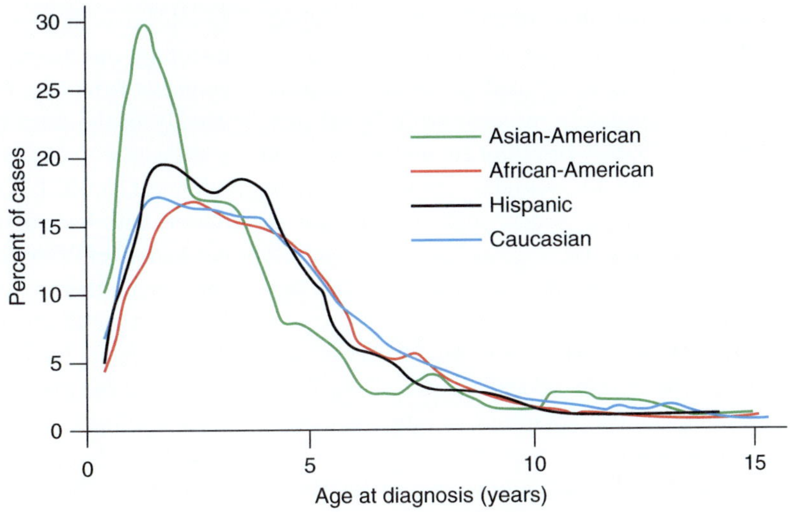

Fig. 13.7 Age distribution of Wilms tumor among patients enrolled on the National Wilms Tumor Study [19]. Data are shown by ethnic group. Note the much higher incidence of disease in the very young across ethnic groups

descent and less common in children of Asian ancestry [104]. Almost uniformly a disease of children, the great majority of Wilms tumors are diagnosed in patients under the age of five with a median age of presentation at just over 3 years (Fig. 13.7) [19, 20, 34]. Wilms tumor is one of the most common tumors associated with pediatric-inherited cancer syndromes, and when it occurs in this context, it tends to occur earlier and has a higher likelihood of involving both kidneys. Thus, the mean age of presentation is between 36 and 42 months for unilateral disease and between 23 and 30 months for bilateral disease [18]. Despite the association between Wilms tumor and various cancer syndromes, however, the great majority of Wilms tumors are sporadic, occurring in patients without recognizable predisposition. Wilms tumor can affect very young infants [53, 66, 115] and has even been diagnosed prenatally [7, 13, 16, 32, 37]. Though Wilms tumor can occur in infants, neonatal Wilms tumor is comparatively rare. One institution reported only 10 % of renal masses occurring in children less than 6 months of age with only a fraction of these being Wilms [53]. In a multicenter National Wilms Tumor Study, only 27 of 3,340 patients (0.8 %) with renal tumors were 30 days old or less, and the majority of those tumors were mesoblastic nephromas [66]. Nonetheless, very young patients with Wilms tumors fare well, with one review of 15 neonatal cases reporting only one death at 31 months [115].

Like other abdominal tumors, Wilms tumors usually come to medical attention through palpation of a hard abdominal mass or because of associated symptoms. In the case of very young infants with Wilms tumors, some may be detected prenatally via ultrasonography [7, 37, 47, 52, 115, 135]. Up to 40 % of unilateral and nearly all bilateral Wilms tumors are thought to arise from precursor lesions in the kidney. These "nephrogenic rests" are intrarenal collections of embryologic kidney cells that normally regress spontaneously by birth or in the postnatal period [40]. Presumably nephrogenic rests represent incompletely malignant but clonally expanded renal cell precursors. In order for cancer (Wilms tumor) to develop, there must be acquisition of a fully malignant phenotype through further genetic or epigenetic changes in one or more cells within the nephrogenic rest. Before the advent of multimodal therapy, Wilms tumor was a uniformly fatal disease. Today, however, the long-term outlook for most Wilms tumor patients is optimistic due to a better understanding of how to combine surgery, chemotherapy, and, in some cases, radiation therapy.

In fact, the major advances in treatment and overall survival for Wilms tumor over the last several decades represent one of the greatest "success stories" for pediatric cancers. Therapy is based on risk stratification of disease which is calculated by staging, histopathology, and genetic features. Wilms tumor staging is fairly standardized, with uniformity across institutions [56]:

- Stage I: Tumor limited to kidney, capsule intact, completely resected with "good margins," no biopsy or tumor rupture/spillage, no involvement of vessels, renal sinuses or regional lymph nodes, and no evidence of metastatic disease.
- Stage II: Tumor infiltration of the renal capsule or vascular invasion.
- Stage III: Residual tumor present after surgery (regional lymph nodes, peritoneal spillage/seeding, unresected tumor, or tumor at margin of resection).
- Stage IV: Distant organ or extraregional lymph node metastasis. The lung is (by far) the most common site of metastasis with liver, bone, and brain involvement possible.
- Stage V: Synchronous involvement of both kidneys.

In addition to stage at diagnosis, histologic characteristics of the disease correlate with outcome. Wilms tumors can be classified as being either "favorable" or "unfavorable" with respect to their histologic characteristics. Favorable histology Wilms tumors display features of their renal tissue of origin. They appear to be more differentiated with prominent renal tubular elements and no sarcomatous features (Fig. 13.6). In contrast, unfavorable histology tumors show evidence of diffuse or focal anaplasia, determined by the presence of hyperdiploid mitotic figures, nuclear enlargement, and/or hyperchromasia (Fig. 13.6). Anaplasia and unfavorable features correlate with more aggressive disease. Among stage III patients, for example, patients with favorable histology tumors had more than 90 % overall survival, whereas those with unfavorable histology tumors had survival rates of roughly 50 % [39]. Unfavorable histology Wilms tumors account for more than 50 % of Wilms tumor deaths despite being found in only 10 % of cases [39]. Fortunately, favorable histology Wilms tumors account for more than 85 % of clinical isolates.

Wilms tumors are treated with surgery and chemotherapy, with or without radiotherapy. Intensity of therapy is determined by stage and histology, with higher stage and/or unfavorable histology disease requiring longer, more intense courses of therapy. Complete surgical resection, usually in the form of total nephrectomy, is the cornerstone of effective treatment for Wilms tumors [116, 123]. While some early-stage Wilms tumors have been treated with surgery alone [57], most cases of Wilms tumors are treated with adjuvant chemotherapy post-nephrectomy to reduce local and metastatic recurrences. Vincristine and dactinomycin (actinomycin D) have been long been used for low-stage favorable disease, while anthracyclines, cyclophosphamide, and etoposide have been incorporated into therapeutic regimens for higher-stage or unfavorable disease [56]. Wilms tumor is radiosensitive and radiation therapy is useful in the setting of stage III or IV disease [56].

Bilateral Wilms tumor, defined by the presence of tumors in both kidneys at diagnosis, accounts for approximately 5 % of cases [92]. As mentioned above, bilateral disease is more common in children with cancer syndromes, and such disorders should be considered in children with bilateral Wilms tumors [62]. Presumed to represent bilateral primary tumor formation rather than metastasis from the contralateral kidney, stage V Wilms is associated with higher morbidity and mortality [45]. When both kidneys are affected, surgical management of disease is not straightforward. Total nephrectomy, commonly done for unilateral disease, is not necessarily the procedure of choice since removal of both kidneys would leave a patient in need of lifelong dialysis or of renal transplantation. Thus nephron-sparing surgery is attempted when feasible to preserve renal function in patients with bilateral disease [118]. Current recommendations for treating stage V Wilms tumor include subtotal nephrectomy and chemotherapy with or without radiation therapy [91]. However, eventual renal failure is not uncommon in patients treated with subtotal nephrectomies. Roughly 15 % of stage V Wilms tumor survivors develop chronic renal failure by age 20 years compared with 1 % of unilateral Wilms tumor patients [21]. Therefore stage V Wilms tumor patients treated with subtotal nephrectomies should avoid nephrotoxic agents and should be closely monitored over time for renal function, preferably with the expert involvement of an experienced pediatric nephrology team.

13.6.3 Clear Cell Sarcoma of the Kidney (CCSK)

Clear cell sarcoma of the kidney (CCSK) was initially distinguished from Wilms tumor because of its propensity to metastasize to the bone and comparatively poorer prognosis when compared to Wilms tumor [86, 95]. Because of its non-epithelioid, sarcomatous histologic features (Fig. 13.6), CCSK probably accounted for a significant proportion of intrarenal malignancies with "unfavorable histology" among tumors registered in early National Wilms Tumor Study Group (NWTSG) clinical trials [14]. CCSK is a relatively rare pediatric malignancy, representing only a small fraction of solid tumors and less than 5 % of renal tumors of infants and children. Roughly 20 cases are diagnosed annually in the United States [103]. The average age of diagnosis is between 1 and 4 years of age [152], and boys seem to be more at risk of disease with a male to female ratio of 2:1 [8]. Though less than 10 % of cases occur in children under 1 year of age, there are at least three reports of CCSK diagnosed in neonates and infants [69, 87, 100].

Even though CCSK has a tendency to metastasize to the bone, less than 5 % of CCSK patients present with evidence of distant metastasis at diagnosis [78]. Rather, the majority of children with CCSK present with either stage II or stage III disease, defined by involvement of local or regional lymph nodes at diagnosis [8]. Bilateral stage V disease involving both kidneys is unusual for CCSK and has only recently been described [85]. In stage IV patients, the bone represents the most common site of distant metastasis, followed by the lung, abdomen, brain, and liver [143]. Most CCSKs are relatively large at presentation (average size of 11.3 cm) and tend to essentially replace the affected kidney.

In contrast to Wilms tumor, CCSK does not seem to be affiliated with familial cancer syndromes [2], and CCSK, unlike Wilms tumor, does not appear to develop from nephrogenic rests [8]. In addition, there are no characteristic genetic abnormalities that define CCSKs, although one recent study reported high expression levels of two tyrosine kinases – the epidermal growth factor receptor (EGFR) and c-Kit – in CCSK [133]. Clinical presentation is similar to Wilms tumor, either detected on radiologic imaging or because of a palpable abdominal mass, hypertension, or hematuria [128]. Diagnosis is confirmed by pathological examination of resected tumor, and staging is achieved with multimodal imaging including CT scanning of the chest, abdomen, and pelvis; nuclear imaging (bone and/or PET scanning); and imaging of the brain [124].

Because of its aggressive phenotype, effective management of CCSK requires more intensified therapy than Wilms tumor. The typical treatment approach involves surgical resection (nephrectomy), adjunct radiation, and chemotherapy for 24 weeks with alternating cycles of vincristine/doxorubicin/cyclophosphamide and cyclophosphamide/etoposide [23, 76, 78, 124]. Positive prognostic factors for CCSK include treatment with doxorubicin, low stage at diagnosis, age between 2 and 4 years at the time of diagnosis, and lack of tumor necrosis on histologic examination [101]. Improvements in staging as well as chemotherapy and medical support have resulted in improved outcomes.

13.6.4 Malignant Rhabdoid Tumor (MRT)

Among the most aggressive cancers of infants and very young children, malignant rhabdoid tumors (MRTs) can arise in the kidney where they are also called rhabdoid tumors of the kidney, in the central nervous system where they are termed atypical teratoid rhabdoid tumors, or in other places in the body as extrarenal rhabdoid tumors [83, 152]. Most MRTs, however, arise in the kidney, where they account for roughly 2 % of renal tumors in infants, ranking behind mesoblastic nephromas and Wilms tumors [137]. They occur most often in infants and very young

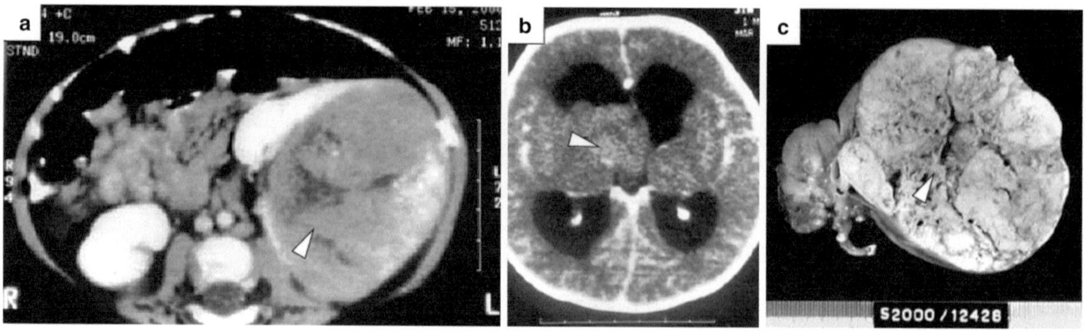

Fig. 13.8 Concurrent malignant rhabdoid tumor of the kidney and brain in a 2-month-old infant who presented with vomiting, abdominal mass, and altered mental status. (**a**) Transverse abdominal CT scan revealing a large left intrarenal mass with evidence of central necrosis (*white triangle*). (**b**) CT scan of the brain of the same patient at diagnosis, showing an AT/RT tumor of the right frontal horn with associated hydrocephalus from obstruction of CSF flow. (**c**) Photograph of the resected renal MRT. Shown is a cut surface of the tumor revealing extensive central hemorrhagic necrosis (*white triangle*) (With kind permission from Springer: Luo et al. [84])

children, with 15 months being the mean age at diagnosis [132]. Although the majority of these tumors are diagnosed in the kidney, metachronous or synchronous disease in more than one site has been observed [1, 49, 136, 149]. In fact, roughly 15 % of patients with MRTs will present with concurrent involvement of the kidney and the CNS (Fig. 13.8) [98]; therefore both anatomic sites must be assessed during a staging workup. Irrespective of tissue of origin, most rhabdoid tumors are characterized by a similar molecular feature – the biallelic inactivating mutation of the *hSNF/INI1* gene on chromosome 22q11.2 [140, 151]. This molecular defect presumably contributes to carcinogenesis through alterations in chromatin remodeling. Molecular testing and immunohistochemical staining for INI1 are available to confirm the diagnosis of MRT [149].

MRTs mainly metastasize to the lungs, but they may also spread to the bone, lymph nodes, and liver [137]. Due to the aggressive clinical nature of the tumor, vague symptoms and young age at presentation, most patients have advanced stages of disease at time of diagnosis [137]. Roughly 60 % of children with intrarenal MRTs present with hematuria since most MRTs are medially positioned in the kidney, invading urinary collecting structures as they grow (Fig. 13.8). In contrast, hematuria occurs only in about 20 % of cases of Wilms tumors, which tend to be laterally positioned in the kidney, growing away from the renal pelvis [6, 114]. Seventy percent of patients with intrarenal MRTs have hypertension, about half manifest fever, and about a quarter have either proteinuria or hypercalcemia. If there is simultaneous disease of the CNS, patients may also present with neurologic symptoms such as seizures, hemiplegia, vomiting, or focal deficits [6, 42].

Grossly, MRTs are solid tumors that often display extensive hemorrhage and necrosis (Fig. 13.8). Highly aggressive, MRTs tend to be infiltrative rather than encapsulated [121]. Histologically, they are characterized by solid sheets of small round cells, some of which resemble rhabdomyoblasts (hence the name "rhabdoid tumor") [132, 149, 151].

Treatment of MRTs involves a combination of surgery, radiotherapy, and chemotherapy, with age, stage at diagnosis, and extent of local control all significantly influencing outcome [132, 152]. Complete nephrectomy is the preferred method of surgical removal of intrarenal MRTs [25, 136]. Although multiple treatment regimens with combined therapies including vincristine, cyclophosphamide, dactinomycin, etoposide, and anthracyclines have been used, clinical outcomes have been poor, with many patients relapsing within a year or suffering toxic events due to their very young age and the intensity of therapy. One study reported a 2-year event free survival of only 15 % and an overall 18-month survival of only 20 % [83]. However, there is hope that new therapeutic options, such as molecularly targeted therapy, will become available as we learn more about the molecular pathways that fuel carcinogenesis of rhabdoid cells.

13.6.5 Renal Cell Carcinoma (RCC)

Mainly a disease of adults, renal cell carcinoma (RCC) accounts for less than 5 % of pediatric renal tumors. Unlike most solid tumors of infancy and childhood, RCC is neither a sarcoma nor an embryonal tumor. Rather, it is an adenocarcinoma with renal tubular differentiation. Less than 2 % of all RCC occurs in the pediatric population [10]; however, it has been described in adolescents [42, 83, 126, 152] as well as in patients as young as 3 months of age [83, 126]. For RCC, younger age is a positive prognostic factor with overall survival rates in children ranging from 64 to 70 %, much higher than those observed in adults with RCC [83, 152]. Distant spread is found in 20 % of patients at diagnosis with the lungs, bone, brain, and liver being the most common sites of metastasis [111]. Stage at diagnosis is highly predictive of outcome. One study found that the 5-year survival rate for children with RCC was 70 % for localized disease and that no child with metastasis at presentation survived beyond 26 months [3].

RCCs frequently present as palpable abdominal masses without associated symptoms. The classic RCC triad in adults – flank pain, palpable mass, and gross hematuria – is much less common in the pediatric population [70, 126]. Rather, pediatric patients may be asymptomatic or simply manifest vague constitutional symptoms such as fatigue, malaise, and fever [130].

RCCs are locally infiltrative and often distort normal renal architecture, sometimes associated with a pseudocapsule [83]. They often exhibit areas of calcification on CT imaging [43, 146]. RCC spreads by lymphatic drainage, and regional retroperitoneal lymph nodes are frequently involved. Roughly a third of childhood RCCs are localized at presentation, almost half exhibit regional lymphatic spread, and about a quarter have evidence of systemic metastases at diagnosis [3, 139]. RCC may be associated with a history of prior malignancy, presumably because of the DNA-damaging nature of various chemotherapeutic agents [106]. RCC may also occur in the context of certain cancer predisposition syndromes, specifically tuberous sclerosis, von Hippel-Lindau syndrome, and Li-Fraumeni syndrome [5, 33, 108].

RCC is highly resistant to chemotherapy and radiotherapy; therefore surgery is the mainstay of therapy. RCC is usually treated with radical nephrectomy and regional lymphadenectomy [9]. Some centers have reported positive outcomes with nephron-sparing surgery in children [24, 26, 126]. Immunotherapy is currently being studied for its role in treatment.

13.6.6 Rhabdomyosarcoma and Sarcoma Botryoides

Among the most common solid tumors of childhood, rhabdomyosarcomas are thought to originate from muscle cells or their mesenchymal progenitors because they express many features of myocytes. Most children with rhabdomyosarcoma are diagnosed between the ages of 1 and 4 years, but between 5 and 10 % of cases occur in infants less than 1 year of age [145]. Rhabdomyosarcomas can occur almost anywhere in the body. The majority –approximately 35–40 % – arise in the head/neck region in parameningeal, parapharyngeal, and orbital sites. The genitourinary system is the second most frequent site of primary disease (approximately 20–25 %), with many tumors arising in or around the bladder, prostate, vagina, uterus, and paratesticular regions [82, 145]. Though rare, rhabdomyosarcoma can even originate in the kidney [110, 127]. The genitourinary tract is frequently the primary site of disease in infants and very young children [109]. Sarcoma botryoides is a special subtype of genitourinary rhabdomyosarcoma, defined by anatomic and histologic features [117]. Derived from the Greek term "botryose" meaning "bunch of grapes," sarcoma botryoides grows in a

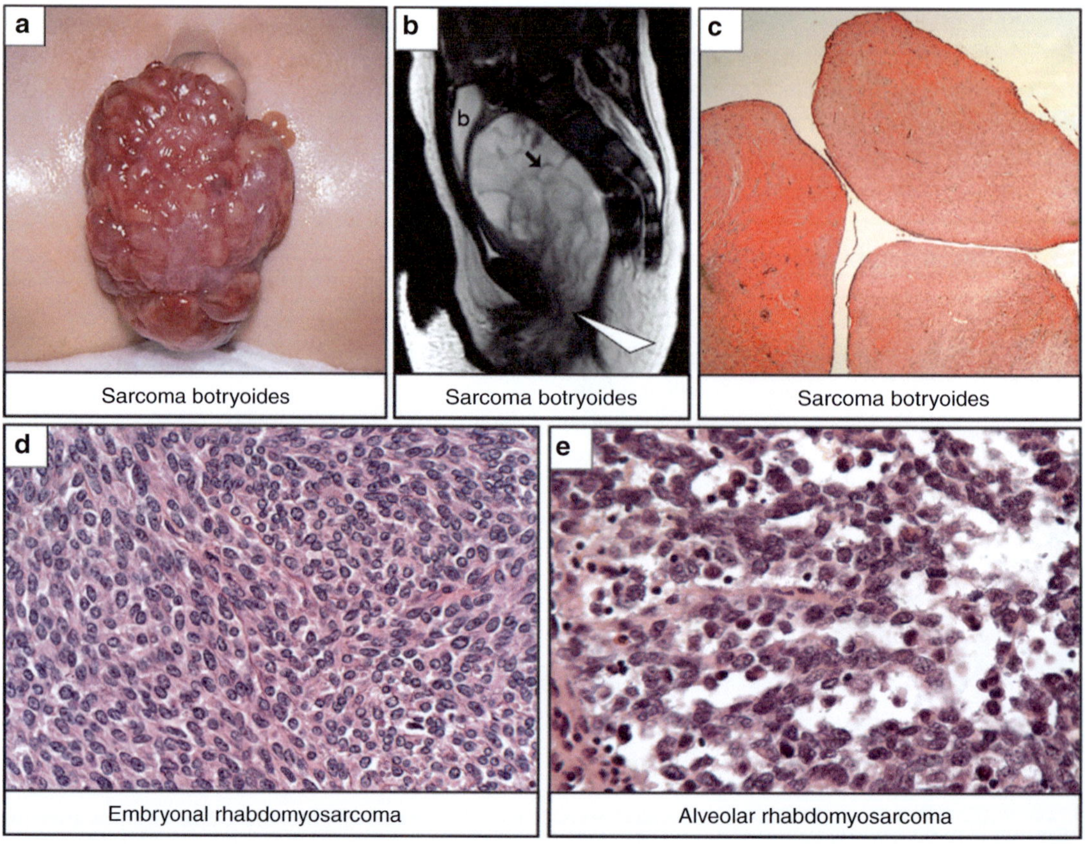

Fig. 13.9 Sarcoma botryoides and rhabdomyosarcoma. Sarcoma botryoides, a subtype of rhabdomyosarcoma characteristically found in the urogenital tract of infants and very young children, has the appearance of a "bunch of grapes" on gross inspection (**a**), on imaging (**b**), and even on histology (**c**). (**a**) A grape-like mass protruding out of the vaginal introitus (This figure was published in Tersak et al. [134]), (**b**) Sagittal magnetic resonance image (*MRI*) showing a large mass with multiple septations (*black arrow*) protruding from the vagina (*white triangle*) and with mass effect anteriorly on the urinary bladder (*b*) (Used with permission from Kobi et al. [74]). (**c**) Low-power view of sarcoma botryoides showing squamous-lined polypoid appearance (20× total magnification). Most sarcoma botryoides and other urinary tract rhabdomyosarcomas of infants exhibit "embryonal" histologic features. (**d**) Characteristic "embryonal" histology of rhabdomyosarcoma – note the abundant stroma and spindle cell appearance (hematoxylin & eosin staining, 200× magnification). (**e**) Alveolar histology of rhabdomyosarcoma – note the increased density with tumor cells arranged along delicate fibrovascular stalks in a pattern somewhat reminiscent of pulmonary alveoli (hematoxylin & eosin staining, 200× magnification)

cluster-like fashion from the walls of hollow, mucosal-lined organs such as the vagina and bladder, protruding into the lumen as it grows (Fig. 13.9). Genitourinary discharge, bleeding, and direct observation of a grape-like tumor mass growing out of the vaginal introitus are common symptoms [17]. Hematuria is common in bladder or renal sites, and rhabdomyosarcoma should be considered in patients with urinary tract tumors having a botryoid appearance on imaging studies [74, 127, 148] (Fig. 13.8).

Rhabdomyosarcomas fall into two broad pathologic subtypes – embryonal or alveolar. Embryonal tumors, associated with young age and lower stage at diagnosis, are characterized histologically by a stroma-rich, spindle cell appearance (Fig. 13.9). Alveolar tumors, on the other hand, tend to be more densely packed with tumor cells deposited in a festooned linear pattern that resembles the pulmonary alveoli (Fig. 13.9). Alveolar histology correlates with older age and higher stage at diagnosis and is often characterized by molecular translocations involving PAX and FKHR genes [102]. In general, genitourinary rhabdomyosarcomas in infants, including sarcoma botryoides, tend to fall into the embryonal category [36, 38, 131].

Prognosis is influenced by pathologic subtype and extent of disease at diagnosis. Rhabdomyosarcoma metastasizes to the local and regional lymph nodes, lung, cortical bone, and bone marrow; thus staging should focus on those sites [145]. Treatment includes surgical resection with lymph node sampling. Postsurgical adjuvant chemotherapy with vincristine and actinomycin and/or anthracyclines is standard. Rhabdomyosarcomas are fairly radiation sensitive; therefore radiotherapy may be an option particularly with unresectable disease.

13.6.7 Anticancer Therapy in Infants

Effective therapy of cancers of the urinary tract usually begins with surgical removal of the tumor. The best chance of long-term cure occurs when the primary tumor can be completely excised [65, 105, 115]. Once local control is achieved, then chemotherapy may be given to prevent local or distant recurrence and to treat any macroscopic or microscopic metastatic tumor foci. Traditional chemotherapy drugs, however, are indiscriminate in their effects. The standard chemotherapy drugs used for most pediatric malignancies target cells and tissues that are actively dividing, regardless of whether those tissues are benign or malignant. Therefore, much of the toxicity of chemotherapy occurs because the medications affect organs in which ongoing cellular proliferation is required for normal function. For a variety of reasons, infants and very young children are more sensitive to the toxic effects of chemotherapy than older children or adults (Table 13.3). Since their brains, organs, and tissues are in active states of development, infants are comparatively more affected by agents that interfere with cell division [125]. The bone marrow is among the most sensitive and important sites of off-target drug effects. Ongoing hematopoiesis is necessary in order to replace the billions of red blood cells, platelets, and white blood cells used up each day by the blood and immune systems, and hematopoiesis depends on proliferative expansion of blood cell precursors in the marrow. Thus, chemotherapeutic agents predictably induce a temporary inhibition of marrow hematopoiesis and reductions in peripheral blood cell counts, leaving cancer patients anemic and prone to bleeding and infections. Infants are at particular risk of bone marrow suppression. Much of the enhanced toxicity of chemotherapy in infants is due to infectious complications. To begin with, infants' immune systems are comparatively immature, making them much more vulnerable to infectious complications even in times of robust bone marrow hematopoiesis. Their infectious risk skyrockets once the marrow is suppressed, particularly during periods of neutropenia following chemotherapy administration. Renal and hepatic metabolic function is also comparatively underdeveloped in the very young, leading to reduction in drug metabolism and detoxification. Thus, chemotherapeutic agents remain active longer and at higher levels when administered to babies [94].

Table 13.3 Factors contributing to enhanced chemotoxicity in infants

Active developmental phase of organs and tissues
Altered drug absorption
Altered pharmacokinetics/pharmacodynamics
Compromised early detection of toxicity in nonverbal patients
Cutaneous sensitivity (diaper area) to chemotherapeutic drugs and skin-irritating metabolites in urine and stool
Higher comparative body surface area leading to higher realized doses of drugs if dosed per m^2
Higher relative content of fat stores in infants
Immature blood-brain barrier
Immature hepatic detoxification mechanisms (prolonged realized dose)
Immature immune system, increasing risk of serious infectious complications (bacterial, fungal, viral)
Immature renal function (delayed renal clearance)
Limited data on drug efficacy and adverse effects in infants
Need for more aggressive therapy for many treatment-resistant infant malignancies (e.g., leukemias)

There have been few appropriately powered clinical studies to address therapeutic and adverse effects of many chemotherapeutic agents in very young patients. Many drugs are used "off-label" and without formal FDA regulation and approval [75]. Nonetheless, some national children's oncology trials have attempted to address issues of safety and efficacy in the very young. In the second National Wilms Tumor Study (NWTS-2), for example, there was a higher frequency of severe toxicity and toxic deaths related to chemotherapy among patients less than 12 months of age. The study then modified the protocol to reduce (by half) doses of chemotherapy given to infants. Dose reductions of actinomycin D, adriamycin, and vincristine resulted in marked reductions in hematologic, pulmonary, and hepatic toxicity without affecting treatment outcome [94]. This and other studies have led to well-accepted guidelines for administration of modified doses chemotherapy to the very young [75]. Chemotherapy dose reductions in infants have, in general, been efficacious but with less toxicity [31]. It is hoped that with further discoveries about carcinogenic molecular mechanisms and the development of more targeted anticancer approaches, infants and children with cancer can be more safely treated.

Conclusion

About a tenth of cancers diagnosed in infants involve the urinary system. Most tumors come to medical attention either prenatally (e.g., by prenatal ultrasonography) or because of symptoms such as the presence of a palpable abdominal mass or hematuria. Many urinary tract tumors, particularly mesoblastic nephromas of the kidney, are actually considered benign. Malignancies that involve the urinary tract of infants and very young children are distinct from the typical carcinomas that affect adults, and they usually respond better to therapy than those in adults. However toxicity of chemotherapy and radiation therapy is comparatively greater in the very young child due to their small size, sensitive developmental stage, and metabolic characteristics. It is important to note that very young presentation of malignancy can be an indication of an inherited cancer predisposition syndrome. Cancer syndromes known to predispose to urinary tract malignancies include von Hippel-Lindau, Li-Fraumeni, and the Wilms tumor syndromes (including Beckwith-Wiedemann and WAGR). The evaluation and management of urinary tract masses is best accomplished by experienced oncologic, surgical, and radiologic clinical teams.

References

1. Agrons GA, Kingsman KD, Wagner BJ, Sotelo-Avila C (1997) Rhabdoid tumor of the kidney in children: a comparative study of 21 cases. AJR Am J Roentgenol 168(2):447–451
2. Ahmed HU, Arya M, Levitt G, Duffy PG, Mushtaq I, Sebire NJ (2007) Part I: Primary malignant non-Wilms' renal tumours in children. Lancet Oncol 8(8):730–737. doi:S1470-2045(07)70241-3 [pii]
3. Al-Shabanah MO, Jenkin DR, Khafaga YO, Al-Zahrani AM, Danjoux C, Greenberg M (2004) Renal cell carcinoma in children. Prognostic factors. Saudi Med J 25(11):1583–1586. doi:20040344 [pii]
4. Alessandri JL, Cuillier F, Ramful D, Ernould S, Robin S, de Napoli-Cocci S, Riviere JP, Rossignol S (2008) Perlman syndrome: report, prenatal findings and review. Am J Med Genet A 146A(19):2532–2537. doi:10.1002/ajmg.a.32391
5. Alrashdi I, Levine S, Paterson J, Saxena R, Patel SR, Depani S, Hargrave DR, Pritchard-Jones K, Hodgson SV (2010) Hereditary leiomyomatosis and renal cell carcinoma: very early diagnosis of renal cancer in a paediatric patient. Fam Cancer 9(2):239–243. doi:10.1007/s10689-009-9306-0
6. Amar AM, Tomlinson G, Green DM, Breslow NE, de Alarcon PA (2001) Clinical presentation of rhabdoid tumors of the kidney. J Pediatr Hematol Oncol 23(2):105–108
7. Applegate KE, Ghei M, Perez-Atayde AR (1999) Prenatal detection of a Wilms' tumor. Pediatr Radiol 29(1):65–67
8. Argani P, Perlman EJ, Breslow NE, Browning NG, Green DM, D'Angio GJ, Beckwith JB (2000) Clear cell sarcoma of the kidney: a review of 351 cases from the National Wilms Tumor Study Group Pathology Center. Am J Surg Pathol 24(1):4–18
9. Asanuma H, Nakai H, Takeda M, Shishido S, Tajima E, Kawamura T, Hara H, Morikawa Y (1999) Renal cell carcinoma in children: experience at a single institution in Japan. J Urol 162(4):1402–1405. doi:S0022-5347(05)68321-8 [pii]
10. Baek M, Jung JY, Kim JJ, Park KH, Ryu DS (2010) Characteristics and clinical outcomes of renal cell carcinoma in children: a single center experience. Int J Urol 17(8):737–740. doi:10.1111/j.1442-2042.2010.02588.x

11. Bayindir P, Guillerman RP, Hicks MJ, Chintagumpala MM (2009) Cellular mesoblastic nephroma (infantile renal fibrosarcoma): institutional review of the clinical, diagnostic imaging, and pathologic features of a distinctive neoplasm of infancy. Pediatr Radiol 39(10):1066–1074. doi:10.1007/s00247-009-1348-9
12. Beckwith JB (1998) Children at increased risk for Wilms tumor: monitoring issues. J Pediatr 132(3 Pt 1):377–379. doi:S0022-3476(98)70001-0 [pii]
13. Beckwith JB (1999) Prenatal detection of a Wilms' tumor. Pediatr Radiol 29(1):64
14. Beckwith JB, Palmer NF (1978) Histopathology and prognosis of Wilms tumors: results from the First National Wilms' Tumor Study. Cancer 41(5): 1937–1948
15. Bolande RP, Brough AJ, Izant RJ Jr (1967) Congenital mesoblastic nephroma of infancy. A report of eight cases and the relationship to Wilms' tumor. Pediatrics 40(2):272–278
16. Bove KE (1999) Wilms' tumor and related abnormalities in the fetus and newborn. Semin Perinatol 23(4):310–318
17. Brand E, Berek JS, Nieberg RK, Hacker NF (1987) Rhabdomyosarcoma of the uterine cervix. Sarcoma botryoides. Cancer 60(7):1552–1560
18. Breslow N, Beckwith JB, Ciol M, Sharples K (1988) Age distribution of Wilms' tumor: report from the National Wilms' Tumor Study. Cancer Res 48(6): 1653–1657
19. Breslow N, Olshan A, Beckwith JB, Green DM (1993) Epidemiology of Wilms tumor. Med Pediatr Oncol 21(3):172–181
20. Breslow NE, Beckwith JB, Perlman EJ, Reeve AE (2006) Age distributions, birth weights, nephrogenic rests, and heterogeneity in the pathogenesis of Wilms tumor. Pediatr Blood Cancer 47(3):260–267. doi:10.1002/pbc.20891
21. Breslow NE, Collins AJ, Ritchey ML, Grigoriev YA, Peterson SM, Green DM (2005) End stage renal disease in patients with Wilms tumor: results from the National Wilms Tumor Study Group and the United States Renal Data System. J Urol 174(5): 1972–1975
22. Breslow NE, Norris R, Norkool PA, Kang T, Beckwith JB, Perlman EJ, Ritchey ML, Green DM, Nichols KE (2003) Characteristics and outcomes of children with the Wilms tumor-Aniridia syndrome: a report from the National Wilms Tumor Study Group. J Clin Oncol 21(24):4579–4585
23. Broecker B (2000) Non-Wilms' renal tumors in children. Urol Clin North Am 27(3):463–469, ix
24. Castellanos RD, Aron BS, Evans AT (1974) Renal adenocarcinoma in children: incidence, therapy and prognosis. J Urol 111(4):534–537
25. Castellino SM, Martinez-Borges AR, McLean TW (2009) Pediatric genitourinary tumors. Curr Opin Oncol 21(3):278–283. doi:10.1097/CCO.0b013e328329f201
26. Chan CH, Cook D, Stanners CP (2006) Increased colon tumor susceptibility in azoxymethane treated CEABAC transgenic mice. Carcinogenesis 27(9):1909–1916
27. Chen WY, Lin CN, Chao CS, Yan-Sheng Lin M, Mak CW, Chuang SS, Tzeng CC, Huang KF (2003) Prenatal diagnosis of congenital mesoblastic nephroma in mid-second trimester by sonography and magnetic resonance imaging. Prenat Diagn 23(11):927–931. doi:10.1002/pd.727
28. Clericuzio CL (1999) Recognition and management of childhood cancer syndromes: a systems approach. Am J Med Genet 89(2):81–90
29. Cohen HL, Haller JO (1987) Diagnostic sonography of the fetal genitourinary tract. Urol Radiol 9(2): 88–98
30. Coppes MJ, Huff V, Pelletier J (1993) Denys-Drash syndrome: relating a clinical disorder to genetic alterations in the tumor suppressor gene WT1. J Pediatr 123(5):673–678
31. Corn BW, Goldwein JW, Evans I, D'Angio GJ (1992) Outcomes in low-risk babies treated with half-dose chemotherapy according to the Third National Wilms' Tumor Study. J Clin Oncol 10(8): 1305–1309
32. Crom DB, Wilimas JA, Green AA, Pratt CB, Jenkins JJ 3rd, Behm FG (1989) Malignancy in the neonate. Med Pediatr Oncol 17(2):101–104
33. Curry S, Ibrahim F, Grehan D, McDermott M, Capra M, Betts D, O'Sullivan M (2011) Rhabdomyosarcoma-associated renal cell carcinoma: a link with constitutional Tp53 mutation. Pediatr Dev Pathol 14(3):248–251. doi:10.2350/10-07-0871-CR.1
34. D'Angio GJ (2007) The National Wilms Tumor Study: a 40 year perspective. Lifetime Data Anal 13(4):463–470. doi:10.1007/s10985-007-9062-0
35. D'Orazio JA (2010) Inherited cancer syndromes in children and young adults. J Pediatr Hematol Oncol 32(3):195–228. doi:10.1097/MPH.0b013e3181ced34c
36. De Giovanni C, Landuzzi L, Nicoletti G, Lollini PL, Nanni P (2009) Molecular and cellular biology of rhabdomyosarcoma. Future Oncol (Lond) 5(9):1449–1475. doi:10.2217/fon.09.97
37. de Oliveira-Filho AG, Carvalho MH, Sbragia-Neto L, Miranda ML, Bustorff-Silva JM, de Oliveira ER (1997) Wilms tumor in a prenatally diagnosed multicystic kidney. J Urol 158(5):1926–1927. doi:S0022-5347(01)64177-6 [pii]
38. Dehner LP, Jarzembowski JA, Hill DA (2011) Embryonal rhabdomyosarcoma of the uterine cervix: a report of 14 cases and a discussion of its unusual clinicopathological associations. Mod Pathol 25(4):602–14. doi:10.1038/modpathol.2011185 [pii]
39. Dome J, Perlman E, Ritchey ML, Coppes M, Kalapurakal J, Grundy PE (2006) Renal tumors. In: Pizzo PA, Poplack DG (eds) Principles and practice of pediatric oncology, 5th edn. Lippincott Williams & Wilkins, Philadelphia, pp 905–932
40. Dome JS, Coppes MJ (2002) Recent advances in Wilms tumor genetics. Curr Opin Pediatr 14(1): 5–11
41. Dome JS, Huff V (1993) Wilms tumor overview. University of Washington, Seattle. doi:NBK1294 [bookaccession]

42. Dome JS, Roberts CWM, Argani P (2009) Pediatric renal tumors. In: Orkin SH, Fisher DE, Look AT, Lux SE, Ginsburg D, Nathan DG (eds) Oncology of infancy and childhood. Saunders Elsevier, Philadelphia, pp 541–573
43. Downey RT, Dillman JR, Ladino-Torres MF, McHugh JB, Ehrlich PF, Strouse PJ (2012) CT and MRI appearances and radiologic staging of pediatric renal cell carcinoma. Pediatr Radiol 42(4):410–417. doi:10.1007/s00247-011-2319-5
44. Drash A, Sherman F, Hartmann WH, Blizzard RM (1970) A syndrome of pseudohermaphroditism, Wilms' tumor, hypertension, and degenerative renal disease. J Pediatr 76(4):585–593
45. Ehrlich PF (2009) Bilateral Wilms' tumor: the need to improve outcomes. Expert Rev Anticancer Ther 9(7):963–973. doi:10.1586/era.09.50
46. Enklaar T, Zabel BU, Prawitt D (2006) Beckwith-Wiedemann syndrome: multiple molecular mechanisms. Exp Rev Mol Med 8(17):1–19
47. Fernbach SK (1991) Imaging of neonatal renal masses. Urol Radiol 12(4):214–219
48. Fischbach BV, Trout KL, Lewis J, Luis CA, Sika M (2005) WAGR syndrome: a clinical review of 54 cases. Pediatrics 116(4):984–988
49. Fort DW, Tonk VS, Tomlinson GE, Timmons CF, Schneider NR (1994) Rhabdoid tumor of the kidney with primitive neuroectodermal tumor of the central nervous system: associated tumors with different histologic, cytogenetic, and molecular findings. Genes Chromosomes Cancer 11(3):146–152
50. Fraumeni JF Jr, Geiser CF, Manning MD (1967) Wilms' tumor and congenital hemihypertrophy: report of five new cases and review of literature. Pediatrics 40(5):886–899
51. Furtwaengler R, Reinhard H, Leuschner I, Schenk JP, Goebel U, Claviez A, Kulozik A, Zoubek A, von Schweinitz D, Graf N (2006) Mesoblastic nephroma–a report from the Gesellschaft fur Padiatrische Onkologie und Hamatologie (GPOH). Cancer 106(10):2275–2283. doi:10.1002/cncr.21836
52. Geirsson RT, Ricketts NE, Taylor DJ, Coghill S (1985) Prenatal appearance of a mesoblastic nephroma associated with polyhydramnios. J Clin Ultrasound 13(7):488–490
53. Glick RD, Hicks MJ, Nuchtern JG, Wesson DE, Olutoye OO, Cass DL (2004) Renal tumors in infants less than 6 months of age. J Pediatr Surg 39(4):522–525. doi:S002234680300928X [pii]
54. Gonzalez KD, Noltner KA, Buzin CH, Gu D, Wen-Fong CY, Nguyen VQ, Han JH, Lowstuter K, Longmate J, Sommer SS, Weitzel JN (2009) Beyond Li Fraumeni Syndrome: clinical characteristics of families with p53 germline mutations. J Clin Oncol 27(8):1250–1256
55. Gormley TS, Skoog SJ, Jones RV, Maybee D (1989) Cellular congenital mesoblastic nephroma: what are the options. J Urol 142(2 Pt 2):479–483, discussion 489
56. Gratias EJ, Dome JS (2008) Current and emerging chemotherapy treatment strategies for Wilms tumor in North America. Paediatr Drugs 10(2):115–124. doi:1026 [pii]
57. Green DM (2004) The treatment of stages I-IV favorable histology Wilms' tumor. J Clin Oncol 22(8):1366–1372. doi:10.1200/JCO.2004.08.008
58. Grundy P, Koufos A, Morgan K, Li FP, Meadows AT, Cavenee WK (1988) Familial predisposition to Wilms' tumour does not map to the short arm of chromosome 11. Nature 336(6197):374–376. doi:10.1038/336374a0
59. Gurney JG (1999) Cancer among infants. http://www.seer.cancer.gov/publications/childhood/
60. Gwin K, Cajaiba MM, Caminoa-Lizarralde A, Picazo ML, Nistal M, Reyes-Mugica M (2008) Expanding the clinical spectrum of Frasier syndrome. Pediatr Dev Pathol 11(2):122–127
61. Haber DA, Buckler AJ, Glaser T, Call KM, Pelletier J, Sohn RL, Douglass EC, Housman DE (1990) An internal deletion within an 11p13 zinc finger gene contributes to the development of Wilms' tumor. Cell 61(7):1257–1269
62. Hamilton TE, Ritchey ML, Haase GM, Argani P, Peterson SM, Anderson JR, Green DM, Shamberger RC (2011) The management of synchronous bilateral Wilms tumor: a report from the National Wilms Tumor Study Group. Ann Surg 253(5):1004–1010. doi:10.1097/SLA.0b013e31821266a0
63. Hampel H, Sweet K, Westman JA, Offit K, Eng C (2004) Referral for cancer genetics consultation: a review and compilation of risk assessment criteria. J Med Genet 41(2):81–91
64. Heaton TE, Liechty KW (2008) Postnatal management of prenatally diagnosed abdominal masses and anomalies. Prenat Diagn 28(7):656–666. doi:10.1002/pd.1933
65. Hendren WH (1973) Pediatric surgery. 3. N Engl J Med 289(11):562–568. doi:10.1056/NEJM197309132891106
66. Hrabovsky EE, Othersen HB Jr, deLorimier A, Kelalis P, Beckwith JB, Takashima J (1986) Wilms' tumor in the neonate: a report from the National Wilms' Tumor Study. J Pediatr Surg 21(5):385–387. doi:S0022346886001823 [pii]
67. Hu JM, Wu TT, Chan SW, Cheng SL, Chen SM, Sheu JN (2006) Congenital mesoblastic nephroma presenting with massive hematuria and hemorrhagic shock: report of one case. Acta Paediatr Taiwan 47(3):135–138
68. Hubbard AM (2003) Ultrafast fetal MRI and prenatal diagnosis. Semin Pediatr Surg 12(3):143–153. doi:S1055858603000313 [pii]
69. Hung NA (2005) Congenital "clear cell sarcoma of the kidney". Virchows Arch 446(5):566–568. doi:10.1007/s00428-005-1253-z
70. Indolfi P, Bisogno G, Cecchetto G, Spreafico F, De Salvo GL, Collini P, Jenkner A, Inserra A, Schiavetti A, di Martino M, Casale F (2008) Local lymph node involvement in pediatric renal cell carcinoma: a report from the Italian TREP project. Pediatr Blood Cancer 51(4):475–478. doi:10.1002/pbc.21652

71. Irsutti M, Puget C, Baunin C, Duga I, Sarramon MF, Guitard J (2000) Mesoblastic nephroma: prenatal ultrasonographic and MRI features. Pediatr Radiol 30(3):147–150
72. Kajbafzadeh AM, Payabvash S, Sadeghi Z, Elmi A, Jamal A, Hantoshzadeh Z, Eslami L, Mehdizadeh M (2008) Comparison of magnetic resonance urography with ultrasound studies in detection of fetal urogenital anomalies. J Pediatr Urol 4(1):32–39. doi:S1477-5131(07)00378-6 [pii]
73. Khashu M, Osiovich H, Sargent MA (2005) Congenital mesoblastic nephroma presenting with neonatal hypertension. J Perinatol 25(6):433–435. doi:7211304 [pii]
74. Kobi M, Khatri G, Edelman M, Hines J (2009) Sarcoma botryoides: MRI findings in two patients. J Magn Reson Imaging 29(3):708–712. doi:10.1002/jmri.21670
75. Koren G, Schechter T (2007) Cancer chemotherapy in young children: challenges and solutions. Pediatr Blood Cancer 49(7 Suppl):1091–1092. doi:10.1002/pbc.21349
76. Kuiper DR, Hoekstra HJ, Veth RP, Wobbes T (2003) The management of clear cell sarcoma. Eur J Surg Oncol 29(7):568–570
77. Kurjak A, Zalud I, Jurkovic D, Alfirevic Z, Tomic K (1989) Ultrasound diagnosis and evaluation of fetal tumors. J Perinat Med 17(3):173–193
78. Kusumakumary P, Mathews A, James FV, Chellam VG, Hariharan S, Varma RR, Nair MK (1999) Clear cell sarcoma kidney: clinical features and outcome. Pediatr Hematol Oncol 16(2):169–174
79. La Quaglia MP (1996) Genitourinary tract cancer in childhood. Semin Pediatr Surg 5(1):49–65
80. Li FP, Fraumeni JF Jr (1969) Soft-tissue sarcomas, breast cancer, and other neoplasms. A familial syndrome? Ann Intern Med 71(4):747–752
81. Linam LE, Yu X, Calvo-Garcia MA, Rubio EI, Crombleholme TM, Bove K, Kline-Fath BM (2010) Contribution of magnetic resonance imaging to prenatal differential diagnosis of renal tumors: report of two cases and review of the literature. Fetal Diagn Ther 28(2):100–108. doi:000313655 [pii]
82. Loughlin KR, Retik AB, Weinstein HJ, Colodny AH, Shamberger RC, Delorey M, Tarbell N, Cassady JR, Hendren WH (1989) Genitourinary rhabdomyosarcoma in children. Cancer 63(8):1600–1606
83. Lowe LH, Isuani BH, Heller RM, Stein SM, Johnson JE, Navarro OM, Hernanz-Schulman M (2000) Pediatric renal masses: Wilms tumor and beyond. Radiographics 20(6):1585–1603
84. Luo CC, Lin JN, Jaing TH, Yang CP, Hsueh C (2002) Malignant rhabdoid tumour of the kidney occurring simultaneously with a brain tumour: a report of two cases and review of the literature. Eur J Pediatr 161(6):340–342. doi:10.1007/s00431-002-0918-8
85. Manchanda V, Mohta A, Khurana N, Gupta CR, Neogi S (2010) Bilateral clear cell sarcoma of the kidney. J Pediatr Surg 45(9):1927–1930. doi:S0022-3468(10)00489-6 [pii]
86. Marsden HB, Lawler W, Kumar PM (1978) Bone metastasizing renal tumor of childhood: morphological and clinical features, and differences from Wilms' tumor. Cancer 42(4):1922–1928
87. Mazzoleni S, Vecchiato L, Alaggio R, Cecchetto G, Zorzi C, Carli M (2003) Clear cell sarcoma of the kidney in a newborn. Med Pediatr Oncol 41(2):153–155. doi:10.1002/mpo.10318
88. McClatchey AI (2007) Neurofibromatosis. Annu Rev Pathol 2:191–216
89. McTaggart SJ, Algar E, Chow CW, Powell HR, Jones CL (2001) Clinical spectrum of Denys-Drash and Frasier syndrome. Pediatr Nephrol 16(4):335–339
90. McVicar M, Margouleff D, Chandra M (1991) Diagnosis and imaging of the fetal and neonatal abdominal mass: an integrated approach. Adv Pediatr 38:135–149
91. Metzger ML, Dome JS (2005) Current therapy for Wilms' tumor. Oncologist 10(10):815–826. doi:10/10/815 [pii]
92. Millar AJ, Davidson A, Rode H, Numanoglu A, Hartley PS, Daubenton JD, Desai F (2005) Bilateral Wilms' tumors: a single-center experience with 19 cases. J Pediatr Surg 40(8):1289–1294. doi:S0022-3468(05)00373-8 [pii]
93. Miller RW, Fraumeni JF Jr, Manning MD (1964) Association of Wilms's Tumor with Aniridia, hemihypertrophy and other congenital malformations. N Engl J Med 270:922–927
94. Morgan E, Baum E, Breslow N, Takashima J, D'Angio G (1988) Chemotherapy-related toxicity in infants treated according to the Second National Wilms' Tumor Study. J Clin Oncol 6(1):51–55
95. Morgan E, Kidd JM (1978) Undifferentiated sarcoma of the kidney: a tumor of childhood with histopathologic and clinical characteristics distinct from Wilms' tumor. Cancer 42(4):1916–1921
96. Moroz V, Machin D, Faldum A, Hero B, Iehara T, Mosseri V, Ladenstein R, De Bernardi B, Rubie H, Berthold F, Matthay KK, Monclair T, Ambros PF, Pearson AD, Cohn SL, London WB (2011) Changes over three decades in outcome and the prognostic influence of age-at-diagnosis in young patients with neuroblastoma: a report from the International Neuroblastoma Risk Group Project. Eur J Cancer 47(4):561–571. doi:S0959-8049(10)01061-0 [pii]
97. Murthi GV, Carachi R, Howatson A (2003) Congenital cystic mesoblastic nephroma. Pediatr Surg Int 19(1–2):109–111. doi:10.1007/s00383-002-0833-0
98. Nagata T, Takahashi Y, Ishii Y, Asai S, Sugahara-Kobayashi M, Nishida Y, Murata A, Yamamori S, Ogawa Y, Nakamura T, Murakami H, Nakamura M, Shichino H, Chin M, Sugito K, Ikeda T, Koshinaga T, Mugishima H (2005) Molecular genetic alterations and gene expression profile of a malignant rhabdoid tumor of the kidney. Cancer Genet Cytogenet 163(2):130–137. doi:10.1016/j.cancergencyto.2005.05.009
99. National Cancer Institute Surveillance Epidemiology and End Results (SEER): International Classification

of Childhood Cancer (ICCC) (2011) http://seer.cancer.gov/iccc/

100. Newbould MJ, Kelsey AM (1993) Clear cell sarcoma of the kidney in a 4-month-old infant: a case report. Med Pediatr Oncol 21(7):525–528
101. Ng A, Jenkinson H, Morland B, Grundy R (2005) Clear cell sarcoma: a dilemma on pathological staging and clinical management. Pediatr Hematol Oncol 22(3):257–261. doi:U7608J2465872708 [pii]
102. Parham DM (2001) Pathologic classification of rhabdomyosarcomas and correlations with molecular studies. Mod Pathol 14(5):506–514. doi:10.1038/modpathol.3880339
103. Parikh SH, Chintagumpala M, Hicks MJ, Trautwein LM, Blaney S, Minifee P, Woo SY (1998) Clear cell sarcoma of the kidney: an unusual presentation and review of the literature. J Pediatr Hematol Oncol 20(2):165–168
104. Parkin DM, Stiller CA, Draper GJ, Bieber CA (1988) The international incidence of childhood cancer. Int J Cancer 42(4):511–520
105. Paya K, Horcher E, Lawrenz K, Rebhandl W, Zoubek A (2001) Bilateral Wilms' tumor–surgical aspects. Eur J Pediatr Surg 11(2):99–104. doi:10.1055/s-2001-13787
106. Perlman EJ (2010) Pediatric renal cell carcinoma. Surg Pathol Clin 3(3):641–651. doi:10.1016/j.path.2010.06.011
107. Plon SE, Malkin D (2006) Childhood cancer and heredity. In: Pizzo PA, Poplack DG (eds) Principles and practice of pediatric oncology, 5th edn. Lippincott Williams & Wilkins, Philadelphia, pp 14–37
108. Poulsen ML, Budtz-Jorgensen E, Bisgaard ML (2010) Surveillance in von Hippel-Lindau disease (vHL). Clin Genet 77(1):49–59. doi:CGE1281 [pii]
109. Ragab AH, Heyn R, Tefft M, Hays DN, Newton WA Jr, Beltangady M (1986) Infants younger than 1 year of age with rhabdomyosarcoma. Cancer 58(12):2606–2610
110. Raney B, Anderson J, Arndt C, Crist W, Maurer H, Qualman S, Wharam M, Wiener E, Meyer W (2008) Primary renal sarcomas in the Intergroup Rhabdomyosarcoma Study Group (IRSG) experience, 1972–2005: a report from the Children's Oncology Group. Pediatr Blood Cancer 51(3):339–343. doi:10.1002/pbc.21639
111. Raney RB Jr, Palmer N, Sutow WW, Baum E, Ayala A (1983) Renal cell carcinoma in children. Med Pediatr Oncol 11(2):91–98
112. Rao A, Rothman J, Nichols KE (2008) Genetic testing and tumor surveillance for children with cancer predisposition syndromes. Curr Opin Pediatr 20(1):1–7
113. Riccio A, Sparago A, Verde G, De Crescenzo A, Citro V, Cubellis MV, Ferrero GB, Silengo MC, Russo S, Larizza L, Cerrato F (2009) Inherited and Sporadic Epimutations at the IGF2-H19 locus in Beckwith-Wiedemann syndrome and Wilms' tumor. Endocr Dev 14:1–9. doi:000207461 [pii]
114. Ritchey M, Daley S, Shamberger RC, Ehrlich P, Hamilton T, Haase G, Sawin R (2008) Ureteral extension in Wilms' tumor: a report from the National Wilms' Tumor Study Group (NWTSG). J Pediatr Surg 43(9):1625–1629. doi:S0022-3468(08)00098-5 [pii]
115. Ritchey ML, Azizkhan RG, Beckwith JB, Hrabovsky EE, Haase GM (1995) Neonatal Wilms tumor. J Pediatr Surg 30(6):856–859. doi:0022-3468(95)90764-5 [pii]
116. Ross JH, Kay R (1999) Surgical considerations for patients with Wilms' tumor. Semin Urologic Oncol 17(1):33–39
117. Rutledge F, Sullivan MP (1967) Sarcoma botryoides. Ann N Y Acad Sci 142(3):694–708
118. Sarhan OM, El-Baz M, Sarhan MM, Ghali AM, Ghoneim MA (2010) Bilateral Wilms' tumors: single-center experience with 22 cases and literature review. Urology 76(4):946–951. doi:S0090-4295(10)00435-8 [pii]
119. Scott J, Cowell J, Robertson ME, Priestley LM, Wadey R, Hopkins B, Pritchard J, Bell GI, Rall LB, Graham CF et al (1985) Insulin-like growth factor-II gene expression in Wilms' tumour and embryonic tissues. Nature 317(6034):260–262
120. Scott RH, Stiller CA, Walker L, Rahman N (2006) Syndromes and constitutional chromosomal abnormalities associated with Wilms tumour. J Med Genet 43(9):705–715
121. Sebire NJ, Vujanic GM (2009) Paediatric renal tumours: recent developments, new entities and pathological features. Histopathology 54(5):516–528. doi:10.1111/j.1365-2559.2008.03110.x
122. Shamberger RC (1999) Pediatric renal tumors. Semin Surg Oncol 16(2):105–120. doi:10.1002/(SICI)1098-2388(199903)16:2<105::AID-SSU4>3.0.CO;2-T [pii]
123. Shamberger RC, Guthrie KA, Ritchey ML, Haase GM, Takashima J, Beckwith JB, D'Angio GJ, Green DM, Breslow NE (1999) Surgery-related factors and local recurrence of Wilms tumor in National Wilms Tumor Study 4. Ann Surg 229(2):292–297
124. Sharma SC, Menon PA (2001) Clear cell sarcoma of the kidney. J Postgrad Med 47(3):206–207
125. Siegel SE, Moran RG (1981) Problems in the chemotherapy of cancer in the neonate. Am J Pediatr Hematol Oncol 3(3):287–296
126. Silberstein J, Grabowski J, Saltzstein SL, Kane CJ (2009) Renal cell carcinoma in the pediatric population: results from the California Cancer Registry. Pediatr Blood Cancer 52(2):237–241. doi:10.1002/pbc.21779
127. Sola JE, Cova D, Casillas J, Alvarez OA, Qualman S, Rodriguez MM (2007) Primary renal botryoid rhabdomyosarcoma: diagnosis and outcome. J Pediatr Surg 42(12):e17–20. doi:10.1016/j.jpedsurg.2007.08.011
128. Sotelo-Avila C, Gonzalez-Crussi F, Sadowinski S, Gooch WM 3rd, Pena R (1985) Clear cell sarcoma of the kidney: a clinicopathologic study of 21 patients with long-term follow-up evaluation. Hum Pathol 16(12):1219–1230

129. Sparago A, Russo S, Cerrato F, Ferraiuolo S, Castorina P, Selicorni A, Schwienbacher C, Negrini M, Ferrero GB, Silengo MC, Anichini C, Larizza L, Riccio A (2007) Mechanisms causing imprinting defects in familial Beckwith-Wiedemann syndrome with Wilms' tumour. Hum Mol Genet 16(3): 254–264
130. Stachowicz-Stencel T, Bien E, Balcerska A, Godzinski J, Synakiewicz A, Perek-Polnik M, Kurylak A, Pietras W, Kuzmicz M, Mizia-Malarz A, Rybczynska A, Nurzynska-Flak J (2011) Diagnosis and treatment of renal cell carcinoma in children: a report from the Polish pediatric rare tumor study group. Klin Padiatr 223(3):138–141. doi:10.1055/s-0031-1275349
131. Stehr M (2009) Pediatric urologic rhabdomyosarcoma. Curr Opin Urol 19(4):402–406. doi:10.1097/MOU.0b013e32832c90c2
132. Sultan I, Qaddoumi I, Rodriguez-Galindo C, Nassan AA, Ghandour K, Al-Hussaini M (2010) Age, stage, and radiotherapy, but not primary tumor site, affects the outcome of patients with malignant rhabdoid tumors. Pediatr Blood Cancer 54(1):35–40. doi:10.1002/pbc.22285
133. Taguchi K, Kojima Y, Mizuno K, Kamisawa H, Kohri K, Hayashi Y (2011) Molecular analysis of clear cell sarcoma with translocation (1;6)(p32.3;q21). Urology 78(3):684–686. doi:S0090-4295(10)02172-2 [pii]
134. Tersak JM, Malatack JJ, Ritchey AK (2007) Hematology and oncology. In: Zitelli BJ, Davis HW (eds) Atlas of pediatric physical diagnosis, 5th edn. Mosby Elsevier, Philadelphia, pp 403–441
135. Vadeyar S, Ramsay M, James D, O'Neill D (2000) Prenatal diagnosis of congenital Wilms' tumor (nephroblastoma) presenting as fetal hydrops. Ultrasound Obstet Gynecol 16(1):80–83. doi:10.1046/j.1469-0705.2000.00169.x
136. van den Heuvel-Eibrink MM, Grundy P, Graf N, Pritchard-Jones K, Bergeron C, Patte C, van Tinteren H, Rey A, Langford C, Anderson JR, de Kraker J (2008) Characteristics and survival of 750 children diagnosed with a renal tumor in the first seven months of life: a collaborative study by the SIOP/GPOH/SFOP, NWTSG, and UKCCSG Wilms tumor study groups. Pediatr Blood Cancer 50(6):1130–1134. doi:10.1002/pbc.21389
137. van den Heuvel-Eibrink MM, van Tinteren H, Rehorst H, Coulombe A, Patte C, de Camargo B, de Kraker J, Leuschner I, Lugtenberg R, Pritchard-Jones K, Sandstedt B, Spreafico F, Graf N, Vujanic GM (2011) Malignant rhabdoid tumours of the kidney (MRTKs), registered on recent SIOP protocols from 1993 to 2005: a report of the SIOP renal tumour study group. Pediatr Blood Cancer 56(5):733–737. doi:10.1002/pbc.22922
138. Varan A (2008) Wilms' tumor in children: an overview. Nephron Clin Pract 108(2):c83–90
139. Varan A, Akyuz C, Sari N, Buyukpamukcu N, Caglar M, Buyukpamukcu M (2007) Renal cell carcinoma in children: experience of a single center. Nephron Clin Pract 105(2):c58–61. doi:97599 [pii]
140. Versteege I, Sevenet N, Lange J, Rousseau-Merck MF, Ambros P, Handgretinger R, Aurias A, Delattre O (1998) Truncating mutations of hSNF5/INI1 in aggressive paediatric cancer. Nature 394(6689): 203–206
141. Vujanic GM, Kelsey A, Perlman EJ, Sandstedt B, Beckwith JB (2007) Anaplastic sarcoma of the kidney: a clinicopathologic study of 20 cases of a new entity with polyphenotypic features. Am J Surg Pathol 31(10):1459–1468. doi:10.1097/PAS.0b013e31804d43a4
142. Wang NJ, Song HR, Schanen NC, Litman NL, Frasier SD (2005) Frasier syndrome comes full circle: genetic studies performed in an original patient. J Pediatr 146(6):843–844
143. Watts KE, Hansel DE, MacLennan GT (2011) Clear cell sarcoma of the kidney. J Urol 185(1):279–280. doi:S0022-5347(10)04813-5 [pii]
144. Weksberg R, Shuman C, Smith AC (2005) Beckwith-Wiedemann syndrome. Am J Med Genet C Semin Med Genet 137C(1):12–23
145. Wexler LH, Meyer WH, Helman LJ (2006) Rhabdomyosarcoma and the undifferentiated sarcomas. In: Pizzo PA, Poplack DG (eds) Principles and practice of pediatric oncology, 5th edn. Lippincott Williams & Wilkins, Philadelphia, pp 971–1001
146. Weyman PJ, McClennan BL, Lee JK, Stanley RJ (1982) CT of calcified renal masses. AJR Am J Roentgenol 138(6):1095–1099
147. Wienk MA, Van Geijn HP, Copray FJ, Brons JT (1990) Prenatal diagnosis of fetal tumors by ultrasonography. Obstet Gynecol Surv 45(10):639–653
148. Woodring JH, Halberg DH, Duff DE (1982) Sarcoma botryoides of the uterus presenting as an abdominal mass. J Clin Ultrasound 10(7):347–349
149. Wu X, Dagar V, Algar E, Muscat A, Bandopadhayay P, Ashley D, Wo Chow C (2008) Rhabdoid tumour: a malignancy of early childhood with variable primary site, histology and clinical behaviour. Pathology 40(7):664–670. doi:10.1080/00313020802436451
150. Xue H, Horwitz JR, Smith MB, Lally KP, Black CT, Cangir A, Takahashi H, Andrassy RJ (1995) Malignant solid tumors in neonates: a 40-year review. J Pediatr Surg 30(4):543–545
151. Yanagisawa S, Kadouchi I, Yokomori K, Hirose M, Hakozaki M, Hojo H, Maeda K, Kobayashi E, Murakami T (2009) Identification and metastatic potential of tumor-initiating cells in malignant rhabdoid tumor of the kidney. Clin Cancer Res 15(9):3014–3022. doi:10.1158/1078-0432.CCR-08-2237
152. Zhuge Y, Cheung MC, Yang R, Perez EA, Koniaris LG, Sola JE (2010) Pediatric non-Wilms renal tumors: subtypes, survival, and prognostic indicators. J Surg Res 163(2):257–263. doi:S0022-4804(10)00298-2 [pii]

14 Cystic Renal Disease

Katherine MacRae Dell

Core Messages

- Cystic kidney disease in neonates often presents with ultrasonography findings of diffusely echogenic kidneys with variable degrees of kidney enlargement rather than discrete cysts.
- Autosomal recessive polycystic kidney disease (ARPKD), autosomal dominant PKD (ADPKD), and diffuse cystic dysplasia can present in the neonate with features that may be indistinguishable from each other.
- With the emergence of modern dialytic therapy, the major contributor to mortality in the neonate with severe cystic kidney disease is respiratory failure (related to oligohydramnios and pulmonary hypoplasia) rather than complications of renal failure.
- Prognosis may be difficult to predict in cystic disease in the newborn, but the presence of oligohydramnios and pulmonary hypoplasia generally is associated with poor long-term renal outcome.

Case Vignette

A male fetus was noted to have large echogenic kidneys on a prenatal ultrasound obtained at 18 weeks gestation. At 28 weeks gestation, oligohydramnios was noted as well as persistence of enlarged kidneys. The infant was born at 38 weeks gestation and developed respiratory distress in the delivery room requiring resuscitation and mechanical ventilatory support. Chest radiograph demonstrated diffuse ground glass opacities within the lungs as well as a right pneumothorax. Physical exam was notable for large palpable bilateral abdominal masses. Postnatal renal ultrasonography showed bilateral markedly echogenic kidneys measuring 7 cm (right) and 6.6 cm (left). No cysts or hydronephrosis was seen. Liver ultrasonography was normal. A chest tube was placed for management of the pneumothorax. The patient was initially oliguric, but urine output improved with initiation of furosemide. On day of life 3, he was extubated and weaned to room air by day of life 5. At 1 week of life, he developed hypertension, requiring treatment with enalapril and continuation of furosemide. He was started on enteral feeds with maternal breast milk. Because of rising serum potassium, sodium-potassium polystyrene resin was added to the feeds

K.M. Dell, MD
Division of Pediatric Nephrology,
Pediatric Kidney Transplant, UHCMC,
UH Rainbow Babies & Children's Hospital,
11100 Euclid Ave, Cleveland, OH 44106, USA
e-mail: katherine.dell@uhhospitals.org

A.S. Chishti et al. (eds.), *Kidney and Urinary Tract Diseases in the Newborn*,
DOI 10.1007/978-3-642-39988-6_14, © Springer-Verlag Berlin Heidelberg 2014

for potassium binding. He was discharged from the nursery at 3 weeks of life. Serum creatinine at that time was 0.65 mg/ dl.

14.1 Introduction

Historically, terms such as "polycystic kidneys" and "infantile polycystic kidney disease" were used to describe a variety of disorders with shared features of cysts evident either radiographically or by pathologic examination [12]. However, as our understanding of modern molecular genetics has continued to expand, it has become evident that many of these disorders have distinct genetic and pathophysiologic features. Cystic kidney disease in neonates is now recognized as representing a spectrum of disorders from those inherited in classic Mendelian fashion (such as ARPKD) to those that occur sporadically (such as multicystic dysplastic kidney, MCDK). With the advent of modern obstetrical ultrasonography, the majority of these disorders are identified prenatally. In many cases the diagnosis of a particular cystic kidney disease is suspected based on the prenatal images. However, even with advanced technology, the findings/diagnosis on prenatal ultrasonography may not be confirmed on postnatal imaging.

Many of the specific diseases addressed in detail in this chapter are uncommon. Taken as a whole, however, they represent important causes of morbidity and mortality in the newborn. It is also important to recognize that even in cases of severe neonatal renal disease, including the more severe forms of cystic kidney disease, renal supportive therapy including infant dialysis is often achievable. However, newborns with a history of severe oligohydramnios and resultant pulmonary hypoplasia may not be viable despite even the most advanced ventilatory support. Thus, the cause of mortality in these patients is usually respiratory, not renal, failure.

14.2 Background

14.2.1 Developmental Considerations

Developmentally, congenital cystic kidney diseases result from one of two general pathways. With the classic polycystic kidneys diseases (such as ARPKD and ADPKD), nephrogenesis occurs normally; then, depending on the underlying genetic disorder, cysts develop along one or more of the nephron segments. In the cystic dysplastic disorders, a defect occurs during nephrogenesis, resulting in primitive nephrons with disorganized and poorly differentiated collecting ducts [45].

14.2.2 Presentation of Cystic Kidney Diseases in the Neonate

Although the polycystic kidney diseases and cystic dysplastic disorders have distinct clinical and pathophysiologic features, they typically present in one of two ways. As the case vignette illustrates, the first presentation is that of diffusely echogenic kidneys (typically quite enlarged) evident ultrasonographically (Fig. 14.1). On physical exam, palpable abdominal masses are evident. Patients with severe bilateral disease (regardless of the underlying etiology) typically have a history of fetal oligohydramnios. This can result in the features of the oligohydramnios sequence, which include Potter's facies (Fig. 14.2), pulmonary hypoplasia, hip dislocation, extremity contractures, and club feet. The second presentation is that of one or more discrete cysts also detected ultrasonographically (Fig. 14.3). Kidneys may be enlarged or normal in size. Palpable abdominal masses are typically not evident in these cases, and a history of oligohydramnios is usually absent. In some instances (such as ADPKD) the presentation can be that of either enlarged echogenic kidneys or discrete cysts with or without kidney enlargement. Similarly, there may be instances where a few small discrete cysts are evident in enlarged echogenic kidneys (e.g., diffuse cystic dysplasia) or instances in which

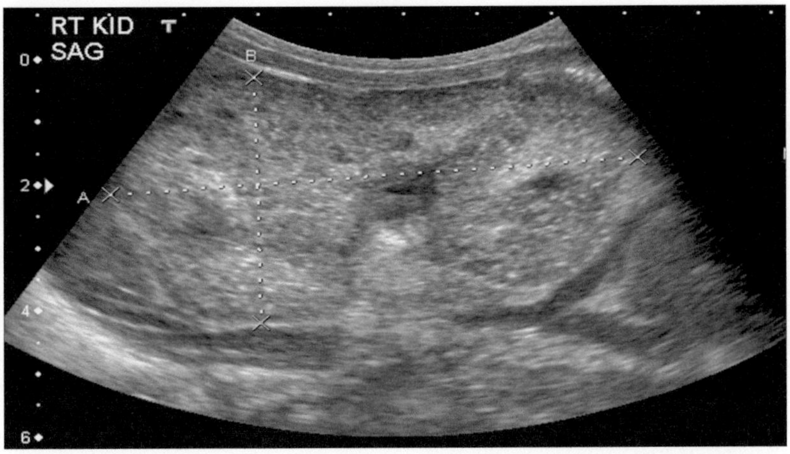

Fig. 14.1 *Enlarged echogenic kidneys*. Ultrasonography of the right kidney from a newborn with ARPKD demonstrates typical kidney enlargement as well as markedly increased echogenicity (brightness when compared to the surrounding liver parenchyma). Similar features were present on the left kidney (not shown). A few very small cysts are evident, which are often absent in neonates with this disease. This ultrasonographic appearance can also been seen in other congenital cystic kidney disease including ADPKD, diffuse cystic dysplasia, and infantile nephronophthisis (Courtesy of Dr. Rashini Parikh, Department of Radiology, University Hospitals Case Medical Center, Cleveland, Ohio)

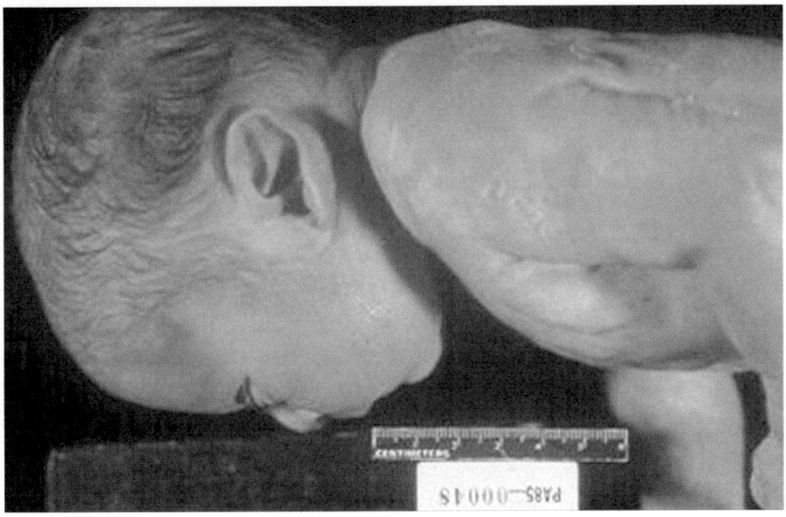

Fig. 14.2 *Potter's facies*. The photograph obtained at autopsy shows a fetus with Potter's facies, a feature of the oligohydramnios sequence. Additional features of the sequence include pulmonary hypoplasia, hip dislocation, and club foot (Courtesy of Dr. Gretta Jacobs, Department of Pathology, University Hospitals Case Medical Center, Cleveland, Ohio)

kidneys are echogenic, but are typically not enlarged (e.g., infantile nephronophthisis).

14.2.3 Differential Diagnosis of Cystic Kidney Diseases

Cystic kidney disorders that present in neonates are outlined in Table 14.1. The typical presentation (enlarged echogenic kidneys, discrete cysts, or either) is indicated by the key below. However, presentations can be variable and considerable overlap can occur, which may make it difficult to determine definitive diagnosis in the newborn period [20]. In one published series, of 93 fetuses with echogenic kidneys (and confirmed nephropathy postnatally), approximately 30 % had visible cysts [9]. In that same series, 33 % of the subjects had ARPKD, 30 % had ADPKD, 12 % had Bardet-Biedl syndrome, 10 % had

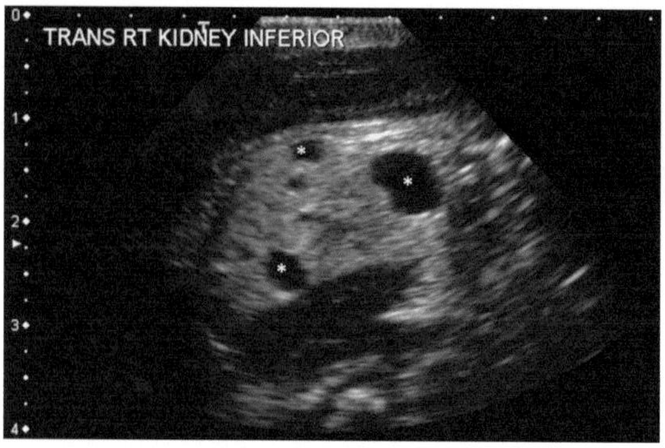

Fig. 14.3 *Renal macrocysts*. Renal ultrasonography of the right kidney from a neonate with ADPKD demonstrates several macroscopic cysts (indicated with *asterisk*). The left kidney demonstrated 2 small cysts (not shown). The kidneys also show mildly increased echogenicity and mild enlargement bilaterally

Meckel-Gruber syndrome, and the remaining 15 % had a variety of other cystic kidney diseases [9]. It should also be noted that congenital obstructive uropathies may sometimes present on prenatal ultrasonography as "cystic kidneys" due to marked dilatation of the collecting systems. On postnatal evaluation, however, the diagnosis of obstructive uropathy is usually evident (see Chaps. 8, 10, and 11).

Table 14.1 Cystic kidney diseases that present in the neonate

Polycystic kidney diseases	Autosomal recessive polycystic kidney disease (ARPKD)[a]
–	Autosomal dominant polycystic kidney disease (ADPKD)[b]
–	ADPKD associated with tuberous sclerosis[c]
–	Glomerulocystic kidney disease[b]
	Juvenile nephronophthisis[a]
Cystic dysplasia	Diffuse cystic dysplasia[a]
	Isolated/sporadic
	Associated with congenital syndromes (e.g., Meckel-Gruber, Bardet-Biedl, Jeune, Beckwith-Wiedemann)
–	Multicystic dysplastic kidney[c]
Other causes of renal cysts in neonates	Simple renal cysts[c]
	Caliceal diverticulum[c]

[a]Typically present with diffusely echogenic kidneys with varying degrees of enlargement
[b]Present with either echogenic kidneys, discrete cysts, or both
[c]Typically present with discrete cysts

14.3 Polycystic Kidney Diseases

Genetics, clinical features, diagnosis, treatment, and prognosis for the inherited polycystic kidney diseases that present in neonates, including ARPKD, ADPKD, glomerulocystic kidney disease, and juvenile nephronophthisis, are discussed below.

14.3.1 Autosomal Recessive Polycystic Kidney Disease (ARPKD)

14.3.1.1 Genetics, Clinical Features, and Diagnosis

ARPKD is a relatively rare disorder, affecting 1:40,000 patients. As the name suggests, it is inherited as an autosomal recessive trait [13]. Males and females are equally affected and all races are affected as well. ARPKD is caused by mutations in the *polycystic kidney and hepatic disease* (*pkhd1*) gene [44]. This gene encodes a very large protein, fibrocystin/polyductin. Mutations are present throughout the gene, with most families having "private" mutations not shared by other kindreds. Genotype-phenotype correlations have not been well established, although it has been proposed that patients with severe mutations that result in little or no protein production may have a very high rate of neonatal mortality [3]. Although the genetics of the disease have been identified, the mechanisms by which the abnormal protein induces pathology remain undefined. Emerging data suggest that alterations in intracellular signaling and mechanosensation mediated through a cellular organelle called the primary cilia are thought to play a major role in the pathophysiology of these diseases [21].

ARPKD primarily affects only the kidneys and liver [13]. The polycystic kidney disease is characterized by microscopic fusiform dilatations affecting all of the collecting tubules (Fig. 14.4).

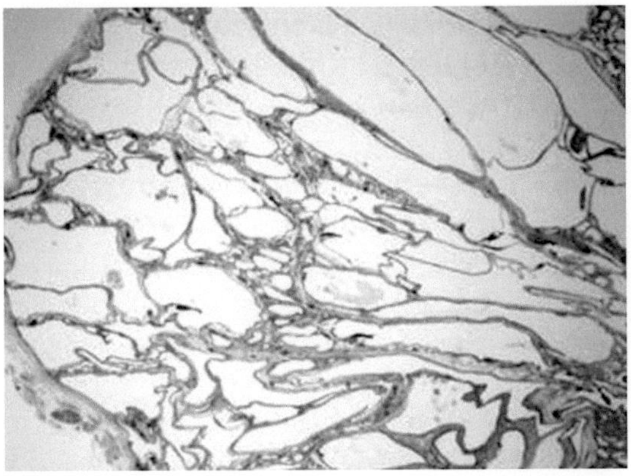

Fig. 14.4 *ARPKD kidney pathology*. Histologic findings in ARPKD kidney disease are shown, including radially oriented, diffuse fusiform dilatations of the collecting tubules (Courtesy Dr. Gretta Jacobs, Department of Pathology, University Hospitals Case Medical Center, Cleveland, Ohio)

These "microcysts" give the radiographic appearance of very enlarged and markedly echogenic kidneys. A few discrete cysts may still be evident in some patients, but this is less common. The liver disease in ARPKD (congenital hepatic fibrosis, CHF, also called Caroli's disease) is a biliary abnormality characterized by proliferation and cystic changes in the bile ducts with accompanying periportal fibrosis [39]. Discrete liver cysts are typically absent. In neonates, the kidney disease predominates, and radiographic or laboratory evidence of hepatic involvement (e.g., echogenic liver) is present in only 40 % [47]. The other signs and symptoms associated with ARPKD, including pulmonary hypoplasia and Potter's facies, are the sequelae of the oligohydramnios sequence rather than a direct result of the mutated gene.

The case vignette highlights the typical presentation of ARPKD in the neonate. Affected infants, particularly those with a history of oligohydramnios, commonly develop respiratory distress in the delivery room and require mechanical ventilation. Respiratory compromise develops not only because of pulmonary hypoplasia but also because the massively enlarged kidneys may prevent adequate diaphragmatic excursion. Renal complications seen in the newborn period include oliguria and elevated serum creatinine (both of which may improve in the short term), hyponatremia, and hypertension [14].

The diagnosis of ARPKD is usually made based on clinical criteria [19, 47]. These include the presence of enlarged echogenic kidneys, absence of cysts in the parents, and one or more of the following: ultrasonographic or histologic evidence of liver disease, parental consanguinity, and/or biopsy proven ARPKD in a sibling/previous pregnancy. Renal imaging of the parents is important in ruling out the possibility of ADPKD, although ADPKD cannot be definitively ruled out unless the parents are older than 30 years of age. Renal or liver biopsies are generally not undertaken for diagnosis purposes, but may be indicated in some patients in whom the diagnosis is unclear.

Genetic testing is generally not necessary in the immediate newborn period because treatment is the same regardless of the underlying cause of the kidney disease. Confirmation of the diagnosis is, however, important for counseling of future pregnancies as well as defining risk (if any) to existing siblings. Thus, families of a child with suspected ARPKD should be referred for genetic counseling. Molecular genetic testing in the form of direct gene sequencing is available for ARPKD and has an accuracy of about 85 % in detecting mutations [3, 38]. For an updated listing of laboratories performing clinical genetic testing for ARPKD and other inherited diseases, see www.geneclinics.org. If a fetus or neonate with suspected cystic kidney disease expires, autopsy should be encouraged in order to definitely establish the diagnosis for counseling of future pregnancies. Consultation with a geneticist should be undertaken in the immediate newborn period if the infant has evidence of syndromic features or extrarenal manifestations other than hepatic disease, as those patients may have diffuse cystic dysplasia associated with a congenital syndrome rather than ARPKD.

14.3.1.2 Treatment and Prognosis

There are currently no disease-specific therapies available in clinical practice. Treatment of ARPKD in the newborn period is primarily focused on respiratory support, fluid and electrolyte balance, and control of hypertension. Consultation with a pediatric nephrologist is essential for the management of these issues. The hypertension can be severe and can occur within the first week of life. Angiotensin converting enzyme inhibitors (ACEI) are considered the treatment of choice, but have not been systematically studied in patients. In addition, acute kidney injury in the newborn period may limit their use in the initial treatment of hypertension in the newborn. Markedly enlarged kidneys contribute to significant feeding intolerance, and achieving adequate nutrition can be very challenging in this population. Based on case reports, some have advocated performing unilateral nephrectomy to relieve both respiratory and feeding difficulties [2]; however, this has not been systematically studied. Rapid growth of the contralateral kidney may eliminate any brief benefit derived from the procedure (unpublished observation).

ARPKD was once considered a uniformly fatal disease for affected infants. With modern neonatal support, this is clearly no longer the case. Nevertheless, mortality in the newborn period is still significant: approximately 30 % of affected infants will die in early infancy, typically from respiratory failure [4]. The long-term complications for infants that survive the newborn period include chronic lung disease, chronic kidney disease (CKD), growth failure, and hepatic complications (varices, portal hypertension, ascending cholangitis) [19]. Approximately 50 % of patients will progress to ESRD within the first decade of life. Based on data generated from the 1950s to the 1990s, 10-year patient survival is 80 % [33]. However, longer-term morbidity and mortality, particularly as it relates to complications of the hepatic disease, are less well defined. The lack of data is due to a number of factors including the more slowly progressive nature of CHF and the fact that many of the children who now survive and undergo kidney transplantation have not yet reached adulthood. Thus, it is likely that complications related to liver disease will become a greater contributor to morbidity and mortality as this population ages.

14.3.2 Autosomal Dominant Polycystic Kidney Disease (ADPKD)

14.3.2.1 Genetics, Clinical Features, and Diagnosis

ADPKD is the most common inherited kidney disease, with a prevalence of 1:1,000 persons [42]. Historically, it was considered a disorder of adulthood; in fact, it has been alternatively named "adult polycystic kidney disease," presumably to distinguish it from ARPKD. While the majority of patients do present in adulthood, it is clear that the disease may present in children, infants, and, rarely, fetuses [10, 41]. ADPKD is inherited as an autosomal dominant trait and is caused by mutations in one of two genes, *PKD1* (85 % of patients) or *PKD2* (15 % of patients) [23]. Consistent with the autosomal dominant inheritance, all patients will develop renal cysts over time. However, there is considerable variation in the disease expression both between families and within members of the same family. Thus, parents of a child with ADPKD may be asymptomatic and unaware that they are affected. In addition, in about 10–15 % of cases, there is no family history of ADPKD and such patients have a new mutation. Because the genes for tuberous sclerosis (*TSC2*) and ADPKD (*PKD1*) lie adjacent to each other on chromosome 16, ADPKD can also be inherited as part of a contiguous gene syndrome [31].

ADPKD is a systemic disease affecting multiple organs. In addition to polycystic kidneys, affected patients can have liver and pancreatic cysts as well as vascular abnormalities, including cerebral and aortic aneurysms and mitral valve prolapse. Young children, however, generally do not show the extrarenal manifestations of ADPKD, and the clinical signs and symptoms of ADPKD can be highly variable. Older children and adults with ADPKD typically present with symptoms such as gross hematuria or elevated blood pressures or are diagnosed after incidental identification of renal cysts while undergoing abdominal imaging for a nonrenal indication. In contrast, newborns with ADPKD are usually identified based on prenatal ultrasonographic findings of one or more discrete cysts (78 % in one series) or with diffusely echogenic kidneys that may be indistinguishable from ARPKD [20, 37]. Clinical signs and symptoms of ADPKD in newborns can be variable [10]. Infants with macrocysts are usually asymptomatic or may have hypertension or urinary tract infection. Infants with diffusely enlarged echogenic kidneys may have clinical features that mirror those of ARPKD, including oliguric acute kidney injury with electrolyte abnormalities, respiratory distress, hypertension, and large palpable abdominal masses on physical exam. Infants with ADPKD as a manifestation of the *PKD1*/*TSC2* contiguous gene syndrome tend to have a severe presentation and may be misdiagnosed as having severe early onset ADPKD alone or ARPKD [34, 40].

Diagnosis of ADPKD in the newborn is generally based on family history and clinical features. The presence of cysts or enlarged echogenic kidneys in a neonate or infant with a parent with ADPKD is considered diagnostic [23]. As noted above, abdominal imaging should be considered in parents of infants with renal cysts or diffuse echogenicity in order to distinguish ADPKD from ARPKD or isolated diffuse cystic dysplasia. However, it should be noted that ADPKD cannot be definitively excluded in parents who are under the age of 40. Because the incidence of simple cysts in children is very low, the presence of several cysts on each kidney is highly suggestive of ADPKD, even in the absence of a positive family history [23]. Genetic testing is available for ADPKD, but is generally not necessary in patients with the classic features of bilateral macroscopic renal cysts. It may be helpful in patients with diffusely echogenic kidneys for whom alternative diagnoses (notably diffuse cystic dysplasia or ARPKD) are not clearly evident. As with ARPKD, parents of newborns with suspected ADPKD should be referred for genetic counseling in order to understand and define the risk for future pregnancies as well as for existing siblings.

14.3.2.2 Treatment and Prognosis

As is the case for ARPKD, there are no disease-specific therapies for ADPKD, although clinical trials in adults with ADPKD are under way [8]. Treatment at all ages is primarily supportive and directed at the specific symptoms (if present). Patients with macroscopic cysts who are otherwise asymptomatic should be monitored for the development of hypertension. Urinary tract infection or gross hematuria may develop rarely in young children. Infants with severe disease should be treated similarly to severely affected ARPKD neonates as outlined above.

Prognosis for patients with very early onset ADPKD (<18 months at presentation) depends, in large part, on the nature of their initial presentation (asymptomatic with macrocysts versus severe symptomatology with enlarged echogenic kidneys). Although it was initially thought that the majority of infants with early onset disease would have a poor prognosis, a recent study suggests that over 90 % of the infants initially identified by screening ultrasonography maintained normal to near-normal kidney function well into childhood [37]. In contrast, infants with ADPKD as part of the *TSC2*/*PKD1* complex generally have a poorer renal prognosis [34]. Importantly, patients with the *TSC2*/*PKD1* complex are also at risk for development of other TS-related complications, such as central nervous system lesions, renal angiomyolipomata, and renal cell carcinoma [40].

14.3.3 Other Inherited Cystic Kidney Diseases

14.3.3.1 Juvenile Nephronophthisis

Juvenile nephronophthisis (JN) is an autosomal recessive disorder characterized by chronic tubulointerstitial nephritis [46]. Although rare, it accounts for up to 10 % of pediatric end-stage renal disease (ESRD). The majority of patients with JN present in childhood and progress to ESRD in later childhood or adolescence. However, approximately 10 % have an "infantile" presentation, with most presenting in the first year of life [43]. Infantile forms of JN are caused by mutations in one of two genes, *nphp2* and *nphp3*, which are part of a large family of genes that encode proteins called nephrocystins [46]. However, a significant proportion (up to 50 %) of patients with infantile JN will not have an identifiable mutation in any of the nephronophthisis genes.

The clinical signs and symptoms of the infantile form are variable. Kidneys may be enlarged, normal sized, or small, but all demonstrate increased echogenicity [25, 43]. Small cysts are present histologically (usually in the corticomedullary region) but are often not visualized by ultrasonography. Common symptoms at presentation include anemia, polyuria, and failure to thrive. Unlike the childhood and adolescent forms, hypertension is a predominant finding in the infantile form. In addition, extrarenal manifestations are common, including cardiac valvular and hepatic disease. Notably congenital hepatic fibrosis (CHF), which is also present in ARPKD, is reported to be evident in 40 % of patients with the infantile form [43].

Diagnosis is based on typical histologic findings on kidney biopsy. Although the presence of CHF may suggest the diagnosis of ARPKD, the majority of patients with infantile JN do not have enlarged kidneys. On the other hand, if the kidneys are small or normal sized, it may be difficult to distinguish infantile JN from cystic dysplasia, particularly the hypoplastic form of glomerulocystic kidney disease.

Treatment is directed at managing the complications of chronic kidney disease (CKD). Unfortunately, rapid progression to ESRD by age 3 years occurs in the vast majority of patients with the infantile JN [43].

14.3.3.2 Glomerulocystic Kidney Disease

Glomerulocystic kidney disease (GCKD) is a descriptive term that was historically based on the histologic appearance cysts in the Bowman's capsule [5]. It is now recognized that this finding may be a manifestation of any number of cystic kidney diseases [7]. These include the polycystic kidney diseases as well as cystic dysplastic disorders associated with congenital malformation syndromes. Specific disorders that are classically associated with glomerular cysts include ADPKD in very young infants and ADPKD that occurs in association with tuberous sclerosis. Glomerular cysts are also a prominent feature of the "hypoplastic" form of glomerulocystic kidney disease, an heritable form of cystic dysplasia that is now known to be caused by inherited mutations in the *hepatocyte nuclear factor-1 beta* (*HNF-1β*) gene. Although less common, glomerular cysts may also be found in certain forms of JN as well as in cases of severe obstructive uropathy that result in dysplasia [7].

14.4 Cystic Kidney Disease Associated with Dysplasia

Cystic dysplasia results from abnormal nephron development and is evident histologically by poorly formed glomeruli, primitive, disorganized tubules and cysts that may be present at any point along the nephron [45]. Cystic dysplasia encompasses a broad range of kidney disorders with variable etiologies, clinical presentations, and prognoses. Cystic dysplasia may be a manifestation of a primary sporadic or inherited congenital kidney disease or may result from secondary insults during prenatal development (such as obstructive uropathy). Cystic dysplasia may be focal (involving only part of the kidney) or diffuse, unilateral or bilateral. The primary focus of this section will be diffuse cystic dysplasia and unilateral multicystic dysplastic kidney (MCDK).

14.4.1 Diffuse Cystic Dysplasia

Diffuse cystic dysplasia typically presents on prenatal ultrasonography as bilateral echogenic kidneys without discrete cysts. Depending on the underlying etiology, kidneys may be small, normal, or enlarged in size. Diffuse cystic dysplasia occurs as a sporadic or inherited disorder or as a component of a well-defined congenital malformation syndrome.

14.4.1.1 Isolated or Familial Diffuse Cystic Dysplasia

The incidence of diffuse cystic dysplasia (not in association with a known congenital syndrome) is not known. In one small case series of seven neonates and two fetuses without syndromic features who were diagnosed with enlarged echogenic kidneys in utero, one had histologic confirmation of diffuse cystic dysplasia [20]. It should be noted, however, that histologic confirmation of the diagnosis underlying diffusely echogenic kidneys is often not available so the true incidence is difficult to estimate.

Historically, many cases of isolated diffuse cystic dysplasia were considered sporadic, i.e., not associated with a known mutation in the patient and without a clear family history of cystic kidney disease. However, recent data has suggested that mutations in the *HNF-1B/TCF2* gene may underlie many cases of both sporadic and familial diffuse cystic dysplasia, including those that present prenatally with diffusely echogenic kidneys [15, 24]. The *HNF-1β* (*TCF2*) gene is located on chromosome 17 and encodes a transcription factor that is broadly expressed in the kidney, liver, pancreas, and genitalia during fetal development [11]. As noted above, it was originally recognized as the cause of familial "hypoplastic" GCKD [6]. This rare autosomal dominant disease is characterized by small echogenic kidneys on ultrasonography and histologic evidence of glomerular cysts. Mutations in HNF-1β also underlie the endocrine disorder, maturity-onset diabetes of the young (MODY), which may be associated with renal cysts. It is now recognized that the phenotype of patients who harbor mutations in HNF-1β is extremely variable, and a family history is often absent [15]. Renal manifestations, however, are the most common feature. Renal cystic kidney disease was present in 57 % of a cohort of 160 patients with HNF-1β mutations [15]. In another series, a prenatal phenotype of hyperechogenic kidneys with normal or moderately enlarged size was found in 34/56 patients with known HNF-1β mutations for whom a prenatal ultrasound was available [24]. Finally, in a series of 62 pregnancies characterized by echogenic fetal kidneys with variable degrees of enlargement, HNF-1β mutations were found in 29 %. These studies suggest that HNF-1β mutations may be a more common cause of isolated diffuse cystic dysplasia than was previously thought.

Because of the variable presentation and disease course of isolated or familial cases of diffuse cystic dysplasia, prognosis is difficult to determine. As with other renal cystic kidney diseases, such as ARPKD and ADPKD, the presence of oligohydramnios and respiratory failure in the newborn is likely to be associated with a poor renal prognosis.

14.4.1.2 Diffuse Cystic Dysplasia Associated with Congenital Malformation Syndromes

Consistent with its developmental origins, diffuse cystic dysplasia is a component of many congenital malformation syndromes. Notable examples include the syndromes of Meckel-Gruber [1], Joubert [32], and Bardet-Biedl [17] and overgrowth syndromes such as Beckwith-Wiedemann [30] and Simpson-Golabi-Behmel [18]. A complete discussion of these and other syndromes associated with cystic dysplasia is beyond the scope of this chapter. For up-to-date detailed genetic and clinical information about syndromes associated with cystic dysplasia (or "polycystic kidneys"), the reader is directed to the NIH-sponsored Online Mendelian Inheritance in Man (OMIM) website, www.ncbi.nlm.nih.gov/omim.

14.4.2 Multicystic Dysplastic Kidney (MCDK)

MCDK is a relatively common entity, occurring in 1:4,300 births, with a slight male gender and left-sided predominance [28, 35]. Most cases are sporadic, although rare familial cases of MCDK have been reported [36]. The genetic basis for the disease is not known, although MCDK has been reported in patients with mutations in one of several developmental genes including EYA1, SIX1, PAX2, and HNF-1β [11, 22].

MCDK is the most severe form of cystic dysplasia, resulting in complete disconnection between the nephron and the collecting system with no functional renal parenchyma [22]. Unlike many of the cystic kidney diseases already discussed, which may present as cysts or diffusely echogenic kidneys, MCDK invariably presents as numerous large cysts present on one kidney. Because MCDK kidneys are nonfunctional, bilateral disease is generally not consistent with viability after birth [35]. Abnormalities in the contralateral kidney and/or the genitourinary tract are common, occurring in 36 % of patients who are diagnosed prenatally [35]. The most common of these abnormalities is vesicoureteral reflux (VUR), which occurs in 20 % of patients. Of those, 60 % have grade I or II (mild) VUR and 40 % have grade III–V (moderate–severe) VUR [35]. Other associated abnormalities include ureteropelvic junction (UPJ) obstruction, ureterovesical junction (UVJ) obstruction, or a variety of genital abnormalities such as Gartner's cysts, seminal cysts, or vaginal malformations [22].

Diagnosis is made based on the typical ultrasonographic appearance. MCDK is distinguished from ADPKD (which can present with unilateral disease) by the numerous large cysts with no apparent normal parenchyma and a contralateral kidney that is generally without cysts, enlargement, or echogenicity. In cases where there is a question of whether functioning parenchyma is present in the MCDK kidney, a radionuclide scan may be helpful [22].

The natural history of most MCDKs is involution over time, with 60 % involution by age 5 [28]. Therefore, surgical resection is generally not required, and medical management involves serial ultrasonography to confirm involution of the affected kidney and appropriate compensatory hypertrophy of the contralateral kidney as well as blood pressure, serum creatinine, and urine protein measurements [22]. In the past, nephrectomy was advocated because of rare reports of hypertension or malignancy. More recent data, however, suggest that there is no increased risk of these complications for patients with MCDK compared to the normal population [22]. Nephrectomy, therefore, is reserved for cases in which involution does not occur over time and/or the MCDK demonstrates rapid growth or the presence of a discrete mass.

Because MCDKs are nonfunctional, prognosis is determined by the status of the contralateral kidney. Those with normal-appearing contralateral kidneys that show appropriate compensatory hypertrophy generally do quite well although an increased risk of proteinuria has been reported [28]. Although long-term data are somewhat limited, those with demonstrated abnormalities in the contralateral kidney appear to have an increased risk of chronic kidney disease and hypertension [22, 28].

14.4.3 Other Causes of Renal Cysts in Neonates

Simple renal cysts occur rarely in childhood, with a reported incidence of 0.2 % [29]. Because of this rare occurrence, it is important to have a high index of suspicion for other cystic kidney disorders. Notably, ADPKD in infants and children can present as an isolated renal cyst in one kidney. In addition, in a patient with a family history of ADPKD, the finding of even one cyst in childhood may be considered diagnostic [14]. Thus, a detailed family history and serial renal ultrasonography to monitor for the development of additional ipsilateral and contralateral cysts are imperative in the evaluation of a neonate found to have a renal cyst.

Another rare cause of a solitary or "simple" renal cyst is a caliceal diverticulum. This disorder is typically unilateral and solitary and may mimic the appearance of a cyst [16, 27]. In instances where ADPKD or suspected isolated renal cyst are suspected, these can be distinguished from caliceal diverticulum either with magnetic resonance urography or computed tomography with delayed images [27]. In one series, 9 % of affected patients have contralateral VUR [16]. Complications of caliceal diverticulum include urinary tract infection and urolithiasis [26]. Management of confirmed caliceal diverticulum is generally guided by pediatric urologists. Various surgical approaches (including percutaneous ablation or marsupialization) have been undertaken in symptomatic patients, whereas asymptomatic patients are generally observed without intervention [16].

Conclusion

Renal cystic diseases in the fetus and newborn encompass a large number of disorders, some of which may be associated with life-threatening complications. It is important to recognize that the presentation of cystic kidney disease in the fetus or newborn may be that of diffusely echogenic kidneys of variable size rather than the discrete cysts typically evident in older children or adults with cystic kidney diseases. The treatment of newborns with severe suspected cystic kidney disease (regardless of the cause) is directed at respiratory support, maintenance of fluid and electrolyte balance, and treatment of hypertension. The diagnostic criteria and long-term prognosis for this heterogeneous group of disorders is variable and depends, in large part, on the nature of the underlying disorder. In general, however, a history of oligohydramnios and the development of respiratory distress from pulmonary hypoplasia suggest a poor long-term renal prognosis.

References

1. Alexiev BA, Lin X, Sun CC et al (2006) Meckel-Gruber syndrome: pathologic manifestations, minimal diagnostic criteria, and differential diagnosis. Arch Pathol Lab Med 130(8):1236–1238
2. Bean SA, Bednarek FJ, Primack WA (1995) Aggressive respiratory support and unilateral nephrectomy for infants with severe perinatal autosomal recessive polycystic kidney disease. J Pediatr 127(2):311–313
3. Bergmann C, Senderek J, Kupper F et al (2004) PKHD1 mutations in autosomal recessive polycystic kidney disease (ARPKD). Hum Mutat 23(5):453–463
4. Bergmann C, Senderek J, Windelen E et al (2005) Clinical consequences of PKHD1 mutations in 164 patients with autosomal-recessive polycystic kidney disease (ARPKD). Kidney Int 67(3):829–848
5. Bernstein J (1993) Glomerulocystic kidney disease–nosological considerations. Pediatr Nephrol 7(4):464–470
6. Bingham C, Bulman MP, Ellard S et al (2001) Mutations in the hepatocyte nuclear factor-1beta gene are associated with familial hypoplastic glomerulocystic kidney disease. Am J Hum Genet 68(1):219–224
7. Bissler JJ, Siroky BJ, Yin H (2010) Glomerulocystic kidney disease. Pediatr Nephrol 25(10):2049–2056, quiz 2056–2049
8. Chang MY, Ong AC (2012) Mechanism-based therapeutics for autosomal dominant polycystic kidney disease: recent progress and future prospects. Nephron Clin Pract 120(1):c25–c34
9. Chaumoitre K, Brun M, Cassart M et al (2006) Differential diagnosis of fetal hyperechogenic cystic kidneys unrelated to renal tract anomalies: a multicenter study. Ultrasound Obstet Gynecol 28(7):911–917
10. Cole BR, Conley SB, Stapleton FB (1987) Polycystic kidney disease in the first year of life. J Pediatr 111(5):693–699
11. Decramer S, Parant O, Beaufils S et al (2007) Anomalies of the TCF2 gene are the main cause of fetal bilateral hyperechogenic kidneys. J Am Soc Nephrol 18(3):923–933
12. Dell KM (2011) The spectrum of polycystic kidney disease in children. Adv Chronic Kidney Dis 18(5):339–347
13. Dell KM, Avner ED (2008) Autosomal recessive polycystic kidney disease. Gene Clinics: Clinical Genetic Information Resource (database online). Copyright, University of Washington, Seattle. Available at http://www.geneclinics.org. Initial posting July 2001, updated 2009
14. Dell KM, McDonald RA, Watkins S et al (2009) Polycystic kidney disease. In: Avner ED, Harmon WE, Niaudet P, Yoshikawa N (eds) Pediatric nephrology, 6th edn. Springer, New York
15. Edghill EL, Bingham C, Ellard S et al (2006) Mutations in hepatocyte nuclear factor-1beta and their related phenotypes. J Med Genet 43(1):84–90
16. Estrada CR, Datta S, Schneck FX et al (2009) Caliceal diverticula in children: natural history and management. J Urol 181(3):1306–1311, discussion 1311
17. Gershoni-Baruch R, Nachlieli T, Leibo R et al (1992) Cystic kidney dysplasia and polydactyly in 3 sibs with Bardet-Biedl syndrome. Am J Med Genet 44(3):269–273
18. Grisaru S, Rosenblum ND (2001) Glypicans and the biology of renal malformations. Pediatr Nephrol 16(3):302–306
19. Guay-Woodford LM, Desmond RA (2003) Autosomal recessive polycystic kidney disease: the clinical experience in North America. Pediatrics 111(5 Pt 1):1072–1080
20. Guay-Woodford LM, Galliani CA, Musulman-Mroczek E et al (1998) Diffuse renal cystic disease in children: morphologic and genetic correlations. Pediatr Nephrol 12(3):173–182
21. Gunay-Aygun M (2009) Liver and kidney disease in ciliopathies. Am J Med Genet C Semin Med Genet 151C(4):296–306
22. Hains DS, Bates CM, Ingraham S et al (2009) Management and etiology of the unilateral multicystic dysplastic kidney: a review. Pediatr Nephrol 24(2):233–241
23. Harris PC, Torres VE (2002) Autosomal dominant polycystic kidney disease. Gene Clinics: Clinical Genetic Information Resource (database online). Copyright,

University of Washington, Seattle. Available at http://www.geneclinics.org. Updated 8 Dec 2011
24. Heidet L, Decramer S, Pawtowski A et al (2010) Spectrum of HNF1B mutations in a large cohort of patients who harbor renal diseases. Clin J Am Soc Nephrol 5(6):1079–1090
25. Hildebrandt F, Zhou W (2007) Nephronophthisis-associated ciliopathies. J Am Soc Nephrol 18(6): 1855–1871
26. Karmazyn B, Kaefer M, Jennings SG et al (2011) Caliceal diverticulum in pediatric patients: the spectrum of imaging findings. Pediatr Radiol 41(11): 1369–1373
27. Kavukcu S, Cakmakci H, Babayigit A (2003) Diagnosis of caliceal diverticulum in two pediatric patients: a comparison of sonography, CT, and urography. J Clin Ultrasound 31(4):218–221
28. Mansoor O, Chandar J, Rodriguez MM et al (2011) Long-term risk of chronic kidney disease in unilateral multicystic dysplastic kidney. Pediatr Nephrol 26(4): 597–603
29. McHugh K, Stringer DA, Hebert D et al (1991) Simple renal cysts in children: diagnosis and follow-up with US. Radiology 178(2):383–385
30. Mussa A, Peruzzi L, Chiesa N et al (2012) Nephrological findings and genotype-phenotype correlation in Beckwith-Wiedemann syndrome. Pediatr Nephrol 27(3):397–406
31. Northrup H, Koenig MK, Au KS (1993) Tuberous sclerosis complex, Gene Reviews™ (Internet). University of Washington, Seattle
32. Parisi MA (2009) Clinical and molecular features of Joubert syndrome and related disorders. Am J Med Genet C Semin Med Genet 151C(4):326–340
33. Roy S, Dillon MJ, Trompeter RS et al (1997) Autosomal recessive polycystic kidney disease: long-term outcome of neonatal survivors. Pediatr Nephrol 11(3):302–306
34. Sampson JR, Maheshwar MM, Aspinwall R et al (1997) Renal cystic disease in tuberous sclerosis: role of the polycystic kidney disease 1 gene. Am J Hum Genet 61(4):843–851
35. Schreuder MF, Westland R, van Wijk JA (2009) Unilateral multicystic dysplastic kidney: a meta-analysis of observational studies on the incidence, associated urinary tract malformations and the contralateral kidney. Nephrol Dial Transplant 24(6): 1810–1818
36. Sekine T, Namai Y, Yanagisawa A et al (2005) A familial case of multicystic dysplastic kidney. Pediatr Nephrol 20(9):1245–1248
37. Shamshirsaz AA, Reza Bekheirnia M, Kamgar M et al (2005) Autosomal-dominant polycystic kidney disease in infancy and childhood: progression and outcome. Kidney Int 68(5):2218–2224
38. Sharp AM, Messiaen LM, Page G et al (2005) Comprehensive genomic analysis of PKHD1 mutations in ARPKD cohorts. J Med Genet 42(4):336–349
39. Shneider BL, Magid MS (2005) Liver disease in autosomal recessive polycystic kidney disease. Pediatr Transplant 9(5):634–639
40. Siroky BJ, Yin H, Bissler JJ (2011) Clinical and molecular insights into tuberous sclerosis complex renal disease. Pediatr Nephrol 26(6):839–852
41. Tee JB, Acott PD, McLellan DH et al (2004) Phenotypic heterogeneity in pediatric autosomal dominant polycystic kidney disease at first presentation: a single-center, 20-year review. Am J Kidney Dis 43(2):296–303
42. Torres VE, Harris PC, Pirson Y (2007) Autosomal dominant polycystic kidney disease. Lancet 369(9569): 1287–1301
43. Tory K, Rousset-Rouviere C, Gubler MC et al (2009) Mutations of NPHP2 and NPHP3 in infantile nephronophthisis. Kidney Int 75(8):839–847
44. Ward CJ, Hogan MC, Rossetti S et al (2002) The gene mutated in autosomal recessive polycystic kidney disease encodes a large, receptor-like protein. Nat Genet 30(3):259–269
45. Winyard P, Chitty LS (2008) Dysplastic kidneys. Semin Fetal Neonatal Med 13(3):142–151
46. Wolf MT, Hildebrandt F (2011) Nephronophthisis. Pediatr Nephrol 26(2):181–194
47. Zerres K, Rudnik-Schoneborn S, Deget F et al (1996) Autosomal recessive polycystic kidney disease in 115 children: clinical presentation, course and influence of gender. Arbeitsgemeinschaft fur Padiatrische, Nephrologie. Acta Paediatr 85(4):437–445

Congenital Nephrotic Syndrome

15

Latawanya D. Pleasant and Stefan G. Kiessling

Core Messages

- Congenital nephrotic syndrome (CNS) is a rare condition diagnosed within the first 3 months of life by high-grade proteinuria, hypoalbuminemia, and edema.
- The most common form of CNS is the Finnish type (CNF), but several other genetic and nongenetic forms do exist and need to be considered in the differential diagnosis.
- Genetic testing is available and should be strongly considered.
- At this point in time, kidney transplantation is the only curative therapy available.
- The management of children with CNS is complex and dependent on the degree of protein losses.

Case Vignette

A female newborn was admitted at 2.5 months of age with lethargy and edema. Her birth weight was 6 lbs 14 oz and her weight at the time of admission was close to 9 lbs. She was born at home as the 4th child of a Mennonite family. She had gained about 1 lbs since she was seen by her pediatrician for an early 2-month check-up. She was exclusively breastfeeding. She seemed to tire much more quickly in the recent past. She was diagnosed with congenital hypothyroidism and received daily Synthroid therapy. She became increasingly mottled, febrile, and floppy and was transferred to the Pediatric Intensive Care Unit at our institution. A blood culture grew Streptococcus pneumoniae. She was noted to have hyponatremia, hypokalemia, and hypoalbuminemia with a serum albumin of 1.2 g/dl. A 24-h urine showed a protein excretion of 650 mg/m^2/h equivalent to about 4 g/day. During the hospitalization, she received several albumin infusions and was started on Lasix, captopril, and enoxaparin. Despite extensive counseling and several family meetings, the parents did agree to neither genetic testing nor possible interventions including nephrectomies, dialysis, or renal transplantation. The child passed away at the family's home 6 weeks later.

L.D. Pleasant, MD, FAAP
Division of Pediatric Nephrology,
Cincinnati Children's Hospital,
3333 Burnet Avenue, Cincinnati,
OH 45229, USA
e-mail: ldplea2@email.uky.edu

S.G. Kiessling, MD, FAAP (✉)
Division of Pediatric Nephrology,
Hypertension and Renal Transplantation,
Kentucky Children's Hospital, University of Kentucky,
William R. Willard Medical Science Building,
800 Rose Street, Room MN-109,
Lexington, KY 40536-0284, USA
e-mail: skies2@email.uky.edu

A.S. Chishti et al. (eds.), *Kidney and Urinary Tract Diseases in the Newborn*,
DOI 10.1007/978-3-642-39988-6_15, © Springer-Verlag Berlin Heidelberg 2014

Eighteen months later, the parents had another child which was admitted at 33 weeks of gestation to the NICU. The child was found to have nephrotic-range proteinuria with a serum albumin of 0.9 g/dl. Despite extensive counseling, the parents requested discharge to comfort care without additional interventions.

15.1 Introduction

Congenital nephrotic syndrome (CNS) is a group of rare conditions that present with high-grade urine protein (albumin) losses, hypoalbuminemia, and edema within the first 3 months of life. It is important to differentiate CNS from other presentations of nephrotic syndrome, mainly the infantile form (4–12 months of age) and childhood nephrotic syndrome (onset after the 1st year of life). Unless treatment is initiated, CNS is universally fatal.

Causes of CNS can be divided into primary and secondary. The most common primary form is CNS of the Finnish type which is inherited in an autosomal recessive fashion and due to mutations of the NPHS1 gene. The gene is located on chromosome 19, and two important mutations have been described (Fin-major and Fin-minor) in over 90 % of the Finnish patients [1]. Other mutations have been reported in non-Finnish patients. Pertinent to our introductory case presentation, a 1481delC mutation is common in Mennonites leading to a truncated form of the nephrin protein [2]. Other primary forms include mutations of the podocin gene (NPHS2) most often leading to focal and segmental glomerulosclerosis and WT1 gene mutations among others as will be discussed later on.

Secondary causes include several infectious etiologies like congenital TORCH infections, hepatitis B and C, HIV, as well as syndrome-associated CNS like Denys-Drash syndrome, Lowe syndrome, or nail-patella syndrome among others [3].

In the more recent past, significant scientific advances have led to a better understanding of the genetics and pathophysiologic factors involved in the disease mechanism (involving the glomerular filtration barrier) of the proteinuric syndromes [4]. Even though the management of children with CNS remains complex and complicated, one certainly hopes that our improved understanding will open new treatment modalities and ultimately translate into improved outcome.

15.2 Pathophysiology

Congenital nephrotic syndrome is distinguished from other forms of nephrotic syndrome by the fact that it compromises a heterogeneous group of renal diseases that results in significant postnatal glomerular permeability that ultimately leads to massive proteinuria and hematuria immediately or shortly after birth.

Each form of primary CNS is part of the large group of the hereditary proteinuric syndromes. Even though pathophysiologically similar, secondary forms of CNS do have identifiable nongenetic causes.

The glomerular filtration barrier is composed of three distinct layers: fenestrated endothelium, glomerular basement membrane, and the podocyte layer which is a composite of distal foot processes and interposed slit diaphragms. The glomerular basement membrane functions as the pre-filtration component while the slit diaphragm functions as the ultrafiltration unit of the filtration barrier. This filtration barrier functions to limit flux of solutes into the urine base and is charge and size selective. Figure 15.1 provides a diagram of the highly specialized filtration apparatus.

The glomerular basement membrane is a precise network of proteins including but not limited to type IV collagen, laminin, nidogen, and proteoglycans which are the proteins responsible for giving the glomerular basement membrane its negative charge. The slit diaphragm – with the exact molecular ultrastructure still being unclear as mentioned by Jalanko – consists of podocyte proteins that form the backbone of the slit diaphragm that interacts with adapter proteins [5]. The adapter proteins are localized in the cytosolic component of the podocyte and connect the slit

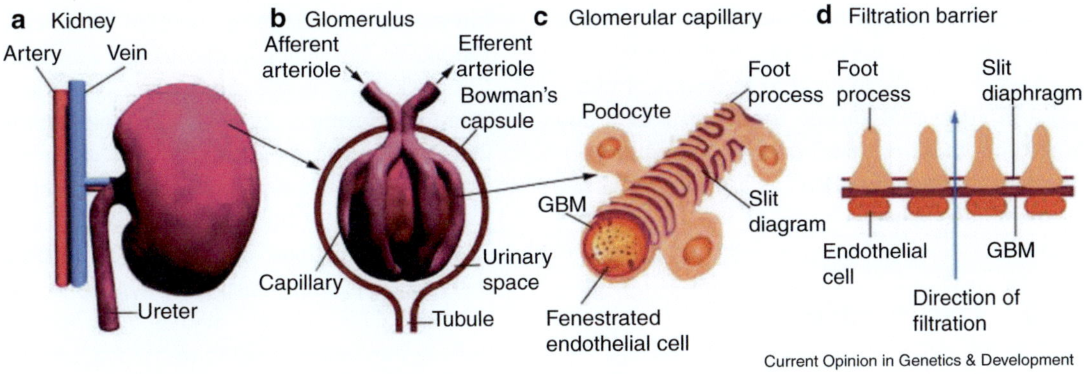

Fig. 15.1 Overview of the renal filtration system (Reprinted from Khoshnoodi and Tryggvason [6], Copyright 2001, with permission from Elsevier)

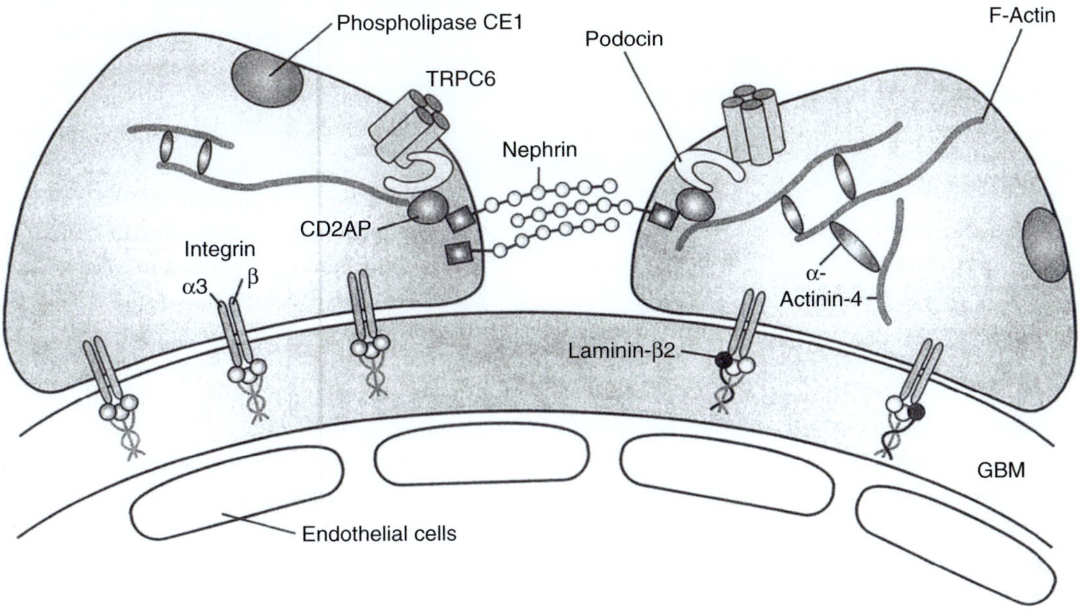

Fig. 15.2 Important components of the glomerular filtration barrier altered by inherited forms of nephrotic syndrome (This figure was published in Weber [56], Copyright Elsevier)

diaphragm with the actin cytoskeleton of the podocyte foot processes and play a pivotal role in signal transduction. Some of those adapter proteins are podocin, CD2AP, and ZO-1. The interaction of the actin cytoskeleton with other surrounding proteins, including α-actinin-4, plays a critical role in the maintenance of the podocyte structure. Figure 15.2 shows a cartoon of some of the most important components of the slit diaphragm and foot processes involved in CNS known today. The slit diaphragm plays a key role in restricting protein content into the ultrafiltrate reaching the Bowman space. Defects in either the slit diaphragms themselves or the structure/function of the podocyte foot processes are the primary reason for the high-grade proteinuria and lipiduria seen in CNS [5, 6]. It is the disruption of this highly intricate and specialized network of proteins that results in loss of the kidney filtration barrier located within the glomerular capillary wall which ultimately leads to CNS or other nephrotic disorders [5]. CNS is a result of excessive leakage of serum proteins into the urine. The exact mechanisms, even though still highly debated, are thought to be results of mutations in genes that encode for the structural and regulatory proteins that form the glomerular capillary wall which functions as a filtration barrier as mentioned above.

15.3 Classification

CNS can be classified as primary when due to a known (or yet unknown) genetic mutation or secondary when it presents in the context of other, often infectious, disease. The primary forms can be divided in mutations involving the nephrin (NPHS1) and podocin gene (NPHS2) mutations as well as other genetic forms oftentimes associated with various syndromes. At least two thirds of newborns and infants diagnosed with CNS have a mutation in one of four genes: NPHS1, NHPS2, WT1, and LAMB2 [7]. The most common nongenetic forms are caused by certain infections or systemic disease:

1. *NPHS1*: NPHS1 refers to nephrotic syndrome type 1 or congenital nephrotic syndrome of the Finnish type which was first described by Ahvenainen et al. in 1956 [8]. It is inherited in an autosomal recessive fashion occurring worldwide but most commonly found in the Finnish population. In 1994, the gene defect has been located on the long arm of chromosome 19, a year later to the exact location 19q13.1 [9, 10]. Affected neonates exhibit massive proteinuria in utero and develop nephrosis shortly after birth. It is due to a mutation in the nephrin gene which is a podocyte protein that is responsible for the slit diaphragm backbone [5]. Nephrin is a type 1 transmembrane protein that belongs in the immunoglobulin superfamily. It consists of eight immunoglobulin-like motifs followed by a fibronectin type III domain, a transmembrane region followed by a cytoplasmic carboxy-terminal part. Nephrin is expressed in multiple areas of the body. In the kidney, nephrin is expressed in the podocytes and exclusively localized in the slit diaphragm [6, 11–13]. NPHS1 is further divided into Fin-major and Fin-minor, with the most common form being Fin-major. Fin-major is due to a 2 base pair (2-bp) deletion in the stop codon on exon 2 (Fin-minor being a nonsense mutation in exon 26), which results in a complete loss of the slit diaphragms and ultimately massive nonselective proteinuria at birth [6, 14]. Recently, several new mutations of NPHS1 have been described including missense mutations and deletions [15]. Classic findings of NPHS1 include intrauterine growth restriction, muscular hypotonia, cardiac hypertrophy, microscopic hematuria with or without normal creatinine, and hyperlipidemia [5]. Most infants are born prematurely with the placenta being significantly enlarged accounting for more than 25 % of the neonate's birth weight. Edema is present immediately at birth or within a few days. Massive proteinuria is accompanied by profound hypoalbuminemia with associated hypogammaglobulinemia. Renal biopsy shortly after birth presents with dilatations of the proximal tubules and microcyst formation with normal glomeruli. Radiographic features include increased cortical echogenicity, loss of corticomedullary differentiation, expansion of the glomerular mesangium, and dilatation of the proximal and distal tubules. Classic microscopic findings include interstitial fibrosis and inflammatory infiltrates, and effacement of the podocyte foot processes. Renal failure occurs most often between 3 and 8 years of age. Finminor is due to a missense mutation in exon 26 [14]. Figure 15.2 provides a diagram of the molecular structure of the glomerular filtration barrier and the role of nephrin.
2. *NPHS2*: Mutations of the NPHS2 gene – which encodes a protein called podocin – are responsible for an autosomal recessive steroid-resistant nephrotic syndrome with often rapid progression to end-stage kidney disease. It is most common in children between 3 months and 5 years of age [6]. Several mutations have been described, the most common one due to a substitution of R138Q in the podocin gene that is a found on chromosome 1q25–q32. This mutation results in the retention of podocin in the endoplasmic reticulum and its inability to

recruit nephrin in the lipid rafts [14, 16]. Podocin is a lipid raft-associated protein at the filtration slit that is exclusively expressed in the podocyte foot process. It interacts with nephrin at the level of the lipid rafts and is responsible for initiating nephrin signaling [14]. Podocin interacts with ion channels and the cytoskeleton [6]. Podocin also interacts with CD2AP, an adapter protein that stabilized contacts between podocytes, thus providing structural integrity and function to the slit diaphragm. This detailed interaction provides maintenance of the glomerular permselectivity [17]. There is wide variability in the degree of proteinuria that occurs with NPHS2. Classical microscopic findings include focal segmental glomerular sclerosis which may ultimately lead to end-stage renal disease. NPHS2 does not typically have any extrarenal manifestations primarily due to lack of expression of podocin in other areas [5]. Figure 15.2 provides a diagram of the molecular structure of the glomerular filtration barrier and the role of nephrin.

3. *Other Genetic Forms of CNS*
   - Abnormalities in the Wilms tumor suppressor gene WT1 can lead to isolated nephrotic syndrome or nephrotic syndrome associated with developmental syndromes including Denys-Drash, Frasier, and WAGR syndromes. WT1 is a transcription factor that is responsible for the embryonic development of the genitourinary system. WT1 controls nephrin expression. Denys-Drash syndrome is defined by the combination of nephrotic syndrome, diffuse mesangial sclerosis, Wilms tumor, and male pseudohermaphroditism [18, 19]. The reason for associated gonadal anomalies is due to WT1 tumor gene is found on chromosome 11p13 and plays a vital role in the transcription of urogenital development. WT1 is highly expressed during embryonic development but in mature kidneys is only expressed in podocytes and epithelial cells of the Bowman's capsule. The WT1 gene product results in the downregulatory effect on transcription factors such as PAX2, PAX8, and NOVH. Mutations ultimately result in absence or reduction in WT1 which leads to overexpression of PAX2 and possible glomerular lesions found in some patients with Denys-Drash syndrome [6]. Frasier syndrome has also been associated with mutations of the WT1 gene and is characterized by the association of male pseudohermaphroditism and progressive glomerulopathy usually due to FSGS. Proteinuria is usually detected between 2 and 6 years of age. Patients with Frasier syndrome typically have a slower progression to end-stage renal disease than those with Denys-Drash syndrome and progress to FSGS [14].
   - Pierson syndrome is a rare autosomal recessive condition caused by deficiency in laminin-β2 expressed in the glomerular basement membrane in which combined ocular and renal abnormalities are found in combination [20, 21]. Laminin-β2 (LAMB2) is responsible for anchoring the podocyte processes to the glomerular basement membrane. It was recently described as a cause of CNS [13].
   - Galloway-Mowat syndrome, first described in 1968, is an autosomal recessive disorder that results in CNS with associated central nervous system abnormalities and hiatus hernia [22]. The gene has not been identified. Central nervous system abnormalities result due to the fact that podocytes consist of similar structure proteins as neuronal cells [5].
   - The loss-of-function mutation causing the autosomal dominant disease hereditary onycho-osteodysplasia (nail-patella syndrome) was first described in 1998 [23]. LAMX1B is primary expressed by podocytes within the kidney and regulates several important proteins involved in the filtration barrier including nephrin, podocin, and the adapter protein CD2AP.
   - A new mutation involving the phospholipase C epsilon 1 (PLCE1, also referred to as NPHS3) gene more recently reported in 2006 [24].
   - Mitochondrial myopathies and mutations in LAMB3 have also been associated with CNS [25, 26].

4. *Nongenetic Forms*: Congenital infections including HIV, CMV, toxoplasmosis, or syphilis can result in congenital proteinuric syndromes [27, 28]. Therefore, newborns with nephrotic-range proteinuria and evidence of CNS should undergo a thorough investigation for transmitted or acquired infections. Also, infantile systemic lupus erythematosus has been reported to be associated with CNS [29, 30]. To our knowledge, CNS has not been associated with neonatal lupus syndrome and it is important to differentiate the two entities [31].

15.4 Epidemiology

CNS is a rare disorder. The exact incidence and prevalence are unknown and most epidemiologic data available refer to congenital nephrotic syndrome of the Finnish type (CNF). With advances in prenatal screening, the prevalence of CNF has been estimated to be 4.2 per 10,000 live births. Due to termination of pregnancy, the incidence has decreased to 0.9 per 10,000 live births [32].

15.5 Clinical Presentation

The majority of patients born with CNS are born prematurely and are small for gestational age, with the placenta usually weighing more than 25 % of the newborn's birth weight [6]. The patients typically have delayed ossification which attributes to widely enlarged sutures. Generalized edema presents within the first week of life for the majority of infants [5]. Typically urine analysis will reveal exclusively proteinuria without any evidence of hematuria which helps differentiate it from other possible etiologies for neonatal edema. The neonates also have profound hypoalbuminemia with associated severe hypogammaglobulinemia. Serum albumin is <10 g/l at presentation and urinary protein concentration is >20 g/l when serum albumin is corrected to >15 g/l [33]. These infants may present septic from lack of gamma globulin and possibly severe thromboembolic complications from excretion of coagulation factors. Infants may have symptoms typically found in hypothyroidism from urinary excretion of thyroxine-binding proteins. Renal sonography demonstrates enlarged hyperechogenic kidneys with lack of corticomedullary differentiation. Elevated creatinine is typically not common initially in the disease process but typically presents between 3 and 8 years of age [5].

15.6 Diagnosis

In CNF, high levels of α-fetoprotein (AFP) in the amniotic fluid and maternal serum can be useful for prenatal diagnosis in selected at-risk families [34, 35]. However, increased levels of α-fetoprotein (AFP) are unspecific and genetic analysis is the preferred method for making the diagnosis [5, 36]. Increased levels of amniotic fluid α-fetoprotein concentration may be used as a marker to distinguish congenital nephrotic syndrome Finnish type from diffuse mesangial sclerosis.

The classic clinical finding of CNS is generalized edema from reduced serum protein content from renal excretion. Clinical signs may not be initially present during the first weeks of life. Patients will present with urinary protein levels greater than 20 g per liter and serum albumin levels are less than 10 g per liter. Renal function is typically normal with all forms of CNS initially. Blood pressure readings are also extremely variable depending on the stage of CNS. Patient with renal failure will have associated hypertension and those with significant untreated proteinuria or hypoalbuminemia may potentially be hypotensive. Diagnostic imaging in the form of a renal ultrasound can be helpful. The kidneys are usually enlarged and echogenic with identifiable loss of corticomedullary differentiation as well as poor visualization of the renal pyramids [37]. Renal biopsy can be a useful tool to confirm the diagnosis in CNS but it does not identify the etiology of CNS due to significant overlap of different disease entities. Specific immunohistochemistry methods to identify expression of podocin or nephrin can be helpful and should be obtained if available. The purpose of a biopsy would be to identify any associated sclerosis or interstitial fibrosis which may guide therapy. Genetic analysis is the optimal method to identify CNS diagnosis. Analysis of NPHS1 and NPHS2 mutations is required for all CNS patients. In cases where NPHS1 and NPHS2 are not identified, WT1 or LAMB2 genetic analysis should be obtained. In some instances NPHS1 may be identified in utero in families with known risk for CNS by obtaining alpha-fetoprotein levels in the amniotic fluid prior to 20 weeks gestation [5].

15.7 Differential Diagnosis

Once CNS is suspected and nephrotic-range proteinuria is confirmed on 24-h collection (urine protein excretion >40 mg/m^2/day), a thorough differential diagnosis needs to be built as outlined earlier in this chapter. The maternal and neonatal history as well as physical exam findings (presence or absence of associated syndromic features) will determine additional serologic and genetic testing of mother and child and aid in establishing a correct diagnosis which is important to determine the degree of necessary interventions as well as the expected course of the disease. For children who do have pathologic proteinuria but do not fit criteria for CNS, the differential diagnosis should include genetic or non-genetic tubular and/or glomerular disorders, and a comprehensive evaluation should be completed depending on associated findings as discussed elsewhere in this book.

15.8 General Aspects of Management

The management of children with CNS can be divided into a medical as well as a surgical component. Both of these have the goal to optimize the child's cognitive and physical growth. The medical component includes treatment of edema by the use of albumin infusions and loop diuretics as well as medications. Surgical care primarily includes native nephrectomy and renal transplantation. Licht et al. have recommended a "stepwise treatment approach" to the disease that continues to be followed by most centers [38]. This stepwise approach has supportive therapies as base, followed by use of medications (ACE inhibitors and Indocin), unilateral nephrectomy, and ultimately bilateral nephrectomy with dialysis before ultimately renal transplantation.

15.8.1 Medical Management

15.8.1.1 Nutrition

Nutrition and growth deficits are particularly common in patients with congenital nephrotic syndrome and need to be minimized under all circumstances [5]. High-protein and high-calorie diets are usually necessary to provide patients with sufficient substrate for basic metabolic needs in addition to growth. Maintaining 120 kcal/kg/day with high-protein diet of 3–4 g/kg/day with a low-sodium diet has provided additional sources of therapy [33]. Breast milk and milk formulas are used first line and additional protein calories are provided using casein-based products [39]. Typical diets should consist of 10–14 % protein, 40–50 % fat, and 40–50 % carbohydrate energy. Monounsaturated and polyunsaturated fatty acids may be substituted with 10–15 ml of rape seed oil and 2 ml of fish oil daily. Initially patients are placed on breast milk and milk formulas that are fortified with additional protein [5]. Many patients may require nasogastric tube feeds to ensure that adequate nutrition is maintained to guarantee their basic metabolic needs. Children should receive additional supplements in magnesium and calcium secondary to deficits in parathyroid hormone which is secondary to excretion of albumin. Recommended magnesium supplement includes 50 mg/day in addition to 500–1,000 mg/day of calcium. Excretion of albumin and thus reduced levels of parathyroid hormone results requirement for vitamin D supplementation. All patients should receive 2,000 IU/day of vitamin D2 and 2.5–3.0 mg/day of rape seed oil in the form of vitamin E. Patients should also receive alphacalcidol pulse therapy to avoid hyperparathyroidism and a calcium carbonate as a phosphate binder. Other nutritional considerations should include

Table 15.1 Treatment recommendations for congenital nephrotic syndrome of the Finnish-type (CNF) patients during their 1st year of life (From Holmberg et al. [33]. With kind permission from Springer Science + Business Media)

Albumin substitution
3–4 g/kg per day i.v. with frusemide 0.5 mg/kg
(in four 2-h infusions during the 1st month and in one 6 to 8-h infusion later)
Nutrition
130 kcal of energy and 4 g protein/kg per day (inaddition to i.v. albumin substitution)
(10 %–14 % protein, 40 %–50 % fat and 40 %–50 % carbohydrate energy)
15 ml rape seed oil and 2 ml fish oil fluids 100–130 mllkg per day vitamin D2 (2,000 IU/day), water-soluble vitamins (according to RDA), magnesium (40–60 mg/day) and calcium (500 mg <6, 750 mg 6–12 and 1,000 mg >12 months of age)
Additional medication
thyroxine (from birth, adjusted according to TSH) sodium warfarin (to keep PTT at 20 %–30 % of normal)
(AT III 50 IU/kg i.v.1 h before surgical or vascular procedures) prompt antibiotic therapy for septic infections

RDA Recommended dietary allowance, *TSH* thyroid-stimulating hormone, *PTT* partial thromboplastin time, *At III* antithrombin III

low-salt diet and possible tube feeding or parenteral alimentation for provision of maximal growth for the ultimate goal of renal transplantation. Table 15.1 provides a list of nutritional recommendations for congenital nephrotic syndrome of the Finnish type during the first year of life.

15.8.1.2 Albumin and Diuretics

The basic problem in children with congenital nephrotic syndrome is the massive urinary loss of protein, 90 % of which is albumin. This loss leads to protein malnutrition, reduced growth, and secondary symptoms of hypoproteinemia [33]. Albumin infusions provide a necessary supplementation for the loss of necessary serum proteins that provide an osmotic gradient for hemodynamic stability, nutrition for growth, coagulation, and protection from infections in the form of immunoglobulin. A common method of substitution includes parenteral albumin infusions with a 20 % albumin solution via a central venous catheter followed by a furosemide bolus. Typical dosing includes 1–5 ml/kg albumin infusions divided into three infusions over 2 h. To guarantee normal growth, serum albumin concentration of 15–20 g/l should be maintained [33]. Maintenance therapy typically may consist of a single albumin infusion of up to 20 ml/kg over 6 h followed by a single Lasix bolus. This substitution only temporarily relieves hypoproteinemia but does not provide complete resolution of the generalized edema [5]. High-protein diets have also played a key role in the medical management of congenital nephrotic syndrome. Maintaining 120 kcal/kg/day with high-protein diet of 3–4 g/kg/day with a low-sodium diet has provided additional sources of therapy [33].

15.8.1.3 Antiproteinuric Therapies

In contrast to childhood nephrotic syndrome, immunosuppressive medications including corticosteroids play no role in the treatment. This certainly makes sense as the disease does not respond with the pathophysiologic process being not immune mediated [40]. The overall goal of therapy is to control generalized edema, maintain renal function, and avoid complications from the loss of anticoagulants and immunoglobulin [5]. Angiotensin-converting enzyme (ACE) inhibitors, used either as monotherapy or in combination with indomethacin, have been shown to be able to control proteinuria and maintain growth and health in some children with CNS [41–43]. Angiotensin-converting enzyme inhibitors lower intraglomerular pressure which ultimately results in a reduction in excretion of protein. Indomethacin exerts its antiproteinuric effects by inhibiting prostaglandin synthetase. With close monitoring of therapy response (as measured by degree of urine protein loss) and renal function, starting doses of 1 mg/kg/day of both captopril and Indocin have been recommended. This dose can be increased to a maximum of about 5 mg/kg/day [38]. In our center, mildly lower starting doses of 0.2–0.5 mg/kg/day with close monitoring of the serum creatinine have been used in the past.

15.8.1.4 Others

Patients with congenital nephrotic syndrome should have TSH and free T4 levels regularly obtained due to risk for hypothyroidism. This seems to be explained by high urinary excretion of thyroid-binding globulin as well as thyroxine and patients may benefit from thyroxine substitution. The hypothyroidism being a result of urinary protein losses is supported by the fact that hypothyroidism usually reverses after bilateral nephrectomies [44]. On laboratory evaluation, serum thyroxine concentrations are always low, TSH may be normal initially, but increase in most patients during the first months. Recommended dosing of thyroxine is typically 6.25 μg/day that should be started from birth and may be adjusted accordingly [33].

Immunoglobulin levels should be monitored due to urinary excretion of gamma globulin and complement factors B and D in patients with congenital nephrotic syndrome. Due to significant urinary excretion of gamma globulin and complement factors, these patients must have a high suspension for significant bacterial infections, specifically capsular organisms such as pneumococci. Parental antibiotics and immunoglobulin should be promptly initiated and admitted to the hospital for a thorough evaluation if at any time they presented with fevers or any other evidence of an infectious process.

Warfarin has been recommended by some centers in patients with NPHS1 [11]. This recommendation is in light of the fact that these patients have significant urinary losses of coagulation factors. Urinary excretion of plasminogen and AT III results in plasma deficiencies, and compensatory protein synthesis may result in increased production of macroglobulins, fibrinogen, thromboplastin, and factors II, V, VII, X, and XIII that result in a hypercoagulable state [33]. Some centers have recommended daily aspirin for all patients with congenital nephrotic syndrome due to this pathophysiology. Patients requiring any surgical procedures are recommended to discontinue warfarin and initiate antithrombin III 50 IU/kg to compensate for urinary losses prior to surgery.

15.8.2 Surgical Management

The role of uni- and bilateral nephrectomies has been investigated in the past [45]. Both methods therefore provide a bridge for the overall goal of renal transplantation [5]. Especially for children with WT1 gene mutations who are progressing quickly toward ESRD or have reached it, bilateral nephrectomy should be considered given the risk for development of Wilms tumor [46]. Some institutions routinely perform unilateral nephrectomies to reduce the amount of protein excretion. Unilateral nephrectomy does not eliminate the need for aggressive nutritional support and albumin infusions. Uremia also develops more often with unilateral nephrectomy [33]. In addition, other institutions perform bilateral nephrectomies and good outcomes have been reported [47]. Even though there are no guidelines, it is preferred to wait with nephrectomies until the patient reaches an acceptable weight and age. Following nephrectomy, the child will be maintained on peritoneal dialysis until renal transplantation becomes an option. In children under the age of 24 months, CNS is a common reason for initiation of peritoneal dialysis [48]. Typically following bilateral nephrectomy, hypoproteinemia dramatically will improve while the patients receive peritoneal dialysis. Most common complications that arise are peritonitis with staphylococci that are readily treated with intraperitoneal vancomycin. Bilateral nephrectomy at an age of 6–10 months and CCPD for 3–4 months provides correction of hypoproteinemia and further improves nutritional status. Subsequently, successful renal transplantation by 2 years of age provides long-term treatment for congenital nephrotic syndrome of any form [33].

Renal transplantation is the overall preferred treatment for congenital nephrotic syndrome. Typical age of renal transplantation is 1–2 years of age using an adult-size kidney if a graft is available [33]. Typical management of patients following transplantation should be maintained. Recurrence of nephrotic syndrome following graft is rare but is possible if anti-nephrin antibodies developed following transplantation.

Typically this may be successfully managed with cyclophosphamide and plasmapheresis [5].

15.9 Prognosis

It is important to distinguish between the different types of nephrotic syndrome. Whereas children with CNF invariably progress toward dialysis- and transplant-dependent renal failure, the clinical course can be different in other forms even with reported spontaneous remission [49]. Several cases of recurrence of proteinuria, nephrotic syndrome, and high risk for graft loss after renal transplantation have been described in patients with CNSF [50, 51]. The pathophysiologic process is thought to be secondary to circulating anti-glomerular and anti-nephrin antibodies. Following transplantation, any patient can potentially develop an immune response to nephrin expressed in the graft which functions as a new antigen, and the anti-nephrin antibodies neutralize the action of nephrin. If proteinuria develops, it is typically observed 2–48 months after the initial transplantation. Several treatments for the recurrent proteinuria have been described, including cyclophosphamide, plasmapheresis, and most recently the anti-CD20 antibody rituximab [52–54]. FSGS has also been found on biopsy of patients with reoccurrence of proteinuria but has been more commonly found in patients who originally had heterozygous mutations in NPHS2. The overall prognosis of congenital nephrotic syndrome is significantly improved if successful renal transplantation is achieved. Reported patient survival in a study including a large number of children with CNF is greater than 90 % at 5 years posttransplant [55]. However, chronic allograft nephropathy is a long-term complication following transplantation that typically results in the need for a second renal transplant [5].

Conclusion

CNS is a rare but extraordinarily complex disease depending on etiology and degree of urine protein losses as well as its high potential for possible complications. Despite our markedly improved understanding of the genetics, pathophysiology, and pathology of the disease, the treatment options are limited and the prognosis remains overall guarded.

15.10 Take-Home Pearls

- Congenital Nephrotic Syndrome (CNS) is defined as nephrotic syndrome presenting within the first 3 months of life. The most common form is the Finnish type (CNF) which usually progresses rapidly toward end-stage renal disease.
- The management is focused on protein substitution and management of edema, optimal nutrition and provision of medications (anticoagulation, thyroxine, antiproteinurics), dialysis, and renal transplantation.
- Recent advances in our understanding of the genetics and associated pathophysiology might at some point improve phenotype recognition, lead to new treatment options, and ultimately translate into improved outcome.
- Careful guidance and education of the families during this process is of extreme importance.

References

1. Kestila M et al (1998) Positionally cloned gene for a novel glomerular protein–nephrin–is mutated in congenital nephrotic syndrome. Mol Cell 1(4):575–582
2. Bolk S et al (1999) Elevated frequency and allelic heterogeneity of congenital nephrotic syndrome, Finnish type, in the old order Mennonites. Am J Hum Genet 65(6):1785–1790
3. Papez KE, Smoyer WE (2004) Recent advances in congenital nephrotic syndrome. Curr Opin Pediatr 16(2):165–170
4. Tryggvason K, Patrakka J, Wartiovaara J (2006) Hereditary proteinuria syndromes and mechanisms of proteinuria. N Engl J Med 354(13):1387–1401
5. Jalanko H (2009) Congenital nephrotic syndrome. Pediatr Nephrol 24(11):2121–2128
6. Khoshnoodi J, Tryggvason K (2001) Congenital nephrotic syndromes. Curr Opin Genet Dev 11(3):322–327
7. Hinkes BG et al (2007) Nephrotic syndrome in the first year of life: two thirds of cases are caused by mutations in 4 genes (NPHS1, NPHS2, WT1, and LAMB2). Pediatrics 119(4):e907–e919

8. Ahvenainen EK, Hallman N, Hjelt L (1956) Nephrotic syndrome in newborn and young infants. Ann Paediatr Fenn 2(3):227–241
9. Kestila M et al (1994) Congenital nephrotic syndrome of the Finnish type maps to the long arm of chromosome 19. Am J Hum Genet 54(5):757–764
10. Mannikko M et al (1995) Fine mapping and haplotype analysis of the locus for congenital nephrotic syndrome on chromosome 19q13.1. Am J Hum Genet 57(6):1377–1383
11. Savage JM et al (1999) Improved prognosis for congenital nephrotic syndrome of the Finnish type in Irish families. Arch Dis Child 80(5):466–469
12. Suh JH et al (2011) Forced expression of laminin beta1 in podocytes prevents nephrotic syndrome in mice lacking laminin beta2, a model for Pierson syndrome. Proc Natl Acad Sci USA 108(37):15348–15353
13. VanDeVoorde R et al (2006) Pierson syndrome: a novel cause of congenital nephrotic syndrome. Pediatrics 118(2):e501–e505
14. Niaudet P (2004) Genetic forms of nephrotic syndrome. Pediatr Nephrol 19(12):1313–1318
15. Heeringa SF et al (2008) Thirteen novel NPHS1 mutations in a large cohort of children with congenital nephrotic syndrome. Nephrol Dial Transplant 23(11): 3527–3533
16. Huber TB et al (2003) Molecular basis of the functional podocin-nephrin complex: mutations in the NPHS2 gene disrupt nephrin targeting to lipid raft microdomains. Hum Mol Genet 12(24):3397–3405
17. Schwarz K et al (2001) Podocin, a raft-associated component of the glomerular slit diaphragm, interacts with CD2AP and nephrin. J Clin Invest 108(11):1621–1629
18. Denys P et al (1967) Association of an anatomopathological syndrome of male pseudohermaphroditism, Wilms' tumor, parenchymatous nephropathy and XX/XY mosaicism. Arch Fr Pediatr 24(7):729–739
19. Drash A et al (1970) A syndrome of pseudohermaphroditism, Wilms' tumor, hypertension, and degenerative renal disease. J Pediatr 76(4):585–593
20. Pierson M et al (1963) An unusual congenital and familial congenital malformative combination involving the eye and kidney. J Genet Hum 12:184–213
21. Zenker M et al (2004) Human laminin beta2 deficiency causes congenital nephrosis with mesangial sclerosis and distinct eye abnormalities. Hum Mol Genet 13(21):2625–2632
22. Galloway WH, Mowat AP (1968) Congenital microcephaly with hiatus hernia and nephrotic syndrome in two sibs. J Med Genet 5(4):319–321
23. Dreyer SD et al (1998) Mutations in LMX1B cause abnormal skeletal patterning and renal dysplasia in nail patella syndrome. Nat Genet 19(1):47–50
24. Hinkes B et al (2006) Positional cloning uncovers mutations in PLCE1 responsible for a nephrotic syndrome variant that may be reversible. Nat Genet 38(12):1397–1405
25. Goldenberg A et al (2005) Respiratory chain deficiency presenting as congenital nephrotic syndrome. Pediatr Nephrol 20(4):465–469
26. Hata D et al (2005) Nephrotic syndrome and aberrant expression of laminin isoforms in glomerular basement membranes for an infant with Herlitz junctional epidermolysis bullosa. Pediatrics 116(4): e601–e607
27. Besbas N et al (2006) Cytomegalovirus-related congenital nephrotic syndrome with diffuse mesangial sclerosis. Pediatr Nephrol 21(5):740–742
28. Shahin B, Papadopoulou ZL, Jenis EH (1974) Congenital nephrotic syndrome associated with congenital toxoplasmosis. J Pediatr 85(3):366–370
29. Dudley J et al (1996) Systemic lupus erythematosus presenting as congenital nephrotic syndrome. Pediatr Nephrol 10(6):752–755
30. Massengill SF, Richard GA, Donnelly WH (1994) Infantile systemic lupus erythematosus with onset simulating congenital nephrotic syndrome. J Pediatr 124(1):27–31
31. Westenend PJ (1995) Congenital nephrotic syndrome in neonatal lupus syndrome. J Pediatr 126(5 Pt 1):851
32. Levy M, Feingold J (2000) Estimating prevalence in single-gene kidney diseases progressing to renal failure. Kidney Int 58(3):925–943
33. Holmberg C et al (1995) Management of congenital nephrotic syndrome of the Finnish type. Pediatr Nephrol 9(1):87–93
34. Seppala M et al (1976) Congenital nephrotic syndrome: prenatal diagnosis and genetic counselling by estimation of amniotic-fluid and maternal serum alpha-fetoprotein. Lancet 2(7977):123–125
35. Wiggelinkhuizen J et al (1976) Alpha fetoprotein in the antenatal diagnosis of the congenital nephrotic syndrome. J Pediatr 89(3):452–455
36. Mannikko M et al (1997) Improved prenatal diagnosis of the congenital nephrotic syndrome of the Finnish type based on DNA analysis. Kidney Int 51(3): 868–872
37. Lanning P et al (1989) Ultrasonic features of the congenital nephrotic syndrome of the Finnish type. Acta Paediatr Scand 78(5):717–720
38. Licht C et al (2000) A stepwise approach to the treatment of early onset nephrotic syndrome. Pediatr Nephrol 14(12):1077–1082
39. Jalanko H, Holmberg C (2009) Congenital nephrotic syndrome. In: Avner ED, Niaudet P, Yoshikawa N (eds) Pediatric nephrology. Springer, Berlin, pp 601–619
40. Kovacevic L, Reid CJ, Rigden SP (2003) Management of congenital nephrotic syndrome. Pediatr Nephrol 18(5):426–430
41. Guez S et al (1998) Adequate clinical control of congenital nephrotic syndrome by enalapril. Pediatr Nephrol 12(2):130–132
42. Heaton PA, Smales O, Wong W (1999) Congenital nephrotic syndrome responsive to captopril and indometacin. Arch Dis Child 81(2):174–175
43. Pomeranz A et al (1995) Successful treatment of Finnish congenital nephrotic syndrome with captopril and indomethacin. J Pediatr 126(1): 140–142

44. Chadha V, Alon US (1999) Bilateral nephrectomy reverses hypothyroidism in congenital nephrotic syndrome. Pediatr Nephrol 13(3):209–211
45. Kim MS, Primack W, Harmon WE (1992) Congenital nephrotic syndrome: preemptive bilateral nephrectomy and dialysis before renal transplantation. J Am Soc Nephrol 3(2):260–263
46. Hu M et al (2004) Prophylactic bilateral nephrectomies in two paediatric patients with missense mutations in the WT1 gene. Nephrol Dial Transplant 19(1):223–226
47. Slaughenhoupt BL et al (1998) Urologic management of congenital nephrotic syndrome of the Finnish type. Urology 51(3):492–494
48. Laakkonen H et al (2008) Peritoneal dialysis in children under two years of age. Nephrol Dial Transplant 23(5):1747–1753
49. Haws RM, Weinberg AG, Baum M (1992) Spontaneous remission of congenital nephrotic syndrome: a case report and review of the literature. Pediatr Nephrol 6(1):82–84
50. Laine J et al (1993) Post-transplantation nephrosis in congenital nephrotic syndrome of the Finnish type. Kidney Int 44(4):867–874
51. Patrakka J et al (2002) Recurrence of nephrotic syndrome in kidney grafts of patients with congenital nephrotic syndrome of the Finnish type: role of nephrin. Transplantation 73(3):394–403
52. Chaudhuri A et al (2011) Rituximab treatment for recurrence of nephrotic syndrome in a pediatric patient after renal transplantation for congenital nephrotic syndrome of Finnish type. Pediatr Transplant 16(5):E183–E187
53. Kuusniemi AM et al (2007) Plasma exchange and retransplantation in recurrent nephrosis of patients with congenital nephrotic syndrome of the Finnish type (NPHS1). Transplantation 83(10):1316–1323
54. Srivastava T et al (2006) Recurrence of proteinuria following renal transplantation in congenital nephrotic syndrome of the Finnish type. Pediatr Nephrol 21(5):711–718
55. Qvist E et al (1999) Graft function 5–7 years after renal transplantation in early childhood. Transplantation 67(7):1043–1049
56. Weber S (2008) Hereditary nephrotic syndrome. In: Geary DF, Schaefer F (eds) Comprehensive pediatric nephrology, 1st edn. Elsevier, Philadelphia

Acute Kidney Injury in the Newborn

16

Jennifer G. Jetton and David Askenazi

Abbreviations

ACE I	Angiotensin-converting enzyme inhibitor
ATN	Acute tubular necrosis
AKI	Acute kidney injury
BUN	Blood urea nitrogen
CAKUT	Congenital anomalies of the kidney and urinary tract
CVVHDF	Continuous venovenous hemodiafiltration
ECMO	Extracorporeal membrane oxygenation
FENa	Fractional excretion of sodium
GFR	Glomerular filtration rate
K	Potassium
kg	Kilogram
L	Liters
Ml	Milliliters
mEq/dl	Milliequivalents per deciliter
Mg/dl	Milligrams per deciliter
Na	Sodium
NGAL	Neutrophil-gelatinase-associated lipocalin
NICU	Neonatal intensive care unit
NSAIDs	Nonsteroidal anti-inflammatory drugs
SCr	Serum creatinine
VLBW	Very low birth weight

J.G. Jetton, MD (✉)
Division of Nephrology,
Dialysis and Transplantation,
Department of Pediatrics,
University of Iowa Children's Hospital,
200 Hawkins Drive, 4035 BT, Iowa City,
IA 52242-1083, USA
e-mail: jennifer-jetton@uiowa.edu

D. Askenazi, MD, MsPH
Division of Pediatric Nephrology,
University of Alabama at Birmingham,
1600 7th Ave South ACC 516,
Birmingham, AL, USA
e-mail: daskenazi@peds.uab.edu

Core Messages

- Acute kidney injury is a common occurrence in neonatal intensive care units with important implications for therapeutic decisions and patient outcomes.
- Acute kidney injury occurs as the result of many different processes that can be categorized as prerenal intrinsic renal, and postrenal (obstructive). Early recognition is key to ameliorating the effects of these processes.
- Care of the neonate with AKI is supportive as there are no proven pharmacologic therapies for treatment or prevention of acute kidney injury. Close attention to assure adequate renal perfusion, prevention of fluid overload, proper dosing (or avoidance) of nephrotoxic medications, and consideration for early initiation of renal replacement therapy will minimize the potential harm and maximize renal support during an acute kidney injury episode.

A.S. Chishti et al. (eds.), *Kidney and Urinary Tract Diseases in the Newborn*,
DOI 10.1007/978-3-642-39988-6_16, © Springer-Verlag Berlin Heidelberg 2014

Case Vignette

A 1-month-old 3 kilogram (kg), former 36-week preterm infant with repaired gastroschisis was preparing for hospital discharge in the nursery when he suddenly became ill with respiratory distress, mottling, and lethargy. He was transferred emergently to the neonatal intensive care unit where he was intubated. He had ongoing hypotension with mean arterial pressure ~20 mmHg. He received fluid resuscitation with crystalloids and blood products. He was also begun on continuous infusions of norepinephrine and dopamine. He received empiric antibiotic coverage with vancomycin and gentamicin. Laparotomy showed a very edematous bowel but no frank areas of necrosis. Within 24 h the blood culture was positive for Group B streptococcus. Within 48 h the infant had received net positive 2.5 liters (L) of fluids. He required conversion to the high-frequency oscillator. He became oligoanuric within 48 h, with only 11 milliliters (ml) of urine output per day. Serum creatinine (SCr) rose from 0.3 milligrams per deciliter (mg/dl) prior to acute decompensation to 0.7 mg/dl within 24 h to 1.1 mg/dl within 48 h. Electrolytes were acceptable with serum sodium (Na) 136 milliequivalents per deciliter (mEq/dl) and potassium (K) 2.9 mEq/dl. Following consultation with the Nephrology Service, the infant underwent placement of an 8 French double-lumen right femoral temporary dialysis catheter at the bedside, and continuous venovenous hemodiafiltration (CVVHDF) was initiated. During the first few days while he remained hypotensive, fluid removal rate was set to keep his fluid balance even each day. Scheduled vancomycin and gentamicin were discontinued, and doses were given when his trough levels dropped to <15.0 mg/dl and <2.0 mg/dl respectively. Once his blood pressure improved, fluid removal rate was increased to achieve a net daily negative fluid balance as tolerated. After several days of fluid removal, his respiratory status improved, and his ventilator settings were decreased. He was subsequently converted to a conventional ventilator. His urine output started to improve about 10 days into his illness. Two days later, it was determined that his urine output was sufficient to maintain euvolemia with adequate nutritional support, and CVVHDF was discontinued. His urine output, renal function, and electrolytes were closely monitored for abnormalities and signs of intravascular volume depletion secondary to excessive urine output and overdiuresis in the recovery period. Once his infection was treated and his anasarca had resolved, he was able to undergo closure of his abdominal wall defect again. He was discharged home from the NICU 1 month later with SCr 0.5 mg/dl, with an appointment scheduled in the Nephrology clinic for kidney function evaluation following this severe AKI event.

16.1 Introduction

Acute kidney injury (AKI) is characterized by a sudden impairment in kidney function that results in the inability to maintain adequate fluid, electrolyte, and waste product homeostasis. It is increasingly recognized as a common and significant event for newborns cared for in the neonatal intensive care unit, with important implications for treatment decisions and clinical outcomes. Indeed, AKI is associated with mortality in critically ill children [2, 87] and adults [14, 25, 52, 66, 79], even after controlling for medical comorbidities, severity of illness scores, and patient demographics. Emerging data suggest a similar association in the neonatal population as well [32, 47, 48], such that kidney injury can no longer be viewed as an incidental finding but rather an important determinant of patient outcomes.

To highlight the importance for early recognition of this dynamic and evolving process, the old description *acute renal failure* has largely been supplanted by the new term *acute kidney injury* by both the Nephrology and Critical Care communities. With this new terminology, the emphasis is on early recognition of the event at the time of *injury* rather than waiting until complete organ *failure* has occurred [55].

The purpose of this chapter is to describe the epidemiology, common etiologies of, and diagnostic and therapeutic approaches to AKI in the neonate in order to guide the clinician in the early identification of this important process as well as clinical decision making.

16.2 Background

16.2.1 Definition of AKI

As stated above, acute kidney injury is a sudden impairment in kidney function that occurs not infrequently in critically ill patients. This complex and clinically heterogeneous disorder occurs with varying degrees of severity in many different clinical situations. The exact incidence of neonatal AKI is difficult to quantify, and reported rates vary widely depending on the patient population evaluated and the AKI definition used (see Table 16.1). In addition, there is great heterogeneity in clinical presentation: patients with AKI may be oliguric or nonoliguric, have few or many electrolyte abnormalities, may be best managed by watchful waiting, or may require initiation of renal replacement therapy. Moreover, we lack a standardized AKI definition for use both at the bedside and in research trials; reported AKI definitions range from oliguria to rise in SCr by 0.3 mg/dl to an arbitrary cutoff of 1.5 mg/dl to need for renal replacement therapy.

Traditionally, AKI has been defined as either a rise in SCr, often in conjunction with a rise in blood urea nitrogen (BUN), or fall in urine output (oliguria, <0.5 ml/kg/h). Each of these – SCr, BUN, and urine output – has limitations in terms of its use as an AKI biomarker, and awareness of these limitations is important when evaluating the neonate who is at risk. For example, many infants have nonoliguric AKI, so urine output cannot be relied upon solely as a marker of AKI. Assessed urine output also depends on accurate urine collection and documentation. BUN levels are affected by a number of factors that are not secondary to an AKI event. These include increases in dietary protein intake (as with changes in the amount of protein in parenteral or enteral feeds), hypercatabolic states, absorption of blood from the gastrointestinal tract as with gastrointestinal bleeds, and use of steroids. SCr too has a number of limitations, even though it is the most widely used and measured biomarker of AKI. One of the most important of these is that SCr rises late in the course of AKI, lagging as much as 24–48 h behind the initial injury. In addition, SCr does not differentiate the nature (e.g., prerenal, nephrotoxic medication exposure, or ischemic acute tubular necrosis) or timing of the kidney insult. SCr is also readily cleared by dialysis such that, once a patient is receiving renal replacement therapy, it can no longer be used as a marker for either further renal injury or renal recovery.

When interpreting SCr levels (and changes in levels) in neonates, several other factors need to be considered. First, after birth, SCr in the newborn reflects maternal creatinine levels. Rather than maintaining a steady state, SCr then declines at varying rates over days to weeks, depending on gestational age, such that changes (or lack of change) in SCr may be difficult to interpret when evaluating for AKI. Second, normal nephrogenesis is complete at 34 weeks' gestation. Preterm infants with wide variation in gestational age will have different rates of maturity in kidney function at the time of birth, leading to different ranges of "normal" or appropriate SCr for a particular patient. Third, depending on laboratory technique used, SCr levels will be affected by hyperbilirubinemia and certain medications (e.g., cephalosporins). Finally, SCr is not always measured on a routine basis in neonates due to concerns about blood loss with frequent lab draws. This is important as the *trend* in SCr levels in the appropriate clinical context provides the best information about whether AKI has occurred given all of the limitations described above.

Table 16.1 Epidemiology of AKI in the neonate: selected articles

Author	Patients	AKI definition	Findings
Asphyxiated infants			
Karlowicz and Adelman [44]	33 infants ≥ 36 weeks GA, 5 min Apgar ≤ 6 with severe asphyxia scores *vs*. 33 infants with moderate asphyxia scores	SCr ≥ 1.5 mg/dl	*AKI incidence:* Severe asphyxia – 61 % Moderate asphyxia – 0 % Nonoliguric AKI – 60 % Oliguric AKI – 5 % Anuric AKI – 15 % ***Asphyxia morbidity score predicted AKI 100% sensitivity, 72% specificity*
Gupta et al. [36]	70 infants, 5 min Apgar ≤ 6 *vs*. 28 healthy controls	UOP < 0.5 ml/kg/h, blood urea > 40 mg/dl, SCr > 1 mg/dl, presence of significant hematuria/proteinuria	*AKI incidence*: Cases – 47.1 % (78 % nonoliguric) Controls – 0 % *Mortality*: Overall mortality – 14.1 % Oliguric AKI – 42.8 % Nonoliguric AKI – 7.7 %
Aggarwal et al. [1]	25 infants ≥ 34 weeks GA, 5 min Apgar ≤ 6 *vs*. 25 matched infants with no asphyxia	SCr > 1.5 mg/dl	*AKI incidence*: Cases – 56 % Controls – 4 %
Infants with sepsis			
Mathur et al. [54]	52 infants with sepsis + AKI *vs*. 146 infants with sepsis + no AKI	BUN > 20 on 2 separate occasions, at least 24 h apart	*AKI incidence*: Entire cohort – 26 % Nonoliguric AKI – 85 % *Mortality*: AKI – 70.2 % No AKI – 25 %
Very low birth weight infants (VLBW ≤ 1,500 g)			
Askenazi et al. [8]	68 VLBW infants who did not survive to hospital discharge *vs*. 127 matched infants (GA, birth weight)	AKIN definition: *Stage 1*: SCr rise 0.3 mg/dl or rise to ≥ 150–200 % baseline value; *Stage 2*:SCr rise ≥ 200–300 % baseline; *Stage 3*:SCr ≥ 300 % baseline	*AKI independently associated with mortality*: 1 mg/dl increase in SCr associated with 3.5-fold increase in odds of death after adjusting for other significant comorbidities
Koralkar et al. [47]	229 VLBW infants prospectively followed from birth until 36 weeks post-menstrual age or hospital discharge	Modified AKIN definition (see Askenazi [8] above)	*AKI incidence*: Overall – 18 % Stage 1–4 % Stage 2–4 % Stage 3–9 % ***AKI was associated with mortality with a crude HR of 9.3 (95% CI, 4.1–21.0). After adjusting for potential confounders, the adjusted HR for AKI was 2.4 (95% CI 0.95–6.04)*

(continued)

Table 16.1 (continued)

Author	Patients	AKI definition	Findings
Infants who received support with extracorporeal membrane oxygenation (ECMO)			
Askenazi et al. [6, 10]	7,941 infants listed in the Extracorporeal Life Support Organization registry	SCr ≥1.5 mg/dl	*AKI incidence*: Non-survivors – 19 % Survivors – 3.9 % *Mortality*: Overall – 27.4 % ***Neonates on ECMO with AKI had 3.2 higher odds of death than those without AKI after adjusting for numerous confounders*
Gadepalli et al. [32]	68 infants with congenital diaphragmatic hernia requiring ECMO	RIFLE criteria: *risk*:1.5x rise in SCr from baseline *injury*: 2x rise *failure*:3x rise	*AKI incidence*: Overall – 71 % AKI "injury" – 22 % AKI "failure" – 49 % *Mortality*: AKI "failure" – 62.7 % Non-AKI – 20 % ***Patients with AKI failure had increased time on ECMO, decreased ventilator free days*
Infants with congenital heart disease			
Krawczeski et al. [48]	35 neonates (total sample 374 infants > 37 weeks GA) with CHD undergoing CPB	0.3 mg/dl increase in SCr from preoperative baseline within 48 h of surgery	*AKI incidence*: Neonates – 23 % *Mortality*: No difference between neonates with and without AKI ***Both plasma and urine NGAL were significant predictors of the development of AKI, rising within 2 h after CPB*
Blinder et al. [19]	430 infants (<90 days age) with CHD undergoing CPB	AKIN definition (as per Askenazi 2009 above + UOP/oliguria)	*AKI incidence*: Overall – 52 % Stage 1–31 % Stage 2–14 % Stage 3–7 % *Mortality*: AKI – 12 % No AKI – 3 % ***Risk of death increased with AKI severity: stage 2 OR 5.1 and stage 3 OR 9.5*

AKI acute kidney injury, *GA* gestational age, *SCr* serum creatinine, *VLBW* very low birth weight, *AKIN* Acute Kidney Injury Network, *ECMO* extracorporeal membrane oxygenation, *CHD* congenital heart disease, *CPB* cardiopulmonary bypass, *UOP* urine output

Table 16.2 Published acute kidney injury definitions/classification systems for *adults*

AKIN			RIFLE	
Stage		Urine output (same for both definitions)	Class	SCr or GFR change
I	↑ SCr ≥ 0.3 mg/dl *or* ↑ SCr ≥ 150–200 % from baseline	<0.5 ml/kg per hour for 6 h	*Risk*	↑ SCr by 150 % *or* GFR decrease by 25 %
II	↑ SCr ≥ 200–300 % from baseline	<0.5 ml/kg per hour for >12 h	*Injury*	↑ SCr by 200 % ≥ *or* GFR decrease by 50 %
III	↑ SCr > 300 % from baseline *or* SCr ≥ 4 mg/dl with an acute rise of ≥0.5 mg/dl *or* receipt of dialysis	<0.3 ml/kg per hour for >24 h *or* anuria >12 h	*Failure*	↑ SCr by 300 % *or* SCr > 4 mg/dl with an acute rise of ≥0.5 mg/dl *or* GFR decrease by 75 %
			Loss	*Failure* > 4 weeks
			ESRD	*Failure* > 3 months

Adapted from Bellomo et al. [18] and Mehta et al. [55]
AKIN Acute Kidney Injury Network, *RIFLE* Risk, Injury, Failure, Loss, and End Stage, *SCr* serum creatinine, *GFR* glomerular filtration rate1854

Table 16.3 Published acute kidney injury definitions/classification systems for *children*

pRIFLE		
Class	eCCl by original Schwartz equation	Urine output
Risk	eCCl decrease by 25 %	<0.5 ml/kg per hour for 8 h
Injury	eCCl decrease by 50 %	<0.5 ml/kg per hour for 16 h
Failure	eCCl decrease by 75 % *or* eCCl < 35 ml/min per 1.73 m²	<0.3 ml/kg per hour for 24 h *or* anuria for 12 h
Loss	*Failure* > 4 weeks	
ESRD	*Failure* > 3 months	

Adapted from Akcan-Arikan et al. [2]
pRIFLE pediatric Risk, Injury, Failure, Loss, and End Stage, *eCCl* estimated creatinine clearance2

Table 16.4 Published acute kidney injury definitions/classification systems for *neonates*

Stage	SCr change	Urine output
0	No change *or* rise < 0.3 mg/dl	<1 ml/kg per hour (*over previous 24 h*)
1	↑ SCr > 0.3 mg/dl *or* ↑ SCr > 150–199 % from baseline[a]	> 0.5 ml/kg per hour but ≤1 ml/kg per hour (*over previous 24 h*)
2	↑ SCr > 200–299 % from baseline	> 0.1 ml/kg per hour but ≤0.5 ml/kg per hour (*over previous 24 h*)
3	↑ SCr > 300 % from baseline *or* SCr ≥ 2.5 mg/dl *or* receipt of dialysis	< 0.1 ml/kg per hour (*over previous 24 h*)

[a]Baseline SCr will be defined as the lowest previous SCr value. *SCr* serum creatinine

Regardless of these limitations, SCr remains the most studied and widely used clinical biomarker for measuring kidney function in patient groups of all ages. *How* SCr is used to define AKI has evolved in the adult and pediatric literature with the development of standardized, categorical AKI classification systems such as the RIFLE (Risk, Injury, Failure, Loss, and End-Stage renal disease) classification [18] and the AKIN (Acute Kidney Injury Network) definition [55] (see Table 16.2). A modification of the RIFLE classification has been proposed for use in the pediatric population (pRIFLE) [2] (see Table 16.3). Similarly, a modification of the AKIN staging system has been proposed for use in the neonatal population (see Table 16.4). Because they do not rely on arbitrary, binary cutoffs (e.g., SCr ≥ 1.5 mg/dl), these modern frameworks allow for improved diagnosis and staging of AKI by severity. Research utilizing these definitions in adult and pediatric populations has demonstrated that AKI severity predicts clinical outcomes such as death and disability, but even changes in SCr as small as 0.3 mg/dl have an independent impact on survival [22, 46]. Similar findings are starting to emerge in the neonatal population as well [6, 10, 19, 32, 47].

The use of an AKI staging system is of somewhat greater importance when it comes to our ability to pool and compare data across research studies. The take-home points for the clinician at the bedside are:

1. Early recognition of and ongoing surveillance for AKI risk factors (described below) is an important part of care as our current biomarkers are late indicators of kidney injury.
2. The trend in SCr levels is important, and SCr should be monitored routinely in at-risk infants.
3. Small changes in serum creatinine (or lack of appropriate downward trend in a newborn) suggest AKI has occurred and should be taken seriously.

16.2.2 Who Is at Risk?

Advancements in intensive care unit technologies and therapies for complex medical conditions have led to a shift in pediatric AKI epidemiology, such that kidney injury secondary to systemic illnesses and/or their treatments (cardiopulmonary bypass, nephrotoxic medications) surpasses primary renal disease as the leading cause of AKI in hospitalized children [41, 81, 84]. In the NICU, while acute or chronic kidney disease may occur in infants with congenital anomalies of the kidney and urinary tract (CAKUT), infants with critical illness and complex nonrenal medical conditions represent a far more prevalent group of AKI sufferers. Certain groups of newborns are recognized as being at increased risk for acute kidney injury. These include the following: infants with perinatal hypoxia [1, 36, 44, 45]; premature and very low birth weight (VLBW) infants [8, 47]; infants with congenital heart disease, especially those requiring cardiopulmonary bypass [19, 48, 63, 76]; infants requiring extracorporeal membrane oxygenation (ECMO) [6, 10, 21, 56, 71, 75, 83]; and infants with sepsis Mathur [55]. These infants warrant close monitoring of kidney function with frequent measurement of SCr, close monitoring of intake/output, and attention to modifiable risk factors such as nephrotoxic medications (see Table 16.5).

16.3 Etiology

The traditional framework of classifying AKI etiologies as prerenal azotemia, intrinsic AKI, and postrenal/obstruction is simple and widely used (see Table 16.5). Because of limitations in current AKI definitions and biomarkers, it is important to identify the conditions listed in Table 16.5 early as AKI *risk factors* and work to correct those that are modifiable *before* kidney injury (and certainly before kidney *failure*) occurs. Moreover, AKI in a newborn in the NICU is frequently multifactorial (e.g., hypotension, nephrotoxic medication exposure, prerenal injury due to large chest tube output), and the risk of AKI increases as the number of prevalent risk factors increases [3, 44, 58]. Finally, newborns may have underlying congenital kidney anomalies not previously identified at the time of presentation. Obviously these infants are at increased risk for kidney injury with additional insults or if their underlying condition is not recognized in a timely fashion and corrected to the extent possible.

16.3.1 Prerenal Azotemia

Prerenal azotemia (increase in BUN concentration, little or no change in SCr) represents an appropriate physiologic response to decreased renal blood flow. A number of autoregulatory mechanisms preserve GFR when conditions of poor renal perfusion occur, with activation of the renin-angiotensin-aldosterone system being one of the most important. Renal hypoperfusion leads to increased sodium and water reabsorption in the renal tubules, stimulated by both angiotensin II and aldosterone [4]. However, newborns, especially premature infants, have relatively immature tubular function and may not be able to conserve sodium and water to the same extent older children and adults do. Thus, oliguria may be less pronounced in these patients, even when they are relatively intravascularly depleted. Correction of the underlying problem with restoration of adequate renal blood flow often results in rapid normalization of renal function and improvement in urine output. However, if renal

Table 16.5 Etiologies of (risk factors for) AKI in the neonate

Prerenal azotemia	*Classically increased BUN, little or no change in SCr* *Secondary to loss of either true or effective circulating blood volume* *Fluid responsive*
Dehydration	Increased insensible losses (radiant warmers, phototherapy, and fever) Poor oral intake Diarrhea Large gastric or chest tube output Excessive diuretic use Underlying renal disease with concentrating defect/salt and water wasting
Capillary leak	Sepsis/systemic inflammatory response Low oncotic pressure/hypoalbuminemia Hydrops
Increased abdominal pressure	Necrotizing enterocolitis Ascites from liver disease, chylous drainage/leaks, or low serum albumin Gastroschisis repair or reduction Omphalocele Hepatosplenomegaly or masses
Decreased cardiac output	Congestive heart failure Coarctation of the aorta Very high mean airway pressures
Blood loss	Perinatal blood loss Hemorrhage for any reason Twin-twin transfusion
Medications	ACE I, NSAIDs
Intrinsic AKI	*Increased BUN and SCr, not easily reversible* *Parenchymal damage though with varying mechanisms depending on underlying etiology* *Requires judicious fluid management with frequent reassessment*
Ischemia/reperfusion	Any of the above "prerenal" causes if prolonged Perinatal asphyxia
Nephrotoxic medications	Aminoglycosides, cephalosporins, amphotericin, vancomycin, intravenous contrast media – *direct tubular injury* ACE I, NSAIDs (indomethacin), diuretics – *decreased renal perfusion* Acyclovir – *tubular obstruction*
Endogenous nephrotoxins	Myoglobin Hemoglobin Uric acid
Sepsis and other infections	Decreased renal blood flow from shock Increased renal blood flow from shock (disease of the microcirculation) Pyelonephritis Bacterial endocarditis Congenital infections
Vascular lesions	Renal vein and artery thrombosis
Postrenal/obstruction	*Requires obstruction of both kidneys; may be a unilateral process if solitary kidney* *Usually correctable with restoration of urinary outflow* *May not be reversible if prolonged or associated with kidney parenchymal abnormalities*

(continued)

Table 16.5 (continued)

Congenital malformations	Posterior urethral valves Prune-belly syndrome Imperforate prepuce Urethral stricture Neurogenic bladder
Extrinsic compression	Hematocolpos Sacrococcygeal teratoma
Intrinsic obstruction	Kidney stones Fungal balls
Other	Occluded or malpositioned Foley catheter Medication-related urinary retention (e.g., morphine)

AKI acute kidney injury, *BUN* blood urea nitrogen, *SCr* serum creatinine, *ACE I* angiotensin-converting enzyme inhibitors, *NSAIDs* nonsteroidal anti-inflammatory drugs

hypoperfusion is severe or prolonged, kidney parenchymal damage (specifically acute tubular necrosis, ATN) may ensue, so prompt recognition is essential.

Causes of prerenal azotemia in neonates include loss of effective circulating blood volume (perinatal blood loss, hemorrhage), dehydration (diarrhea, transepidermal free water losses as with radiant warmers or phototherapy for hyperbilirubinemia, poor intake, gastric or chest tube losses, underlying renal disease with salt and water wasting), capillary leak (hydrops, infection, or hypoalbuminemia), increased abdominal pressure (necrotizing enterocolitis, ascites, repair or reduction of gastroschisis, omphalocele), or decreased cardiac output (congestive heart failure, aortic coarctation). Certain medications, most importantly nonsteroidal anti-inflammatory drugs (NSAIDs) such as indomethacin and angiotensin-converting enzyme inhibitors (ACE I) such as captopril, can decrease renal blood flow, leading to a state of renal hypoperfusion because of their effects on prostaglandins and angiotensin II, respectively. If given when a prerenal state already exists, these medications have the potential to cause severe ischemic injury as well (see Table 16.5).

16.3.2 Intrinsic Acute Kidney Injury

Causes of intrinsic AKI in the newborn include hypoxic-ischemic injury, nephrotoxic exposures (both exogenous medications and endogenous toxins such as myoglobin and hemoglobin), and infection-/sepsis-associated AKI. Infants, more so than older children and adults, are also prone to vascular insults such as renal vein and artery thrombosis. This type of event occurs either before or just after birth and is often associated with a history of perinatal asphyxia, dehydration, infection, prematurity and maternal diabetes, and possibly an underlying hypercoagulable state in the infant [20]. The classic triad for renal vein thrombosis includes microscopic or gross hematuria, palpable flank mass, and thrombocytopenia. Newborns are also more susceptible to cortical necrosis and irreversible kidney injury, with the outcome in some cases being end-stage renal disease and need for lifelong renal replacement therapy (dialysis or transplant).

Of note, it is important to remember that not all AKI etiologies within this intrinsic AKI category are the result of the same underlying mechanisms. Hypoxic-ischemic AKI, nephrotoxic medication exposure, and sepsis all have distinct pathophysiologic pathways with different potential therapeutic targets and potentially different outcomes. New insights into sepsis-associated AKI suggest that this condition is not just due to renal hypoperfusion but from dysfunction of the microcirculation as well. These distinctions will become more important in the future once specific goal-directed AKI therapies become available.

Because they are two of the most common categories of AKI in the neonate, hypoxic-ischemic AKI and nephrotoxin-related AKI are described in further detail here.

16.3.2.1 Ischemic AKI (Ischemia/Reperfusion Injury)

As said before, any of the processes described in the "prerenal AKI" section, if prolonged or severe, can result in ischemic parenchymal damage. In contrast to prerenal azotemia, renal function abnormalities in intrinsic AKI are not immediately reversible once damage to the renal tubules occurs. Intrinsic AKI may range from mild tubular dysfunction to renal infarction and irreversible cortical necrosis [27].

The course of ischemic AKI may be subdivided into the prerenal, initiation, extension, maintenance, and recovery phases [50, 78]. It is important to recognize that the kidney is vulnerable to additional injury throughout this process, so ongoing vigilance is essential. If renal blood flow is adequately restored during the prerenal phase, then renal function may return quickly to normal. However, if the insult is prolonged, tubular injury with resulting dysfunction ensues (maintenance phase). The duration of the maintenance phase depends, at least in part, on the severity and duration of the initial insult. The recovery phase is characterized by the gradual restoration of GFR and tubular functions which can take days to months to occur. Again, preventing additional kidney insults and maintaining adequate renal perfusion during this process will shorten time to recovery of kidney function.

Hypoxic-ischemic injury results in endothelial as well as tubular cell damage. Endothelial and tubular cell damage leads to not only dysfunction within the kidney but to a systemic inflammatory response as well that may trigger distant organ dysfunction. This inflammatory dysregulation is due (at least in part) to dysfunctional immune, inflammatory, and soluble mediator metabolism [50]. Thus, AKI can lead not only to renal dysfunction but to pulmonary inflammation (independent of fluid overload), brain injury, and cardiac dysfunction [12, 76], with distant organ effects having important implications for overall outcomes including survival.

16.3.2.2 Nephrotoxic Acute Kidney Injury

Pharmacologic agents are among the most common causes of AKI in neonates and therefore deserve special mention here. Endogenous substances (hemoglobin, myoglobin, and uric acid) may also be toxic to the kidney but are much less common. Nephrotoxic medications can cause neonatal AKI by decreasing renal perfusion (NSAIDs, diuretics, ACE inhibitors), causing direct tubular injury (aminoglycosides, cephalosporins, amphotericin B, vancomycin, NSAIDs, contrast media, myoglobin/hemoglobin), triggering an episode of interstitial nephritis (rare), or causing tubular obstruction (acyclovir). Below is a description of the mechanisms of some of the more commonly used nephrotoxins in the NICU.

Indomethacin, a prostaglandin inhibitor used to treat patent ductus arteriosus in premature infants, can cause severe, although usually transient, nephrotoxicity. Because neonatal renal function is more dependent on local prostaglandin production than that of the older patients (especially in the context of intravascular volume depletion as with fluid restriction, increased capillary leak, and transepidermal water losses in the preterm infant with patent ductus arteriosus), indomethacin administration is commonly associated with elevated SCr concentrations, decreased urine output, and hyponatremia [23].

Amphotericin B has a direct effect on tubular function, resulting in renal tubular acidosis and increased urinary potassium excretion. Although these nephrotoxic effects are most often reversible, cases of fatal neonatal renal failure due to amphotericin B toxicity have been reported [15]. Amphotericin B lipid complex, with its higher affinity to fungal rather than mammalian structures, may be a safer alternative than traditional amphotericin [11], though close monitoring of kidney function is still warranted.

Gentamicin, an aminoglycoside, is one of the most commonly used medications for the treatment of suspected or proven neonatal sepsis. Aminoglycosides lead primarily to proximal tubular cell damage [34]. Aminoglycosides should be used with caution in any patient with renal dysfunction, concomitant nephrotoxic medication use, or poor renal perfusion (e.g., with volume depletion, hypoalbuminuria, heart failure). Because aminoglycoside toxicity is usually *nonoliguric*, serial monitoring of SCr values and gentamicin levels is necessary, especially during prolonged administration of this medication.

Acyclovir is an antiviral agent that is renally excreted though nearly insoluble in the urine. Intravenous high-dose acyclovir treatment may lead to crystal precipitation and tubular obstruction. Acyclovir-related nephrotoxicity can be limited by avoiding its use in those with renal insufficiency or intravascular volume depletion, infusing the drug slowly (over several hours), and by assuring adequate hydration to maintain high urinary flow rate [42].

Finally, use of certain medications such as NSAIDs or ACE inhibitors in the pregnant mother may cause combined ischemic and nephrotoxic renal injury in the fetus, resulting in the clinical presentation of AKI after birth. NSAIDs prescribed for tocolysis – both nonselective and selective cyclooxygenase inhibitors such as indomethacin or ketoprofen [16, 62] – may lead to severe AKI in the newborn. ACE inhibitors, when taken during the first and second trimesters, may cause catastrophic kidney injury by their effects on the renin-angiotensin-aldosterone system that is critical for maintaining GFR in the fetal kidney.

16.3.3 Postrenal/Obstruction

Kidney injury from urinary tract obstruction requires obstruction of both kidneys, though a unilateral process like a ureteral stone may cause similar injury if the patient has a solitary kidney. The most common causes for obstructive nephropathy in the newborn are congenital malformations including imperforate prepuce, urethral stricture, prune-belly syndrome, and posterior urethral valves. Other causes of acute obstruction include neurogenic bladder, extrinsic compression (e.g., hematocolpos, sacrococcygeal teratoma), and intrinsic obstruction from renal calculi or fungal balls. Occluded or malpositioned Foley catheters as well as morphine-related urinary retention may also be culprits. Prompt recognition and restoration of urinary flow, either by Foley catheter or nephrostomy tube placement, is critical for normalization of kidney function. Obstruction that occurs early in fetal development (e.g., posterior urethral valves) or that has been severe and prolonged may not completely reverse. Obstructive uropathy is covered in Chaps. 10 and 11.

16.4 Diagnostic Evaluation

16.4.1 History and Risk Factors

A careful history should include a search for any of the events described in the preceding sections, with attention to the fact that often more than one of these conditions will exist in the same patient. Evaluate for important prenatal findings and events including any documentation of abnormal urinary tract anatomy on prenatal ultrasound, amniotic fluid levels (especially oligohydramnios), maternal medication use (ACE I, illicit drugs), perinatal complications including nonreassuring fetal status, placental abruption, twin-twin transfusion, and the type of resuscitation received. The need for chest compressions, vasoactive medications, and nephrotoxic medication exposure suggest that the infant may be at risk for AKI going forward.

16.4.2 Physical Examination

A primary focus of the physical examination is assessment of volume status in order to determine whether a condition of renal hypoperfusion exists so that fluid management strategies may be optimized. Vital signs provide important clues: tachycardia and hypotension suggest intravascular volume depletion, whereas tachypnea and worsening oxygenation status may suggest fluid overload and the development of pulmonary edema. Physical examination findings suggestive of dehydration include sunken fontanel, sunken eyes, or dry mucous membranes. Findings suggestive of fluid overload include clinical edema (chest wall, dependent areas such as the posterior scalp, scrotum, and labia), tachypnea, escalating oxygen requirements, or escalation of ventilatory support.

The cumulative fluid balance based on recorded intake/output in conjunction with the daily weight trend (if available) is critical for quantifying the degree of either volume depletion or fluid overload, as estimates based on the physical examination alone may be difficult to make. Ensure that all inputs are recorded (flushes, intermittently dosed medications) as these seemingly small volumes may add up to significant input for the smallest of infants. Similarly, ensure that all losses are accounted for, such as chest tube output and silo drainage from an infant with gastroschisis. Infants receiving phototherapy have large insensible losses that will not be accounted for in the I/O totals but should be considered when assessing the patient.

Finally, assessment should be made of the quantity of urine output as well as trend in urine output volume over the last several hours and days. Determine whether the amount of daily urine output is sufficient given the amount of fluid the baby is receiving. For example, if a 3 kg infant is receiving ~150 ml/kg/day (total 450 ml/day), 2 ml/kg/h of urine output (total 144 ml/day) may not be sufficient for preventing fluid accumulation even though the baby does not appear to be "oliguric." With this I/O, over the course of 5 days, the baby will have received 2,250 ml fluid, with only 720 ml urine out. Accounting for insensible losses of 40 cm^3/kg/day, this infant would have a positive total fluid balance positive of 1.2 l (or 40 % fluid overload). To lend perspective, 40 % fluid overload in a 70 kg adult would equal 28 l of fluid. A growing number of studies suggest that even 10 % fluid overload is an independent risk factor for mortality in critically ill children and adults [5, 31, 38, 39, 59, 70, 80]. Similar studies in neonates have yet to be performed.

16.4.3 Laboratory and Radiology Findings

Laboratory values to be monitored in the infant with AKI include serum sodium, potassium, chloride, bicarbonate, calcium, phosphorus, magnesium, urea, creatinine, albumin, uric acid, glucose, blood gases, hemoglobin, and platelets. Remember that SCr often does not rise immediately after an injury; thus, monitoring these values for several days after the inciting event is necessary to determine if AKI has occurred and whether the process is resolving, remaining stable, or worsening over time.

If urine is available, a urinalysis, urine culture, and a spot urine sample for sodium, creatinine, and osmolality should be sent and may be helpful in differentiating prerenal azotemia from intrinsic AKI. When hypoperfused, the kidney will avidly retain sodium and water to preserve appropriate intravascular volume status. Thus, the fractional excretion of sodium (FENa) should be low in a prerenal state. Normal FENa in a term newborn is <2 % in prerenal states and >3 % with ATN or intrinsic kidney dysfunction. However, preservation of urine sodium and water depends on the integrity and maturity of tubular dysfunction. FENa is difficult to interpret in preterm newborns who have varying degrees of tubular immaturity. Normal FENa in preterm infants born at less than 32 weeks of gestation is usually higher than 3 % [26]. Moreover, FENa is not valid when an infant is receiving diuretics.

A renal and bladder ultrasound should be performed immediately if an obstructive process is suspected and to determine if congenital renal abnormalities are present. If hematuria or hypertension (or both) is present, the possibility of renal vascular insult should also be considered, and Doppler ultrasound of the renal vessels should be performed.

16.5 Medical Management of AKI in the Neonate

There are currently no specific medical therapies for the treatment or prevention of AKI, such that our management of kidney injury in neonates (as with all other patient groups) remains supportive. Keys to managing the infant with AKI include identifying and correcting any modifiable risk factors/AKI etiologies (e.g., replacement of large chest tube fluid losses) and minimizing additional kidney insults going forward (e.g., substituting potentially nephrotoxic medications with a suitable, less nephrotoxic alternative if one exists). Determination of AKI etiology is based on clinical interpretation of history, physical examination, laboratory, and radiology findings. As mentioned before, SCr does not provide information about the nature or exact timing of the kidney insult.

If obstruction of the urinary outflow is discovered, interventions to establish urinary drainage, via either the urethra or percutaneous nephrostomy tubes, should be undertaken immediately. In addition, plans for definitive surgical correction should be discussed with a pediatric urologist. Polyuria with electrolyte losses may occur following the relief of the obstruction. Thus, close monitoring of serum electrolytes (especially sodium, potassium, and bicarbonate) is necessary – every 2–4 h in some cases – with replacement of these as needed.

If the suspicion for renal hypoperfusion is high, an appropriate fluid challenge with 10–20 ml/kg of isotonic fluids (usually normal saline) should be given. Several boluses may be necessary, with careful prescription of fluid volume for the next 24 h. Large chest tube and gastrointestinal tract losses may need to be replaced using an appropriate fluid determined by the electrolyte composition of the losses. Ensure adequate oncotic pressure by measuring serum albumin levels, with target minimum serum albumin >2.0 mg/dl and preferably >2.5 mg/dl. Be sure to consider whether the infant has congestive heart failure or a urinary outlet obstruction prior to giving multiple fluid boluses. Frequent reassessment of the patient is key to achieving appropriate restoration of intravascular volume and avoiding excessive fluid administration that may lead to volume overload.

Fluid management in the critically ill neonate with AKI can be very difficult, especially when the infant is oliguric. These infants may require large volumes of fluid to maintain adequate nutrition and hematologic indices and for pharmacologic treatment of their underlying condition. In an oliguric/anuric child, these fluids can be detrimental and lead to congestive heart failure, chest wall edema, and pulmonary failure. Severe fluid restriction limiting intake to insensible, gastrointestinal, and renal losses is sometimes required but at a heavy price in the form of inadequate nutrition. At this point (or as soon as this situation is anticipated), renal replacement therapy should be considered.

16.5.1 Electrolyte and Mineral Homeostasis

Electrolyte abnormalities can vary depending on the cause of AKI, and infants with AKI may have no, few, or many of these. For example, severe oliguric/anuric AKI may lead to marked hyponatremia, hyperkalemia, hyperphosphatemia, and hypocalcemia, whereas nonoliguric AKI and proximal tubular dysfunction as occuring with aminoglycoside toxicity may result in hypokalemia and hypomagnesemia. The key to medical management of electrolyte disorders includes attention to electrolyte intake during initial course of AKI (e.g., review the electrolyte content of all IV fluids and parenteral nutrition prescription), with frequent reevalution and adjustment of fluids as necessary.

Hyponatremia may occur during the course of AKI and is more often the result of total body volume overload rather than total body sodium depletion. Attention to fluid status is critical when determining the cause and proper treatment of hyponatremia. In cases of non-symptomatic hypervolemic hyponatremia (serum sodium concentrations usually between 120 and 130 mEq/l), restriction of free water intake is recommended. If hyponatremia at this level results in clinical signs and symptoms (lethargy, seizures) or serum sodium concentration falls below 120 mEq/l, use of NS or 3 % sodium chloride according to the following formula should be considered:

$$\mathrm{Na^+}_{\text{required}}\,(\mathrm{mEq}) = \left(\left[\mathrm{Na^+}\right]_{\text{desired}} - \left[\mathrm{Na^+}\right]_{\text{actual}}\right) \times \text{body weight}\,(\mathrm{kg}) \times 0.8$$

Potential complications of hypertonic saline administration include congestive heart failure, pulmonary edema, hypertension, intraventricular hemorrhage, and periventricular leukomalacia. Care should be taken not to increase serum sodium concentration more rapidly than 0.5 mEq/h [7, 9].

Severe hyperkalemia is a life-threatening medical emergency. Frequent review of the electrolyte composition of all fluids being given is critical for preventing this situation. If an infant becomes anuric, then potassium should be removed from all intravenous fluids. Enteral formulas as well should be reviewed for their potassium content. Options available for the treatment of hyperkalemia include measures to remove potassium from the body, such as oral or rectal sodium polystyrene (Kayexalate®), loop diuretics to enhance urinary potassium excretion (if not anuric), and dialysis. Other options include maneuvers to shift potassium from the extracellular to the intracellular compartment including albuterol inhalation, sodium bicarbonate, and insulin/glucose. Adequate ionized calcium levels for cardioprotection should be ensured.

Hyperkalemia unresponsive to medical management is one of the most common indications for renal replacement therapy in the newborn [24, 43].

Hyperphosphatemia is common in AKI due to impaired renal excretion of phosphorus, and serum phosphate levels should be monitored regularly. The dietary prescription should be evaluated for phosphorus intake and adjusted accordingly. Enteral feeding options low in phosphorus (as well as potassium) relative to other infant formulas include breast milk, Similac® 60/40 and Nestle® Good Start. Calcium carbonate may be used as a phosphate-binding agent in those whose phosphorous intake exceed excretion in spite of dietary adjustments. Formula or breast milk may also be pretreated with phosphate-binding agents such as sevelamer hydrochloride prior to being given to the infant [28]. In some rare but severe cases, removal by hemodialysis may be required. Significant elevations in serum phosphate may promote the development of extraskeletal calcifications of the heart, blood vessels, and kidneys in the newborn, especially when the calcium-phosphorus product exceeds 70 [71]. Close follow-up with a NICU and/or renal dietician is an important part of care for these patients.

Hypocalcemia may develop in neonates with severe and prolonged AKI, especially in those with impaired ability to convert 25-hydroxyvitamin D to 1,25-dihydroxyvitamin D. Ionized calcium should be measured in those with low total calcium levels as concurrent hypoalbuminemia can affect total calcium levels. Calcium may be replaced by either enteral or IV routes depending on the clinical situation. Infants with prolonged severe AKI may also require treatment with calcitriol to supplement deficient 1,25-dihydroxyvitamin D levels. In these infants, serum levels of intact parathyroid hormone should also be monitored.

16.5.2 Acid-Base Homeostasis

Non-anion gap metabolic acidosis is a common finding in infants with AKI as normal acid-base homeostasis depends on the kidneys' ability to reabsorb bicarbonate. Base supplementation with either bicarbonate or acetate is indicated in those with AKI and metabolic acidosis. In infants with severe respiratory failure, large doses of bicarbonate should be avoided as they can culminate in increased carbon dioxide retention. Metabolic acidosis should be treated aggresively in those with severe pulmonary hypertension, as an acidic environment can worsen this condition.

16.5.3 Nutrition

Nutritional goals in infants with AKI are similar to those of infants without AKI, with adjustments needed most commonly for potassium, sodium, and phosphorus content. The total volume required to deliver adequate nutrition is often of concern, especially in oliguric/anuric patients. Commonly, parental nutrition and/or enteral feeds will need to be concentrated to avoid excessive fluid gains. If nutritional goals are unable to be achieved due to oliguria/ongoing fluid overload, then initiation of renal replacement therapy should be considered taking into account the potential risks associated with dialysis therapy compared with those associated with prolonged, inadequate caloric and protein intake.

16.5.4 Therapeutics

Several therapies including dopamine, diuretics, and fenoldopam are used in the management of the patient with AKI in spite of the fact that little evidence is available to support their use in this regard. Dopamine has been studied and is widely used in the neonatal population for support of systemic blood pressure in both preterm and term infants [72–74]. In terms of low-dose or "renal-dose" dopamine as a therapy for AKI prevention, however, well-powered randomized controlled studies [17] and several meta-analyses [30, 40, 53] in adults with AKI have shown that low-dose dopamine does not improve survival, shorten hospital stay, or limit dialysis use when compared to placebo. These studies have not been performed in children or neonates.

Diuretics are commonly used to augment urine output in critically ill neonates, especially given the technical difficulties associated with providing renal replacement therapy to very small infants. However, no studies in neonates, children, or adults have shown that diuretics are effective in preventing AKI or improving outcomes once AKI occurs [13, 17]. Nonetheless, loop diuretics may be used in oliguric neonates in an attempt to improve urine output. In these cases, continuous intravenous infusion of furosemide may be superior to larger intermittent doses, with smaller total quantities of medication delivered [51]. The potential toxicity of long-term and aggressive furosemide therapy, including ototoxicity, interstitial nephritis, osteopenia, nephrocalcinosis, hypotension, and persistence of patent ductus arteriosus, should be taken into consideration, especially in the preterm newborns [43].

Fenoldopam is a selective dopamine-1 receptor agonist whose effects include vasodilation of renal and splanchnic vasculature, increased renal blood flow, and increased GFR. It is approved for the treatment of severe hypertension in adults but is not clinically approved for the treatment of AKI. Nonetheless, its use in neonates with AKI has been explored in several single-center analyses, with some data suggesting that urine output is increased with this medication in a select group of neonates [57, 85]. Its use has been explored in two prospective studies of infants undergoing cardiopulmonary bypass, with no benefit seen in terms of AKI incidence, fluid balance, or time to sternal closure using low-dose fenoldopam (0.1 mcg/kg/min) [68] and some modest benefit seen with high-dose fenoldopam (1 mcg/kg/min) [67]. Currently there is not enough data to support the routine use of fenoldopam as a treatment or prevention strategy for neonates with AKI.

16.5.5 Other Medications

In a neonate with AKI, careful assessment of medication dosing is imperative. Because many drugs are excreted in the urine, impaired metabolism or clearance from the kidneys can cause drug accumulation and adverse side effects. Consultation with pharmacists and nephrologists familiar with drug dosing in renal failure is essential when caring for the infant with AKI. Medication lists should be reviewed frequently to ensure correct dosing has been prescribed based on the level of renal failure. In addition, consideration should be given for stopping potentially nephrotoxic medications and substituting with a suitable, less nephrotoxic alternative if one exists.

16.5.6 Dialysis

Indications for the initiation of renal replacement therapy are the same as for other patients (e.g., severe hyperkalemia). However, it is important to remember that these indications are based on our experience in patients with end-stage renal disease. Waiting for these late indicators of severe renal dysfunction to occur is likely not appropriate for the infant with AKI, and thus consideration for renal replacement therapy should occur earlier in the course of illness [82]. For example, marked edema creates significant technical difficulties for dialysis access placement and makes support of the infant much more difficult. Data on fluid overload in pediatric and adult patients show that those with higher fluid overload at the time of dialysis initiation have worse survival even when controlling for severity of illness scores [29, 33, 35, 77]. These data suggest that prevention of fluid overload and/or early initiation of renal support therapy with dialysis could improve outcomes in those with AKI. See Chapter 17 for a complete discussion of the provision of renal replacement therapies for infants.

16.6 Novel Biomarkers

As discussed previously, SCr-based AKI definitions have multiple shortcomings, especially in the neonatal population. Of the most important, SCr estimates glomerular function, not damage, and takes days to rise after an injury has occurred. Thus, the focus has been to find better AKI biomarkers to diagnose this process earlier in the course, allow for the development of interventions, and ultimately improve outcomes. Urinary biomarkers show great promise in this regard. Studies in VLBW infants [6, 10, 49], infants who undergo cardiopulmonary bypass surgery [37, 48, 60, 61, 64, 86][65], and other sick newborns admitted to a neonatal intensive care unit [7, 9] suggest that these biomarkers can detect those infants who will later have a rise in SCr and may also predict hard clinical endpoints such as mortality. Currently, bedside tests for serum and urine neutrophil-gelatinase-associated lipocalin and kidney injury biomarker-1 (KIM-1) are available in Europe and are undergoing rigorous testing and are under review by the FDA.

In premature infants, it is very important to recognize that normal levels of these urine biomarkers will differ by gestational age, probably due to different degrees of tubular immaturity. Controlling for this important variable is critical as we aim to identify better AKI biomarkers.

16.7 Future Directions

Over the last few years, our understanding of neonatal AKI has grown and we now have clear data that suggest that AKI is common and is associated with mortality. However, better understanding of risk factors, preventive strategies, and management strategies are greatly needed. In addition, technologic advances have been made such that dialysis machines made specific for neonates have been made and are undergoing testing [69]. Maximizing the efficiency and safety of renal support therapies with these machines could change our approach to the neonate with AKI.

In order for us to improve outcomes of infants with AKI, neonatologists and nephrologists must work together to develop better definitions of AKI using newer biomarkers, perhaps in conjunction with SCr, urine output, and clinical criteria. In order to accomplish this task, large-scale observational multicenter studies in which these biomarkers are tested against hard clinical endpoints (such as need for dialysis provision, mortality, lengths of stay, and long-term evidence of chronic kidney disease) must be performed. In addition, AKI prevention studies that use novel biomarkers to define AKI are needed. If an intervention is shown to reduce AKI incidence or severity (as defined by AKI biomarkers), it would lend support to that biomarker's clinical utility. More importantly, studies are needed in which AKI biomarkers are used to identify AKI early in the disease process, and once AKI is identified, randomized interventions can be tested.

Conclusion

Acute kidney injury is a common and complex process with important outcome implications for critically ill neonates. It is associated with an increased risk in morbidity and mortality for these patients. Our current AKI definitions and biomarkers are limited and have limited advancements in treatment strategies. For now, anticipating who may be at risk is an important part of management. Early identification of AKI risk factors, close monitoring of serum creatinine levels, attention to fluid balance (for signs of both renal hypoperfusion and fluid overload), avoidance of additional nephrotoxic exposures whenever possible, and frequent reassessment are all critical aspects in the care of these patients. Early consultation with a pediatric nephrologist is often warranted. Advancements in the care of these patients and improvement in survival will depend on close collaboration between the Neonatology and Nephrology communities.

References

1. Aggarwal A, Kumar P, Chowdhary G, Majumdar S, Narang A (2005) Evaluation of renal functions in asphyxiated newborns. J Trophic Pediatr 51(5): 295–299. doi:10.1093/tropej/fmi017
2. Akcan-Arikan A, Zappitelli M, Loftis LL, Washburn KK, Jefferson LS, Goldstein SL (2007) Modified RIFLE criteria in critically ill children with acute kidney injury. Kidney Int 71(10):1028–1035. doi:10.1038/sj.ki.5002231
3. Andreoli SP (2002) Acute renal failure. Curr Opin Pediatr 14(2):183–188
4. Andreoli SP (2004) Acute renal failure in the newborn. Semin Perinatol 28(2):112–123
5. Arikan AA, Zappitelli M, Goldstein SL, Naipaul A, Jefferson LS, Loftis LL (2012) Fluid overload is associated with impaired oxygenation and morbidity in critically ill children*. Pediatr Crit Care Med 13(3):253–258. doi:10.1097/PCC.0b013e31822882a3
6. Askenazi DJ, Ambalavanan N, Hamilton K, Cutter G, Laney D, Kaslow R, Georgeson K, Barnhart DC, Dimmitt RA (2011) Acute kidney injury and renal replacement therapy independently predict mortality in neonatal and pediatric noncardiac patients on extracorporeal membrane oxygenation. Pediatr Crit Care Med 12(1):e1–6. doi:10.1097/PCC.0b013e3181d8e348
7. Askenazi DJ, Furth S, Warady B (2012) Acute and chronic kidney failure. In: Gleason CA, Devaskar S (eds) Avery's diseases of the newborn, 9th edn. Elsevier, Philadelphia
8. Askenazi DJ, Griffin R, McGwin G, Carlo W, Ambalavanan N (2009) Acute kidney injury is independently associated with mortality in very low birthweight infants: a matched case-control analysis. Pediatr Nephrol 24(5):991–997. doi:10.1007/s00467-009-1133-x
9. Askenazi DJ, Koralkar R, Hundley HE, Montesanti A, Parwar P, Sonjara S, Ambalavanan N (2012) Urine biomarkers predict acute kidney injury in newborns. J Pediatr 161(2):270–275. doi:10.1016/j.jpeds.2012.02.007
10. Askenazi DJMA, Hunley H, Koralkar R, Pawar P, Shuaib F, Liwo A, Devarajan P, Ambalavanan N (2011) Urine biomarkers predict acute kidney injury and mortality in very low birth weight infants. J Pediatr 159(6):907–12.e1
11. Auron A, Auron-Gomez M, Raina R, Viswanathan S, Mhanna MJ (2009) Effect of amphotericin B lipid complex (ABLC) in very low birth weight infants. Pediatr Nephrol 24(2):295–299. doi:10.1007/s00467-008-1017-5
12. Awad AS, Okusa MD (2007) Distant organ injury following acute kidney injury. Am J Physiol Renal Physiol 293(1):F28–29
13. Bagshaw SM, Delaney A, Haase M, Ghali WA, Bellomo R (2007) Loop diuretics in the management of acute renal failure: a systematic review and meta-analysis. Crit Care Resusc 9(1):60–68
14. Bagshaw SM, George C, Bellomo R (2007) Changes in the incidence and outcome for early acute kidney injury in a cohort of Australian intensive care units. Crit Care 11(3):R68. doi:10.1186/cc5949. cc5949 [pii]
15. Baley JE, Kliegman RM, Fanaroff AA (1984) Disseminated fungal infections in very low-birth-weight infants: therapeutic toxicity. Pediatrics 73(2):153–157
16. Bannwarth B, Lagrange F, Pehourcq F, Llanas B, Demarquez JL (1999) (S)-ketoprofen accumulation in premature neonates with renal failure who were exposed to the racemate during pregnancy. Br J Clin Pharmacol 47(4):459–460
17. Bellomo R, Chapman M, Finfer S, Hickling K, Myburgh J (2000) Low-dose dopamine in patients with early renal dysfunction: a placebo-controlled randomised trial. Australian and New Zealand Intensive Care Society (ANZICS) Clinical Trials Group. Lancet 356(9248):2139–2143
18. Bellomo R, Ronco C, Kellum JA, Mehta RL, Palevsky P, Acute Dialysis Quality Initiative w (2004) Acute renal failure – definition, outcome measures, animal models, fluid therapy and information technology needs: the Second International Consensus Conference of the Acute Dialysis Quality Initiative (ADQI) Group. Crit Care 8(4):R204–212. doi:10.1186/cc2872
19. Blinder JJ, Goldstein SL, Lee VV, Baycroft A, Fraser CD, Nelson D, Jefferies JL (2012) Congenital heart surgery in infants: effects of acute kidney injury on outcomes. J Thorac Cardiovasc Surg 143(2):368–374. doi:10.1016/j.jtcvs.2011.06.021
20. Brandao LR, Simpson EA, Lau KK (2011) Neonatal renal vein thrombosis. Semin Fetal Neonatal Med 16(6):323–328. doi:10.1016/j.siny.2011.08.004
21. Cavagnaro F, Kattan J, Godoy L, Gonzales A, Vogel A, Rodriguez JI, Faunes M, Fajardo C, Becker P (2007) Continuous renal replacement therapy in neonates and young infants during extracorporeal membrane oxygenation. Int J Artif Organs 30(3):220–226
22. Chertow GM, Burdick E, Honour M, Bonventre JV, Bates DW (2005) Acute kidney injury, mortality, length of stay, and costs in hospitalized patients. J Am Soc Nephrol 16(11):3365–3370. doi:10.1681/ASN.2004090740
23. Cifuentes RF, Olley PM, Balfe JW, Radde IC, Soldin SJ (1979) Indomethacin and renal function in premature infants with persistent patent ductus arteriosus. J Pediatr 95(4):583–587
24. Coulthard MG, Vernon B (1995) Managing acute renal failure in very low birthweight infants. Arch Dis Child Fetal Neonatal Ed 73(3):F187–F192
25. Cuhaci B (2009) More data on epidemiology and outcome of acute kidney injury with AKIN criteria: benefits of standardized definitions, AKIN and RIFLE classifications. Crit Care Med 37(9):2659–2661. doi:10.1097/CCM.0b013e3181ad76c200003246-200909000-00031 [pii]
26. Ellis EN, Arnold WC (1982) Use of urinary indexes in renal failure in the newborn. Am J Dis Child 136(7):615–617
27. Feld LG, Springate JE, Fildes RD (1986) Acute renal failure. I. Pathophysiology and diagnosis. J Pediatr 109(3):401–408

28. Ferrara E, Lemire J, Reznik VM, Grimm PC (2004) Dietary phosphorus reduction by pretreatment of human breast milk with sevelamer. Pediatr Nephrol 19(7):775–779. doi:10.1007/s00467-004-1448-6
29. Foland JA, Fortenberry JD, Warshaw BL, Pettignano R, Merritt RK, Heard ML, Rogers K, Reid C, Tanner AJ, Easley KA (2004) Fluid overload before continuous hemofiltration and survival in critically ill children: a retrospective analysis. Crit Care Med 32(8):1771–1776
30. Friedrich JO, Adhikari N, Herridge MS, Beyene J (2005) Meta-analysis: low-dose dopamine increases urine output but does not prevent renal dysfunction or death. Ann Intern Med 142(7):510–524
31. Fulop T, Pathak MB, Schmidt DW, Lengvarszky Z, Juncos JP, Lebrun CJ, Brar H, Juncos LA (2010) Volume-related weight gain and subsequent mortality in acute renal failure patients treated with continuous renal replacement therapy. ASAIO J 56(4):333–337. doi:10.1097/MAT.0b013e3181de35e4
32. Gadepalli SK, Selewski DT, Drongowski RA, Mychaliska GB (2011) Acute kidney injury in congenital diaphragmatic hernia requiring extracorporeal life support: an insidious problem. J Pediatr Surg 46(4):630–635. doi:10.1016/j.jpedsurg.2010.11.031
33. Gillespie RS, Seidel K, Symons JM (2004) Effect of fluid overload and dose of replacement fluid on survival in hemofiltration. Pediatr Nephrol 19(12):1394–1399. doi:10.1007/s00467-004-1655-1
34. Giuliano RA, Paulus GJ, Verpooten GA, Pattyn VM, Pollet DE, Nouwen EJ, Laurent G, Carlier MB, Maldague P, Tulkens PM et al (1984) Recovery of cortical phospholipidosis and necrosis after acute gentamicin loading in rats. Kidney Int 26(6):838–847
35. Goldstein SL, Somers MJ, Baum MA, Symons JM, Brophy PD, Blowey D, Bunchman TE, Baker C, Mottes T, McAfee N, Barnett J, Morrison G, Rogers K, Fortenberry JD (2005) Pediatric patients with multi-organ dysfunction syndrome receiving continuous renal replacement therapy. Kidney Int 67(2):653–658. doi:10.1111/j.1523-1755.2005.67121.x
36. Gupta BD, Sharma P, Bagla J, Parakh M, Soni JP (2005) Renal failure in asphyxiated neonates. Indian Pediatr 42(9):928–934
37. Hall IE, Koyner JL, Doshi MD, Marcus RJ, Parikh CR (2011) Urine cystatin C as a biomarker of proximal tubular function immediately after kidney transplantation. Am J Nephrol 33(5):407–413. doi:10.1159/000326753. 000326753 [pii]
38. Hayes LW, Oster RA, Tofil NM, Tolwani AJ (2009) Outcomes of critically ill children requiring continuous renal replacement therapy. J Crit Care 24(3):394–400. doi:10.1016/j.jcrc.2008.12.017
39. Heung M, Wolfgram DF, Kommareddi M, Hu Y, Song PX, Ojo AO (2012) Fluid overload at initiation of renal replacement therapy is associated with lack of renal recovery in patients with acute kidney injury. Nephrol Dial Transplant 27(3):956–961. doi:10.1093/ndt/gfr470
40. Hoste EA, Clermont G, Kersten A, Venkataraman R, Angus DC, De Bacquer D, Kellum JA (2006) RIFLE criteria for acute kidney injury are associated with hospital mortality in critically ill patients: a cohort analysis. Crit Care 10(3):R73
41. Hui-Stickle S, Brewer ED, Goldstein SL (2005) Pediatric ARF epidemiology at a tertiary care center from 1999 to 2001. Am J Kidney Dis 45(1):96–101
42. Izzedine H, Launay-Vacher V, Deray G (2005) Antiviral drug-induced nephrotoxicity. Am J Kidney Dis 45(5):804–817
43. Karlowicz MG, Adelman RD (1992) Acute renal failure in the neonate. Clin Perinatol 19(1):139–158
44. Karlowicz MG, Adelman RD (1995) Nonoliguric and oliguric acute renal failure in asphyxiated term neonates. Pediatr Nephrol 9(6):718–722
45. Kaur S, Jain S, Saha A, Chawla D, Parmar VR, Basu S, Kaur J (2011) Evaluation of glomerular and tubular renal function in neonates with birth asphyxia. Ann Trop Paediatr 31(2):129–134. doi:10.1179/1465328 11X12925735813922
46. Kellum JA, Angus DC (2002) Patients are dying of acute renal failure. Crit Care Med 30(9):2156–2157. doi:10.1097/01.CCM.0000026731.62424.B3
47. Koralkar R, Ambalavanan N, Levitan EB, McGwin G, Goldstein S, Askenazi D (2011) Acute kidney injury reduces survival in very low birth weight infants. Pediatr Res 69(4):354–358. doi:10.1203/PDR.0b013e31820b95ca
48. Krawczeski CD, Woo JG, Wang Y, Bennett MR, Ma Q, Devarajan P (2011) Neutrophil gelatinase-associated lipocalin concentrations predict development of acute kidney injury in neonates and children after cardiopulmonary bypass. J Pediatr 158(6):1009–1015 e1001. doi:10.1016/j.jpeds.2010.12.057
49. Lavery AP, Meinzen-Derr JK, Anderson E, Ma Q, Bennett MR, Devarajan P, Schibler KR (2008) Urinary NGAL in premature infants. Pediatr Res 64(4):423–428. doi:10.1203/PDR.0b013e318181b3b2
50. Li X, Hassoun HT, Santora R, Rabb H (2009) Organ crosstalk: the role of the kidney. Curr Opin Crit Care 15(6):481–487. doi:10.1097/MCC.0b013e328332f69e
51. Luciani GB, Nichani S, Chang AC, Wells WJ, Newth CJ, Starnes VA (1997) Continuous versus intermittent furosemide infusion in critically ill infants after open heart operations. Ann Thorac Surg 64(4):1133–1139
52. Macedo E, Castro I, Yu L, Abdulkader RR, Vieira JM, Jr. (2008) Impact of mild acute kidney injury (AKI) on outcome after open repair of aortic aneurysms. Ren Fail 30(3):287–296. doi:10.1080/08860220701857522. 791578002 [pii]
53. Marik PE (2002) Low-dose dopamine: a systematic review. Intensive Care Med 28(7):877–883
54. Mathur NB, Agarwal HS, and Maria A (2006) Acute renal failure in neonatal sepsis. Indian J Pediatrics 73(6):499–502
55. Mehta RL, Kellum JA, Shah SV, Molitoris BA, Ronco C, Warnock DG, Levin A, Acute Kidney Injury Network (2007) Acute Kidney Injury Network: report

of an initiative to improve outcomes in acute kidney injury. Crit Care 11(2):R31. doi:10.1186/cc5713
56. Meyer RJ, Brophy PD, Bunchman TE, Annich GM, Maxvold NJ, Mottes TA, Custer JR (2001) Survival and renal function in pediatric patients following extracorporeal life support with hemofiltration. Pediatr Crit Care Med 2(3):238–242
57. Moffett BS, Mott AR, Nelson DP, Goldstein SL, Jefferies JL (2008) Renal effects of fenoldopam in critically ill pediatric patients: a retrospective review. Pediatr Crit Care Med 9(4):403–406
58. Moghal NE, Brocklebank JT, Meadow SR (1998) A review of acute renal failure in children: incidence, etiology and outcome. Clin Nephrol 49(2):91–95
59. National Heart Lungs, Blood Institute Acute Respiratory Distress Syndrome Clinical Trials Network, Wiedemann HP, Wheeler AP, Bernard GR, Thompson BT, Hayden D, deBoisblanc B, Connors AF Jr, Hite RD, Harabin AL (2006) Comparison of two fluid-management strategies in acute lung injury. N Engl J Med 354(24):2564–2575. doi:10.1056/NEJMoa062200
60. Nguyen MT, Dent CL, Ross GF, Harris N, Manning PB, Mitsnefes MM, Devarajan P (2008) Urinary aprotinin as a predictor of acute kidney injury after cardiac surgery in children receiving aprotinin therapy. Pediatr Nephrol 23(8):1317–1326. doi:10.1007/s00467-008-0827-9
61. Parikh CR, Devarajan P, Zappitelli M, Sint K, Thiessen-Philbrook H, Li S, Kim RW, Koyner JL, Coca SG, Edelstein CL, Shlipak MG, Garg AX, Krawczeski CD (2011) Postoperative biomarkers predict acute kidney injury and poor outcomes after pediatric cardiac surgery. J Am Soc Nephrol 22(9):1737–1747. doi:10.1681/ASN.2010111163. ASN.2010111163 [pii]
62. Peruzzi L, Gianoglio B, Porcellini MG, Coppo R (1999) Neonatal end-stage renal failure associated with maternal ingestion of cyclo-oxygenase-type-1 selective inhibitor nimesulide as tocolytic. Lancet 354(9190):1615
63. Picca S, Principato F, Mazzera E, Corona R, Ferrigno L, Marcelletti C, Rizzoni G (1995) Risks of acute renal failure after cardiopulmonary bypass surgery in children: a retrospective 10-year case-control study. Nephrol Dial Transplant 10(5):630–636
64. Portilla D, Dent C, Sugaya T, Nagothu KK, Kundi I, Moore P, Noiri E, Devarajan P (2008) Liver fatty acid-binding protein as a biomarker of acute kidney injury after cardiac surgery. Kidney Int 73(4):465–472. doi:10.1038/sj.ki.5002721. 5002721 [pii]
65. Ramesh G, Krawczeski CD, Woo JG, Wang Y, Devarajan P (2010) Urinary netrin-1 is an early predictive biomarker of acute kidney injury after cardiac surgery. Clin J Am Soc Nephrol 5(3):395–401. doi:10.2215/CJN.05140709. CJN.05140709 [pii]
66. Ricci Z, Cruz D, Ronco C (2008a) The RIFLE criteria and mortality in acute kidney injury: a systematic review. Kidney Int 73(5):538–546. doi:10.1038/sj.ki.5002743. 5002743 [pii]
67. Ricci Z, Luciano R, Favia I, Garisto C, Muraca M, Morelli S, Di Chiara L, Cogo P, Picardo S (2011) High-dose fenoldopam reduces postoperative neutrophil gelatinase-associated lipocaline and cystatin C levels in pediatric cardiac surgery. Crit Care 15(3):R160. doi:10.1186/cc10295
68. Ricci Z, Stazi GV, Di Chiara L, Morelli S, Vitale V, Giorni C, Ronco C, Picardo S (2008) Fenoldopam in newborn patients undergoing cardiopulmonary bypass: controlled clinical trial. Interact Cardiovasc Thorac Surg 7(6):1049–1053. doi:10.1510/icvts.2008.185025
69. Ronco C, Davenport A, Gura V (2011) The future of the artificial kidney: moving towards wearable and miniaturized devices. Nefrologia 31(1):9–16. doi:10.3265/Nefrologia.pre2010.Nov.10758
70. Sakr Y, Vincent JL, Reinhart K, Groeneveld J, Michalopoulos A, Sprung CL, Artigas A, Ranieri VM, Sepsis Occurrence in Acutely Ill Patients Investigator (2005) High tidal volume and positive fluid balance are associated with worse outcome in acute lung injury. Chest 128(5):3098–3108. doi:10.1378/chest.128.5.3098
71. Sell LL, Cullen ML, Whittlesey GC, Lerner GR, Klein MD (1987) Experience with renal failure during extracorporeal membrane oxygenation: treatment with continuous hemofiltration. J Pediatr Surg 22(7):600–602
72. Seri I (1995) Cardiovascular, renal, and endocrine actions of dopamine in neonates and children. J Pediatr 126(3):333–344
73. Seri I, Abbasi S, Wood DC, Gerdes JS (1998) Regional hemodynamic effects of dopamine in the sick preterm neonate. J Pediatr 133(6):728–734
74. Seri I, Abbasi S, Wood DC, Gerdes JS (2002) Regional hemodynamic effects of dopamine in the indomethacin-treated preterm infant. J Perinatol 22(4):300–305
75. Shaheen IS, Harvey B, Watson AR, Pandya HC, Mayer A, Thomas D (2007) Continuous venovenous hemofiltration with or without extracorporeal membrane oxygenation in children. Pediatr Crit Care Med 8(4):362–365
76. Sorof JM, Stromberg D, Brewer ED, Feltes TF, Fraser CD Jr (1999) Early initiation of peritoneal dialysis after surgical repair of congenital heart disease. Pediatr Nephrol 13(8):641–645
77. Sutherland SM, Zappitelli M, Alexander SR, Chua AN, Brophy PD, Bunchman TE, Hackbarth R, Somers MJ, Baum M, Symons JM, Flores FX, Benfield M, Askenazi D, Chand D, Fortenberry JD, Mahan JD, McBryde K, Blowey D, Goldstein SL (2010) Fluid overload and mortality in children receiving continuous renal replacement therapy: the prospective pediatric continuous renal replacement therapy registry. Am J Kidney Dis 55(2):316–325. doi:10.1053/j.ajkd.2009.10.048
78. Sutton TA, Fisher CJ, Molitoris BA (2002) Microvascular endothelial injury and dysfunction during ischemic acute renal failure. Kidney Int 62(5):1539–1549

79. Uchino S (2008) Outcome prediction for patients with acute kidney injury. Nephron Clin Pract 109(4): c217–223. doi:10.1159/000142931. 000142931 [pii]
80. Upadya A, Tilluckdharry L, Muralidharan V, Amoateng-Adjepong Y, Manthous CA (2005) Fluid balance and weaning outcomes. Intensive Care Med 31(12):1643–1647. doi:10.1007/s00134-005-2801-3
81. Vachvanichsanong P, Dissaneewate P, Lim A, McNeil E (2006) Childhood acute renal failure: 22-year experience in a university hospital in southern Thailand. Pediatrics 118(3):e786–791. doi:10.1542/peds.2006-0557
82. Walters S, Porter C, Brophy PD (2009) Dialysis and pediatric acute kidney injury: choice of renal support modality. Pediatr Nephrol 24(1):37–48. doi:10.1007/s00467-008-0826-x
83. Weber TR, Connors RH, Tracy TF Jr, Bailey PV, Stephens C, Keenan W (1990) Prognostic determinants in extracorporeal membrane oxygenation for respiratory failure in newborns. Ann Thorac Surg 50(5):720–723
84. Williams DM, Sreedhar SS, Mickell JJ, Chan JC (2002) Acute kidney failure: a pediatric experience over 20 years. Arch Pediatr Adolesc Med 156(9):893–900
85. Yoder SE, Yoder BA (2009) An evaluation of off-label fenoldopam use in the neonatal intensive care unit. Am J Perinatol 26(10):745–750
86. Zappitelli M, Krawczeski CD, Devarajan P, Wang Z, Sint K, Thiessen-Philbrook H, Li S, Bennett MR, Ma Q, Shlipak MG, Garg AX, Parikh CR (2011) Early postoperative serum cystatin C predicts severe acute kidney injury following pediatric cardiac surgery. Kidney Int 80(6):655–662. doi:10.1038/ki.2011.123ki2011123 [pii]
87. Zappitelli M, Parikh CR, Akcan-Arikan A, Washburn KK, Moffett BS, Goldstein SL (2008) Ascertainment and epidemiology of acute kidney injury varies with definition interpretation. Clin J Am Soc Nephrol 3(4):948–954. doi:10.2215/CJN.05431207. CJN.05431207 [pii]

17 Hemodialysis and Continuous Renal Replacement Therapy

Megan M. Lo and Timothy E. Bunchman

Core Messages

- Renal replacement therapy through vascular means in neonates is significantly more complicated than in older patients. A higher level of vigilance and attention to detail with staff familiar with neonates and neonatal hemodialysis are necessary.
- Vascular access is one of the most important components of hemodialysis and continuous renal replacement therapy success. Placement in the right internal jugular vein is preferred for flow and recirculation concerns.
- Because most of the equipment and supplies have been developed for larger patients, clearance, anticoagulation, ultrafiltration, and blood flow are different for neonates.
- Data on neonatal vascular renal replacement therapy remains limited, and outcomes remain guarded for these smallest of patients who need to start dialysis at such an early age.

Case Vignette

You are called to the NICU for a 32-week, 1.7-kg premature male who had oligohydramnios and was receiving amnioinfusion therapy in utero. The baby is intubated and respiratory status is stabilized on low ventilation settings. However, he is anuric and renal ultrasound shows bilateral renal agenesis. The family would like to proceed with all possible courses of action to save their baby. Despite his small size, peritoneal dialysis is initiated and proceeds with multiple complications. After 2 months, he has peritoneal membrane failure and is changed to hemodialysis. A temporary 7-French left subclavian catheter is used emergently due to the presence of a tunneled right internal jugular Broviac. Blood primes are used with frequent monitoring of vital signs with dopamine needed to

M.M. Lo (✉)
Department of Pediatric Nephrology, VCU School of Medicine, McGuire Hall Annex 1112 East Clay St., Richmond, VA 23298, USA
e-mail: mlo@mcvh-vcu.edu

T.E. Bunchman
Department of Pediatric Nephrology, Children's Hospital of Richmond, VCU School of Medicine, Sanger Hall 12-024C1101 East Marshall St, 980498, Richmond, VA 23298, USA
e-mail: tbunchman@mcvh-vcu.edu

A.S. Chishti et al. (eds.), *Kidney and Urinary Tract Diseases in the Newborn*, DOI 10.1007/978-3-642-39988-6_17, © Springer-Verlag Berlin Heidelberg 2014

support blood pressure. Dialysis is only used for the first hour of each session with ultrafiltration only for the remainder due to the high clearance rates on a small baby. Ativan boluses are used to improve fluid removal. Flow and clotting complications occur with his subclavian catheter, and his Broviac is exchanged for a tunneled 8-French hemodialysis catheter. Chronic hemodialysis proceeds until the patient is transplanted with a kidney from his mother.

17.1 Introduction

Neonatal hemodialysis (HD) for acute or chronic renal failure is a rare but important component of pediatric nephrological care. The needs for dialysis in infants are usually related to three different indications. Cause can be related to end-stage renal disease (ESRD), acute kidney injury (AKI), and finally inborn error of metabolism [2]. In larger children and rarely in infants, the other indication for renal replacement therapy is intoxication [9]. Because of the rarity of this cause in neonates, it will not be addressed in this chapter.

Data from the North American Pediatric Renal Trials and Collaborative Studies database (NAPRTCS) estimates the incidence of dialysis-treated (all modalities) neonatal ESRD as 0.32 cases per 100,000 live births [13]. This number probably underestimates the total, however, as NAPRTCS is a voluntary reporting system and patients in smaller centers have been missed. Alternatively, larger centers may be too busy to report on all incidences. The general trend over time has been to move to peritoneal dialysis (PD) due to access and feasibility concerns. However, certain situations still require the use of hemodialysis such as the presence of a hostile abdomen or the need for rapid clearance. These smallest of patients suffer from a lack of appropriately sized equipment (partially dictated by physics) as well as increased risk of complications. Their management, therefore, is different from that of a general pediatric dialysis patient. This chapter will not focus on peritoneal dialysis, for it is discussed in another chapter, but will address the use of extracorporeal therapies including hemodialysis and the use of continuous renal replacement therapy (CRRT).

17.2 Indications

Very few neonatal series exist regarding dialysis at all and hemodialysis specifically. However, the therapy has been used in this age group at least as far back as the 1970s. Initial indications were mostly for acute kidney injury. All five patients under 1 month of age had "medical ATN" (acute tubular necrosis) as the indication for hemodialysis in a single-center analysis from 1978 [25]. Out of ten patients dialyzed starting at age 13 weeks at the oldest, six patients had indications of "acute renal failure," mostly from sepsis and one for posttransplantation [26].

In more recent reports, indications for starting dialysis varied by study, at least partially a consequence of variable practice preferences and type of referral center. Infants were more likely to have dysplasia/hypoplasia (7/20 patients) compared to older children (up to age 36 months at the start of dialysis) who tended to have diffuse mesangial sclerosis (7/14 patients). Infants were more likely to start with PD (16/20 versus 4/14 patients age 13–36 months). Nine of those 16 transitioned to HD due to PD failure [20]. The preference for non-HD in this age group was supported by NAPRTCS data. Hemodialysis was less likely to be the chosen modality, occurring in 2.1 % of patients compared to 9.5 % of patients up to 24 months of age. The most likely indication for neonatal dialysis of any modality was dysplasia (37 %) [13].

In contrast, in a series of 33 patients between 1980 and 1991, 18 were dialyzed for acute kidney injury, seven had primary renal disease, and eight had hyperammonemia. AKI was associated with the need for extracorporeal membrane oxygenation therapy (11 patients) or with hemodynamic compromise from other causes [35]. Other studies have also shown that as much as 25 % of infants will have some degree of AKI in the neonatal intensive care unit [1]. AKI in this population is often related to a catastrophic illness of sepsis or hypoxia-ischemia. Most of these infants do not need to undergo renal replacement therapy.

In terms of ESRD, the etiology in infants is often related to congenital renal abnormalities. This can run the gamut of obstructive uropathy, polycystic kidney disease, (either recessive or dominant), or the rarer forms of nephrotic syndrome. Furthermore, children who suffer catastrophic illness in the first few days of life from hypoxia-ischemia can develop cortical necrosis and loss of kidney function, resulting in AKI-induced need for chronic dialysis.

Hyperammonemia is a definitive indication for hemodialysis as this modality has been shown to be more rapidly effective in inborn errors of metabolism [16, 37]. Additional steps include starting a glucose infusion while planning management with genetics. These are classically infants who show up between day two and five of life who have cardiovascular collapse associated with a significant metabolic acidosis, Kussmaul ventilation, and evidence of significantly high and lethal levels of ammonia. Time is of the essence as prolonged exposure to high ammonium levels leads to prolonged neurological damage [31]. Therefore, hemodialysis and CRRT by CVVHD or CAVHD are first-line modalities unless limited by surgical or dialysis nursing expertise locally. If HD is not available immediately, PD is a reasonable alternative while further medical interventions are proceeding to decrease ammonium production.

Another case report included a 1,220-g ex-28-week-gestational-age infant successfully treated with hemodialysis for theophylline toxicity at 8 days of life. The patient had seizures with a serum level of 82 mg/L at the start of dialysis and decreased to 11.8 mg/L after 2 h, with resolution of seizure activity 15 min after starting [22].

17.3 Location of Therapy

Initiation and performance of hemodialysis or CRRT must occur where the physician, hemodialysis nurses, and support staff have the experience and expertise to safely manage these patients. Rapid interventions such as fluid boluses, code drugs, and accessibility of the pediatric nephrologist, critical care physician, anesthesia, and ancillary staff at bedside are critical. Regardless of the location chosen to perform the procedures, consistency is vital to progressive success. Many programs treat less than 10–15 children per year on CRRT. Therefore, the lack of ongoing experience makes this a relatively higher risk and higher anxiety-producing maneuver. With these considerations, although the patients are neonates, due to the infrequent nature of these procedures, the pediatric (rather than neonatal) intensive care unit may be the better choice dialysis/CRRT site to concentrate incidences. Wherever the chosen venue, all neonatal sessions should be performed there, with the patients taken care of by a core group of intensive care and dialysis/CRRT nurses. This will allow the core group of caregivers to develop adequate experience with these patients and situations that are relatively few and far between.

17.4 Vascular Access

Access is one of the most important factors to dialysis success. If the initial catheter location fails, then that major blood vessel may become unusable for future access attempts. Therefore, it is very important to obtain the highest blood flow possible, lest the attempt be wasted. Given that flow is proportional to radius to the 4th power, an 8-French double-lumen catheter would have a per-lumen flow rate approximately three times higher than a 6-French double lumen of the same length. In a study of CRRT patients, 5-French catheters had significantly decreased survival times compared to any other catheter. Although not specified, these were presumably double-lumen catheters for CRRT. Internal jugular placement conferred a significant advantage [23]. Catheter tips ending in the right atrium tended to demonstrate more consistent blood flow rates [35]. Care must be taken to avoid placements which are too deep and risk arrhythmias. Therefore, the patient should start with a 7- to 8-French catheter at a minimum, placed in the

Table 17.1 Possible hemodialysis catheters for neonates

Company	Size (Fr)	Length (cm)	Cuffed	Design	Material
Medcomp: Soft-Line	7	7, 10	No	Coaxial	Polyurethane
Soft-Line	9	12, 15	No	Coaxial	Polyurethane
Hemo-Cath ST	8	12	No	Coaxial	Silicone
DuoFlow	9	12, 15	No	Coaxial	Polyurethane
Hemo-Cath LT	8	18	Yes	End ports	Silicone
Pediatric Split Cath	10	15	Yes	Split offset	Polyurethane
Mahurkar	8	9, 12, 15	No	Double-D	Polyurethane
Arrow	8	11	No	Coaxial	Polyurethane

Not all catheters may be available in all areas. In general a catheter at least 8Fr in size will provide better flow. Shorter lengths also reduce resistance as long as tip reaches superior vena cava-atrial junction at least. Cuff presence may be determined by expected length of treatment needed, although cuffed catheters may provide improved line survival (See text)

right internal jugular vein, and end just inside the atrium for the best chance at long-term success. Femoral catheters should be avoided if possible due to decreased longevity [23] and to prevent the risk to future transplant vascular access sites.

Uncuffed catheters may be used in the acute setting; however the duration of therapy is not always immediately obvious. Neonates pose a particular challenge with their relatively short necks and frequent manipulations in an intensive care setting. Therefore, a cuffed catheter may be the correct choice even for what appears to be an AKI. In a review of patients who were dialyzed (by HD alone or with PD) for at least 6 months, cuffed catheters lasted 5.7 ± 2.2 months versus only 1.3 ± 0.8 months for uncuffed catheters [20]. Medcomp (Harleysville, PA) and Cook Critical Care (Bloomington, IN) both make 7-French 10-cm uncuffed catheters. This catheter is still longer than these patients need, but shorter catheters are not commonly available. Medcomp also makes 8-French 12- and 18-cm catheters that could be used in children as small as 2.5–3 k as a source of chronic vascular access. Table 17.1 summarizes the catheters which are currently available.

The size of neonatal vessels relative to that of the cannulas, in conjunction with low blood flows, makes recirculation more likely. Mechanistically, using a double-lumen catheter with a distal end-hole return and a proximal side-hole arterial draw would appear to reduce this problem. Single-lumen access (using a Y-connector near the access point) has been proposed as an option to increase the available flow rate. A variable amount of recirculation (depending on the design of the tubing) will occur distal to the Y-connector. Limitations of this method include the need for a machine compatible with single-needle dialysis.

Two separate 5-French catheters in the umbilical veins have been used previously but have shown a higher complication rate, most likely due to the pliability of the catheters (personal experience).

Shunts and fistulas are not an option for a variety of reasons, but there was a report on three infants, with a maximum longevity of 60 days [26].

Lastly, there is no established cutoff on minimal size criteria for initiating HD, this decision depending more upon the patient's comorbidities, available surgical expertise, and familiarity of the dialysis staff. Babies as small as 1.6 kg have been reported although not with good outcomes [26].

Between treatments, the catheter should be closed with heparin (1,000 units/mL), 4 % sodium citrate, or tissue plasminogen activator (TPA, 1 mg/mL) to maintain patency [30]. Our practice is to reserve TPA for signs of catheter malfunction. The volume of the solutions is equal to the priming volume of each catheter lumen, which is often written on the hub. Only experienced dialysis personnel who know to withdraw the packing solution first, rather than flush the lines as other central lines are treated, should access these dialysis catheters under sterile conditions. Pushing these solutions into a neonate could have severe consequences. Some programs suggest "overfilling" the lumens by adding an additional 0.1–0.2 mL of the packing solution. However, we do not recommend this practice as this procedure could result in delivery of a significant drug dose unintentionally.

The dialysis catheter should not be used for any purposes other than dialysis to minimize infection or clotting complications that could impair proper blood flow. Only dialysis nurses or nephrologists familiar with these lines should access them.

17.5 Specifics of Hemodialysis

17.5.1 Dialysis Filters and Machines

A dialysis machine that accounts for the special needs of small infant patients is preferable and would include features such as proper pump speeds for small circuit lines and very tight tolerances on ultrafiltration errors. The latter concern can be a difference of as much as 50 mL/h, leading to possibly 150 mL over a 3-h treatment [6]. For a 3-kg infant, this would be 5 % difference and even larger in smaller patients. Volumetric ultrafiltration monitoring systems (which continuously monitor the actual volume removed rather than relying on calculated or expected volumes) reduce this error. All sources of fluid input (parenteral nutrition, intravenous fluids, gastric feeds, medications, etc.) and output (urine, nasogastric suction, diarrhea if very watery, surgical drains, blood draws, etc.) must be taken into account. The patient must be weighed using the same scale with as little external equipment, bedding, and clothing as possible just before and after each dialysis session. One must keep in mind that even "minimum UF" can be 100 ml/h, a significant amount for a baby.

The smallest artificial kidney currently available is the Gambro Polyflux 2H and has a priming volume of 17 mL and 0.2-m^2 triple-layer polymer surface; this product is not approved in the USA, however. The smallest one available in the USA is the Fresenius F3 and has a 24-mL priming volume with 0.4-m^2 surface area for contact using polysulfone fibers. These small-volume dialyzers are not high flux and rightly should not be, as the small ultrafiltration rates could lead to backflow of dialysate. The lowest priming volume for tubing is still 32 mL giving a total volume of 56 mL. At 80-mL/kg blood volume and a maximum of 10 % of this blood in the extracorporeal space, this means that the smallest patient on hemodialysis who would not need a blood prime would be 7 kg, which is well outside of the neonatal range. Therefore, to minimize antigen exposure from the blood primes, 1 unit of donor blood should be split and leukoreduced. The blood should be diluted from the baseline hematocrit of about 70–35 %. Depending on the storage time of the blood, significant amounts of potassium may be contained as well. Unless the patient needs to be transfused, the patient should not receive a "blood return" at the end of dialysis as this would give the patient the excess volume and red cells. If the transfusion is desired, it must be returned slowly (5–10 mL/min maximum) with close monitoring of hemodynamic changes from a rapid volume infusion. Development of a gallop rhythm warrants immediate cessation of blood flow and possibly removal of the excess volume [15]. The saline used to flush the blood out of the line can also constitute a large volume relative to the patient which must be accounted for in the ultrafiltration target. An air return, with a slow blood pump rate drawing in air instead of saline, would decrease the volume infusion, but extreme care must be taken to prevent air emboli.

Other considerations in neonates include settings on machines which are not adapted for low body weight patients. For example, until recently, the neonatal lines on the Gambro dialysis machine required a blood flow rate setting of four times the desired speed (i.e., setting the rate at 160 mL/min to achieve a true flow rate of 40 mL/min – this has since been remedied with a software upgrade). Heat loss is also of special concern due to the large proportion of extracorporeal volume and suboptimal thermoregulation in small infants. The dialysate temperature can be increased to compensate, but alternative methods must be used if the patient is running in ultrafiltration only mode.

A manual system that used two syringes to shift blood back and forth through the filter until adequate ultrafiltration was achieved was described in three infants under 1,000 g. However, all three infants died of comorbidities within 4 months [14]. The last report from this group was from 2007, at which time seven patients had been treated with this system for clearance needs as well [18, 19]. However, as of this writing there appear to be no further updates, and this mechanism has not been approved for use in the USA.

17.5.2 Water Supply

Regardless of the brand of dialysis equipment used for chronic or portable HD, the dialysate water supply must conform to standards set by the Association for the Advancement of Medical Instrumentation (AAMI). The details of these requirements are beyond the scope of this chapter, but the latest update from 2012 can be found and purchased on the AAMI website.

17.5.3 Prescriptions

The frequency of dialysis will be determined by the patient's needs. Polyuric renal failure may require less frequent dialysis (3–4 times a week for 3 h per session) for clearance rather than fluid removal. Anuric renal failure will likely require at least 4–5 sessions per week with longer runs each time. Determination of frequency and length of therapy should be based on solute clearance and fluid removal in the acute patient and proper growth in the chronic patient. Nutrition should never be decreased or withheld due to inadequate dialysis, but rather dialysis must be increased to meet nutritional demands.

Frequent if not constant vital signs monitoring in the form of temperature, heart rate, blood pressure, and pulse oximetry is essential. Neonates can suffer rapid heat loss from the extracorporeal volume. Supportive measures such as oxygen, ventilatory equipment, pressor agents, and isotonic or colloid fluids must be readily at hand to respond to hemodynamic changes. This generally means the procedure must be carried out in an intensive care setting. Staff familiar with neonatal signs of distress (heart rate changes, irritability, color changes, emesis) is needed.

17.5.4 Blood and Dialysate Flow Rates

Blood flow rates used have been reported at as high as 25–50 mL/min [35]. A blood flow rate of 20 mL/min was sufficient to achieve the targeted 15 mL/min of BUN clearance using older parallel-plate dialyzers [26]. A general guideline of at least 3–5 mL/kg/min blood flow rate can be used; however, a minimum of 20 mL/min may be needed to maintain circuit patency. Dialysate flow rates should be kept as low as possible (generally 500 mL/min) as this provides high clearance relative to the blood flow rates. Electrolyte composition will be determined by patient needs. Phosphorus may need to be added due to the blood flow/dialysate flow mismatch, and more frequent sessions are often needed.

17.5.5 Anticoagulation

Heparin can be of special concern in the premature population due to the risk of cerebral hemorrhage. Although the slow flow rates increase the risk of circuit clots, attempts can be made initially to run the dialysis using saline flushes only. When heparin is used, the dosing is 10–20 units/kg to load and then a maintenance dose of 10–20 units/kg/h depending on patient response on the circuit and bleeding risk factors. If heparin is contraindicated, regional anticoagulation with citrate, calcium-free dialysate, and a separate intravenous calcium infusion has also been used [27]. Target circuit post-filter ionized calcium levels have been reported to be less than 0.3 mM [27]. However, higher levels up to 0.5mM are used successfully in continuous veno-venous hemofiltration, which requires longer anticoagulation times and hence greater risk of circuit loss [5]. Therefore, if citrate is to be used, we recommend tolerating the higher target levels to decrease the risk of complications. Patient's ionized calcium levels should be kept in the 1.1- to 1.3-mM range. Certain centers have also rarely used calcium-free dialysate without citrate, as the latter is not always available. For any of these methods involving calcium manipulation, immediate ionized calcium level results must be available throughout the dialysis run to prevent dangerous systemic hypocalcemia. Lastly, anticoagulation is not always necessary; we have had success with chronic hemodialysis using only saline flushes (accounting for this volume in the UF) and a blood flow rate of 40 mL/min in a 4-kg patient.

17.5.6 Complications of Therapy

17.5.6.1 Clotting/Blood Loss

Despite the use of anticoagulation, blood volume can still be lost in clotted circuits. The frequency is not well reported. Given that most neonates require blood primes on circuits available at this time, this does not translate into worsening anemia necessarily but does increase antigen exposure and the possibility of catheter malfunction. Blood loss due to other aspects of HD care was estimated in chronic HD patients up to 1 year of age. The estimated residual blood volume in the circuit was 15.7 mL/kg/month. Higher heparin doses can decrease this residual. An additional 12.1 ± 5.9 mL/kg/month was lost due to blood draws. This led to an average transfusion rate of 25 ± 17 mL/kg/month in the first 3 months of therapy. These volumes decreased as patients grew and generally stabilized [20]. The use of erythropoiesis-stimulating agents has also decreased transformation needs.

Blood priming is of special concern for antigen exposure and dialysis management (see above in Dialysis Filters and Machines).

17.5.6.2 Disequilibrium and Hypotension

As for all dialysis patients, disequilibrium syndrome can be of concern, especially in the face of a small infant patient dialyzed against a filter and dialysate flow rate with a large (relative to the patient) clearance. Signs can include agitation, irritability, vomiting, or skin discoloration. A high-glucose (up to 700 mg/dL for BUN levels over 100 mg/dL) dialysate bath with a mannitol infusion (1 g/kg) was used to help prevent disequilibrium, and no apparent episodes were noted with this plan. Additionally, clearance was limited to 2–3 mL/min/kg of BUN to prevent rapid shifts [26].

Approximately 60–70 % of patients can have an episode of hypotension during a hemodialysis session [35]. Intradialytic hypotension may occur if the volume to be removed is greater than 5 % of the patient's weight. This risk can be reduced with the use of sodium modeling (increasing dialysate sodium concentration to as high as 150 mEq/L by the end of therapy) or the infusion of colloid such as mannitol (no more than once weekly) or albumin (remembering to account for these excess volumes in the targeted ultrafiltration). These measures can also help with disequilibrium [15].

17.5.6.3 Electrolytes

As with HD on any size patient, electrolyte abnormalities are a risk if there is a mistake or machine error in the dialysate bath. Contrary to older patients who generally need to be more severely restricted, infants often require higher levels of potassium, calcium, and phosphorus for growth. Renal dietary formulas tend to be low in these components. Phosphorus levels (obtained pre-dialysis), specifically were very dependent on food intake and binder use. A dialysate bath containing phosphorus has been recommended [26].

17.5.7 Outcomes

The outcome of infants initiating dialysis early in life is generally dismal and has not improved significantly over time. All nine patients in a series from 1973 died, of which only two were able to discontinue dialysis before dying of other causes. None of the deaths were attributed to the dialysis procedure; however, one patient died at the end of the first session, and intracranial hemorrhage ("of many days duration") was found on autopsy. Another died at the second session, no reason given. The three patients dialyzed for chronic kidney disease died after transplantation [26]. All five infants who were started on hemodialysis due to "medical ATN" from meconium aspiration, pneumonia, RSD, or cardiac abnormalities died in a 1978 case review [25].

When compared to patients who started dialysis at age 1–24 months in the self-reported NAPRTCS database, those who started dialysis under 1 month of age were slightly more likely to die (11 versus 8 %), less likely to be transplanted (46.5 versus 57.7 %), and more likely to recover native kidney function (15 versus 4 %). There was no difference in the hazard ratio for death or transplant when comparing patients from 1992 to1998 versus 1999 to 2005; there was a trend for patients of the more recent cohort to go to transplant slightly sooner, but the difference was not significant [13]. Again, these numbers do not give the complete picture due to the nature of the database, but 193 neonates were included in this review. In a much smaller series, during a follow-up of 3 years, only one of eight patients who initiated any dialysis in the first month of life received a kidney transplant but subsequently died. Five out of the eight patients died during a follow-up of 3 years. This was not significantly different from patients who initiated dialysis before 1 year of life [20].

17.5.8 Growth

Studies in older children have suggested that growth on PD is better than growth on HD [33]. However, long-term studies on patients initiating dialysis in infancy have not been done. No difference was observed in height and weight SDS changes between PD and HD in 6 months of follow-up [20]. Two out of nine patients in a prior series had dialysis long enough to study their growth and development. Both made gains but at significantly decreased rates from expected [26].

17.6 Specifics of Continuous Renal Replacement Therapy (CRRT)

17.6.1 CRRT Machines

CRRT is used in an ICU setting for critically ill infants. These machines can offer either convective clearance in CVVH mode (continuous veno-venous hemofiltration) or diffusive clearance in CVVHD mode (continuous veno-venous hemodialysis). Additionally, one can undergo both convective and diffusive clearance using CVVHDF, which is continuous veno-venous hemodiafiltration. The question of whether convective or diffuse clearance is better is an ongoing question. Work by Maxvold and colleagues in 2000 identified that clearance of small molecular weight proteins such as urea or citrate is identical whether one is in a convective or a diffusive mode [28]. High molecular weight or high-protein binding solutes have preferential clearance in convective versus diffusive mode. Studies by Flores and colleagues showed that in highly catabolic stem cell transplant patients, survival is improved with the use of convective clearance [21]. In unpublished studies by our group, we identified improved solute clearance of cytokines in convective versus diffusive mode.

Often the decision of convection or diffusion is made by available local solutions. Physiologic solutions have been bicarbonate based since 2000 in North America and have been used earlier throughout the world. In the USA, the Food and Drug Administration (FDA) identifies any medication that goes in the vascular space as a drug. Therefore, those solutions that are used in a convective mode whether it is pre-filter or post-filter are considered a drug. The FDA has then identified any medication that goes outside the vascular space as a device. Therefore, those solutions that are used as dialysate solutions are considered device. Experience has identified that the companies that make both convective and diffusive solutions have similar products with different labels. Both of these solutions are sterile and have physiologic levels of solute. Further, in the solutions that are used in the diffusive mode, one has to know there is some degree of back filtration at the level of the membrane; therefore, diffusive solutions will still enter the vascular space. Going back to the question of which is better, convection or diffusion, it may not only be based on the metabolic needs of the patient but also may be based on the clinical indication and local availability of solutions. Specifically in septic or otherwise highly catabolic patients, there is an advantage based on data mentioned above in the use of convective solutions. In patients with inborn errors of metabolism, no studies to date have identified whether diffusion or convection is superior to one or the other. Personal experience has identified that each of these are equal and therefore the modality does not matter.

17.6.2 Solutions Used for CRRT

As mentioned, since the year 2000, solutions are now available in the USA that are bicarbonate based. Historically, many programs used solutions mixed through in-house pharmacies instead of using industry-made solutions. Work by Barletta et al identified catastrophic complications including death using pharmacy-made solutions for CRRT [3]. Suspected causes may include repeated compounding in the pharmacy rather than batch processing from industry sources, increasing the number of possible chances for error. Given the immediate need of pharmacy solutions when ordered, there is also no confirmation testing of the products prior to use. Therefore, since the advent of industry-made solutions, pharmacy-made solutions should no longer be considered.

Many companies make both a convective and diffusive solution. Often the choice of the solution will be based on what type of anticoagulation is done. In patients receiving systemic heparinization, a normal physiologic calcium solution is reasonable. In patients receiving citrate anticoagulation, a zero-calcium solution is needed to avoid clotting of the circuit. As metabolic alkalosis is a possible complication of citrate use, a lower bicarbonate solution is preferable. Otherwise these solutions essentially contain a normal physiologic level of sodium, chloride, and magnesium, with bicarbonate levels ranging between 22 and 40 mEq/L. Specific compositions of the numerous solutions available can be obtained from each manufacturer.

The amount of potassium in the solution is based on the needs of the patient. In patients with intoxication or inborn error of metabolism, these patients need to have a normal physiologic potassium level. In patients with AKI, perhaps starting with a lower potassium bath initially and then adjusting up to normal physiologic potassium concentrations would be in order.

Presently, in the USA as well as many other parts of the world, phosphorus is not commonly placed in solutions by industry. Phosphorus over time is cleared very easily by CRRT; therefore replacing phosphorus either enterally, intravenously, or through the convective or diffusive mode is important. Personal experience for over a decade shows that one can place a potassium phosphate in a calcium-free bath either in a diffusive or convective mode in order to maintain physiologic levels of phosphorus and avoid hypophosphatemia.

17.6.3 Anticoagulation

Anticoagulation choices between heparin and citrate differ across programs. What is clear is that the smaller the child is, the smaller the vascular access becomes. The smaller vascular access is associated with slower blood flows; this in turn is associated with a higher incidence of clotting, and so maintaining proper anticoagulation becomes very important.

Heparin-based protocols have commonly been used for the last two decades. Heparin dosing has targeted an activated clotting time (ACT) of about 200 s on HD which is a common protocol also used in extracorporeal membrane oxygenation [8]. This requires a bolus of heparin typically at 20 units/kg per dose and a continuous infusion of heparin anywhere between 10 and 40 units/kg/h in order to target the same level of ACT. The benefit of heparin-based anticoagulation is the ease of its use. The risk is systemic heparinization to the patient. Historical adult-based protocols have used protamine post-filter pre-patient in order to rescue the patient from the anticoagulation. This not only resulted in no improvement of circuit life but also rebound hypercoagulability or hypocoagulability in the patient, causing more complications.

Since the early 2000s, these authors as well as others have developed the use of citrate anticoagulation used in infants and children [10]. Citrate protocols are based on giving citrate to chelate ionized calcium in the circuit, preventing the coagulation cascade. The target ionized calcium in the circuit is one-third of the normal physiologic level. Then calcium, preferably in the form of calcium chloride, is infused back to the patient separate from the dialysis catheter. The calcium is titrated back to the patient for physiologic normal levels. Table 17.2 provides a suggested titration protocol. The recommended starting rate for citrate is 1.5 times the blood flow rate but in mL per hour, e.g., for a blood flow rate of 100 mL/min, the initial citrate rate is 150 mL/h. Initiation of calcium chloride is 40 % the citrate rate; hence, for the current example, the calcium chloride would start at 0.4×150 mL/h which is 60 mL/h. Monitoring schedules vary but it is reasonable to check an initial ionized calcium within half an hour of starting the circuit to ensure that the patient is not becoming hypocalcemic. Further checks can then be spaced out to as far as every 4–6 h, depending on patient stability and whether any infusion rate adjustments have been needed.

This is now a common practice in up to 70 % of programs throughout North America. Younger patients often metabolize citrate poorly, leading to a higher risk of citrate accumulation. This may result in high physiologic levels of total calcium ("citrate lock") with rebound hypercalcemia as one discontinues CRRT, the citrate is broken down, and the calcium is released. Therefore, even in experienced hands, the use of citrate anticoagulation in premature infants, small infants, or those with liver dysfunction is very difficult requiring significant attention to detail. The additive advantage of citrate anticoagulation is the attention to maintaining an adequate ionized calcium to children, especially if they have some degree of cardiac compromise or sepsis. Calcium is a reasonable inotrope and can improve cardiac output.

Table 17.2 Citrate and calcium titration protocols

Titrate the citrate infusion according to the citrate sliding scale below:		
Prisma ionized Ca++ (mmol/L)	Citrate infusion adjustment >20 kg	<20 kg
<0.35	↓ rate by 10 ml/h	↓ rate by 5 ml/h
0.35–0.5 (optimum range)	No adjustment	
0.5–0.6	↑ rate by 10 ml/h	↑ rate by 5 ml/h
>0.6	↑ rate by 20 ml/h	↑ rate by 10 ml/h
Notify MD if citrate infusion rate >200 ml/h		
Titrate the calcium infusion according to the calcium sliding scale below:		
Patient ionized Ca++ (mmol/L)	Calcium infusion adjustment >20 kg	<20 kg
>1.3	↓ rate by 10 ml/h	↓ rate by 5 ml/h
1.1–1.3 (optimum range)	No adjustment	
0.9–1.1	↑ rate by 10 ml/h	↑ rate by 5 ml/h
<0.9	↑ rate by 20 ml/h	↑ rate by 10 ml/h
Notify MD if calcium infusion rate >200 ml/h		

Source: Pediatric Continuous Renal Replacement Therapy website (www.pCRRT.com). Used with permission

Studies by Brophy et al identified that citrate and heparin result in identical CRRT circuit life in older children [5]. There have been very limited experience and clearly no direct study using heparin versus citrate as a source of anticoagulation in infants to date. Therefore, each program will have to decide the best use of anticoagulation for the child.

17.6.4 CRRT Prescription

A prescription for CRRT for AKI is based on local standard of practice. Work by Maxvold and colleagues has suggested that a blood flow rate of roughly about 4 mL to 5 mL/kg/min along with either a diffusive or convective clearance at 2,000 mL/1.73 m^2/h would result in roughly about 30 % urea clearance [28]. Work by Ronco and colleagues in adults identified that 40 mL/kg/h of convective clearance results in improved survival in adults with AKI [34]. The 40 m/kg/h equates to roughly about 2,500 to 3,000 mL/1.73 m^2/h of either convective or diffusive clearance.

In reality, the optimal prescription is based on:

1. The blood flow. The blood flow is maximized based on the vascular access. The higher the blood flow, the less the likelihood of clotting. The higher blood flow will not result in hemodynamic compromise.
2. Whether one is using convective or diffusive clearance, one should target based on the catabolic needs of the patient. Thus, using 2,000 to 3,000 mL/1.73 m^2/h would be a reasonable starting point, and then one would titrate the solution exposure upward or downward based on the needs of the patient.

Net ultrafiltration rates are based on the hemodynamics of the patient. Classically, urine output is 0.5–2 mL/kg/h. If one uses that as the standard, then that may be a target that may be best obtained in the patient. This author's experience has suggested that for the first 6–12 if not 24 h of initiation of CRRT, the net ultrafiltration should be zero unless there is pulmonary compromise. This means that the ultrafiltration rate set should equal to the patient's hourly intake from medications and nutrition. This will allow for a maximal solute clearance and then slowly begin fluid removal as tolerated. Vasopressor agents may need to be increased or decreased based on the ultrafiltration needs of the patient. Therefore, many programs will increase the direct use of vasopressor agents as a way to support hemodialysis in order to "dry out" the patient.

17.6.5 Complications

Complications of CRRT in infants are similar to those in older children. This includes hypotension associated with the extracorporeal membrane. The hypotension can be associated with a large extracorporeal volume compared to the intravascular blood volume of the patient. Historically, in chronic hemodialysis, one was always taught not to have more than 10 % of blood extracorporeal to the patient. This data, which is no longer valid in the outpatient chronic hemodialysis world, has been extrapolated to the inpatient CRRT world. This comparison is not valid because one is comparing hemodynamically stable outpatients to hemodynamically unstable inpatients.

What is known is that the larger extracorporeal volume at the initiation of CRRT, the more chance of causing some degree of hypotension. Therefore, the use of blood priming may be necessary if one has 5, 10, 15, or even 20 % of blood volume extracorporeal. The use of blood priming is primarily based on the hemodynamics of the patient. The risks of blood priming are twofold. One is related to the acidotic, hypocalcemic, and hyperkalemic composition of the blood itself, and the second is the potential of a significant membrane reaction associated with the AN-69 membrane which is made by Gambro. A study by Brophy and colleagues identified that the acidotic milieu (pH of 6.2), elevated potassium (up to 40 mEq/L), and low ionized calcium (down to 0.02 mM due to the citrate to prevent clotting) of banked blood can interact with the AN-69 membrane and cause anaphylaxis when post-filter blood returns to the patient [4]. This is related to a pH-dependent bradykinin reaction. Studies by Brophy as well as Hackbarth have identified methods to avoid this reaction [24]. Other membranes such as polysulfone are not associated with these problems.

Other complications in children are related to thermic instability. Because of the large extracorporeal blood volume and the relatively slow blood flow rate, blood may be extracorporeal to the patient for 3–4 min. This allows for significant cooling and puts the child at risk for hypothermia and masking fevers.

The other two major complications of CRRT in infants are related to nutritional losses, as well as drug dosing. Maxvold and colleagues identified that roughly 15–35 % of parenteral TPN amino acids may be lost through CRRT [28]. Therefore, many programs including this author will titrate the protein load to keep the patient at a BUN of roughly 40–60 mg/dL. Experiences show that some infants require 8–9 g/kg/day of TPN protein in order to have a BUN of 20–30 mg/dL for adequate protein load. Work by Zappitelli and colleagues have identified that standard practice still usually orders about 2.5 g/kg/day, which is usually insufficient for children and even more so for infants on CRRT [38]. Further work by Zappitelli and colleagues has identified trace elements as well as vitamins being removed by CRRT system [39]. Therefore, overall attention to detail with nephrology input is very important to compensate for the nutritional stealing that occurs on the CRRT machine.

Medication dosing in children on CRRT is very difficult. Smaller molecular weight and less-protein-bound drugs have higher levels of clearance. Given the continuous nature of CRRT, however, many medications which do not fit that profile are still significantly cleared over time. To determine relative clearance on CRRT, vasopressor agent use and levels of antibiotics such as aminoglycosides or vancomycin can help. Vancomycin is about 1,500 Da and about 75 % protein bound. It is not unusual that infants or children on CRRT require normal dosing of vancomycin with normal kinetics. This experience with vancomycin then can allow one to identify how to dose other medications in general. Vasopressor agents such as epinephrine, norepinephrine, and dopamine have small molecular weight and are poorly protein bound. Therefore, it is imperative to know that at the initiation of CRRT, these medications are cleared quite rapidly and doses may need to be increased over time to give adequate hemodynamic control.

Lastly, the placement of vascular access in these children is important in relation to other points of access. If the tip of another central venous line delivering vasopressor agents is in immediate proximity to the CRRT dialysis catheter (as they often are due to the nature of these medications), there may be an immediate loss of these medications at the initiation of CRRT.

17.6.6 Tandem Therapies

Patients with inborn errors of metabolism can undergo hemodialysis or CRRT. Work by Picca and others has identified that optimally, hemodialysis and CRRT are superior to peritoneal dialysis for removal of ammonia [32]. Recent work by our group has identified the use of sequential hemodialysis followed by CRRT as the optimal way to take care of infants with inborn errors of metabolism [7]. Furthermore, a recent paper by Eding and colleague has identified the use of transitioning blood from the hemodialysis machine to the CRRT machine not only to avoid membrane reactions associated with AN-69 filters but also to avoid extra blood exposure to that patient [17]. In contrast to the dialysate used in AKI which may be low in phosphorus, and potassium, the bath used in inborn errors of metabolism needs to be physiologic.

Like intoxications, the duration for hemodialysis or CRRT in inborn error of metabolism would be targeted based on the clearance of ammonia. Recent studies identified that the "cocktail" that is used in the treatment of hyperammonemia is cleared easily on CRRT. Work done by McBryde and colleagues has shown that arginine is easily cleared [29]. Phenylacetate and benzoate are easily cleared on CRRT but not at the compromise of improving ammonia in the patient [7].

17.6.7 Outcome

There is a paucity of data on the outcome of infants on CRRT. Most studies combined modalities as well as patient ages, involving both pediatric and infant groups together [11, 12]. In a multicenter retrospective database study looking at survival in children less than 10 kg, there was an overall survival of 40 %. In those less than 3 kg, the mortality was roughly 25 %, pointing out that even in experienced hands, this is a very difficult population to effectively dialyze [36].

In essence, CRRT is a commonly used therapy in children with AKI and intoxications and less commonly used in infants. The typical difficulties are usually around the issues of vascular access and the complications related to a large extracorporeal circuit. Developments out of Europe identified smaller and smaller extracorporeal therapies for CRRT in infants perhaps making this an easier therapy to use in this population.

17.7 Social Supports

The importance of supporting the family during this time cannot be stressed enough. Caregivers must be careful not to impose their value system on families while at the same time guiding parents in what, for them, is an extraordinary situation that they have likely never prepared for. Given the complications and unsure outcomes discussed above, some families may choose never to start renal replacement therapy in the first place, and caregivers must be prepared to discuss and possibly accept these decisions with the family.

Conclusion

Neonatal renal replacement therapy using HD or CRRT has many indications and may need to be modality of choice for some ESRD patients. The prognosis remains grim for many of these patients, and much work remains to be done to improve their outcome. In the meantime, careful attention to detail regarding vascular access, location of therapy, core staff members, access placement, vigilant monitoring during each session, preparation ahead of time for possible complications, and the care and management of non-dialysis factors such as nutrition and family support are vital to increasing the chances of success for these vulnerable patients.

References

1. Askenazi DJ, Ambalavanan N et al (2009) Acute kidney injury in critically ill newborns: what do we know? What do we need to learn? Pediatr Nephrol 24(2):265–274
2. Barletta GM, Bunchman TE (2004) Acute renal failure in children and infants. Curr Opin Crit Care 10(6):499–504
3. Barletta JF, Barletta GM et al (2006) Medication errors and patient complications with continuous renal replacement therapy. Pediatr Nephrol 21(6): 842–845
4. Brophy PD, Mottes TA et al (2001) AN-69 membrane reactions are pH-dependent and preventable. Am J Kidney Dis 38(1):173–178
5. Brophy PD, Somers MJ et al (2005) Multi-centre evaluation of anticoagulation in patients receiving continuous renal replacement therapy (CRRT). Nephrol Dial Transplant 20(7):1416–1421
6. Bunchman TE (1995) Chronic dialysis in the infant less than 1 year of age. Pediatr Nephrol 9(Suppl): S18–22
7. Bunchman TE, Barletta GM et al (2007) Phenylacetate and benzoate clearance in a hyperammonemic infant on sequential hemodialysis and hemofiltration. Pediatr Nephrol 22(7):1062–1065
8. Bunchman TE, Donckerwolcke RA (1994) Continuous arterial-venous diahemofiltration and continuous veno-venous diahemofiltration in infants and children. Pediatr Nephrol 8(1):96–102
9. Bunchman TE, Ferris ME (2011) Management of toxic ingestions with the use of renal replacement therapy. Pediatr Nephrol 26(4):535–541
10. Bunchman TE, Maxvold NJ et al (2003) Pediatric convective hemofiltration: normocarb replacement fluid and citrate anticoagulation. Am J Kidney Dis 42(6):1248–1252
11. Bunchman TE, Maxvold NJ et al (1995) Continuous venovenous hemodiafiltration in infants and children. Am J Kidney Dis 25(1):17–21
12. Bunchman TE, McBryde KD et al (2001) Pediatric acute renal failure: outcome by modality and disease. Pediatr Nephrol 16(12):1067–1071
13. Carey WA, Talley LI et al (2007) Outcomes of dialysis initiated during the neonatal period for treatment of end-stage renal disease: a North American Pediatric Renal Trials and Collaborative Studies special analysis. Pediatrics 119(2):e468–473
14. Coulthard MG, Sharp J (1995) Haemodialysis and ultrafiltration in babies weighing under 1000 g. Arch Dis Child 73(3):F162–165
15. Donckerwolcke RA, Bunchman TE (1994) Hemodialysis in infants and small children. Pediatr Nephrol 8(1):103–106
16. Donn SM, Swartz RD et al (1979) Comparison of exchange transfusion, peritoneal dialysis, and hemodialysis for the treatment of hyperammonemia in an anuric newborn infant. J Pediatr 95(1):67–70
17. Eding DM, Jelsma LR et al (2011) Innovative techniques to decrease blood exposure and minimize interruptions in pediatric continuous renal replacement therapy. Crit Care Nurse 31(1):64–71
18. Everdell NL (2007) A haemodialysis system for the treatment of acute renal failure and metabolic disorders in neonates. Med Eng Phys 29(4):516–524
19. Everdell NL, Coulthard MG et al (2005) A machine for haemodialysing very small infants. Pediatr Nephrol 20(5):636–643
20. Feinstein S, Rinat C et al (2008) The outcome of chronic dialysis in infants and toddlers–advantages and drawbacks of haemodialysis. Nephrol Dial Transplant 23(4):1336–1345
21. Flores FX, Brophy PD et al (2008) Continuous renal replacement therapy (CRRT) after stem cell transplantation. A report from the prospective pediatric CRRT Registry Group. Pediatr Nephrol 23(4): 625–630

22. Gitomer JJ, Khan AM et al (2001) Treatment of severe theophylline toxicity with hemodialysis in a preterm neonate. Pediatr Nephrol 16(10):784–786
23. Hackbarth R, Bunchman TE et al (2007) The effect of vascular access location and size on circuit survival in pediatric continuous renal replacement therapy: a report from the PPCRRT registry. Int J Artif Organs 30(12):1116–1121
24. Hackbarth RM, Eding D et al (2005) Zero balance ultrafiltration (Z-BUF) in blood-primed CRRT circuits achieves electrolyte and acid-base homeostasis prior to patient connection. Pediatr Nephrol 20(9): 1328–1333
25. Hodson EM, Kjellstrand CM et al (1978) Acute renal failure in infants and children: outcome of 53 patients requiring hemodialysis treatment. J Pediatr 93(5): 756–761
26. Kjellstrand CM, Mauer SM et al (1973) Haemodialysis of premature and newborn babies. Proc Eur Dial Transplant Assoc 10:349–362
27. Kreuzer M, Ahlenstiel T et al (2010) Management of regional citrate anticoagulation in pediatric high-flux dialysis: activated coagulation time versus post-filter ionized calcium. Pediatr Nephrol 25(7):1305–1310
28. Maxvold NJ, Smoyer WE et al (2000) Amino acid loss and nitrogen balance in critically ill children with acute renal failure: a prospective comparison between classic hemofiltration and hemofiltration with dialysis. Crit Care Med 28(4):1161–1165
29. McBryde KD, Kudelka TL et al (2004) Clearance of amino acids by hemodialysis in argininosuccinate synthetase deficiency. J Pediatr 144(4):536–540
30. Moran JE, Ash SR (2008) Locking solutions for hemodialysis catheters; heparin and citrate–a position paper by ASDIN. Semin Dial 21(5):490–492
31. Msall M, Batshaw ML et al (1984) Neurologic outcome in children with inborn errors of urea synthesis. Outcome of urea-cycle enzymopathies. N Engl J Med 310(23):1500–1505
32. Picca S, Dionisi-Vici C et al (2001) Extracorporeal dialysis in neonatal hyperammonemia: modalities and prognostic indicators. Pediatr Nephrol 16(11): 862–867
33. Potter DE, San Luis E et al (1986) Comparison of continuous ambulatory peritoneal dialysis and hemodialysis in children. Kidney Int Suppl 19:S11–14
34. Ronco C, Bellomo R et al (2000) Effects of different doses in continuous veno-venous haemofiltration on outcomes of acute renal failure: a prospective randomised trial. Lancet 356(9223):26–30
35. Sadowski RH, Harmon WE et al (1994) Acute hemodialysis of infants weighing less than five kilograms. Kidney Int 45(3):903–906
36. Symons JM, Brophy PD et al (2003) Continuous renal replacement therapy in children up to 10 kg. Am J Kidney Dis 41(5):984–989
37. Wiegand C, Thompson T et al (1980) The management of life-threatening hyperammonemia: a comparison of several therapeutic modalities. J Pediatr 96(1):142–144
38. Zappitelli M, Goldstein SL et al (2008) Protein and calorie prescription for children and young adults receiving continuous renal replacement therapy: a report from the Prospective Pediatric Continuous Renal Replacement Therapy Registry Group. Crit Care Med 36(12):3239–3245
39. Zappitelli M, Juarez M et al (2009) Continuous renal replacement therapy amino acid, trace metal and folate clearance in critically ill children. Intensive Care Med 35(4):698–706

18 Peritoneal Dialysis in the Newborn

Joshua J. Zaritsky and Bradley A. Warady

Core Messages

- Peritoneal dialysis (PD) has long been considered an effective treatment modality for neonates with severe acute kidney injury (AKI) and is the modality of choice when treating neonates with end-stage renal disease (ESRD) needing chronic renal replacement therapy. Its popularity and success largely derive from its simplicity and effectiveness in even the smallest patients.
- A clear advantage of prompt PD initiation in cases of severe AKI and ESRD is the ability to help meet the nutritional demands of the neonate through the effective removal of solute and fluid. The substantial nutritional demands of this patient population are intended to address the marked increases in height, weight, and brain development that the neonate/young infant is experiencing in the setting of impaired kidney function.
- Historically, the morbidity and mortality rate of neonates treated with chronic PD has been quite poor, with the presence of nonrenal disease being the most important predictor of mortality. Over the last decade, however, there has been steady improvement in the quality and rate of patient survival with recent studies showing no differences in mortality rates between PD patients who initiated dialysis at less than 1 month old versus 2–24 months of age.

Case Vignette

A 38-week male infant is born and quickly intubated due to severe respiratory distress. The prenatal history is notable for oligohydramnios. On exam, the baby is noted to have a distended abdomen with absent abdominal musculature and undescended

J.J. Zaritsky
David Geffen School of Medicine at UCLA, Los Angeles, CA, USA
e-mail: jzaritsky@mednet.ucla.edu

B.A. Warady, MD (✉)
Department of Pediatrics, Children's Mercy Hospitals and Clinics, University of Missouri-Kansas City School of Medicine, Kansas City, MO 64108, USA

Pediatric Nephrology, Children's Mercy Hospitals and Clinics, 2401 Gillham Road, Kansas City, MO 64108, USA

Dialysis and Transplantation, Children's Mercy Hospitals and Clinics, 2401 Gillham Road, Kansas City, MO, 64108, USA
e-mail: bwarady@cmh.edu

A.S. Chishti et al. (eds.), *Kidney and Urinary Tract Diseases in the Newborn*,
DOI 10.1007/978-3-642-39988-6_18, © Springer-Verlag Berlin Heidelberg 2014

testes. An abdominal ultrasound reveals highly echogenic and small kidneys, characteristic of renal dysplasia, along with dilated ureters and a dilated bladder with a thickened wall.

Over the next 7 days, ventilatory support is able to be progressively decreased, but the infant is noted to develop progressive fluid overload despite the aggressive use of diuretics. Although nutrition has been limited due to fluid restriction, the infant is mildly hyperkalemic and hyperphosphatemic. The serum creatinine has been steadily rising and is currently 4.2 mg/dL. After consultation with the attending neonatologist and nephrologist, along with several members of the neonatal multidisciplinary team, the family agrees with plans to place a peritoneal dialysis catheter along with a gastrostomy tube and to initiate peritoneal dialysis.

18.1 Introduction

Peritoneal dialysis (PD) has long been considered an effective treatment modality for neonates with severe acute kidney injury (AKI) and is the modality of choice when treating neonates with end-stage renal disease (ESRD) needing chronic renal replacement therapy. Its popularity and success largely derive from its simplicity and effectiveness as a means of removing solute and fluid in even the smallest patients. In its most basic terms, the removal of plasma solutes (solute clearance) is achieved by diffusion of the solute down a concentration gradient between dialysate and blood and across the semipermeable peritoneal membrane. Fluid removal (ultrafiltration) is achieved by the osmolarity of the dialysate creating an osmotic gradient along which fluid moves across the membrane and is drained from the patient. Access for PD can be achieved easily and even emergently in the unstable patient with AKI at the bedside, and the continuous and gradual provision of both solute clearance and ultrafiltration aims to mimic the function of the native kidney.

18.2 The Acute Setting: Acute Kidney Injury

18.2.1 Etiology and Incidence of AKI and the Need for Acute Peritoneal Dialysis

There is limited literature documenting the etiology of AKI that results in the need for acute PD in the neonatal population. However, some generalizations can be made. In most cases, congenital malformations such as renal dysplasia or posterior urethral valves do not compromise kidney function so severely that dialysis is required in the newborn period. Instead, acquired renal disorders, usually related to perinatal asphyxia, hypoxia, sepsis, or hypovolemia, make up the majority of insults that mandate acute replacement therapy [1, 2]. Very rarely, acute vascular events such as renal artery or renal vein thrombosis are to blame but usually have to affect both kidneys to result in AKI requiring dialysis.

It its estimated that AKI severe enough to require dialysis occurs in less than 1 % of admissions to neonatal intensive care units [2, 3]. A retrospective, single-center study from Turkey found that 20 of 4,036 neonates (0.5 %) received PD [4]. Since the indication for PD in half of the cases was an inborn error of metabolism, the actual incidence of AKI resulting in PD was significantly lower. An older study from the same center found that 45 out 1,311 (3.4 %) neonates were diagnosed with AKI, with only 10 (0.7 %) requiring dialysis [5].

It is important to recognize that there will be variations in the etiology and incidence of AKI based on the institution, with more specialized centers likely seeing higher AKI rates and presumably higher utilization of dialysis due to surgical complications of extremely ill neonates. This is particularly evident in centers in which complex cardiac surgery is performed. One recent single-center retrospective study documented that 95 of 1,510 neonates (6.5 %) undergoing cardiac surgery had AKI that required PD [6]. In some centers, routine care of complex cardiac surgery cases includes the placement of a PD catheter in case dialysis is needed [7].

18.2.2 Indications for the Initiation of Acute PD

In general, most of the indications for acute PD in the neonatal period mirror that seen in older children (Table 18.1). Although the majority of cases of AKI can be managed conservatively, severe metabolic disturbances, particularly hyperkalemia that is not responsive to medical management, mandate prompt initiation of dialysis. Additionally, inborn errors of metabolism, which usually are not accompanied by AKI, can require dialysis for optimal management (see below). There is accumulating evidence that fluid overload in the setting of AKI is associated with adverse outcomes, particularly in the pediatric population [8–12]. A multicenter, prospective study of children demonstrated that the percent fluid accumulation prior to starting continuous renal replacement therapy (CRRT) was significantly lower in survivors versus non-survivors [11]. Although this has not been examined prospectively in the neonatal population, fluid overload in the neonate takes on special significance in the face of an often precarious respiratory status and may benefit from the early initiation of PD.

Table 18.1 Indications for dialysis in neonates

Volume overload
Hyperkalemia, hyperphosphatemia
Severe metabolic acidosis
Inborn errors of metabolism (hyperammonemia)
Uremia with encephalopathy or bleeding
Improved nutritional support

Additionally, PD can typically be performed safely and effectively in patients with cardiovascular instability as a result of the inherent gradual and continuous provision of both ultrafiltration and solute clearance characteristic of the procedure.

The shift in older children away from PD and toward CRRT is likely the result of improved CRRT techniques and technology [13, 15]. However, the small blood volume of neonates can present a challenge, despite the use of current day CRRT devices. The use of a blood prime of the extracorporeal circuit is regularly required to initiate therapy, and maintenance of a complication-free central venous access can be problematic. Additionally, outcomes associated with the use of CRRT in this age group, although consistent over the past decade, remain significantly lower than in older children with patients <3 kg tending to have a particularly poor survival [16, 17]. Finally, PD offers the additional advantage of not requiring systemic anticoagulation, in contrast to hemodialysis (HD) and CRRT .

Despite these technical challenges, CRRT and HD are viable alternative acute renal replacement therapy options and in most situations, provide superior clearance of metabolic toxins such as ammonia in neonates with inborn errors of metabolism [18, 19]. Additionally, there are rare absolute contradictions to PD in neonates such as omphalocele, diaphragmatic hernia, or gastroschisis, all scenarios in which there is essentially the lack of a functional peritoneal cavity. Relative contraindications to PD include the presence of severe pulmonary disease since the increased intra-abdominal pressure associated with PD could further compromise pulmonary function [20] or a history of extensive abdominal surgery because of the possibility of adhesions and

18.2.3 Peritoneal Dialysis as a Renal Replacement Modality for AKI

Peritoneal dialysis has long been considered an effective dialysis modality in the setting of AKI. Despite the growing popularity of CRRT, survey results of pediatric nephrologists provide evidence that PD remains the predominant dialysis modality for children <2 years of age [7, 13]. As mentioned above, access can be placed emergently at the bedside in patients who are too unstable to undergo a surgical procedure [6, 14].

a compromised peritoneal cavity. The presence of a vesicostomy or colostomy or the diagnosis of polycystic kidney disease is not a contraindication [21]. With these issues in mind and given the lack of prospective trials comparing the outcomes of neonates with AKI stratified by dialysis modality, the decision regarding dialysis modality selection always needs to factor in local resources and expertise along with the patient's clinical status.

18.2.4 Peritoneal Dialysis Access in AKI

The two most commonly placed accesses for acute PD are the percutaneously placed Cook catheter and the surgically placed Tenckhoff catheter (Figs. 18.1 and 18.2). The Cook catheter offers the advantage of bedside placement by a nephrologist or intensivist via the Seldinger technique. Since only local anesthesia is required, it can be placed promptly, even in an unstable patient [14, 22]. However, its use is hampered by a very high rate of complications such as leakage of dialysis fluid from the catheter entry site on the abdominal wall and obstruction. Chadha et al. [23], in a single-center retrospective study of infants and young children with AKI, found that by day 6 of dialysis, only 46 % of Cook catheters were functioning without complications. In comparison, they found that over 90 % of surgically placed Tenckhoff catheters were free of complications at the same time point. Thus, the authors suggested that if dialysis is expected to be required for more than 5 days, either a Tenckhoff catheter should be placed initially or elective replacement of the Cook catheter with a Tenckhoff catheter be performed in a timely manner. Recently, a multipurpose percutaneous catheter (Cook Mac-Loc multipurpose drainage catheter) showed promising results in a small cohort of infants with AKI with a mean complication-free survival of approximately 11 days [22]. It continues to be used with good success at one of the author's centers; additional data on this experience is forthcoming.

Methods to decrease the risk of dialysate leakage are particularly important when dialysis is to be initiated emergently, soon after placement of the access. There is preliminary evidence that the application of fibrin sealant (glue) at the peritoneum can be used to treat leaks that occur soon after placement of a Tenckhoff catheter and the implementation of PD. Rushoven et al. demonstrated in eight infants, ages 0.8–57 months, that fibrin glue applied to part of the subcutaneous catheter tunnel through the exit site, as close to the cuff as possible, was able to successfully treat leaks that occurred within 48 h of starting therapy while using a single-cuff straight Tenckhoff catheter [24]. Additionally, Sojo et al. were able to show in an open-label, prospective randomized study that application of

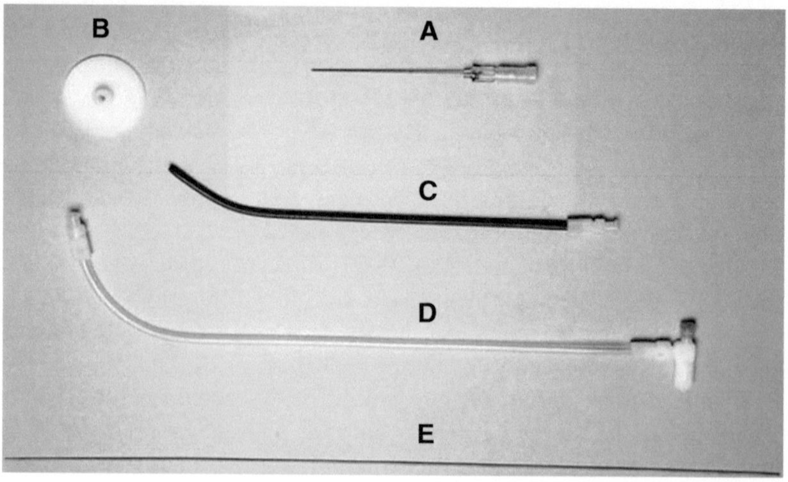

Fig. 18.1 A Cook catheter set for PD, inserted by the Seldinger (guidewire) technique. (*A*) Needle for insertion of the guidewire. (*B*) Flange for securing the catheter to the abdominal wall. (*C*) Catheter. (*D*) Tube for attaching the catheter to the dialysis set. (*E*) Guidewire (Reprinted from Haycock [2], Copyright 2003, with permission from Elsevier)

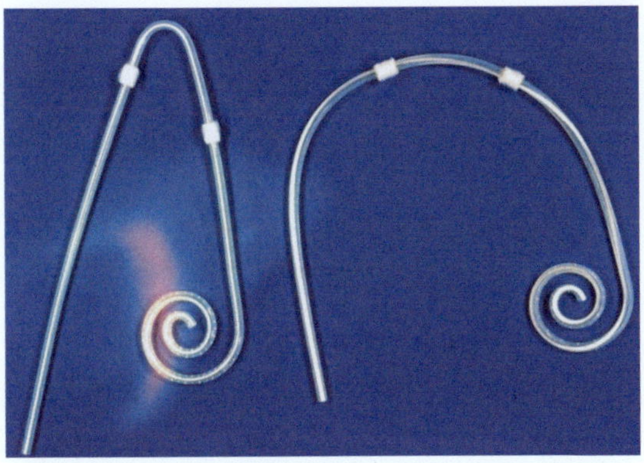

Fig. 18.2 Tenckhoff catheters

fibrin glue to the peritoneal cuff suture at time of implantation reduced the incidence of leakage in the early postoperative period [25]. Dialysate leakage only occurred in 9 % of the fibrin glue group versus 57 % of the control group.

The most important consideration for the successful placement and function of a Tenckhoff catheter in the neonate is the experience of the surgeon [26]. This can be particularly problematic at centers caring for a small number of patients overall, where the need to provide dialysis to a very young infant may be a rare event. Because of the importance of the access and the desire for the outcome of placement to be complication-free, the surgical placement should be limited to only a few surgeons per center, and on rare occasion, it may be preferable to refer the patient to another, more experienced center for access placement, in a manner similar to what has been recommended for vascular access [27].

There are a variety of configurations of neonatal-sized Tenckhoff catheters available from several manufactures (Baxter, USA; Medionics, Canada; Covidien, USA). Although there is limited data available to permit determination of the "best" configuration, data from the North American Pediatric Renal Trials and Collaborative Studies (NAPRTCS) pertaining to chronic PD suggests that a dual-cuffed, swan-neck (allows for downward facing exit site) catheter is associated with a reduction in infectious complications compared to other catheter configurations (see below) [28].

18.2.5 Prescription Considerations for AKI

In the acute setting, the prescription of PD is guided by the need for low dialysate exchange volumes to prevent dialysate leakage and to keep the intraperitoneal pressures as low as possible to avoid any respiratory embarrassment [20]. Typically, initial dialysis exchange volumes should be 10–20 mL/kg body weight (300–600 mL/m^2) and are increased as clinically warranted and tolerated. Because these low volumes result in a rapidly diminished osmotic gradient and resultant limited ultrafiltration, dwell times of one hour or less are frequently utilized. Dwell times as short at 20 min have also been used in neonates when rapid removal of small solutes is desired [29]. Despite the inefficiency introduced by using low dialysate volumes, adequate solute clearance and ultrafiltration rates can be achieved if exchanges are performed around the clock. Golej et al. [30] reported a case series of 116 neonatal and pediatric patients who underwent low-volume PD in whom the mean ultrafiltration rate was 2.8 mL/kg/h. A negative fluid balance was accomplished in 53 % of patients, despite the presence of hemodynamic instability in a majority of the subjects. Several patients with hyperkalemia and metabolic acidosis did require the use of higher dwell volumes to adequately control the biochemical abnormalities.

In extreme cases of hyperphosphatemia or hyperammonemia, continuous-flow PD (CFPD) has been employed [31, 32]. CFPD requires placement of two intraperitoneal catheters, with one catheter used for influx and another for efflux of dialysate. In this manner, the transport potential of the peritoneal membrane is maximized by maintaining the highest possible solute concentration gradient. Dialysate flow rates of up to 300 mL/h in patients as small as 3 kg have been described using this technique [31].

The lower dialysate dwell volume employed in the neonate generally necessitates the use of manual exchanges early in the course of PD in contrast to an automated cycling device. Advantages of manual exchanges include the low expense and technical simplicity. Neonatal or

PICU nurses can be trained rapidly to perform manual exchanges which avoids the need for a dialysis nurse to continuously supervise therapy. Indeed, the combination of simplicity, low cost, and efficacy makes PD with the use of manual exchanges in the neonatal setting an attractive option for centers with limited resources. There are several commercially available manual exchange sets (Baxter, USA; Fresenius, USA; Gesco International, USA; Medionics International, CA; Utah Medical Products, USA) which minimize the risk of contamination and allow for the warming of dialysate before it is instilled into the patient.

In contrast to manual exchanges, there are automated cyclers that permit the accurate delivery of an exchange volume as low as 60 mL with low-flow drainage modes to avoid unnecessary alarms (Home Choice Pro, Baxter). Practically, automated peritoneal dialysis (APD) can be performed using the cycling device without a substantial recirculation volume in the dialysis tubing when the exchange volume is more than 100 mL. The volume of tubing to the patient using a "low-volume" set is approximately 19 ml.

Standard commercially available dialysate solutions are employed in the acute setting with the choice of dextrose concentration [1.5, 2.5, or 4.25] driven by the need for ultrafiltration. The choice of PD solutions is also largely dependent upon their availability in different regions of the world. In the United States, only lactate-buffered solutions are available, whereas bicarbonate-buffered solutions, which are presumably more biocompatible, are available in Europe and other geographic regions. Lactate-based solutions should be avoided in neonates with severe acidemia as lactate needs to be converted by the liver to the effective base. Thus, if PD is to be used in a neonate with severe acidosis in the USA, the local hospital pharmacy will often provide a custom dialysate solution which is bicarbonate based. Vigilance with respect to monitoring the accuracy of the electrolyte content of pharmacy-made solutions is mandatory if severe disturbances (e.g., hypo- or hypernatremia) are to be prevented.

In the acute setting, there are no definitive parameters for determining the "adequacy of dialysis" in terms of solute or fluid removal. Given that these patients are rarely in a steady state and tend to be hypercatabolic, the utility of urea kinetic modeling (Kt/V) is questionable and has not been validated. Since there are no consensus recommendations on what levels of solute (e.g., urea, creatinine) removal are adequate or optimal when treating patients with AKI, there has been a tendency to fall back on recommendations for patients on chronic PD in some centers [33, 34]. However, adequacy in the acute setting is primarily based upon the ability to achieve fluid and electrolyte balance while ideally having the capacity to provide the patient with their required medications and nutrition. Whether or not the fluid targets recently recognized to be associated with improved outcomes in the treatment of AKI in older children are applicable to the neonatal population will require further study [8–10].

18.2.6 PD Complications and Outcome in AKI

Despite significant advances in care, morbidity remains high in neonates receiving acute PD. Most complications seen early in the course of dialysis are technical in nature, such as catheter malfunction and/or dialysate leakage which predisposes the patient to infectious complications such as catheter-related infections and peritonitis. As mentioned above, the complication rate is highest with temporary catheters, effectively limiting their use to no more than a 6-day period. Other less frequent surgical complications can include bowel perforation, hemoperitoneum, or hydrothorax [6]. Rarely but more commonly in the neonate versus older children, metabolic complications such as hyperglycemia (due to the use of dextrose as the osmotic agent in the dialysate), hypokalemia, and hyponatremia can occur and require early correction.

Published data describing outcomes in neonates receiving PD for treatment of AKI is sparse and is limited to single-center reports. Given the considerable variation in patient characteristics, etiology of renal disease, indications for dialysis, and dialysis methodology, it is not surprising that reported outcomes describe a wide range of mortality rates from 35 to 73 % [30, 35]. There is recent evidence which suggests that the timing of PD initiation may affect outcome. In a single-center report, Bojan et al. found that the initiation of PD within 1-day post-cardiac surgery in infants (including 1,510 neonates) with AKI was associated with a 40 % decrease in mortality when compared to the outcome of patients who initiated PD later [6]. Finally, there have not been any prospective trials comparing outcomes with different dialysis modalities in neonates or older children with severe AKI.

18.3 The Chronic Setting: ESRD

18.3.1 Incidence and Etiology of ESRD in Neonates/Infants

Despite an increased awareness of the capacity to care for neonates with end-stage renal disease (ESRD), the need for long-term renal replacement therapy (RRT) in this age group, which consists almost universally of chronic peritoneal dialysis, remains rare. Actual neonatal incidence data regarding the use of PD is limited with much of the published data examining the management of ESRD patients in the broader age range of birth to 24 months. Carey et al. [36] using data from the dialysis registry of the NAPTRCS estimated an incidence of only 0.045 cases of dialysis-treated neonates with ESRD per million population per year or 0.32 cases per 100,000 live births. This is substantially lower than the overall incidence of ESRD during the first 4 years of life as the United States Renal Data System (USRDS) reported an incidence of approximately ten cases per million population in the 0–4-year age group over the last decade [37]. This difference likely reflects the fact that the most common cause of chronic kidney disease in the neonatal period (see below), congenital renal dysplasia, does not typically compromise kidney function so severely that dialysis is required in the newborn period. The incidence of ESRD resulting in chronic dialysis in the neonatal age group also appears to vary regionally with a recent report of the International Pediatric Peritoneal Dialysis Network (IPPN) suggesting that centers in low-income countries (gross national income <$12,000) offer PD to fewer young patients, with only 8 % of their dialysis patients being <3 years old [38].

Table 18.2 Diagnosis of neonates with ESRD

Diagnosis	*n* (%)
Renal dysplasia	72 (37.3)
Obstructive uropathy	39 (20.2)
ARPKD	23 (11.9)
Congenital nephrotic syndrome	3 (1.5)
Other	56 (29)

Adapted from Carey et al. [36]

The list of disorders that result in kidney disease requiring chronic dialysis in the neonatal period is short. In the cohort of neonatal patients ($n = 193$) examined by Carey et. al., the most frequent renal disorders resulting in the need for chronic dialysis were congenital renal hypoplasia/dysplasia and obstructive uropathy (e.g., posterior urethral valves) [28, 36] (Table 18.2). Similarly, Warady and Martz reviewed the causes of ESRD in 85 neonates who were entered into the NAPRTCS database from 2000 to 2010 and found the same two diagnoses predominant [39]. These and other structural abnormalities of the urinary tract account for nearly 60.0 % of cases of neonatal dialysis, with the next most common diagnosis being polycystic kidney disease. Compared to relatively older infants and children (1–24 months of age at dialysis initiation), Carey et al. found a reduced incidence of congenital nephrotic syndrome (1.5 % vs. 10.7 %) in the group of neonates who received dialysis.

18.3.2 Ethical Considerations

Clearly, one of the most difficult issues that families and pediatric nephrology teams are confronted with is the decision regarding when and if chronic dialysis therapy should be initiated for the neonate with ESRD. Despite advances in dialysis technology and clinical expertise that now makes it possible to provide dialysis to this patient population safely and effectively, the concept of proceeding with a lifetime of ESRD care is unavoidably complex. Comorbidities such as neurocognitive delay, growth delay, and the almost universal need for supplemental tube feeding and multiple hospitalizations contribute to the ethical dilemma experienced by many. Often complicating the situation is the presence of significant nonrenal abnormalities, such as pulmonary hypoplasia, which are present in up to one-third of infants with ESRD and which are associated with an increased risk for mortality [40]. In fact, the mortality rate of the youngest infants (0–2 years) who have received chronic dialysis has historically been quite poor, with 2-year mortality rates as high as 30 %; however, more recent data has revealed significantly better outcomes (see below) [36, 41].

In adult patients, the four principles of medical ethics, autonomy, beneficence, non-maleficence, and justice, are characteristically applied to decisions on whether to withhold or withdraw dialysis [42]. However, in the case of infants, the wishes of the parents, who are entitled to make decisions on the medical care their children receive, must also be taken into consideration. This ethical dilemma is not all that uncommon in the neonatal intensive care unit and occurs in other situations, such as in the case of the neonate with hypoplastic left heart syndrome [43, 44]. Ideally, the decision of whether to provide or withhold dialysis represents a consensus opinion of the parents, nephrologist, neonatologist, and other members of a multidisciplinary team, determined only after a thorough review of the patient's status and the family's status is conducted, along with a review of the limited data that exists within the medical literature on the outcome of young infants with ESRD. Despite the best efforts to this end, there remains substantial potential for disagreement regarding the best course of action to take because of the multiple patient and social factors that often exist, along with the different prior experiences of health-care team members with similar patient scenarios. All of this can result in an emotionally charged environment. It is, nonetheless, most desirable for all nephrology team members that are involved in the patient's care to have the opportunity to weigh in on the decision process. Whereas the nephrology team and family members most often come to a conclusion that is agreeable to all, on occasion, a hospital ethics committee may be consulted for their opinion.

More than a decade ago, Geary and colleagues surveyed the opinions of pediatric caregivers from around the globe regarding the decision process surrounding the initiation of chronic dialysis in infants <1 year of age [45]. In that survey, a substantial percentage (50 %) of physicians responded that it was usually acceptable for parents to refuse dialysis for children less than 1 month of age in contrast to the situation when children were 1–12 months of age at presentation, at which time dialysis refusal was less acceptable. Factors felt to be most influential by the physicians with respect to their opinions regarding withholding dialysis were the presence of "coexistent serious medical abnormalities" and the "anticipated morbidity for the child." As a follow-up to that survey, Teh et al. and many of the same authors recently reported on the results of a similar multination survey of both nephrologists and nurses on this topic to determine if the perspectives of health-care providers had changed over the subsequent decade in association with the advances in care that had taken place and additional personal and published experiences [46]. Of note, only thirty percent (30 %) of the 270 nephrologists indicated that they offer chronic dialysis therapy to all children less than 1 month of age and 50 % to all children aged 1–12 months. The figure of 30 % was decreased from the figure of 41 % reported in the prior survey. Ninety-eight percent of physicians who responded to the recent survey stated they would offer dialysis to some infants less than 1 month of age compared to 93 % 10 years ago. In the recent assessment, a minority of physicians (27 %) believed that the parents should not be given the option to refuse dialysis for infants less than 1 month of age, a figure which increased to 50 % for children aged 1–12 months. Not surprisingly and as was reported in the initial survey, the most influential factor on the decision to not offer dialysis was the presence of a coexisting nonrenal abnormality. One additional and potentially troubling finding in terms of generating the all important consensus within the health-care team was the presence of significant differences in the responses of physicians and nurses with respect to dialysis initiation in the neonate. Specifically, nurses were more likely to consider the presence of oliguria or anuria as a contraindication to initiating dialysis, and they placed more emphasis on the parent's right to decide.

The topic of ethics is undoubtedly in need of additional study, supported by the accumulation of data from clinicians and affected family members. The influence of advances in dialysis care, more recent data on short- and long-term patient outcomes, and cultural differences must be considered in any future analysis.

18.3.3 Peritoneal Dialysis as a Renal Replacement Modality for ESRD

Many of the same considerations that favor PD as a renal replacement modality for AKI apply in the setting where long-term dialysis is needed. The high rates of both infectious and mechanical complications of HD when provided to the youngest infants make its use over long periods of time impractical in most situations. For patients receiving HD for extended periods, access revision rates for young infants are estimated at 40 % [47]. Couple these issues with recognition that long-term HD access in a neonate consists of a central venous catheter, a practice that is accompanied by a significant potential for stenosis of central veins and the resultant inability to create a fistula in the future for patients who face a lifetime of ESRD care, one can fully understand the preferential selection of PD as the chronic dialysis modality for neonates/infants.

Chronic PD is particularly advantageous compared to HD for the neonatal patient for reasons other than access. Meeting the nutritional needs of neonates can be challenging, especially with the severely oliguric/anuric patient who must receive formula volumes as high as 150 mL per kg of body weight per day. The relative ease with which the fluid status can be managed with PD on a daily basis precludes the fluctuations of body volume and potentially, blood pressure inherent to intermittent HD. Multiple studies have also suggested that better growth rates can be achieved in patients on PD compared to HD [48–50]. Current NAPRTCS data does show improvements in height SDS scores at 24 month follow-up of patients who initiated PD at less than 1 year of age, while SDS scores remain unchanged for those on HD [51]. Finally, PD promotes gradual expansion of the abdominal cavity in preparation for successful renal transplantation. This takes on added importance when one considers that although transplantation is the ideal renal replacement therapy for children, technical aspects limit the feasibility of the procedure in the first year of life. Thus, dialysis is used as a bridge to successful early transplantation with PD the modality of choice.

18.3.4 Peritoneal Dialysis Access for ESRD

Long-term PD mandates the surgical placement of a Tenckhoff catheter. As with AKI, the most important consideration for its successful placement and function in the neonate is the experience of the surgeon [26]. If complications such as dialysate leakage are to be avoided, placement of the catheter 2–3 weeks before its eventual use is ideal. The provision of fibrin sealant at the peritoneum as a means of achieving a tight closure when a delay in PD initiation is not possible has been practiced, as discussed above. Additional considerations in the chronic setting are the orientation of the subcutaneous tunnel of the catheter, the exit-site orientation and location, the potential need for an omentectomy, and the timing of placement with respect to concurrent or future placement of a gastrostomy tube (G-tube).

Observational data from the NAPRTCS suggests that Tenckhoff catheters with a downward pointed exit site are associated with the best peritonitis rates, a characteristic (along with the possible preference for two cuffs) that should be considered for all PD catheters placed in infants and young children because of their increased rates of peritonitis compared to older children [28, 52]. The catheter exit site should also be placed outside of the diaper area and away from any potential ostomy site with the superficial cuff located approximately 2 cm from the skin surface [28, 52]. Occasionally, this necessitates placement of the exit site in the chest wall [53]. Given the small size of the neonatal/infant patient, these requirements can be difficult to accommodate and, as noted above, require a very skilled and experienced surgeon.

One somewhat controversial aspect of Tenckhoff catheter placement is the decision of whether to routinely perform an omentectomy. A survey of pediatric surgeons indicated that an omentectomy is performed routinely in 53 % of pediatric centers at the time of PD catheter placement [54]. The basis for its performance in children is that catheter obstruction (usually due to the presence of omentum in the holes of the dialysis catheter) is second only to peritonitis in terms of major catheter complications in this age group [55]. Ironically, although children appear to be at higher risk for omental obstruction compared to adults, most of the data in support of omentectomy comes from the adult literature [56]. There are no well-designed studies in neonates/infants/children addressing this topic. One retrospective study of children by Cribs et al. did demonstrate a decrease risk of early catheter failure in patients who underwent an omentectomy at the time of catheter placement, and Rinaldi et al. noted improved catheter survival (especially in children <2 years) in association with a higher frequency of omentectomy based on data collected by the Italian Registry of Pediatric Chronic Peritoneal Dialysis [57, 58]. Additionally, in a retrospective study of 92 pediatric patients (mean age 5 years), Conlin et al. demonstrated that the rate of outflow obstruction was 5 % in patients who received an omentectomy versus 10 % in patients who did not [59]. In contrast, however, Lewis et al. calculated that 11 omentectomies would be required to prevent two omental PD catheter obstructions [60].

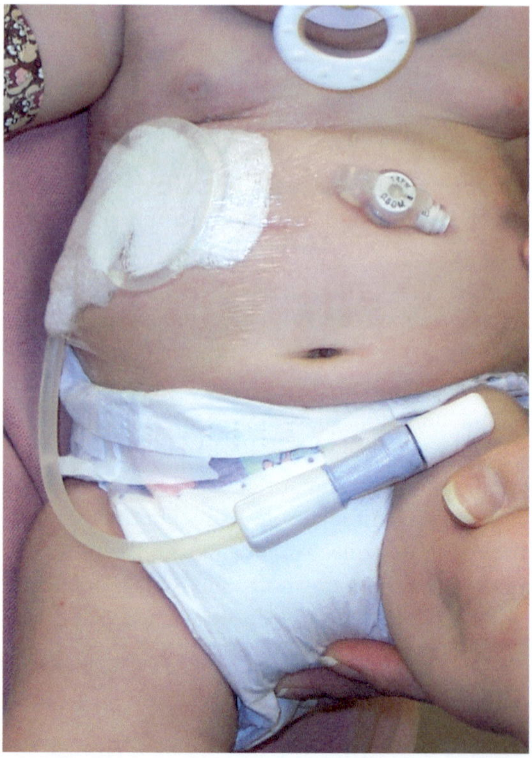

Fig. 18.3 Ideal placement of a PD catheter with G-tube on contralateral side

As suggested above, one additional unique consideration in the neonatal age group is the timing and location of catheter placement relative to G-tube placement in order to accommodate nutritional requirements (see below). The catheter exit site should ideally be placed at a distance (often the contralateral side) from the site of a current or potential gastrostomy to decrease the risk of contamination and possible peritonitis (Fig. 18.3). Likewise, it is recommended that when possible, the PD catheter be placed either simultaneously with or after placement of a G-tube to avoid contamination of the peritoneum from gastric contents concurrent with the use of dextrose containing dialysate [52, 61]. When the catheter placement precedes G-tube placement, the latter procedure should take place under prophylactic antibiotic and antifungal therapy.

18.3.5 Prescription Considerations in ESRD

Historically, the prescription of PD in infants was based on the perception that the pediatric peritoneal membrane, especially in infants, had different solute transport properties than that of an adult. This was in large part based on the results of early studies in which dialysis exchange volumes were based on body weight. When scaled to body weight, the surface area of the infant peritoneal membrane is almost twice that of a 70 kg adult. Thus, the use of weight-based volumes results in a relatively low fill volume which, in turn, results in more rapid solute equilibrium and the inaccurate perception of an inherent increased solute transport capacity. In contrast, the provision of an exchange volume in young children scaled to body surface area (BSA) takes into consideration the age independent relationship of BSA to peritoneal surface area and makes possible the accurate assessment of membrane transport capacity. Indeed, when Warady et al. based fill volumes on BSA, peritoneal membrane transport capacity in children was similar across the pediatric age range and to adults [62].

Thus, the prescribed exchange volume for the neonate on PD should be scaled to BSA rather than weight in order to avoid the use of a small volume which could lead to rapid solute equilibration and resultant inadequate ultrafiltration. Equally important is the need not to provide too large a volume that may lead to an excessive increase in intraperitoneal pressure (IPP) (>18 cm H_2O) [63]. The latter development can result in reduced dialysis efficiency due to enhanced lymphatic uptake, in addition to poor tolerance by the patient [64–66]. Accordingly, the recommended maintenance exchange volume for patients below the age of 2 years is limited by patient tolerance and is generally 600–800 mL/m^2 [67]. This is in contrast to a volume of approximately 1,200 mL/m^2 that is recommended for older children and adolescents [67]. As mentioned earlier, a smaller, manually delivered volume is typically used when the neonate is started on dialysis and is progressively increased to the limits noted above.

In the chronic setting, an initial empiric dwell time of 1 h is often used in infants, although consideration has to be made for clearance of larger molecules which would be favored by longer dwell times. Phosphate removal is less of a consideration in these patients compared to older children, as neonates characteristically receive formula with a low phosphorus content or breast milk and may actually require supplemental phosphorus. As in older children and adults, the final determination of dwell time should take into account the characteristics of the individual's peritoneal membrane via standardized testing of solute transport capacity (peritoneal equilibration testing), as well as clinical and laboratory measures of dialysis adequacy [68].

As in the acute setting, the choice of PD solutions is largely dependent upon their availability. Despite the lack of firm data, there is a concern that the standard lactate-buffered solutions with glucose may have negative consequences on long-term membrane performance due to their low pH and the presence of glucose degradation products (GDPs). Given that these patients have many years of ESRD therapy in their future, the use of the new, more biocompatible dialysis solutions may prove to be particularly beneficial to the pediatric patient population [69]. Data in neonates and young children on the subject is very limited (see Canepa et al. for a recent review [70]).

Icodextrin (Extraneal®), a colloidal osmotic agent that is employed in place of dextrose, is available in the USA in contrast to other new solutions but is rarely used in infants. Whereas Boer et al. showed that in 11 children (median age 10.3 years) a 12-h exchange with 7.5 % icodextrin produced ultrafiltration comparable to a 3.86 % dextrose solution [71], Dart et al. reported poor ultrafiltration in very young children (median age 2.8 years) with its use [72]. This poor efficacy was due to enhanced absorption of icodextrin across the peritoneal membrane with half of the patients showing substantial absorption even when dwell times were reduced from

10 to 6 h. Van Hoeck also noted that the use of a long exchange with icodextrin could place a child into a negative amino acid balance [73].

As in the acute setting, it can be difficult to precisely determine the efficiency or "adequacy" of dialysis with chronic PD. Although small molecule clearance measurements in the form of urea kinetic modeling (Kt/V_{urea}) are widely used, it must be emphasized that the current National Kidney Foundation K/DOQI guidelines on PD adequacy which recommend a total Kt/V_{urea} of ≥1.8 for children are largely opinion based. Because a large, prospective study correlating solute removal and clinical outcome in pediatric patients treated with PD has not been conducted [67], care must always be taken to individualize therapy, even in cases of "adequate" or even high urea clearance. This is particularly true for the neonatal/infant patient population. Parameters that should be taken into consideration include linear growth and weight gain, increase in head circumference, and neurocognitive/psychomotor development. Additional qualitative targets of dialysis adequacy are the avoidance of hypovolemia and sodium depletion (see below), because of their significant influence on growth [74].

18.3.6 Nutrition in the Neonate with ESRD

In the setting of ESRD, the provision of adequate nutrition takes on particular importance because the neonatal period is typically characterized by accelerated brain growth and a very high linear growth rate of nearly 25 cm/year. Remarkably, ½ of postnatal brain growth takes place in the 1st year of life, and 1/3 of the normal final adult height is achieved during the initial 2 years of life [75, 76].

Infants with ESRD can lose more than 2 SD of height and forever impact their final height if their clinical status is compromised by suboptimal care and/or complications of their disorder [77, 78]. One single-center retrospective study by Karlberg et al. of 71 children with early-onset ESRD found that one-third of the reduction in height occurred during the first postnatal months [78]. There is also data linking poor growth with mortality in children with ESRD. Both Wong et al. and Furth et al. demonstrated an independent association between a decrease in height standard deviation score and an increased risk of death, with impaired growth likely serving as a surrogate of overall well-being [79, 80].

Table 18.3 Recommended parameters and frequency of nutritional assessment for neonates and infants with ESRD

Measure	Minimal interval (months)
Dietary intake	0.5–2
Height or length velocity-for-age percentile or SDS	0.5–1
Height or length-for-age percentile or SDS	0.5–1
Estimated dry weight and weight for age	0.25–1
BMI-for-height-age percentile or SDS	0. 5–1
Head circumference-for-age percentile or SDS	0.5–1

Adapted from KDOQI Work Group [74]

Most noteworthy is the fact that this early period of growth is primarily dependent upon the provision of optimal nutrition, with the growth hormone/insulin-like growth factor (IGF) axis having less importance when compared to later in life. Updated KDOQI pediatric nutrition guidelines have recently been published that provide recommendations for the monitoring of growth and nutritional status in infants/young children with CKD (Table 18.3) and recommend that patients with ESRD receive 100 % of the estimated energy requirements (EER) for chronological age, with adjustments based on changes in either weight or linear growth [74, 81].

There are several additional nutritional considerations that need to be addressed when PD is conducted. Specifically, neonates and infants can experience excessive losses of protein via PD with studies demonstrating average losses of 250 mg of protein per Kg of body weight or almost twice the peritoneal protein losses seen in older children [82]. In order to avoid the negative consequences of protein depletion, current guidelines recommend an allowance for protein of 1.8 g/kg/day for the first 6 months of life, taking into account the dietary reference intakes (DRI) and peritoneal losses [74]. Of note, protein losses can be higher with the use of alternative PD regimens such tidal PD [34].

Infants receiving PD also experience excessive sodium losses across the peritoneal membrane due to the need for high ultrafiltration rates in relation to body weight. Both breast milk and standard formulas contain 7–8 mmol of sodium per liter which is inadequate for replacement of ongoing losses. Without adequate supplementation (~3–5 mEq/kg/day), the consequences of the resultant hyponatremia and low intravascular volume can be catastrophic and include both blindness due to anterior ischemic optic neuropathy and cerebral edema [83, 84].

In most cases, the nutritional targets defined by the guidelines for neonates on PD are not achievable without the implementation of either nasogastric (NG) or gastrostomy tube feeding. Children with ESRD suffer from poor appetite and early satiety that may be, in part, due to elevated circulating cytokines [85, 86]. No doubt, the generation of increased intraperitoneal pressure secondary to the presence of dialysis fluid also plays a role. Compounding the problem is a high rate of poor gastrointestinal motility and gastroesophageal reflux which can lead to the loss of up to 1/3 of feedings via emesis [47, 86–88]. In turn, the provision of nocturnal feedings by slow, continuous drip per tube along with intermittent bolus feedings during the day is very often required to meet the nutritional goals (Table 18.4).

Data from single-center studies have repeatedly shown that tube feeding facilitates both weight gain and growth. Ramage et al. demonstrated that the use of enteral feedings in eight infants receiving PD arrested the decline in height SDS traditionally reported [89]. Similarly, Ledermann et al. demonstrated that enteral feeding resulted in significant improvements in weight, height, and head circumference SDS at both 1 and 2 years of age in 12 infants receiving PD [49]. Kari et al., in a review of 81 tube-fed infants with a GFR less than 20 mL/min/1.73 m^2 during the first 6 months of life or placed on dialysis during the first 2 years of life, found that 81 % achieved a normal height SDS after 1 year of follow-up [77]. Subsequent evaluation of this same population 10 years later revealed that the intensive feeding regimen combined with early transplantation resulted in a normal mean adult height in those patients without comorbidities [90]. Data from the International Pediatric Peritoneal Dialysis Network (IPPN) have recently provided further evidence of the benefit of supplemental tube feedings in terms of height and weight gain in children <2 years and on PD, with marked global variation in the use of tube feedings during infancy [91].

Historically, NG tubes were preferentially used because of the simplicity of placement (although not necessarily simple from the perspective of the parent and patient) and with no disruption of any ongoing PD. However, frequently associated complications of this approach to therapy, in addition to the unsightly appearance, include recurrent emesis, nasal trauma associated with tube replacement, and inhibition of the normal development of oral motor skills [92–94]. The latter problem needs to be addressed with oral and occupational therapy. On the other hand, gastrostomy tubes/buttons, which were championed early on by Watson and Coleman, are not as frequently associated with the development of altered oral motor skills, are not regularly associated with emesis, and are not visible. They also offer the advantage of being available for prolonged use into the post-renal transplant period where they can be essential to ensure proper hydration and enhance medication administration in the young infant [95]. It is for these reasons that gastrostomy tubes/buttons have supplanted NG tubes as the preferred route of enteral tube support in many centers.

Table 18.4 Suggested rates for initiating and advancing tube feedings for neonates and infants with ESRD

Method	Initial hourly infusion	Daily increases	Goal
Continuous feedings	1–2 mL/kg/h	1 mL/kg/h	6 mL/kg/h
Bolus feedings	10–15 mL/kg/feed	20–40 mL q 4 h	20–30 mL/kg/feed

Adapted from KDOQI Work Group [74]

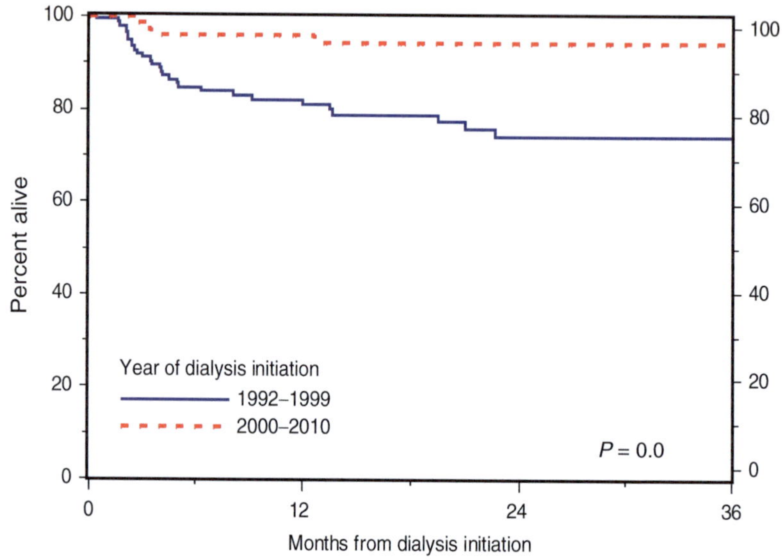

Fig. 18.4 Neonatal patient survival during initial course of dialysis (From Warady and Martz [39])

As mentioned above, a G-tube should ideally be placed prior to or simultaneously with placement of the PD catheter. Ideally, percutaneous placement while on PD should not be performed due to the high risk of infection and mechanical failure [96]. Placement via an open Stamm gastrostomy procedure in the patient already on PD is, however, possible if sufficient precautions are taken, specifically the use of prophylactic antibiotic and antifungal therapy. Conversely, PD catheter placement is possible in the setting of a well-established G-tube with no increased risk of bacterial or fungal peritonitis [49, 97, 98].

18.3.7 Complications and Outcome in ESRD

Even with surgically placed Tenckhoff catheters, chronic catheter survival remains suboptimal. Data from the Italian PD registry reported a 50 % 1-year catheter survival rate in patients less than 6 months of age versus an 83.7 % 1-year catheter survival rate for those 6–24 months of age [58]. Infectious complications including exit-site infections and peritonitis also occur at a higher rate in neonates. While peritonitis rates for patients 0–2 years of age have improved from an annualized rate of 1–0.79 over the last decade, they remain higher than the rate of 0.6 seen in older children [28, 99, 100].

Much of the limited data on the outcome of neonates with ESRD treated with dialysis comes from the analysis of the NAPRTCS database by Carey et al. of 193 infants who initiated dialysis at <1 month of age [36]. As noted above, the vast majority of these infants were treated with PD (98 %). The most frequent cause of dialysis termination in this cohort was renal transplantation (46 %). Termination due to death or recovery of renal function accounted for 10.8 and 14.6 % of patients, respectively. A more recent report of NAPRTCS data from 2000 to 2010 identified 85 neonates who initiated dialysis at <30 days of life. In comparison to Carey et al., there were a similar percentage of patients who terminated dialysis due to transplant (45 %), but termination due to death or recovery of renal function was 4.7 and 8.2 %, respectively [39]. Infant (0–1 year at dialysis initiation) survival during their initial course of dialysis was significantly improved compared to historical data with a 3-year patient survival of 86.6 % (personal communication, K. Martz). Neonatal patient survival during the initial course of dialysis was >90 % at 3 years and significantly greater than the experience a decade earlier ($p>0.002$) (Fig. 18.4). Finally, two recent studies have shown no differences in mortality rates between PD patients who initiated dialysis

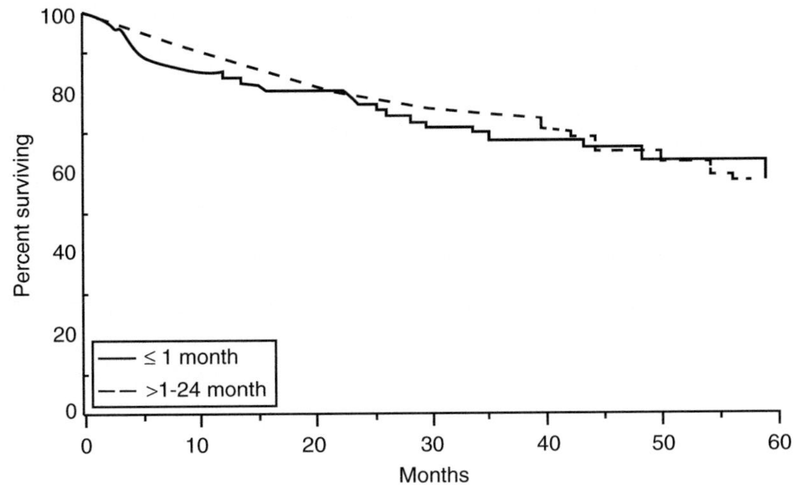

Fig. 18.5 Kaplan-Meier survival curve for neonates versus older children. Both groups had similar survival within 5 years of dialysis initiation (Carey et al. [36], Copyright 2007 by the AAP)

at less than 1 month old versus 2–24 months of age [36, 101] (Fig. 18.5). Importantly, this data is complemented by the fact that the transplant outcome of our young patients is the best among the pediatric population with a 10-year survival of 86.5 and 80.6 % for those transplanted at ages <1 or 1–5 years, respectively [102]. What persists, however, is the finding that the most important predictor of mortality in this PD patient age group remains the presence of nonrenal disease [77, 103–105]. Wood et al. clearly showed that comorbidities such as anuria, pulmonary hypoplasia, and severe development delay were associated with the greatest risk of mortality in infants undergoing dialysis [103]. A recent publication of the IPPN examining 1,830 patients aged 0–19 years found that the presence of at least one comorbidity was associated with a 4-year survival of 73 % versus 90 % survival in those without a comorbidity ($p<0.001$) [40]. Data on the influence of comorbidities on survival is likely impacted by regional difference as countries with a lower gross national income appear to be more restrictive in terms of making PD available to very young patients and those with significant extrarenal complications [38].

Conclusion

The last two decades have witnessed tremendous advances in the care of the neonate requiring renal replacement therapy. Peritoneal dialysis, due to its simplicity and effectiveness, remains a popular modality for neonates with severe AKI and is the dialytic modality of choice when treating neonates with ESRD. There have been notable improvements in patient survival, although complications remain high, especially in those infants with comorbidities. Thus, dialysis initiation must also factor in ethical considerations. All of these issues highlight the need for a multifaceted approach to care to minimize or prevent complications and in turn promote growth, development, and readiness for transplant.

References

1. Gouyon JB, Guignard JP (2000) Management of acute renal failure in newborns. Pediatr Nephrol 14(10–11):1037–1044
2. Haycock GB (2003) Management of acute and chronic renal failure in the newborn. Semin Neonatol 8(4):325–334
3. Askenazi DJ, Ambalavanan N, Hamilton K, Cutter G, Laney D, Kaslow R, Georgeson K, Barnhart DC, Dimmitt RA (2011) Acute kidney injury and renal replacement therapy independently predict mortality in neonatal and pediatric noncardiac patients on extracorporeal membrane oxygenation. Pediatr Crit Care Med 12(1):e1–e6
4. Unal S, Bilgin L, Gunduz M, Uncu N, Azili MN, Tiryaki T (2012) The implementation of neonatal peritoneal dialysis in a clinical setting. J Matern Fetal and Neonatal Med 25(10):2111–2114

5. Agras PI, Tarcan A, Baskin E, Cengiz N, Gurakan B, Saatci U (2004) Acute renal failure in the neonatal period. Ren Fail 26(3):305–309
6. Bojan M, Gioanni S, Vouhe PR, Journois D, Pouard P (2012) Early initiation of peritoneal dialysis in neonates and infants with acute kidney injury following cardiac surgery is associated with a significant decrease in mortality. Kidney Int 82:474–481
7. Kidney Disease: Improving Global Outcomes (KDIGO) Acute Kidney Injury Work Group (2012) KDIGO clinical practice guideline for acute kidney injury. Kidney Int 2(Suppl. 2012):1–138
8. Arikan AA, Zappitelli M, Goldstein SL, Naipaul A, Jefferson LS, Loftis LL (2011) Fluid overload is associated with impaired oxygenation and morbidity in critically ill children. Pediatr Crit Care Med 13(3):253–258
9. Goldstein SL (2009) Overview of pediatric renal replacement therapy in acute kidney injury. Semin Dial 22(2):180–184
10. Goldstein SL, Devarajan P (2012) Pediatrics: acute kidney injury leads to pediatric patient mortality. Nat Rev Nephrol 6(7):393–394
11. Sutherland SM, Zappitelli M, Alexander SR, Chua AN, Brophy PD, Bunchman TE, Hackbarth R, Somers MJ, Baum M, Symons JM, Flores FX, Benfield M, Askenazi D, Chand D, Fortenberry JD, Mahan JD, McBryde K, Blowey D, Goldstein SL (2011) Fluid overload and mortality in children receiving continuous renal replacement therapy: the prospective pediatric continuous renal replacement therapy registry. Am J Kidney Dis 55(2):316–325
12. Payen D, de Pont AC, Sakr Y, Spies C, Reinhart K, Vincent JL (2008) A positive fluid balance is associated with a worse outcome in patients with acute renal failure. Crit Care 12(3):R74
13. Warady BA, Bunchman T (2000) Dialysis therapy for children with acute renal failure: survey results. Pediatr Nephrol 15(1–2):11–13
14. Bunchman TE (1996) Acute peritoneal dialysis access in infant renal failure. Perit Dial Int 16(Suppl 1):S509–S511
15. Goldstein SL (2011) Continuous renal replacement therapy: mechanism of clearance, fluid removal, indications and outcomes. Curr Opin Pediatr 23(2):181–185
16. Zobel G, Ring E, Kuttnig M, Grubbauer HM (1991) Five years experience with continuous extracorporeal renal support in paediatric intensive care. Intensive Care Med 17(6):315–319
17. Symons JM, Brophy PD, Gregory MJ, McAfee N, Somers MJ, Bunchman TE, Goldstein SL (2003) Continuous renal replacement therapy in children up to 10 kg. Am J Kidney Dis 41(5):984–989
18. Picca S, Dionisi-Vici C, Abeni D, Pastore A, Rizzo C, Orzalesi M, Sabetta G, Rizzoni G, Bartuli A (2001) Extracorporeal dialysis in neonatal hyperammonemia: modalities and prognostic indicators. Pediatr Nephrol 16(11):862–867
19. Wong KY, Wong SN, Lam SY, Tam S, Tsoi NS (1998) Ammonia clearance by peritoneal dialysis and continuous arteriovenous hemodiafiltration. Pediatr Nephrol 12(7):589–591
20. Bunchman TE, Meldrum MK, Meliones JE, Sedman AB, Walters MB, Kershaw DB (1992) Pulmonary function variation in ventilator dependent critically ill infants on peritoneal dialysis. Adv Perit Dial 8:75–78
21. Geary DF, Schaefer F (2008) Comprehensive pediatric nephrology. Mosby/Elsevier, Philadelphia, xvii, 1099 p
22. Auron A, Warady BA, Simon S, Blowey DL, Srivastava T, Musharaf G, Alon US (2007) Use of the multipurpose drainage catheter for the provision of acute peritoneal dialysis in infants and children. Am J Kidney Dis 49(5):650–655
23. Chadha V, Warady BA, Blowey DL, Simckes AM, Alon US (2000) Tenckhoff catheters prove superior to cook catheters in pediatric acute peritoneal dialysis. Am J Kidney Dis 35(6):1111–1116
24. Rusthoven E, van de Kar NA, Monnens LA, Schroder CH (2004) Fibrin glue used successfully in peritoneal dialysis catheter leakage in children. Perit Dial Int 24(3):287–289
25. Sojo ET, Grosman MD, Monteverde ML, Bailez MM, Delgado N (2004) Fibrin glue is useful in preventing early dialysate leakage in children on chronic peritoneal dialysis. Perit Dial Int 24(2):186–190
26. Watson AR, Gartland C (2001) Guidelines by an Ad Hoc European Committee for elective chronic peritoneal dialysis in pediatric patients. Perit Dial Int 21(3):240–244
27. NKF-K/DOQI Clinical Practice Guidelines for Vascular Access: update 2000. Am J Kidney Dis, 2001. 37(1 Suppl 1):S137–S181
28. Annual Report of the North American Pediatric Renal Trials and Collaborative Studies (NAPRTCS) (2008) [cited 7/9/2010]. Available from https://web.emmes.com/study/ped/annlrept/Annual%20Report%20-2008.pdf
29. Alarabi AA, Petersson T, Danielson BG, Wikstrom B (1994) Continuous peritoneal dialysis in children with acute renal failure. Adv Perit Dial 10:289–293
30. Golej J, Kitzmueller E, Hermon M, Boigner H, Burda G, Trittenwein G (2002) Low-volume peritoneal dialysis in 116 neonatal and paediatric critical care patients. Eur J Pediatr 161(7):385–389
31. Kostic D, Rodrigues AB, Leal A, Metran C, Nagaiassu M, Watanabe A, Ceccon ME, Tannuri U, Koch VH (2010) Flow-through peritoneal dialysis in neonatal enema-induced hyperphosphatemia. Pediatr Nephrol 25(10):2183–2186
32. Arbeiter AK, Kranz B, Wingen AM, Bonzel KE, Dohna-Schwake C, Hanssler L, Neudorf U, Hoyer PF, Buscher R (2010) Continuous venovenous haemodialysis (CVVHD) and continuous peritoneal dialysis (CPD) in the acute management of 21 children with inborn errors of metabolism. Nephrol Dial Transplant 25(4):1257–1265
33. McNiece KL, Ellis EE, Drummond-Webb JJ, Fontenot EE, O'Grady CM, Blaszak RT (2005)

Adequacy of peritoneal dialysis in children following cardiopulmonary bypass surgery. Pediatr Nephrol 20(7):972–976
34. Chitalia VC, Almeida AF, Rai H, Bapat M, Chitalia KV, Acharya VN, Khanna R (2002) Is peritoneal dialysis adequate for hypercatabolic acute renal failure in developing countries? Kidney Int 61(2):747–757
35. Flynn JT (2002) Choice of dialysis modality for management of pediatric acute renal failure. Pediatr Nephrol 17(1):61–69
36. Carey WA, Talley LI, Sehring SA, Jaskula JM, Mathias RS (2007) Outcomes of dialysis initiated during the neonatal period for treatment of end-stage renal disease: a North American Pediatric Renal Trials and Collaborative Studies special analysis. Pediatrics 119(2):e468–e473
37. Atlas of ESRD: United States Renal Data System (USRDS) (2010) [cited 7/8/2010]. Available from http://www.usrds.org/2010/pdf/v2_08.pdf
38. Schaefer F, Borzych D, Azocar M, Munarriz RL, Sever L, Aksu N, Barbosa LS, Galan YS, Xu H, Cocia PA, Szabo A, Wong W, Salim R, Vidal E, Pottoore S, Warady BA (2012) Impact of global economic disparities on practices and outcomes of chronic PD in children: insights from the International Pediatric Peritoneal Dialysis Network (IPPN) Registry. Perit Dial Int 32:399–409
39. Warady BA, Martz K (2011) Providing or withholding dialysis for neonates: a report of the NAPRTCS. Presented at the Pediatric Academic Societies annual meeting, Denver
40. Neu AM, Sander A, Borzych-Dużałkac D, Watson AR, Vallése PG, Ha IS, Patel H, Askenazi D, Bałasz-Chmielewskac I, Lauroneni J, Groothoffj JW, Feber J, Schaefer F, Warady BA (2012) Co-morbidities in chronic pediatric peritoneal dialysis patients: a report of the International Pediatric Peritoneal Dialysis Network (IPPN). Perit Dial Int 32:410–418
41. Brunner FP, Fassbinder W, Broyer M, Oules R, Brynger H, Rizzoni G, Challah S, Selwood NH, Dykes SR, Wing AJ (1988) Survival on renal replacement therapy: data from the EDTA Registry. Nephrol Dial Transplant 3(2):109–122
42. Beauchamp TL, Childress JF (2001) Principles of biomedical ethics, 5th edn. Oxford University Press, Oxford/New York, xi, 454 p
43. Mavroudis C, Mavroudis CD, Farrell RM, Jacobs ML, Jacobs JP, Kodish ED (2011) Informed consent, bioethical equipoise, and hypoplastic left heart syndrome. Cardiol Young 21(Suppl 2):133–140
44. Zeigler VL (2003) Ethical principles and parental choice: treatment options for neonates with hypoplastic left heart syndrome. Pediatr Nurs 29(1):65–69
45. Geary DF (1998) Attitudes of pediatric nephrologists to management of end-stage renal disease in infants. J Pediatr 133(1):154–156
46. Teh JC, Frieling ML, Sienna JL, Geary DF (2011) Caregivers' attitude to management of end-stage renal disease in infacbrsnts. Perit Dial Int 31:459–465
47. Rees L (2007) Long-term peritoneal dialysis in infants. Perit Dial Int 27(Suppl 2):S180–S184
48. Kaiser BA, Polinsky MS, Stover J, Morgenstern BZ, Baluarte HJ (1994) Growth of children following the initiation of dialysis: a comparison of three dialysis modalities. Pediatr Nephrol 8(6):733–738
49. Ledermann SE, Spitz L, Moloney J, Rees L, Trompeter RS (2002) Gastrostomy feeding in infants and children on peritoneal dialysis. Pediatr Nephrol 17(4):246–250
50. Shroff R, Wright E, Ledermann S, Hutchinson C, Rees L (2003) Chronic hemodialysis in infants and children under 2 years of age. Pediatr Nephrol 18(4):378–383
51. Annual Report of the North American Pediatric Renal Trials and Collaborative Studies (NAPRTCS) (2011) [cited 6/20/2012]. Available from https://web.emmes.com/study/ped/annlrept/Annual%20Report%20-2008.pdf
52. Warady BA, Bakkaloglu S, Newland J, Cantwell M, Verrina E, Neu AM, Chadha V, Yap H, Schaefer F (2012) Consensus guidelines for the prevention and treatment of catheter-related infections and peritonitis in pediatric patients receiving peritoneal dialysis: 2012 update. Perit Dial Int 32:S32–S86
53. Chadha V, Jones LL, Ramirez ZD, Warady BA (2000) Chest wall peritoneal dialysis catheter placement in infants with a colostomy. Adv Perit Dial 16:318–320
54. Neu AM, Kohaut EC, Warady BA (1995) Current approach to peritoneal access in North American children: a report of the Pediatric Peritoneal Dialysis Study Consortium. Adv Perit Dial 11:289–292
55. White CT, Gowrishankar M, Feber J, Yiu V (2006) Clinical practice guidelines for pediatric peritoneal dialysis. Pediatr Nephrol 21(8):1059–1066
56. Nicholson ML, Burton PR, Donnelly PK, Veitch PS, Walls J (1991) The role of omentectomy in continuous ambulatory peritoneal dialysis. Perit Dial Int 11(4):330–332
57. Cribbs RK, Greenbaum LA, Heiss KF (2010) Risk factors for early peritoneal dialysis catheter failure in children. J Pediatr Surg 45(3):585–589
58. Rinaldi S, Sera F, Verrina E, Edefonti A, Gianoglio B, Perfumo F, Sorino P, Zacchello G, Cutaia I, Lavoratti G, Leozappa G, Pecoraro C, Rizzoni G (2004) Chronic peritoneal dialysis catheters in children: a fifteen-year experience of the Italian Registry of Pediatric Chronic Peritoneal Dialysis. Perit Dial Int 24(5):481–486
59. Conlin MJ, Tank ES (1995) Minimizing surgical problems of peritoneal dialysis in children. J Urol 154(2 Pt 2):917–919
60. Lewis MA, Smith T, Postlethwaite RJ, Webb NJ (1997) A comparison of double-cuffed with single-cuffed Tenckhoff catheters in the prevention of infection in pediatric patients. Adv Perit Dial 13:274–276

61. Rees L, Brandt ML (2010) Tube feeding in children with chronic kidney disease: technical and practical issues. Pediatr Nephrol 25(4):699–704
62. Warady BA, Alexander SR, Hossli S, Vonesh E, Geary D, Watkins S, Salusky IB, Kohaut EC (1996) Peritoneal membrane transport function in children receiving long-term dialysis. J Am Soc Nephrol 7(11):2385–2391
63. Fischbach M, Desprez P, Terzic J, Lahlou A, Mengus L, Geisert J (1996) Use of intraperitoneal pressure, ultrafiltration and purification dwell times for individual peritoneal dialysis prescription in children. Clin Nephrol 46(1):14–16
64. Durand PY (2000) Optimization of fill volumes in automated peritoneal dialysis. Perit Dial Int 20(6):601–602
65. Fischbach M, Terzic J, Menouer S, Bergere V, Ferjani L, Haraldsson B (2000) Impact of fill volume changes on peritoneal dialysis tolerance and effectiveness in children. Adv Perit Dial 16:321–323
66. Fischbach M, Terzic J, Menouer S, Haraldsson B (2000) Optimal volume prescription for children on peritoneal dialysis. Perit Dial Int 20(6):603–606
67. Clinical practice recommendations for peritoneal dialysis adequacy. Am J Kidney Dis, 2006. 48(Suppl 1):S130–S158
68. Golper TA (2001) A summary of the 2000 update of the NKF-K/DOQI clinical practice guidelines on peritoneal dialysis adequacy. Perit Dial Int 21(5):438–440
69. Fischbach M, Warady BA (2009) Peritoneal dialysis prescription in children: bedside principles for optimal practice. Pediatr Nephrol 24(9):1633–1642; quiz 1640, 1642
70. Canepa A, Verrina E, Perfumo F (2008) Use of new peritoneal dialysis solutions in children. Kidney Int Suppl 108:S137–S144
71. de Boer AW, Schroder CH, van Vliet R, Willems JL, Monnens LA (2000) Clinical experience with icodextrin in children: ultrafiltration profiles and metabolism. Pediatr Nephrol 15(1–2):21–24
72. Dart A, Feber J, Wong H, Filler G (2005) Icodextrin re-absorption varies with age in children on automated peritoneal dialysis. Pediatr Nephrol 20(5): 683–685
73. van Hoeck KJ, Rusthoven E, Vermeylen L, Vandesompel A, Marescau B, Lilien M, Schroder CH (2003) Nutritional effects of increasing dialysis dose by adding an icodextrin daytime dwell to Nocturnal Intermittent Peritoneal Dialysis (NIPD) in children. Nephrol Dial Transplant 18(7):1383–1387
74. KDOQI Work Group (2009) KDOQI Clinical Practice Guideline for Nutrition in Children with CKD: 2008 update. Executive summary. Am J Kidney Dis 53(3 Suppl 2):S11–104
75. Reed RB, Stuart HC (1959) Patterns of growth in height and weight from birth to eighteen years of age. Pediatrics 24:904–921
76. Lowrey G (1978) Growth and development of children, 7th edn. Year Book Medical Publishers, Chicago
77. Kari JA, Gonzalez C, Ledermann SE, Shaw V, Rees L (2000) Outcome and growth of infants with severe chronic renal failure. Kidney Int 57(4):1681–1687
78. Karlberg J, Schaefer F, Hennicke M, Wingen AM, Rigden S, Mehls O (1996) Early age-dependent growth impairment in chronic renal failure. European Study Group for Nutritional Treatment of Chronic Renal Failure in Childhood. Pediatr Nephrol 10(3):283–287
79. Furth SL, Stablein D, Fine RN, Powe NR, Fivush BA (2002) Adverse clinical outcomes associated with short stature at dialysis initiation: a report of the North American Pediatric Renal Transplant Cooperative Study. Pediatrics 109(5):909–913
80. Wong CS, Hingorani S, Gillen DL, Sherrard DJ, Watkins SL, Brandt JR, Ball A, Stehman-Breen CO (2002) Hypoalbuminemia and risk of death in pediatric patients with end-stage renal disease. Kidney Int 61(2):630–637
81. Food and Nutrition Board (2002) Dietary reference intakes for energy, carbohydrate, fiber, fat, fatty acids, cholesterol, protein, and amino acids (macronutrients). National Academies, Food and Nutrition Board Washington, DC
82. Quan A, Baum M (1996) Protein losses in children on continuous cycler peritoneal dialysis. Pediatr Nephrol 10(6):728–731
83. Lapeyraque AL, Haddad E, Andre JL, Bremond-Gignac D, Taylor CM, Rianthavorn P, Salusky IB, Loirat C (2003) Sudden blindness caused by anterior ischemic optic neuropathy in 5 children on continuous peritoneal dialysis. Am J Kidney Dis 42(5):E3–E9
84. Bunchman TE (1995) Chronic dialysis in the infant less than 1 year of age. Pediatr Nephrol 9(Suppl): S18–S22
85. Bellisle F, Dartois AM, Kleinknecht C, Broyer M (1995) Alteration of the taste for sugar in renal insufficiency: study in the child. Nephrologie 16(2): 203–208
86. Mak RH, Cheung W, Cone RD, Marks DL (2006) Leptin and inflammation-associated cachexia in chronic kidney disease. Kidney Int 69(5):794–797
87. Daschner M, Tonshoff B, Blum WF, Englaro P, Wingen AM, Schaefer F, Wuhl E, Rascher W, Mehls O (1998) Inappropriate elevation of serum leptin levels in children with chronic renal failure. European Study Group for Nutritional Treatment of Chronic Renal Failure in Childhood. J Am Soc Nephrol 9(6):1074–1079
88. Ruley EJ, Bock GH, Kerzner B, Abbott AW, Majd M, Chatoor I (1989) Feeding disorders and gastroesophageal reflux in infants with chronic renal failure. Pediatr Nephrol 3(4):424–429
89. Ramage IJ, Geary DF, Harvey E, Secker DJ, Balfe JA, Balfe JW (1999) Efficacy of gastrostomy feeding in infants and older children receiving chronic peritoneal dialysis. Perit Dial Int 19(3):231–236
90. Mekahli D, Shaw V, Ledermann SE, Rees L (2010) Long-term outcome of infants with severe chronic kidney disease. Clin J Am Soc Nephrol 5(1):10–17

91. Rees L, Azocar M, Borzych D, Watson AR, Buscher A, Edefonti A, Bilge I, Askenazi D, Leozappa G, Gonzales C, van Hoeck K, Secker D, Zurowska A, Ronnholm K, Bouts AH, Stewart H, Ariceta G, Ranchin B, Warady BA, Schaefer F (2011) Growth in very young children undergoing chronic peritoneal dialysis. J Am Soc Nephrol 22(12): 2303–2312
92. Dello Strologo L, Principato F, Sinibaldi D, Appiani AC, Terzi F, Dartois AM, Rizzoni G (1997) Feeding dysfunction in infants with severe chronic renal failure after long-term nasogastric tube feeding. Pediatr Nephrol 11(1):84–86
93. Warady BA, Kriley M, Belden B, Hellerstein S, Alan U (1990) Nutritional and behavioural aspects of nasogastric tube feeding in infants receiving chronic peritoneal dialysis. Adv Perit Dial 6:265–268
94. Warady BA, Weis L, Johnson L (1996) Nasogastric tube feeding in infants on peritoneal dialysis. Perit Dial Int 16(Suppl 1):S521–S525
95. Wong H, Mylrea K, Cameron A, Manion I, Bass J, Feber J, Filler G (2005) Caregiver attitudes towards gastrostomy removal after renal transplantation. Pediatr Transplant 9(5):574–578
96. von Schnakenburg C, Feneberg R, Plank C, Zimmering M, Arbeiter K, Bald M, Fehrenbach H, Griebel M, Licht C, Konrad M, Timmermann K, Kemper MJ (2006) Percutaneous endoscopic gastrostomy in children on peritoneal dialysis. Perit Dial Int 26(1):69–77
97. Ramage IJ, Harvey E, Geary DF, Hebert D, Balfe JA, Balfe JW (1999) Complications of gastrostomy feeding in children receiving peritoneal dialysis. Pediatr Nephrol 13(3):249–252
98. Warady BA, Bashir M, Donaldson LA (2000) Fungal peritonitis in children receiving peritoneal dialysis: a report of the NAPRTCS. Kidney Int 58(1): 384–389
99. Neu AM, Ho PL, McDonald RA, Warady BA (2001) Chronic dialysis in children and adolescents. The 2001 NAPRTCS annual report. Pediatr Nephrol 17(8):656–663
100. Annual Report of the North American Pediatric Renal Trials and Collaborative Studies (NAPRTCS) (2011) [cited 6/30/2011]. Available from https://web.emmes.com/study/ped/annlrept/annualrept2011.pdf
101. Wedekin M, Ehrich JH, Offner G, Pape L (2010) Renal replacement therapy in infants with chronic renal failure in the first year of life. Clin J Am Soc Nephrol 5(1):18–23
102. Annual Report of the U.S. Organ Procurement and Transplantation Network and the Scientific Registry of Transplant Recipients: Transplant Data 1994–2009. Department of Health and Human Services, Health Resources and Services Administration, Healthcare Systems Bureau, Division of Transplantation, Rockville; United Network for Organ Sharing, Richmond; University Renal Research and Education Association, Ann Arbor, 2010
103. Wood EG, Hand M, Briscoe DM, Donaldson LA, Yiu V, Harley FL, Warady BA, Ellis EN (2001) Risk factors for mortality in infants and young children on dialysis. Am J Kidney Dis 37(3):573–579
104. Ledermann SE, Scanes ME, Fernando ON, Duffy PG, Madden SJ, Trompeter RS (2000) Long-term outcome of peritoneal dialysis in infants. J Pediatr 136(1):24–29
105. Shroff R, Rees L, Trompeter R, Hutchinson C, Ledermann S (2006) Long-term outcome of chronic dialysis in children. Pediatr Nephrol 21(2):257–264

Transplant Considerations in the Newborn

19

Alun Williams

Core Messages

- Established renal failure in newborns is uncommon, and uropathies are commoner in children than adults with established renal failure.
- Early attention to growth and nutrition is important.
- Dialysis access in infants is tenuous.
- Vascular and urological workup in preparation for transplant is vital.
- A transplant is the gold standard treatment of established renal failure.

Case Vignette

A baby boy was born after spontaneous labor at 32 weeks' gestation with antenatally detected bilateral hydroureteronephrosis and worsening oligohydramnios. He had a palpable bladder, and in view of the antenatal history, had a suprapubic tube placed on the neonatal intensive care unit. After his diuresis had settled, an antegrade cystourethrogram showed posterior urethral valves. He underwent transurethral resection at term corrected gestational age.

His growth was slow, augmented with nasogastric feeds and recombinant growth hormone. By 2 years of age, his creatinine and urea were climbing, and he had worsening lassitude and growth failure.

In preparation for transplant, he underwent videourodynamics which showed a very small bladder (<30 mL capacity), high filling pressures (>40 cm H_2O) with leakage of urine, overactive contractions, and reflux into very dilated ureters bilaterally. An ultrasound scan showed bilateral small kidneys, and DMSA scan showed nonfunction of the right kidney. He underwent a right nephrectomy, ureterocystoplasty using the massively dilated right ureter, and an appendiceal Mitrofanoff.

Doppler imaging of the abdominal vessels showed patent iliocaval veins and a normal abdominal aorta.

At 3 years of age at a weight of 14 kg, he underwent a preemptive intra-abdominal (because of his previous major abdominal surgery) living-related kidney transplant, his father being the donor. He had immediate graft function.

A. Williams, MD
Department of Paediatric Urology, Queen's Medical Centre, E Floor, Nottingham NG7 2UH, UK
e-mail: alunrwilliams@mac.com

A.S. Chishti et al. (eds.), *Kidney and Urinary Tract Diseases in the Newborn*, DOI 10.1007/978-3-642-39988-6_19, © Springer-Verlag Berlin Heidelberg 2014

19.1 Introduction

Established renal failure (ERF) in newborns and infants is uncommon. In the most recent report of the UK Renal Registry, the prevalence of children undergoing renal replacement therapy (RRT) in the United Kingdom was 65 per million age-related population (pmarp), with an incidence of 9.3 pmarp. Although incidence and prevalence data for the newborn population are not recorded for this discrete group, the prevalence of RRT in the under-twos is 21.6 pmarp. Six percent of children receiving RRT are born prematurely [1].

The commonest cause of ERF remains renal dysplasia, including associated vesicoureteric reflux (VUR), making up 34 % of prevalent cases. Glomerular diseases (about 17 % of the prevalent population) and obstructive uropathies (16 %) complete the top three causes of ERF in childhood. Obstructive uropathies continue to feature much more prominently in the major causes of ERF in childhood compared with the adult population, making urological assessment and management of this group all the more important.

Almost all children will be potential transplant recipients at some stage. This is in contrast to the dialysis population as a whole including adults where far fewer (perhaps only a third overall) will be suitable for activation on the transplant waiting list usually as a result of general fitness.

Transplantation as a modality of RRT remains very uncommon under the age of 2 years however. In the UK review, only one of 497 children had a transplant under the age of 2 years. There have been reported cases of successful kidney transplantation in infancy, and a recent review suggests that outcomes are good in small children [2, 3] although the children transplanted within the first year of life remain in a minority within this already very small group.

There is inevitably a period of time required for adequate workup of a potential transplant recipient. A thorough cardiorespiratory assessment is required, and cardiorespiratory status needs to be maximized. The UK review [1] confirms that increasingly children undergoing RRT have significant comorbidity, and it is logical to maximize the potential for long-term graft survival by maximizing the recipient's fitness for a transplant. Likewise vaccinations against infectious disease are needed in anticipation of lifelong immunosuppression. Crucially also, establishment of growth and nutrition is a prerequisite, and this is discussed in more detail below. The preponderance of uropathies needs to be considered, and some intervention (operative or otherwise) may be needed in the workup to transplantation. Finally there are physical constraints on the actual placement of an allograft: recipient size may not be felt to be as important as before in light of the above case series, but there still needs to be adequate space to place the organ and adequate recipient blood vessels to provide inflow and outflow for the graft.

A major rate limiting step in kidney transplantation is the availability of a donor organ. The counsel of perfection is a preemptive transplant. This avoids dialysis access and the complications of access and those of dialysis. It has been proposed that avoiding dialysis may confer a survival advantage to the transplant [4, 5]. At present, on average between 20 and 30 % of children receive a preemptive kidney transplant [6]. The median wait for a deceased donor transplant for children in the UK for registrations up to the end of 2006 was 277 days [7]. In the USA in 2003, the median wait for ages 1–5 years was 360 days [8]. A living donor transplant may be more expedient but still requires a period of intensive workup for the prospective donor.

The availability of dialysis removes the immediate urgency of transplantation, and we know that peritoneal dialysis (PD) and hemodialysis (HD) are feasible and effective even in very small newborns [9–11]. There are also the sometimes poorly evidenced psychosocial aspects of ERF. New parents can find that their baby born with a congenital abnormality is difficult to care for. This is compounded by the prospect of a chronic condition needing complex treatment. We know that children can achieve good psychosocial, developmental, and cognitive outcomes and that we are doing better than we were, but there remain significant challenges [12].

The following outline does not attempt to consider the minutiae of medical workup of the potential kidney transplant recipient. Rather it considers the issues arising in the newborn and infant periods during workup to transplantation.

19.2 Nutrition and Growth

It has been recognized for many years that growth in children with chronic kidney disease (CKD) is poor. This is compounded by the metabolic disturbances with evolving kidney failure and further compounded with commencement of dialysis.

A recent multicenter analysis (involving 18 countries) reported 153 children starting peritoneal dialysis under the age of 2 years [13]. Growth slowed starting dialysis but improved with augmentation of nutrition. Particularly important is that demand feeding was associated with a decrease in age-related body mass index (BMI), but nasogastric or gastrostomy feeds increased the BMI. Clearly appetite is suppressed significantly with ERF. Nearly all of the gastrostomy-fed children were accounted for by the cohorts from North America and the UK. Children fed by gastrostomy had high length measurements over time. There was also significant regional variation in the nutritional status of children. The study reported that 50 % of Turkish children were malnourished at last observation compared with the 26 % of North American children who were reported as obese.

Recombinant human growth hormone (rhGH) is also associated with an increase in linear growth in both the CKD population in general [14] and in those on dialysis [13]. A recent Cochrane review shows an appreciable increase in height velocity above untreated children with CKD. Concerns about possible adverse effects on individual patients or on their subsequent transplants as a result of rhGH have not been borne out in the short term. However, the studies are too short in timescale to extrapolate these results until the cohort of patients can be followed.

We know gastrostomy feeding is advantageous as it avoids the complications of nasogastric feeds and removes the difficulty in persisting with oral feeds when they are tolerated poorly by uremic infants and children. At the author's unit, we have advocated early gastrostomy feeds [15] especially in the population approaching ERF requiring dialysis. The timing of placement of peritoneal dialysis tubes and gastrostomies is more debatable however. One review recognized an increased peritonitis rate if percutaneous endoscopic gastrostomies (PEG) were placed in children already on PD [16] and documented the course of children who also frequently required fundoplication for gastroesophageal reflux.

At the author's unit, we have routinely placed gastrostomy tubes synchronously with peritoneal dialysis catheters, initially with open surgery and latterly using laparoscopic assistance [17]. Withholding PD early in the postoperative recovery seems to have circumvented problems with leak and infection. If elective intraperitoneal surgery is required on PD, a useful strategy is to place a temporary hemodialysis catheter and suspend PD. It is usually possible to restart PD within a few days of surgery.

19.3 Dialysis Access

Establishing and maintaining dialysis access in newborn babies and infants is a formidable challenge [9]. PD is a convenient modality for dialysis in children of all ages (as well as in adults). It allows preservation of vessels in the first instance, crucial as the majority of pediatric recipients will become adults in need of retransplantation or further dialysis access in the form of peripheral arteriovenous fistula. It avoids rapid hemodynamic changes which can go with hemodialysis (HD). In newborns and small infants, their low intravascular volume is an important consideration for dead space volume in HD circuits where a very significant volume is extracorporeal. PD is also more usually amenable to home dialysis (which can be overnight) which allows a more normal existence for the child compared with trips on a frequent basis to a dialysis unit.

HD is possible even in very tiny babies although there are particular mechanical challenges [11]. Whether on PD or HD, catheter problems are frequent. We have found that catheter longevity is better in the PD population than in the HD population [10] but mortality is low. Parents need to be made aware of this.

It is important to avoid the lower body circulation for vascular access as far as possible. This will inevitably be the site of allograft implantation and technically easier into vessels not previously manipulated, narrowed, or lost to catheter thrombosis.

A useful principle in redo vascular access is to reutilize vessels as far as possible. Improvements in interventional radiological techniques have made this a viable proposition, with steerable guidewires and the ability to access central veins via small tributaries (e.g., the azygos system) and the ability to recanalize or dilate stenotic veins.

19.4 Blood Vessel Imaging

Imaging of vessels is important in revision dialysis access, and the section above outlines some of the techniques which can be used by interventional radiologists. However, in preparation for transplantation, blood vessel imaging is important, especially in small children, or if the lower body vessels have been instrumented or mobilized (for vascular access or during abdominopelvic surgery, e.g., nephrectomy or urological surgery) or if there has been previous abdominal surgery.

At the author's unit, we have found Doppler ultrasound to be reliable for demonstrating the aortoiliac and iliocaval systems, but when technical reasons dictate or there is uncertainty about the configuration of vessels, the imaging modality of choice is a magnetic resonance angiogram. Direct angiography is used less and less, partly as a consequence of improved magnetic resonance images, and partly as this usually involves instrumenting the vessels directly.

Children with anorectal malformations in particular require detailed assessment of their abdominopelvic vessels. Arterial and venous anatomy can be highly abnormal in these patients [18] and a "road map" is mandatory before planning transplantation.

19.5 Pretransplant Management of the Urinary Tract

An abnormal urinary tract's effect on native kidneys is well documented: Maguire's seminal work on native urinary tracts, spinal dysraphism, and hydronephrosis remains a reference point [19]. A urethral leak point pressure of greater than 40 cm H_2O represents a lower tract considered to be "unsafe." There is a suggestion that in children, a "safe" pressure may be 30 cm H_2O or less [20].

Pretransplant urodynamics are mandatory in children born with a uropathy. In the author's unit, we extend the indications for urodynamics to include those children with lower urinary tract symptoms, known vesicoureteric reflux, and recurrent urinary infections, although invasive formal urodynamics are always preceded by noninvasive studies to demonstrate bladder capacity, flow rate and efficiency, and emptying to completion.

The commonest single condition in the uropathic ERF population is posterior urethral valves (PUV). A paradoxical situation in managing the newborn with PUV is that urodynamics change and probably evolve over time [21]. Thus, it is more appropriate to undertake urodynamic studies in the immediate time before listing for transplantation rather than early in the newborn period.

With the urodynamic findings in mind, appropriate measures can be implemented to lower pressures, correct reflux if necessary, and provide capacity and drainage (by means of augmentation cystoplasty with or without Mitrofanoff drainage or by diversion).

Several studies have demonstrated that transplantation into an abnormal urinary tract is safe with good outcomes, so long as appropriate follow-up is in place. Likewise, transplantation into a reconstructed urinary tract is safe [22–28]. It is generally appreciated that reconstructive surgery is more conveniently and safely and logically done before transplantation [29] and that this then obviates the anxiety about reconstructive urinary tract surgery in the face of immunosuppression. Some authors have, however, commented that the so-called dry augment can be problematic [30], and care should be exercised in reconstructing the urinary tract of an anuric patient. The decision to undertake major reconstruction early in life of course also needs to depend on the support for teaching and learning intermittent catheterization and bladder irrigation and vigilance for complications such as stones.

Transplantation into an enteric diversion is safe [31], and there is always the prospect of a growing child or adolescent opting for an undiversion in time. Anecdotally, we have implanted an allograft ureter onto a bladder diverted by ureterostomy or suprapubic cystostomy with good outcome in the short term, mindful of the prospects for reconstruction at a later date.

VUR is a risk factor for urinary tract infection (UTI). UTI is the single commonest infectious complication to follow a kidney transplant and is commoner still in children with an underlying uropathy [32]. If recurrent UTI is a problem, this is a valid reason for considering an antireflux procedure in the workup for transplantation. It is crucial to consider the effects of VUR on the overall capacity of the urinary tract however: a significant contribution to overall capacity might be made by dilated ureters. This can, of course, be turned to the surgeon's advantage (as in the vignette) by using dilated ureters as a means of augmentation cystoplasty.

In boys with recurrent UTI, circumcision alone [33] may lower the subsequent risk or may be combined with another procedure. In the author's practice, the merits of circumcision at the time of PUV ablation, for example, are discussed with patients' families.

Pretransplant native nephrectomy is indicated for a number of reasons, including malignancy, refractory hypertension, and refractory protein loss. Recurrent infection, stones, and high-grade VUR have also been included among the indications, but a recent review of the author's center's cumulative practice has identified a trend towards more conservative management of the native kidneys [34]. The arguments for preservation of the native upper tracts include more straightforward fluid management of patients with ERF, preservation of native biochemical and endocrine function, as well as avoiding surgery in the workup to transplantation.

19.6 The Transplant

The choice of incision and approach for the transplant is largely a matter of surgeon choice and experience. In small children, traditionally the transperitoneal route to the aorta and inferior vena cava has been used. A recent report (admittedly not referring to recipients in the newborn or early infant period) does suggest that the extraperitoneal route if possible is reasonable and may even be preferable for graft outcome [35]. Closure of the abdomen, irrespective of the route to the large vessels, can be challenging. It is certainly reasonable to leave the abdomen open and return for a secondary closure, although experience is reported with prosthetics to achieve primary closure [36, 37].

Graft survival post-transplant has improved over the years [8]. For a living donor transplant, it is reasonable to quote graft survivals of 95, 90, and 85 % at 1, 3, and 5 years post-transplant, respectively. There is a suggestion that pediatric recipients may benefit from transplantation from a pediatric donor [38]. However, it is a virtual certainty that a pediatric recipient will inevitably require a retransplant (and possibly further transplants) over the course of a lifetime. This makes a more compelling case for as rigorous a pretransplant workup as possible.

Transplant outcomes and in particular complications [39] are dealt with more comprehensively elsewhere, but worthwhile is a mention of transplant thrombosis.

19.7 Vascular Thrombosis

One review summarizes recent literature [40] where the highest incidences of venous (up to 7 %) and arterial thromboses (up to 7.5 %) occur in pediatric recipients. There are donor and recipient factors, although the literature remains divided and undoubtedly is evolving. Traditionally, kidneys from very small donors have been considered to be at higher risk of thrombosis, although a recent paper describing a single center's experience of en bloc transplants from mean 11.4 kg donors may challenge this [41]. These would not be grafts suitable for implantation into very small recipients however. Donor age above 60 years may also increase the risk of thrombosis, although this may reflect atherosclerosis, itself a risk factor for thrombosis.

Recipient risk factors are difficult to tease out but may include small age (or size) per se, a previous thrombotic tendency, technical problems with the anastomosis, and perioperative hemodynamic instability. The latter are crucially important for very small recipients.

Conclusion

Established renal failure in newborns is uncommon, but attention to detail around the general condition, growth, nutrition and development of the baby is vital to promoting an ideal environment for a transplant. The value of a transplant done very early is debatable, and cases of kidney transplantation within the first few months of life are still rare. Nonetheless renal replacement therapy in the run up to transplantation can be very morbid itself. Sometimes, the need for a successful transplant can override the need to optimize factors like reconstruction of the urinary tract, if dialysis access becomes very tenuous or end stage. Fortunately the need for an urgent kidney transplant is still rare at this stage of life and the months of infancy can be spent optimizing the workup for transplantation while maximizing growth, somatic, cognitive, and psychosocial development of the baby.

References

1. Sinha M, Castledine C, von Schalkurgh D et al (2011) UK Renal Registry 13th Annual Report (Dec 2010) Chapter 5: demography of UK paediatric renal replacement therapy population 2009. Nephron Clin Pract 119(Suppl 2):C97–C106
2. Velak F, Butt K, Moel D et al (1977) Successful renal transplantation in infancy. J Pediatr Surg 12(8): 1075–1078
3. Herthelius M, Celsi G, Edstrom Halling S et al (2012) Renal transplantation in infants and small children. Pediatr Nephrol 27(1):145–150
4. Mahmoud A, Said M, Dawarha M et al (1997) Outcome of preemptive renal transplantation and pretransplantation dialysis in children. Pediatr Nephrol 11:537–541
5. Ishitani M, Isaacs R, Norwood V et al (2000) Predictors of graft survival in pediatric living-related kidney transplant recipients. Transplantation 70:288–292
6. Vats A, Donaldson L, Fine R, Chavers B (2000) Pretransplant dialysis status and outcome of renal transplantation in North American children: a NAPRTCS study. Transplantation 69:1414–1419
7. http://www.organdonation.nhs.uk:8001/ukt/about_transplants/waiting_time_to_transplant/waiting_time_to_transplant.asp. Accessed 29 July 2012
8. NAPRTCS Annual Report 2006. Available at web.emmes.com/study/ped/annlrept/annlrept2006.pdf. Accessed 30 July 2012
9. Laakkones H, Holtla T, Lonnqvist T (2008) Peritoneal dialysis in children under two years of age. Nephrol Dial Transplant 23(5):1747–1753
10. Paul A, Fraser N, Manoharan S et al (2011) The challenge of maintaining dialysis lines in the under twos. J Pediatr Urol 7(1):48–51
11. Everdell N, Coulthard M, Crozier J, Keir M (2005) A machine for haemodialyzing very small infants. Pediatr Nephrol 20(5):636–643
12. Madden S, Ledermann S, Guerrero-Blanco M (2003) Cognitive and psychosocial outcome of infants dialysed in infancy. Child Care Health Dev 29(1): 55–61
13. Rees L, Azocar M, Borzyck D et al (2011) Growth in very young children undergoing chronic peritoneal dialysis. J Am Soc Nephrol 22(12):2303–2312
14. Hodson E, Willis N, Craig J (2012) Growth hormone for children with chronic kidney disease. Cochrane Database Syst Rev 2, CD003264
15. Watson A (2006) Gastrostomy feeding in children on chronic peritoneal dialysis. Perit Dial Int 26(1):41–42
16. Ledermann S, Spitz L, Maloney J et al (2002) Gastrostomy feeding in infants and children on peritoneal dialysis. Pediatr Nephrol 17(4):246–250
17. Lindley RM, Williams AR, Fraser N, Shenoy MU (2012). Synchronous laparoscopic-assisted percutaneous endoscopic gastrostomy and peritoneal dialysis catheter placement is a valid alternative to open surgery. J Pediatr Urol 8(5):527–530
18. Dykes E, Oesch I, Ransley P, Hendren W (1993) Abnormal aorta and iliac arteries in children with urogenital abnormalities. J Pediatr Surg 28(5): 696–700

19. McGuire EJ, Woodside JR, Borden TA, Weiss RM (1981) Prognostic value of urodynamic testing in myelodysplastic patients. J Urol 126: 205–209
20. Houle AM, Gilmour RF, Churchill BM et al (1993) What volume can a child normally store in the bladder at a safe pressure? J Urol 149:561–564
21. De Gennaro M, Capitanucci M, Mosiello G et al (2000) The changing urodynamic pattern from infancy to adolescence in boys with posterior urethral valves. BJU Int 85(9):1004–1008
22. Rigamonti W, Capizzi A, Zacchello G et al (2005) Kidney transplantation into bladder augmentation or urinary diversion: long-term results. Transplantation 80:1435–1440
23. Mendizabal S, Estornell F, Zamora I et al (2005) Renal transplantation in children with severe bladder dysfunction. J Urol 173:226–229
24. Ali-El-Dein B, Abol-Enein H, El-Husseini A et al (2004) Renal transplantation in children with abnormal lower urinary tract. Transplant Proc 36: 2968–2973
25. Adams J, Mehls O, Wiesel M (2004) Pediatric renal transplantation and the dysfunctional bladder. Transpl Int 17:596–602
26. Neild GH, Dakmish A, Wood S et al (2004) Renal transplantation in adults with abnormal bladders. Transplantation 77:1123–1127
27. Luke PP, Herz DB, Bellinger MF et al (2003) Long-term results of pediatric renal transplantation into a dysfunctional lower urinary tract. Transplantation 76:1578–1582
28. Crowe A, Cairns HS, Wood S et al (1998) Renal transplantation following renal failure due to urological disorders. Nephrol Dial Transplant 13: 2065–2069
29. Taghizadeh A, Desai D, Ledermann S et al (2007) Renal transplantation or bladder augmentation first? A comparison of complications and outcomes in children. BJU Int 100(6):1365–1370
30. Alfrey EJ, Salvatierra O, Tanney DC et al (1997) Bladder augmentation can be problematic with renal failure and transplantation. Pediatr Nephrol 11: 672–675
31. Surange R, Johnson R, Tavakoli A et al (2003) Kidney transplantation into an ileal conduit: a single center experience of 59 cases. J Urol 170(5):1727–1730
32. John U, Everding AS, Kuwertz-Broking E et al (2006) High prevalence of febrile urinary tract infections after paediatric renal transplantation. Nephrol Dial Transplant 21:3269–3274
33. Singh-Grewal D, Macdessi J, Craig J (2005) Circumcision for the prevention of urinary tract infection in boys: a systematic review of randomised trials and observational studies. Arch Dis Child 90: 853–858
34. Fraser N, Lyon C, Williams A et al (2013) Native nephrectomy in pediatric transplantation – less is more! J Pediatr Urol 9(1):84–89
35. Heap S, Webb N, Kirkman M et al (2011) Extraperitoneal renal transplantation in small children results in a transient improvement in early graft function. Pediatr Transplant 15(4):362–366
36. Nguan CY, Beasley KA, McAlister VC, Luke PP (2007) Treatment of renal transplant complications with a mesh hood fascial closure technique. Am J Surg 193:119–121
37. Pentlow A, Smart N, Richards S et al (2008) The use of porcine dermal collagen implants in assisting abdominal wall closure of pediatric renal transplant recipients with donor size discrepancy. Pediatr Transplant 12(1):20–23
38. Pape L, Hoppe J, Becker T et al (2006) Superior long-term graft function and better growth of grafts in children receiving kidneys from paediatric compared with adult donors. Nephrol Dial Transplant 21:2596–2600
39. Williams A (2008) Kidney transplantation. In: Wilcox D, Godbole P, Koyle M (eds) Pediatric urology: surgical complications and management. Blackwell, Oxford, pp 247–254
40. Keller AK, Jorgensen TM, Jespersen B (2012) Identification of risk factors for vascular thrombosis may reduce early renal graft loss: a review of recent literature. J Transplant. doi:10.1155/2012/793461. Epub 2012
41. Sharma A, Fisher R, Cotterell A et al (2011) En block kidney transplantation from pediatric donors: comparable outcomes with living donor kidney transplantation. Transplantation 92(5):564–569

Neonatal Hypertension

20

René G. VanDeVoorde and Mark M. Mitsnefes

Core Messages

- Healthy, full-term neonates rarely have hypertension. Preterm and ill newborns are at increased risk of developing hypertension, especially if they have chronic lung disease, patent ductus arteriosus, intracranial bleeding, need for ECMO, umbilical artery catheter placement, or coexistent renal disease.
- The etiology of neonatal hypertension is best evaluated by a thorough history, including prenatal, perinatal, and postnatal findings. The highest-yield laboratory and radiologic studies are a renal panel, urinalysis, and renal ultrasound which aid in determining the presence of renovascular and renal parenchymal diseases.
- Treatment options for neonatal hypertension should start with treating any reversible causes. Pharmacotherapy options are varied and none have been systematically studied in this population.

Case Vignette

A former premature (27 weeks gestational age) male infant is scheduled for NICU discharge in the coming week and the parents have questions about his home care. At 6 weeks of age, he was noted to have blood pressure readings of 115/70 for three consecutive days. Shortly after birth, he was intubated for 2 weeks and currently requires oxygen by nasal cannula which has been difficult to wean over the last 2 weeks. He has no other comorbidities noted during this admission, and there was no history of umbilical catheters being placed. His initial evaluation for hypertension included a normal electrolyte panel, normal serum creatinine, normal appearing kidneys on ultrasound, and normal echocardiogram. To control his blood pressure, he was started on chlorothiazide and has had good blood pressure readings over the ensuing 3 weeks. While on the same dose of chlorothiazide, he has been appropriately gaining weight with stable electrolytes. His parents are wondering about his expected course of hypertension, including his long-term need for medication and what it means for his long-term health.

R.G. VanDeVoorde • M.M. Mitsnefes, MD, MS (✉)
Division of Nephrology and Hypertension,
Cincinnati Children's Hospital Medical Center,
3333 Burnet Avenue, Cincinnati, OH 45229, USA
e-mail: mark.mitsnefes@cchmc.org

A.S. Chishti et al. (eds.), *Kidney and Urinary Tract Diseases in the Newborn*,
DOI 10.1007/978-3-642-39988-6_20, © Springer-Verlag Berlin Heidelberg 2014

20.1 Introduction

Since its first cited description in the 1970s [2], there has been a greater awareness of neonatal hypertension amongst neonatologists and pediatric nephrologists. Advances have been made in the ability to accurately assess blood pressure (BP) in neonates as well as increased knowledge of normal BP values and trends in newborns with lower birth weights and shorter gestational age, thus allowing better identification of neonates who are at risk for hypertension. Despite progress in these areas, there are others (pathogenesis, threshold for treatment, comparative trials of therapies) that have advanced much more slowly. Fortunately, overall outcomes in neonates with hypertension remain very good.

20.2 Blood Pressure Measurement in Neonates

20.2.1 Proper Measurement of Blood Pressure in Neonates

The criterion standard for measurement of blood pressure in neonates has long been intra-arterial analysis via arterial catheter and pressure transducer of the pulse pressure waveform. Studies have shown good correlation of measurements in neonates with either central (umbilical) or peripheral artery catheters [11], unlike in older children. However, the inherent risks (thrombosis, perforation, arteritis, compromised peripheral perfusion, …) with arterial catheters should restrict their use for blood pressure measurement to those neonates who have other issues of cardiorespiratory compromise necessitating their use, as they should not be used solely to monitor blood pressure. Unlike in children, measuring blood pressure by auscultation in neonates is generally not recommended, as hearing Korotkoff sounds in the brachial artery is very difficult, especially in the NICU setting, so as to make this method impractical. Likewise, accurate palpation of a brachial or radial systolic pulse pressure is also difficult, and thus impractical, in small neonates. Ultrasonic Doppler assessment had long been used as an accurate noninvasive means to measure blood pressure [17]. However, it can be slightly more labor-intensive to perform as it requires proper positioning of the probe throughout the measurement [20] and has largely been replaced in most nurseries and NICUs.

Automated oscillometric methods of blood pressure measurement are the most widely used technique in neonates currently. They measure the mean arterial pressure and, through algorithms unique to each machine manufacturer, calculate the systolic and diastolic blood pressure. Studies have shown a good correlation between this technique and intra-arterial and Doppler measurements [20, 42], while others have noted some overestimations of blood pressure, especially in the face of hypotension, using this technique [33, 44]. However, this technique does not appear to underestimate blood pressure readings and therefore is reasonable to use when screening for hypertension in newborns. Oscillometric devices are practical to use, giving rapid and reproducible measures, and allow for following BP readings over time. However, the initial readings by the device when first turned on may be less accurate, as the cuff may initially inflate to higher preset values and deflate by greater intervals [15].

There are several variables that may affect the accuracy of blood pressure measurement in newborns. Like in older children, cuff size can affect readings, as too large a cuff may underestimate blood pressure, while smaller cuffs may overestimate readings [27]. It is recommended that the cuff bladder should cover at least 2/3 of the upper arm or thigh and encircle 80–100 % of the circumference of the extremity. Also, measurements are most accurate when the cuff width to circumference ratio is 0.44–0.55 [27, 40]. Unlike in older children, studies have shown that lower extremity blood pressure values are not necessarily elevated compared to upper extremity readings [36].

The neonate's state of alertness and calmness can also have great effect on its blood

Table 20.1 Features of a standard protocol for blood pressure measurement in the newborn [32]

1. Oscillometric measurement
2. Appropriately sized cuff – smallest cuff size that covered at least two-thirds of the upper arm and encircled the entire arm
3. Measured in the right upper arm
4. Infant lying prone or supine
5. Measured at least 90 min following their last feeding or any medical intervention
6. After cuff placement, the infants is left undisturbed for at least 15 min
7. Infant is sleeping or quietly awake
8. Three successive readings done 2 min apart

pressure. Studies have shown elevation in blood pressure readings when newborns are crying or agitated, feeding or sucking, have their head elevated, or even when their abdomen is being compressed [4, 15]. It has even been noted that blood pressure is elevated in newborns in the supine versus the prone position [32] though this may not be clinically relevant. A study evaluating a standardized protocol for blood pressure management in neonates <2,500 g compared to "routine" nursing measurement of vital signs showed that the protocol gave significantly lower BP measurements with significantly less variation in their results [32]. The authors also noted that first BP measurements were significantly higher than subsequent measures, similar to decreases seen in older children, though they did not feel this difference was clinically significant. This protocol, as highlighted in Table 20.1, has been recommended as a reasonable nursing standard for blood pressure measurement in NICUs [15], though the need for repeated measures and averaging of values is debatable from a practicality standpoint.

20.2.2 Normative Values of Blood Pressure in Neonates

Defining of normal blood pressure in newborns is a complicated matter and uniform values cannot be easily applied across the board to all neonates. The predominant variables that may affect BP include gestational age, postnatal age, and birth weight.

Normal values for full-term neonates have been investigated by different groups and there seems to be little variation in values based off of gestational age [21, 25]. Values first reported by the Brompton study from 1980 [14] were incorporated by the pediatric task force on blood pressure control in children. This longitudinal study of 1,800 term newborns measured BP with the Doppler technique and found that mean BP increases 1–2 mmHg per day during the first week of life, then rises only 1–2 mmHg per week over the subsequent several weeks [13]. A similar pattern, with slowing of the rise in BP after the first several days of life, was noted using oscillometric measurements as well [21]. Term infants that are small for gestational age have been shown to have a slightly higher increase in BP over the first weeks of life [28], such that all term infants seem to have a similar BP pattern by 1 month of life.

Large-scale data on preterm infants, similar to that of term infants, had been lacking for a long period of time. A study of >300 infants admitted on their initial day of life to several NICUs measured BP serially by the oscillometric method and were able to define mean as well as upper and lower confidence limits in this varied population [46]. This analysis showed a clear correlation of higher normal BP values with increased gestational age and birth weight which has been confirmed in subsequent studies [35]. Similar to term infants, preterm infants have a more rapid increase in systolic and diastolic blood pressure over the first few days of life with subsequent slowing of the rate of increase in the following weeks [35, 46]. Despite the complexities of differing baseline blood pressure and rates of increase based off of gestation, neonatal BP measures have been shown to correlate to postconceptual age [46]. This allows for the longitudinal evaluation of blood pressure for all neonates, irrespective of their gestational age. Recently, a reference table of 95th and 99th

Table 20.2 Neonatal blood pressure parameters for postconceptual age

Postconceptual age	50th percentile	95th percentile	99th percentile
44 weeks			
SBP	88	105	110
DBP	50	68	73
MAP	63	80	85
42 weeks			
SBP	85	98	102
DBP	50	65	70
MAP	62	76	81
40 weeks			
SBP	80	95	100
DBP	50	65	70
MAP	60	75	80
38 weeks			
SBP	77	92	97
DBP	50	65	70
MAP	59	74	79
36 weeks			
SBP	72	87	92
DBP	50	65	70
MAP	57	72	77
34 weeks			
SBP	70	85	90
DBP	40	55	60
MAP	50	65	70
32 weeks			
SBP	68	83	88
DBP	40	55	60
MAP	49	64	69
30 weeks			
SBP	65	80	85
DBP	40	55	60
MAP	48	63	68
28 weeks			
SBP	60	75	80
DBP	38	50	54
MAP	45	58	63
26 weeks			
SBP	55	72	77
DBP	30	50	56
MAP	38	57	63

From Dionne et al. [15]. With kind permission from Springer Science + Business Media

BP percentiles for all neonates [16] has been published, as shown in Table 20.2. This table is to be applied for newborns after 2 weeks of age and encompasses data from the published studies to date, accounting for the variables of gestational age and appropriateness of size for gestation.

20.3 Prevalence of Hypertension in Neonates

With a lack of consistent normative data, the definition of hypertension in neonates has varied over time. An early, and often cited, definition was BP greater than 90/60 for term newborns or greater than 80/50 in preterm infants [2], while others have used a single measure, systolic blood pressure (>113 mmHg) [19] or mean arterial pressure (>70 mmHg) [39], as standards. Currently, with better normative data, hypertension is often defined by three readings above the 95th percentile for gestational age and birth weight [37].

The prevalence of hypertension is considered to be very rare in healthy full-term neonates, as low as 0.2 %, such that routine blood pressure screening is not recommended for this group [6]. However, newborns that require monitoring in the intensive care unit have been shown to have a higher incidence of hypertension throughout the years. This prevalence has varied, with differing definitions of hypertension, from 0.81 to 3.2 % [10, 38, 39]. More recent prevalence studies, citing the 95th percentile standards, have reported rates of 1.0–1.3 % [9, 37].

Several risk factors for neonatal hypertension have been identified through these cohort studies. The prevalence of hypertension was as high as 9 % in infants with bronchopulmonary dysplasia (BPD), patent ductus arteriosus (PDA), intraventricular hemorrhage, or with umbilical artery catheter usage in one study [38]. Other risk factors for increased prevalence include antenatal steroid use, use of ECMO, and coexistent renal disease [9, 37]. A recent multivariate analysis of a large national pediatric hospital database found the odds ratio for hypertension to be highest in patients with greater severity of illness, defined by the All-Patient Refined Diagnosis Related Groups subclass. It is apparent that the most ill of neonates are indeed at the highest risk for hypertension.

20.4 Etiologies of Neonatal Hypertension

There are numerous potential causes of hypertension in the neonate, as cited in Table 20.3. However, a clear etiology may be ascertained in less than half of all hypertensive newborns [10, 19]. The pathophysiology of hypertension in neonates is typically secondary to common pathways with elevations in renin-angiotensin-aldosterone, catecholamines, and/or sodium and fluid. The more common causes, as listed in Table 20.3, are disorders of the renovasculature, renal parenchyma, aortic coarctation, and bronchopulmonary dysplasia.

Early studies cited renovascular disease as the most common cause of hypertension [4, 10, 38], though this may not be as true with current neonatal practices. This high incidence was attributable to the use of umbilical artery catheters (UACs), as they were associated with a high rate of thrombus formation. It is thought that disruption of the vascular endothelium of the umbilical artery, likely at time of UAC placement, leads to thrombus formation and risk of embolism to the renal arteries, local infarction, and release of renin. A Cochrane review showed that there was no difference in hypertension rates comparing "high" versus "low" placed catheters [8], so it is the presence of the catheter altogether, not its location, which places patients at risk. In patients with prothrombotic risk, renal vein thrombosis may also lead to hypertension, but it is often a later finding. However, with less regular use of UACs, the incidence of renovascular etiologies of hypertension may be decreasing altogether.

Outside of thrombosis, other renovascular causes of hypertension are still common. Renal artery stenosis from congenital narrowing may often occur, with stenoses often present in distal branched vessels and not as easily identified on ultrasound. Mechanical compression of the renal artery can occur with renal tumors, perirenal hematomas, or massive hydronephrosis. Rarely, there may be infiltration of the vessel wall from either hematoma, calcification, or oligosaccharides.

Congenital renal parenchymal disorders are often cited as the second most common cause of neonatal hypertension. Autosomal recessive

Table 20.3 Different etiologies of neonatal hypertension

Renovascular
Renal artery thrombosis (secondary to umbilical artery catheterization)
Renal artery stenosis
Congenital (fibromuscular dysplasia, congenital rubella)
Intramural hematoma
Secondary to external compression (tumor, perirenal hematoma)
Renal vein thrombosis
Invasive vascular disease (idiopathic arterial calcification, galactosialidosis)
Renal parenchymal disease
Polycystic kidney disease (autosomal recessive or dominant)
Renal hypoplasia/dysplasia
Unilateral multicystic dysplasia kidney (MCDK)
Renal outflow obstruction
Anatomic (ureteropelvic or ureterovesical junction, bladder outlet)
Acquired (stones, tumor)
Acute tubular or cortical necrosis
Acute interstitial nephritis
Hemolytic uremic syndrome
Cardiopulmonary
Coarctation of the aorta
Bronchopulmonary dysplasia
Extracorporeal membrane oxygenation (ECMO)
Endocrine
Congenital adrenal hyperplasia
11-β hydroxylase deficiency
17-α hydroxylase deficiency
Hyperaldosteronism
Hyperthyroidism
Monogenic disorders behaving like hyperaldosteronism
Liddle syndrome
Glucocorticoid-remedial aldosteronism
Pseudohypoaldosteronism type 2 (Gordon syndrome)
Neoplastic
Wilms tumor
Mesoblastic nephroma
Neuroblastoma
Pheochromocytoma
Neurologic
Pain
Neonatal withdrawal syndrome
Intracranial hypertension
Seizures
Familial dysautonomia

(continued)

Table 20.3 (continued)

Medications	
	Dexamethasone
	Methylxanthines (caffeine, theophylline)
	Adrenergic agents (bronchodilators, vasopressors)
	Pancuronium
	Phenylephrine ophthalmic drops
	Vitamin A or D intoxication
	Maternal cocaine or heroin use
Miscellaneous	
	Closure of abdominal wall defects
	Bladder exstrophy repair
	Iatrogenic overload of fluid or sodium
	Hypercalcemia
	Adrenal hemorrhage

polycystic kidney disease often manifests with early onset hypertension, at a mean of 16 days of life [23], which can be quite pronounced and difficult to control. Alternatively, autosomal dominant disease typically manifests in adulthood but has been associated with hypertension in the newborn period. Renal dysplasia is a much more prevalent parenchymal disorder; however, hypertension is not ubiquitous in dysplasia. The tubular wasting of salt and fluids in dysplasia typically does not allow for blood pressure elevation, but renin-induced hypertension can be seen. This is also thought to be the mechanism of hypertension in unilateral multicystic dysplastic kidney, as abnormalities may often be present in the contralateral kidney. Urologic abnormalities, such as renal outflow obstruction, have also been associated with hypertension, with prevalence rates as high as 19 % [26]. The mechanism is again thought to be alteration of the renin-angiotensin system, as correction of the obstruction does not always lead to resolution of the hypertension. Lastly, acquired renal parenchymal disorders, such as tubular necrosis, interstitial nephritis, and hemolytic uremic syndrome, are very uncommon but have been seen in neonates, with accompanying hypertension likely from sodium and volume overload along with hyperreninism.

Aortic coarctation causes BP elevation in the upper extremities primarily by renin induction from inadequately perfused kidneys. It was commonly cited in many early cohort studies [10, 38] and often presented with congestive heart failure, following closure of a patent ductus. Hypertension has been known to persist even after surgical correction of the coarctation [34] though not always readily apparent in the neonatal period. Bronchopulmonary dysplasia has been associated with increasing risk of hypertension, with rates reported from 12 to 45 % and correlation seen with more severe pulmonary disease [1, 5]. Although this association has been noted for over 30 years, little is known as to the pathophysiologic cause of the hypertension. Some of the medications used in chronic lung disease, like steroids and bronchodilators, may contribute to BP elevation. It has been speculated that hypoxemia may modify either plasma renin activity or catecholamine secretion. However, the development of hypertension in chronic lung disease often occurs later, months after delivery and sometimes noted even after discharge from the NICU [38]. Conversely, patients requiring ECMO often become hypertensive within weeks of discontinuation of therapy. The pathophysiology is again unclear but may be related to altered sodium and fluid handling by the kidneys or derangement to the atrial baroreceptors that control volume status.

Endocrinologic causes of hypertension are rare to begin with, and the more common etiologies (congenital adrenal hyperplasia and hyperthyroidism) may first be identified by neonatal screening before manifesting with hypertension. Extremely rare are the monogenic disorders which may cause hypertension. Liddle syndrome is caused by a mutation to the β or γ subunits of the aldosterone-responsive sodium channel (ENaC), causing the channels to be constitutively activated and increased sodium resorption. Glucocorticoid-remedial aldosteronism occurs when the adrenal gland produces a protein with aldosterone synthase activity, such that aldosterone secretion becomes linked to cortisol secretion. Gordon syndrome is secondary to increased expression of the WNK kinases distally, which causes increased activity of the thiazide-sensitive co-transporter. There is increased sodium resorption in the distal tubule but also an inability to excrete potassium and acid in the collecting duct. These three rare autosomal dominant disorders are associated with suppressed renin levels.

Congenital renal tumors, such as mesoblastic nephroma and Wilms tumor, have been shown to cause increased renin production, though it is unclear if this is purely secondary to renal vessel displacement or from aberrant production by the tumor tissue. Neuroblastoma may produce vasoactive catecholamines, while there are case reports of pheochromocytomas diagnosed in the newborn period. Similarly, centrally mediated hypertension may be seen with pain, neonatal withdrawal, or seizures. Intracranial hypertension may be seen with subdural hematomas or other causes of intracranial bleeding. Familial dysautonomia is a rare disorder, more commonly seen among Ashkenazi Jews, with episodic hypertension or hypotension along with temperature dysregulation.

Numerous medications given to neonates have been associated with hypertension. Antenatal steroids and bronchodilators used to treat chronic lung disease have both been associated with hypertension in newborns. Stimulants like caffeine or aminophylline, to treat for apnea of newborns, may also have undesired effects on blood pressure, while phenylephrine eye drops have been associated with systemic symptoms. Prolonged use of pancuronium can cause catecholamine release. Also, the ordered fluid and electrolyte solutions given to newborns could cause iatrogenic hypertension from volume overload or hypercalcemia.

Lastly, there have been reports of hypertension seen following certain types of surgery which are unique to newborns, with the hypertension seeming to be independent of pain. Repair of abdominal wall defects, omphaloceles more so than gastroschisis, has been associated with hypertension, possibly from increased intra-abdominal pressure and its effect on renal perfusion. However, the associated hypertension is often very transient and seems not to require any intervention [12]. Hypertension has also been seen with bladder exstrophy repairs and is thought to be related to traction on the nerves [24].

20.5 Diagnostic Evaluation

20.5.1 Signs, Symptoms, and Physical Exam Findings

Most neonates with hypertension are completely asymptomatic, and the hypertension is detected because of routine monitoring. There are no classic symptoms of neonatal hypertension but nonspecific findings such as feeding difficulties, lethargy, irritability, tachypnea, and apnea may be seen. More severe hypertension may cause encephalopathy (vomiting and seizures), while long-standing hypertension may result in congestive heart failure (weight gain, pulmonary edema, hepatomegaly), though these presentations are uncommon. Additionally, because hypertension is often asymptomatic, it is also important to determine if the patient truly has persistent BP elevation and not just normal variation because of pain or agitation from other sources.

The first steps in evaluating neonatal hypertension is a detailed medical history, including the obstetrical history, delivery events, and subsequent medical history, as well as a thorough list of medications being given to the newborn. The prenatal history should include any abnormal results from routine care as well as any maternal drug exposures, both of prescribed and illicit medications. Maternal ACE inhibitor use in the first trimester is associated with abnormal fetal renal development, while recent cocaine exposure or heroin withdrawal may also cause hypertension in the newborn. Birth asphyxiation at the time of delivery can lead to acute kidney injury and hypertension, while chronic lung disease, need for ECMO, cerebral hemorrhage, placement of UAC, and other surgeries following delivery have all been associated with hypertension (See Table 20.3). Newborn medication history should include any corticosteroids, stimulants, vasopressors, and intravenous fluids, as well as any opioid exposure that could lead to withdrawal. Family history tends to have less pertinence in neonates, though inquiring specifically about polycystic kidney disease or prior infants with hypertension may assist with some of the less common etiologies of hypertension.

Table 20.4 Pertinent physical exam findings in the hypertensive infant

Finding	Possible etiology of hypertension
Edema, fluid overload	Acute Kidney Injury (Acute tubular necrosis, interstitial nephritis, HUS); iatrogenic excess of fluid or sodium
Bulging fontanelle	Intracranial hypertension (hemorrhage, hydrocephalus)
Tachycardia	Pain; withdrawal; catecholamine excess (neuroblastoma, pheochromocytoma); hyperthyroidism
Abdominal bruit	Renal artery stenosis
Flank Mass	
Bilateral	Polycystic kidney disease
Unilateral	Renal vein thrombosis; UPJ obstruction; tumor (mesoblastic nephroma, Wilms tumor, neuroblastoma)
Hepatomegaly	Neuroblastoma
Diminished femoral pulses	Coarctation of the aorta
Ambiguous genitalia	Congenital adrenal hyperplasia

The physical exam should focus on identifying any associated findings that may elucidate the etiology of the hypertension, as listed in Table 20.4. Blood pressure should be checked in all four extremities to rule out coarctation of the aorta and the abdomen should be thoroughly palpated for any masses. The cardiac exam should mainly focus on any signs of heart failure, rather than the etiology of the hypertension, though significant tachycardia in the face of hypertension may call into question whether excess catecholamines or other stimulants are present.

20.5.2 Laboratory and Radiologic Evaluation

In many instances, the laboratory and radiologic studies needed to evaluate is fairly limited, as the etiology may be suggested by the patient's history. However, there should not be a delay in the evaluation for hypertension as the opportunity to properly identify the etiology may be reduced as time passes, as thromboses may resolve radiographically.

Table 20.5 Laboratory and radiologic testing of neonatal hypertension

Generally recommended	Useful in selected situations
Serum electrolytes	Plasma renin activity
BUN, serum creatinine	Aldosterone
Urinalysis	Urine sodium, potassium, and creatinine
Serum calcium	Thyroid studies
Renal ultrasound with Doppler	Cortisol
Chest X-ray	Urine VMA/HVA
	Urine steroid metabolites
	Head ultrasound or CT scan
	Renal angiography

BUN blood urea nitrogen, *CT* computed tomography, *HVA* homovanillic acid, *VMA* vanillylmandelic acid

A list of generally recommended studies and other studies to consider obtaining is given in Table 20.5.

Those studies which are generally recommended are able to give high yields of information about various etiologies. Serum electrolytes, BUN, and creatinine can give a sense of overall renal function and assist with determining whether there is renal parenchymal injury. Additionally, elevated serum sodium and decreased serum potassium levels may suggest whether hyperaldosteronism is present and other investigation is needed. Urinalysis findings of hematuria or proteinuria may also assist with determining if renal parenchymal injury is present. Serum calcium levels are also easily checked, often with the serum electrolytes, to help rule out hypercalcemia as an etiology. Renal ultrasound with Doppler can help evaluate for renal parenchymal injury, anatomical abnormalities of the genitourinary tract, arterial and venous thrombosis, renal tumors, and sometimes renal artery narrowing. Additionally, a thorough ultrasonographer may also look at the adrenal glands and other surrounding structures to pick up on potential evidence of adrenal hemorrhage or other abdominal tumors. Lastly, a chest X-ray will be limited in determining the etiology of the hypertension but may be helpful in determining whether there is evidence of heart failure secondary to the hypertension.

Plasma renin activity levels have been recommended by others as part of the standard work-up in the hypertensive newborn, but the difficulties with this testing limit its general utility. There is limited data on normal values of plasma renin in infants, especially in premature infants [41]. Plasma renin levels can be elevated in hypovolemia, respiratory distress, and with the use of methylxanthines. They may also be altered by the use of some antihypertensive medications, so levels need to be obtained prior to treatment of the hypertension for greatest validity. Lastly, the test also has limited sensitivity as it is not always elevated peripherally in verified conditions of hyperreninism, such as renal artery stenosis or thrombosis. Its use should be considered in patients with severe hypertension without other etiologies or those patients with hypernatremia or hypokalemia to suggest alteration in the renin-angiotensin-aldosterone axis.

Other serum and urine studies that may be useful in selected situations include evaluation for excess catecholamines or endocrinopathies. Imaging of the brain, by ultrasound or computed tomography, should be considered in patients at risk for central hypertension. Renal angiography, to look for distal arterial stenosis, may be considered in the newborn with severe hypertension but the risks of the procedure in someone that small must be weighed against the true benefits of positive findings. Unfortunately, noninvasive angiography (CT or MR) is limited from identifying branch stenoses in smaller renal vessels.

20.6 Treatment

The initial step for treatment of neonatal hypertension is correction of any reversible causes of elevated blood pressure. This would include treating seizures, pain, or withdrawal; correcting any endocrinopathies or hypercalcemia; removal of umbilical artery catheters; discontinuing any causative medications that is feasible; and limiting fluid and sodium in iatrogenic overload. If the primary cause of hypertension is not as easily identifiable or treated, one must then question at what level of BP elevation should be treated. The answer is not as straightforward in other age groups, as no antihypertensive medications have been routinely tested in neonates.

In the absence of overt findings of end-organ injury (heart failure, encephalopathy), it has been recommended to consider treatment if the blood pressure remains above the 99th percentile for adjusted age [15, 18]. This threshold certainly seems reasonable, given the lack of long-term outcome data in this age group. A review of a national database of children's hospitals showed that only 58 % of NICU patients diagnosed with hypertension were given antihypertensives, excluding diuretics [9], supporting this concept that not all hypertension needs to be treated.

Newborns with severe hypertension or critically ill with hypertension are best treated with intravenous continuous infusions of antihypertensive medication to allow for rapid changes in dosing depending on clinical needs. The goal would be to lower blood pressure gradually while avoiding too rapid of a correction, as this may place the already susceptible infant at risk for cerebral and renal ischemia. A list of commonly used antihypertensive agents, both intravenous and oral forms, is given in Table 20.6. For continuous infusion, nicardipine use has been most recently reported on as an effective agent used in neonates, including premature newborns [22, 29]. Nitroprusside use may be limited to less than 72 h, or shorter periods if renal insufficiency, because of the risk of thiocyanate toxicity. For patients with renal failure or volume overload, the total volume of continuously infused medication may be a limitation. Intermittently dosed intravenous medications should also be considered [43] as their use is not limited by oral tolerability or variation in absorption.

Certain medications deserve special mention, either because of their associated risks or benefits. Diuretics are often very effective agents for treating hypertension related to volume overload or associated with chronic lung disease. Loop diuretics are especially efficacious; however, they also cause increased urinary calcium excretion, putting newborns at risk for nephrocalcinosis. Therefore, their use should ideally be intermittent or closely monitored. Thiazide

Table 20.6 Neonatal antihypertensive agents (grouped by class of agent)

Drug	Dosing/comments
ACE inhibitors:	
Captopril	Oral: 0.01–0.65 mg/kg/dose given tid
Enalapril	Bolus: 5–15 mcg/kg/dose given daily to tid Oral: 0.08–0.6 mg/kg/day divided daily or bid
Lisinopril	Oral: 0.07–0.6 mg/kg/day given once daily
Beta-blockers:	
Carvedilol	Oral: 0.1–0.5 mg/kg/dose given bid (also α-antagonist)
Esmolol	Cont: 100–500 mcg/kg/min
Labetalol	Bolus: 0.2–1 mg/kg/dose every 4–6 h (also α-antagonist) Cont: 0.25–3 mg/kg/h Oral: 0.5–5 mg/kg/dose given bid
Propranolol	Oral: 0.5–3.3 mg/kg/dose given tid
Calcium channel blockers (vasodilators):	
Amlodipine	Oral: 0.05–0.6 mg/kg/day divided daily or bid
Isradipine	Oral: 0.05–0.2 mg/kg/dose given qid
Nicardipine	Cont: 0.5–4 mcg/kg/min
Nifedipine	Oral: 0.25–0.5 mg/kg/dose every 4–6 h
Diuretics:	
Chlorothiazide	Bolus: 5–10 mg/kg/dose given bid Oral: 5–10 mg/kg/dose given bid
Furosemide	Bolus: 0.5–2 mg/kg/dose given bid to qid Oral: 0.5–6 mg/kg/dose given daily to qid (may give high doses once daily to see if responds in oliguria, but would not dose regularly because of ototoxicity risk)
Hydrochlorothiazide	Oral: 1–3 mg/kg/day divided daily or bid
Metolazone	Oral: 0.2–0.4 mg/kg/day divided daily or bid
Spironolactone	Oral: 1–3 mg/kg/day divided daily or bid (potassium sparing)
Vasodilators:	
Diazoxide	Bolus: 2–5 mg/kg/dose (rapid injection)
Hydralazine	Bolus: 0.2–1 mg/kg/dose given every 4 h Cont: 0.75–5 mcg/kg/min Oral: 0.25–1.8 mg/kg/dose given tid–qid
Minoxidil	Oral: 0.1–0.2 mg/kg/dose given daily to bid
Nitroprusside	Cont: 0.2–10 mcg/kg/min (risk of thiocyanate toxicity)
Miscellaneous:	
Clonidine	Oral: 5–25 mcg/kg/day divided bid or tid (α-agonist with central action, may cause sedation)

Bolus intermittent intravenous dosing, *Cont* continuous intravenous infusion rate

diuretics are effective chronic therapy, as they do not have the calciuric effect of loop diuretics. However, because of their mechanism of action and the immaturity of tubular function in neonates, they do put the patient at risk for hyponatremia, hypokalemia, and metabolic alkalosis so serum electrolytes should be monitored. Using salt and fluid restriction in combination with diuretics may limit the risk of hyponatremia. Also, the potassium-sparing effects of spironolactone allows for its combined use with other diuretics to minimize the risk of hypokalemia while maintaining diuresis.

Angiotensin-converting enzyme (ACE) inhibitor use has been shown to be effective in lowering blood pressure in neonates [45] and should be considered a first-line agent for renovascular hypertension. However, renal hemodynamics are especially dependent on the renin-angiotensin system during the perinatal and early postnatal period. Nephrogenesis continues until about 36 weeks gestation, even occurring after birth in premature or low birth weight infants [30]. Therefore, ACE inhibitors should be avoided altogether until at least 36 weeks postconceptual age or possibly even later. Also, newborns may be particularly susceptible to ACE inhibitor effects so even low doses may have significant effects. Therefore, it is recommended to start dosing lower than normal in patients while routinely monitoring urine output, serum potassium, and creatinine levels when first dosing.

Beta-blockers may be particularly effective because of an increased sensitivity to catecholamines in the neonatal kidney [30], but their use may be contraindicated in patients with chronic lung disease. Vasodilators, including calcium channel blockers, can cause tachycardia and fluid retention. Diazoxide is a historically used intravenous vasodilator that could be given by rapid injection; however, its variation in duration has made it a less desirable option. Clonidine is an α-agonist that may be especially effective in centrally mediated hypertension; however, it can cause rebound hypertension if its use is abruptly discontinued.

Some general recommendations regarding the choice of antihypertensive are to first choose an agent that may directly address the primary etiology of the hypertension. Dosing should start at the lowest dosage and then be gradually increased until the desired antihypertensive effect. Therefore, it may be desirable to maximize dosing of a single agent before adding another, though one may consider using agents in combination which may cancel out the others' side effects, such as a beta-blocker with a vasodilator to negate effects on heart rate. In the national hospital database review, 45 % of all treated hypertensive neonates received two or more medications [9] though this did not include diuretics. Developing experience with just one or two agents in each antihypertensive class will allow the flexibility to treating multiple different etiologies while permitting familiarity with the potential pitfalls of each medication.

Lastly, surgical correction may be necessary in certain etiologies. Surgery may be the primary treatment for aortic coarctation, obstructions of the urinary tract, and abdominal or renal tumors. However, surgery should not be the primary approach to correct hypertension from renal artery thrombosis, arterial stenosis, or multicystic dysplastic kidney as medical management is preferred. Autosomal recessive polycystic kidney disease also may require surgical correction (bilateral nephrectomy) if the hypertension is refractory to medications.

20.7 Outcomes

Initial reports of outcomes of neonatal hypertension in the 1970s were quite grim with one-third of patients dying either of severe uncontrolled hypertension or associated problems [4]. However, with improved recognition and treatment amongst neonatologists, the overall morbidity and mortality of neonatal hypertension has improved significantly. Renovascular hypertension secondary to UAC use typically resolves over time, such that antihypertensive medications are not needed after a few months [3], but growth impairment of the involved kidney may be seen in nearly half of all patients. Hypertension associated with chronic lung disease also tends to resolve with time, with antihypertensive needs often mirroring the need for supplemental oxygen [7]. However, hypertension secondary to neurologic or renal parenchymal disease seems less likely to spontaneously resolve. Hypertension has been known to recur after surgical correction in patients with aortic coarctation and congenital renal artery stenosis, so that continued monitoring is needed outside of the neonatal period. Likewise, de novo development of hypertension for high-risk neonates outside of the NICU has been reported at a fairly high prevalence of 2.6 % in an early report [19]. There has not been replication of these results but it is recommended that BP monitoring be done in routine follow-up for all former NICU patients [31].

A more recent study with short-term NICU follow-up found only 41 % of infants that developed hypertension needed treatment upon hospital discharge and 15 % still needing treatment at 3–6 months of age [37]. A large-scale review of NICU antihypertensive prescribing practices showed that the median duration of exposure was just 10 days [9] so that long-term therapy is typically not indicated. There are currently no large-scale, long-term follow-up studies of neonates with hypertension to see about more remote outcomes in patients.

References

1. Abman SH, Warady BA, Lum GM et al (1982) Systemic hypertension in infants with bronchopulmonary dysplasia. J Pediatr 104:928–931
2. Adelman RD (1978) Neonatal hypertension. Pediatr Clin North Am 25:99–110
3. Adelman RD (1987) Long-term follow-up of neonatal renovascular hypertension. Pediatr Nephrol 1:35–41
4. Adelman RD (1988) The hypertensive neonate. Clin Perinatol 15:567–585
5. Alagappan A, Malloy MH (1998) Systemic hypertension in very low-birth weight infants with bronchopulmonary dysplasia: incidence and risk factors. Am J Perinatol 15(1):3–8
6. American Academy of Pediatrics Committee on Fetus and Newborn (1993) Routine evaluation of blood pressure, hematocrit, and glucose in newborns. Pediatrics 92:474–476
7. Anderson AH, Warady BA, Daily DK et al (1993) Systemic hypertension in infants with severe bronchopulmonary dysplasia: associated clinical factors. Am J Perinatol 10(3):190–193
8. Barrington KJ (2010) Umbilical artery catheters in the newborn: effects of position of the catheter tip. Cochrane Database Syst Rev 1:CD 000505. doi:10.102/14658188
9. Blowey DL, Duda PJ, Stokes P et al (2011) Incidence and treatment of hypertension in the neonatal intensive care unit. J Am Soc Hypertens 5:478–483
10. Buchi KF, Siegler RL (1986) Hypertension in the first month of life. J Hypertens 4(5):525–528
11. Butt WW, Whyte H (1984) Blood pressure monitoring in neonates: comparison of umbilical and peripheral artery catheter measurements. J Pediatr 105(4): 630–632
12. Cachat F, Van Melle G, McGahren ED et al (2006) Arterial hypertension after surgical closure of omphalocele and gastroschisis. Pediatr Nephrol 21(2): 225–229
13. DeSwiet M, Fayers P, Shinebourne EA (1976) Blood pressure survey in a population of newborn infants. BMJ 2:9–11
14. DeSwiet M, Fayers P, Shinebourne EA (1980) Systolic blood pressure in a population of infants in the first year of life: the Brompton Study. Pediatrics 65:1028–1035
15. Dionne JM, Abitbol CL, Flynn JT (2012) Hypertension in infancy: diagnosis, management and outcome. Pediatr Nephrol 27(1):17–32
16. Dionne JM, Abitbol CL, Flynn JT (2012) Erratum to: Hypertension in infancy: diagnosis, management and outcome. Pediatr Nephrol 27(1):159–160
17. Dweck HS, Reynolds DW, Cassady G (1974) Indirect blood pressure measurements in newborns. Am J Dis Child 127:492–494
18. Feld GF, Waz WR (1997) Pharmacologic therapy of hypertension. In: Feld GF (ed) Hypertension in children. Butterworth-Heinemann, Boston
19. Friedman AL, Hustead VA (1987) Hypertension in babies following discharge from a neonatal intensive care unit. Pediatr Nephrol 1:30–34
20. Friesen RH, Lichtor JL (1981) Indirect measurement of blood pressure in neonates and infants utilizing an automatic non-invasive oscillometric monitor. Anesth Analg 60(10):742–745
21. Gemelli M, Manganaro R, Mami C et al (1990) Longitudinal study of blood pressure during the first year of life. Eur J Pediatr 149:318–320
22. Gouyon JB, Geneste B, Semana DS et al (1997) Intravenous nicardipine in hypertensive preterm infants. Arch Dis Child 76:F126–F127
23. Guay-Woodford LM, Desmond RA (2003) Autosomal recessive polycystic kidney disease: the clinical experience in North America. Pediatrics 111(5 Pt 1): 1072–1080
24. Husmann DA, McLorie GA, Churchill BM (1993) Hypertension following primary bladder closure for vesical exstrophy. J Pediatr Surg 28(2):239–241
25. Kent AL, Kecskes Z, Shadbolt B et al (2007) Normative blood pressure data in the early neonatal period. Pediatr Nephrol 22(9):1335–1341
26. Lanzarini VV, Furusawa EA, Sadeck L et al (2006) Neonatal arterial hypertension in nephrological malformations in a tertiary care hospital. J Hum Hypertens 20:679–683
27. Lum LG, Jones MD (1977) The effect of cuff width on systolic blood pressure measurements in neonates. J Pediatr 91:963–966
28. Lurbe E, Garcia-Vicent C, Torro I et al (2007) First-year blood pressure increase steepest in low birthweight newborns. J Hypertens 25:81–86
29. Milou C, Debuche-Benouachkou V, Semana DS et al (2000) Intravenous nicardipine as a first-line antihypertensive drug in neonates. Intensive Care Med 26:956–958
30. Nafday SM, Brion LP, Benchimol C et al (2005) Renal disease. In: McDonald MB, Mullett MD, Seshia MMK (eds) Avery's neonatology, 6th edn. Lippincott Williams & Wilkins, Philadelphia
31. National High Blood Pressure Education Program Working Group on High Blood Pressure in Children and Adolescents (2004) The fourth report on the diagnosis, evaluation, and treatment of high blood pressure in children and adolescents. Pediatrics 114:555–576
32. Nwankwo MU, Lorenz JM, Gardiner JC (1997) A standard protocol for blood pressure measurement in the newborn. Pediatrics 99(6):e10
33. O'Shea J, Dempsey EM (2009) A comparison of blood pressure in newborns. Am J Perinatol 26(2): 113–116
34. O'Sullivan JJ, Derrick G, Darnell R (2002) Prevalence of hypertension in children after early repair of coarctation of the aorta: a cohort study using casual and 24 hour blood pressure measurement. Heart 88:163–166
35. Pejovic B, Peco-Antic A, Marinkovic-Eric J (2007) Blood pressure in non-critically ill preterm and full-term neonates. Pediatr Nephrol 22:249–257

36. Piazza SF, Chandra M, Harper RG et al (1985) Upper vs lower limb systolic blood pressure in full term normal newborn. Am J Dis Child 139:797–799
37. Seilem WA, Falk MC, Shadbolt B et al (2007) Antenatal and postnatal risk factors for neonatal hypertension and infant follow-up. Pediatr Nephrol 22:2081–2087
38. Singh HP, Hurley RM, Myers TF (1992) Neonatal hypertension. Incidence and risk factors. Am J Hypertens 5(2):51–55
39. Skalina MEL, Kliegman RM, Fanaroff AA (1986) Epidemiology and management of severe symptomatic neonatal hypertension. Am J Perinatol 3:235–239
40. Sonesson SE, Broberger U (1987) Arterial blood pressure in the very low birthweight neonate. Evaluation of an oscillometric technique. Acta Paediatr Scand 76(2):338–341
41. Stephenson TJ, Broughton Pipkin F, Elias-Jones AC (1991) Factors influencing plasma renin and renin substrate in premature infants. Arch Dis Child 66: 1150–1154
42. Takci S, Yigit S, Korkmaz A et al (2012) Comparison between oscillometric and invasive blood pressure measurements in critically ill premature infants. Acta Paediatr 101:132–135
43. Thomas CA, Moffett BS, Wagner JL et al (2011) Safety and efficacy of intravenous labetalol for hypertensive crisis in infants and small children. Pediatr Crit Care Med 12(1):28–32
44. Wareham JA, Haugh LD, Yaeger SB et al (1987) Prediction of arterial blood pressure in the premature neonate using the oscillometric method. Am J Dis Child 141(10):1108–1110
45. Wells TG, Bunchman TE, Kearns GL (1990) Treatment of neonatal hypertension with enalaprilat. J Pediatr 117:664–667
46. Zubrow AB, Hulman S, Kushner H et al (1995) Determinants of blood pressure in infants admitted to neonatal intensive care units: a prospective multicenter study. Philadelphia Neonatal Blood Pressure Study Group. J Perinatol 15(6): 470–479

Erratum

Kidney and Urinary Tract Diseases in the Newborn

Aftab S. Chishti, Shumyle Alam, and Stefan G. Kiessling
Editors

ISBN 978-3-642-39987-9
ISBN 978-3-642-39988-6 (eBook)

Figure (10.3 on page 204) was published with permission by Dr. Curtis Sheldon, Cincinnati Children's Hospital Medical Center and the University of Cincinnati, Cincinnati, Ohio, USA

A.S. Chishti et al. (eds.), *Kidney and Urinary Tract Diseases in the Newborn*,
DOI 10.1007/978-3-642-39988-6_21, © Springer-Verlag Berlin Heidelberg 2014

Index

A.S. Chishti et al. (eds.), *Kidney and Urinary Tract Diseases in the Newborn*,
DOI 10.1007/978-3-642-39988-6, © Springer-Verlag Berlin Heidelberg 2014

F

G

MIX
Papier aus verantwortungsvollen Quellen
Paper from responsible sources
FSC® C105338

If you have any concerns about our products,
you can contact us on
ProductSafety@springernature.com

In case Publisher is established outside the EU,
the EU authorized representative is:
Springer Nature Customer Service Center GmbH
Europaplatz 3, 69115 Heidelberg, Germany

Printed by Libri Plureos GmbH
in Hamburg, Germany